ASSESSING MEDICAL TECHNOLOGIES

Committee for Evaluating Medical Technologies
in Clinical Use

Division of Health Sciences Policy

Division of Health Promotion and Disease Prevention

INSTITUTE OF MEDICINE

NATIONAL ACADEMY PRESS
Washington, D.C. 1985

National Academy Press • 2101 Constitution Avenue, NW • Washington, DC 20418

NOTICE: The project that is the subject of this report was approved by the Governing Board of the National Research Council, whose members are drawn from the councils of the National Academy of Sciences, the National Academy of Engineering, and the Institute of Medicine. The members of the committee responsible for the report were chosen for their special competencies and with regard for appropriate balance.

This report has been reviewed by a group other than the authors according to the procedures approved by a Report Review Committee consisting of members of the National Academy of Sciences, the National Academy of Engineering, and the Institute of Medicine.

The Institute of Medicine was chartered in 1970 by the National Academy of Sciences to enlist distinguished members of the appropriate professions in the examination of policy matters pertaining to the health of the public. In this, the Institute acts under both the Academy's 1863 congressional charter responsibility to be an advisor to the federal government and its own initiative in identifying issues of medical care, research, and education.

This study was supported by the Henry J. Kaiser Family Foundation, Kaiser Foundation Hospitals, the National Research Council Fund, and by the Office of Medical Applications of Research, National Institutes of Health, Contract No. ASU000001-03.

The National Research Council Fund is a pool of private, discretionary, nonfederal funds that is used to support a program of academy-initiated studies of national issues in which science and technology figure significantly.

Library of Congress Cataloging-in-Publication Data

Institute of Medicine (U.S.). Division of Health
Science Policy.
Assessing medical technologies.
Outgrowth of a conference held by the Institute of
Medicine in 1980.
Prepared by the Committee for Evaluating Medical
Technologies in Clinical Use.
Includes bibliographies and index.
1. Medical care—United States. 2. Technology
assessment—United States. 3. Medical technology—
United States—Evaluation. 4. Medical care. 5. Technology assessment. 6. Medical technology—Evaluation.
I. Institute of Medicine (U.S.). Division of Health
Promotion and Disease Prevention. II. Institute of
Medicine (U.S.). Committee for Evaluating Medical
Technologies in Clinical Use. III. Title. [DNLM:
1. Evaluation Studies. 2. Technology Assessment,
Biomedical. 3. Technology, Medical—standards.
WB 365 I59a]
RA445.I58 1985 610'.28 85-15284
ISBN 0-309-03583-X

Printed in the United States of America

Committee for Evaluating Medical Technologies in Clinical Use

FREDERICK MOSTELLER
Roger I. Lee Professor, Harvard School of Public Health, Boston, Massachusetts (*Chairman*)

H. DAVID BANTA
Deputy Director, Pan American Health Organization, Washington, D.C.

STUART BONDURANT
Professor of Medicine and Dean, University of North Carolina School of Medicine, Chapel Hill, North Carolina

MORRIS F. COLLEN
Former Director, Technology Assessment, Department of Medical Methods Research, Kaiser Permanente Medical Care Program, Oakland, California

JOANNE E. FINLEY
Fellow, Department of Psychiatry, University of Pennsylvania Graduate Hospital Division (Former New Jersey State Commissioner of Health)

BARBARA J. McNEIL
Professor of Radiology and Clinical Epidemiology, Harvard Medical School, and Director, Center for Cost-Effective Care, Brigham and Womens Hospital Boston, Massachusetts

LAWRENCE C. MORRIS, JR.
Senior Vice President, Health Benefits Management, Blue Cross and Blue Shield Association, Chicago, Illinois

LINCOLN E. MOSES
Professor of Statistics, Stanford University, Stanford, California

SEYMOUR PERRY
Senior Fellow and Deputy Director, Institute for Health Policy Analysis Georgetown Medical Center, Washington, D.C.

DOROTHY P. RICE
Regent's Lecturer, Department of Social and Behavioral Sciences, School of Nursing, University of California, San Francisco, California

HERMAN A. TYROLER
Alumni Distinguished Professor, Department of Epidemiology, School of Public Health, University of North Carolina, Chapel Hill, North Carolina

DONALD A. YOUNG
Executive Director, Prospective Payment Assessment Commission, Washington, D.C.

Study Staff

ENRIQUETA C. BOND, Study Director and Director, Division of Health Promotion and Disease Prevention

BARBARA FILNER, Director, Division of Health Sciences Policy

CAREN CARNEY, Research Assistant

CLIFFORD GOODMAN, National Research Council Fellow

LINDA DePUGH, Administrative Secretary

NAOMI HUDSON, Administrative Secretary

WALLACE K. WATERFALL, Editor

Acknowledgments

As with many reports issued by the Institute of Medicine (IOM), this report represents the collaborative efforts of the committee, a number of IOM members, the project staff, and many persons outside the IOM. The individuals listed below drafted sections of the report, wrote background papers for committee consideration, reviewed drafts, submitted suggestions for improving technology assessment, and, in general, gave their active assistance and collaboration. In Appendix B are collected a number of papers written or contributed to the project as furthering our undertaking of technology assessment. We wish especially to express our gratitude to National Research Council Fellow, Clifford Goodman, who has worked closely with the committee for the past 2 years. The major contributors to each chapter are further identified in appropriate sections of the report.

John Bailar, Harvard School of Public Health
John Ball, American College of Physicians
Benjamin Barnes, Harvard School of Public Health
*Jeremiah A. Barondess, Cornell University Medical College
*Lionel M. Bernstein, Knowledge Systems, Inc.
Jonathan Brown, Harvard School of Public Health
*Thomas C. Chalmers, Mount Sinai Medical Center
David Cohen, Cleveland Metropolitan General Hospital
*Jerome R. Cox, Jr., St. Louis School of Engineering and Applied Sciences, Washington University
Betty L. Dooley, Center for Health Policy Studies
Jack Dunn, Employee Benefit Specialist, Ford Motor Company

* Denotes IOM member

*David Eddy, Duke University
*Richard H. Egdahl, Boston University Medical Center
Penny H. Feldman, Harvard School of Public Health
*Harvey V. Fineberg, Harvard School of Public Health
G.D. Friedman, The Permanente Medical Group
Clifton R. Gaus, Foundation for Health Services Research
George Greenberg, U.S. Department of Health and Human Services
Paul F. Griner, The Henry J. Kaiser Family Foundation
*Ruth S. Hanft, Consultant
Richard J. Havlik, National Heart, Lung, and Blood Institute
Paul Jones, Case Western Reserve University School of Medicine
*Albert R. Jonsen, University of California, San Francisco
Edward H. Kass, Harvard Medical School
Jeffrey P. Koplan, Centers for Disease Control
John Laszlo, Duke University Medical Center
*Robert H. Moser, American College of Physicians
*Duncan B. Neuhauser, Case Western Reserve University School of Medicine
Joel J. Nobel, ECRI (formerly the Emergency Care Research Institute)
*Gerald T. Perkoff, University of Missouri-Columbia School of Medicine
Michael R. Reich, Harvard School of Public Health
Janet Reis, Northwestern University Center for Health Services and Policy Research
Stanley J. Reiser, The University of Texas Health Science Center at Houston
Pierre F. Renault, National Institutes of Health
J. Sanford Schwartz, University of Pennsylvania
*Sam Shapiro, The Johns Hopkins University
Donald Shepard, Harvard School of Public Health
Herbert Sherman, Harvard School of Public Health
Jonathan Showstack, University of California, San Francisco
*Reuel A. Stallones, University of Texas Health Science Center at Houston
C. Frank Starmer, St. Louis School of Engineering and Applied Sciences, Washington University
Seymour Sudman, University of Illinois
Bruce Vladeck, United Hospital Fund of New York
Milton C. Weinstein, Harvard School of Public Health
*Frank Young, Food and Drug Administration

* Denotes IOM member

Preface

Twentieth century advances in scientific knowledge have been responsible for profound improvements in human health. Many diseases have been eradicated and others now can be successfully treated or prevented. However, new technologies and procedures have developed so rapidly—and there are such economic and social incentives to use them—that the evaluation of their safety, efficacy, and cost-effectiveness as well as the consideration of their social and ethical consequences has lagged far behind. This situation does not serve the patient, the physician, or our society well, and there is an increasing conviction that we need a coordinated system for medical technology assessment and a national program of support for it.

This study was the outgrowth of a 1980 Institute of Medicine conference on linking the clinical use of biomedical technologies and the collection of evaluative data.* The conferees considered several methods for evaluating biomedical technologies and for applying the information obtained to physician education, clinical practice, resource allocation, quality assurance, and reimbursement. They also considered such issues as the funding of evaluative research and translating research findings on safety, efficacy, and cost-effectiveness into policy and practice.

This study was undertaken to address in greater detail the following questions raised at the conference:

• What are the strengths and limits of methods for technology assessment and how can it be improved? This question is primarily considered in Chapter 3 of the report. Useful methods do exist for assessing medical technologies.

* Supported by the Charles H. Revson Foundation.

• How does knowledge from technology assessment translate into better clinical care? This issue is discussed in Chapter 4, which indicates that we have much to learn in this area.

• What gaps exist in the current system for technology assessment? Chapter 2 explores the terrain of technology assessment, identifying who is doing it, how much they are spending on it, and for what purposes. These considerations are carried further in Chapters 6 and 7.

• Who should pay for technology assessment? The stage for this important question is set in Chapters 2 and 5. The question is also examined in Chapter 7, along with the recommendations of the study committee.

PROCEDURE FOR THE STUDY

Primary responsibility for conducting the study was vested in a committee of 12 experts in the fields of technology assessment, biostatistics, epidemiology, public health policy, clinical practice, and third-party payment mechanisms. Committee members defined the task more precisely in preliminary meetings and then enrolled the assistance of outside experts in drafting materials for their review and incorporation into the report. Committee members, staff, and outside experts worked collaboratively to complete the report.

Dr. Enriqueta Bond led the staff, organized much of the committee's work, and tirelessly wrote parts of and contributed to the editing of the report. Clifford Goodman contributed much beyond the sections signed by him and wrote Appendix A to this book, which gives basic systematic information about many of the institutions performing technology assessment. Wallace Waterfall aided the committee enormously by editing a massive manuscript flowing from many hands. Without the excellent secretarial assistance of Naomi Hudson and Linda DePugh, the book would never have been completed.

AUDIENCE FOR THE STUDY

Various chapters of the report are expected to be of particular interest to one or another segment of the total audience. To facilitate the reader's choosing his or her own path through the text, each chapter is intended to include enough information from the others to keep at hand the context of the whole. First, the book is a terrain map of medical technology assessment that can serve as a textbook for students and educators. Second, researchers and funding agencies can find a research agenda developed throughout the book, but especially in Chapters 3, 4, and 7. Next, those who carry out and use the results of technology assessment will find value in the scope of technology assessment described in Chapter 2 and Appendix A, the methods identified in Chapter 3, and recommendations for developing a better system of technology assessment outlined in Chapter 7. Policymakers will also be interested in these recommendations as well as the Summary, Chapter 2, and Appendix A. Finally, the book should serve as a resource to the Institute of

Medicine in its efforts to contribute to the nation's system for technology assessment by the establishment of a Council for Technology as defined by P.L. 98-551.

Recommendations in this report are of three types. Most of the individual chapters include recommendations very specific to the chapter topics. Chapter 7 has recommendations pertinent to establishing a system of technology assessment. And the text in several chapters has sentences that are highlighted in boldface type as contributions to a research agenda for technology assessment.

Appendix B of this report presents a selection from among the many papers prepared for the committee. Paper titles and authors are as follows: Guide to Comparative Clinical Trials, by Clifford S. Goodman; Information Needs for Technology Assessment, by Morris F. Collen; Toward Evaluating Cost-Effectiveness of Medical and Social Experiments, by Frederick Mosteller and Milton C. Weinstein; Technology Assessment in Prepaid Group Practice, by Morris F. Collen; A Randomized Controlled Trial to Evaluate the Effects of an Experimental Prepaid Group Practice on Medical Care Utilization and Cost, by Gerald T. Perkoff; The Metro Firm Trials: An Innovative Approach to Ongoing Randomized Clinical Trials, by David I. Cohen and Duncan Neuhauser; Values and Preferences in the Delivery of Health Care, by Barbara J. McNeil; New Federalism and State Support of Technology Assessment, by George D. Greenberg and Penny H. Feldman; and Government Payers for Health Care, by Donald A. Young.

FREDERICK MOSTELLER
Chairman

Contents

Summary

Medical care has changed dramatically in recent decades. It has become more ambitious and much more effective, but it also has become more costly. The cost both strains our financial resources and attracts attention to other aspects of medical care—safety, efficacy, quality, and ethical implications. All these considerations make it increasingly necessary that we be able to choose knowledgeably the health care technologies to be made available and the conditions of availability.

One might hope that such selection processes would be guided by an orderly, well-conceived, unified system of testing and assessing the new, comparing it with the old, and moving forward as warranted by valid, reliable, evaluative information. At present that hope is only partially fulfilled.

The nation requires a systematic approach for technology assessment. We need to have a strategy and an organization for setting priorities. Given the priorities, we need mechanisms for actually making the assessments and implementing the findings. And finally, we need a method for paying for many of the needed assessments. As with any large-scale technological enterprise, we need to maintain a strong body of professional personnel to carry out the assessments, and they must be encouraged to conduct work of high quality and develop new techniques as required. Although some parts of this overall process are in place and are contributing well to the health of Americans, the system as a whole has major gaps and deficiencies.

The questions of who should carry out assessments, how they should be done, and who should pay for them are complicated and political and have no simple answers. Consequently, a committee of the Institute of Medicine was established to study these issues. This report addresses the present state of the assessment of medical technology; gives attention to processes, problems, interested parties, and successes and failures; and finally points to some needs and opportunities for improving the present system of medical technology assessment.

Medical technology is a term that embraces a wide range of activities. For consistency we shall follow the usage of the Congress's Office of Technology Assessment (OTA), which employs the term to refer to "techniques, drugs, equipment, and procedures used by health-care professionals in delivering medical care to individuals, and the systems within which such care is delivered."

We shall use the term assessment of a medical technology to denote any process of examining and reporting properties of a medical technology used in health care, such as safety, efficacy, feasibility, and indications for use, cost, and cost-effectiveness, as well as social, economic, and ethical consequences, whether intended or unintended.

Technology assessment ideally would be comprehensive and include evaluation not only of the immediate results of the technology but also of its long-term consequences. A comprehensive assessment of a medical technology—after assessment of its immediate effects—may also include an appraisal of problems of personnel training and licensure, new capital expenditures for equipment and buildings, and possible consequences for the health insurance industry and the social security system. Technology assessment provides a form of policy analysis that includes as potential components the narrower approaches to technology evaluation. Most assessments stop with a partial effort. Not all technologies warrant the full assessment, nor is it feasible to provide comprehensive assessments for all technologies. As we shall see, various participants in the health care system find different properties to be salient.

THE SCOPE OF U.S. MEDICAL TECHNOLOGY ASSESSMENT

Heightened interest in medical technology assessment has prompted a wide variety of responses in recent years as one or another organization tries to meet its needs for assessment information. The scope of these responses is given in Chapter 2. Since 1977, the National Institutes of Health (NIH) have conducted 50 consensus development conferences on a variety of biomedical problems and technologies. Each consensus was widely reported. The American College of Cardiology, the American Hospital Association, the American College of Physicians, and the American Medical Association are among those professional and provider associations that have instituted new assessment programs. The independent medical device evaluator ECRI (formerly the Emergency Care Research Institute) has an implant registry and a device-experience reporting network and is expanding its assessment services with new publications. More drug companies are instituting permanent drug surveillance and cost analysis programs.

Many organizations arrange for the exchange of assessment information. Blue Cross and Blue Shield Association and other major insurers increasingly seek assistance from medical associations such as the American College of Physicians, the American College of Radiology, and the American College of Surgeons in formulating coverage policies. At congressional request, the Office of Technology Assessment has in recent years produced more than 60 reports and case studies of medical technology that have been widely circulated and cited throughout government, industry, and the public. The Department of Health and Human Services (DHHS), NIH, and the Veterans Administration are among those agencies that have instituted coordinating committees to enhance the exchange of information about technology assessment and to make recommendations regarding their assessment policies. The U.S. General Accounting Office issues an increasing number of reports touching on technology assessment in federal programs. The Stevenson-Wydler Technology Innovation Act of 1980 (P.L. 96-480) requires DHHS to report annually to the Department of Commerce regarding its health technology assessment and transfer activities.

But the recent flurry of attention to assessment has not been accompanied by a fitting increase in new assessment information. Notwithstanding the national investment in health care and the diversity and scope of assessment needs, current assessment activities are inconsistent in quality and are poorly funded. Organizations are scrambling for limited available information and are relying heavily upon expert opinion to fill wide gaps in the data. The bulk of all resources allocated for technology assessment is in premarketing tests of drugs for safety and efficacy. Although current premarketing assessment of drugs and devices appears adequate, insufficient attention is given to postmarketing studies. Even less attention is paid to evaluating medical and surgical procedures for safety and effectiveness. Among all technologies, existing assessment activities are concentrated on the new technologies and not on those that are widely accepted and possibly outmoded. Assessments of cost-effectiveness and cost-benefit are few; assessments for ethical, legal, and other social implications are rare.

Varieties and Expense of Assessment

Medical technology assessment can be described according to many different aspects, including the type of technology, its application, the stage of diffusion, the concerns of assessment, the methods of assessment, and the assessors. Various combinations of these aspects account for the great diversity among assessment programs. Some programs devote most of their assessment resources to one type of technology, such as ECRI for medical devices; others may address a variety of technologies, as does the congressional Office of Technology Assessment.

The total dollar level of effort in technology assessment—including clinical trials, health services research, and synthesis activities such as consensus development conferences, state-of-the-art workshops, and formulation of coverage decisions—is small compared with the national effort in research and development (R&D) of technologies. In fact, assessment spending can be lost in the rounding error for national health expenditures, as is evident in the relative magnitudes of the following estimates for 1984.

National Health Care	$384.3 billion
Health R&D	11.8 billion
All Health Technology Assessment	1.3 billion
Clinical trials	1.1 billion
Health services research	under 0.2 billion
Other technology assessment	under 0.05 billion

Federal Government The federal government conducts and supports medical technology assessment to serve its functions in biomedical research, health services research, health care delivery, payment, regulation, legislation, and defense. Federal government expenditures for medical technology assessment were approximately $450 million in 1984. That included $280 million for clinical trials (primarily NIH support), roughly $100 million–150 million for health services research, and $30 million for other assessment activities, including consensus development conferences and other syntheses and special studies by many agencies. Federal expenditures for medical technology assessment—including health services research expenditures—constitute about 7 percent of federal health R&D expenditures and 0.4 percent of federal health care expenditures.

Drug Industry Data are lacking for direct estimates of drug industry expenditures devoted to technology assessment activities such as clinical trials and postmarketing surveillance; company budgets do not generally show line items for such activities. However, indirect estimates can be made from survey data.

Based on a recent survey of its members, the Pharmaceutical Manufacturers Association (PMA) estimated that clinical evaluation (including controlled and uncontrolled trials in phases I, II, and III and in phase IV postmarketing studies) accounts for 23.1 percent of R&D expenditures. Adjusting for non-PMA firms that may devote a smaller proportion of their R&D dollar to clinical trials would mean that $700 million–$750 million of the $3.3 billion human-use drug R&D in 1984 was devoted to clinical evaluation, including postmarketing studies. (Members of the association number about 130 of the more than 1,000 U.S. drug companies and primarily are the larger, brand name drug firms, accounting for more than 90 percent of total U.S. drug sales.) A rough estimate of expenditures for postmarketing studies is $100 million per year, most of which is spent by industry.

Premarketing assessment of drugs for safety and efficacy in the United States, regulated by the Food and Drug Administration (FDA), is perhaps the most comprehensive and well-funded area of medical technology assessment in the world today.

Medical Device Industry Medical device industry expenditures for clinical evaluation (Chapter 2) were probably on the order of $35 million in 1984, or about 4 percent of the industry's R&D expenditures. At least half of this amount may be accounted for by clinical trial expenditures associated with devices submitted for FDA premarket approval application (PMAA). Clinical evaluation costs other than those for devices submitted under PMAA include costs for devices tested under investigational device exemptions but not carried through the entire premarket approval process and for those few thousand devices that annually bypass the PMAA process because they are substantially equivalent to devices already on the market. However, few of these entail costly, if any, clinical evaluation.

PMAA is a comparatively new and infrequently used regulatory pathway. Based on an FDA survey of 20 manufacturers of various types of medical devices, the cost of bringing a new device to market through the PMAA process—including device development, clinical trials, manufacturing and controls, application preparation, and other activities conducted during review—ranges from $370,000 to $1,025,000.

Medical device assessment has yet to emerge from a shakedown period, partly because of the relative newness of the 1976 Medical Device Amendments (as compared with the 1962 amendments to the Food, Drug, and Cosmetic Act) and the great diversity of devices subject to regulation. Many thousands of devices—from implantable, programmable, dual-chamber cardiac pacemakers and diagnostic reagents using monoclonal antibodies to snakebite kits, ice bags, and bed boards—must be properly classified and regulated so as to protect consumers and to be responsive to provider needs and manufacturers' concerns.

Rigorous clinical evaluation of medical devices largely is confined to the final regulatory step of premarket approval. As is the case for drugs, resources for device assessment are limited and too narrowly focused. Device assessment rarely extends beyond safety and efficacy to matters of cost-effectiveness and broader social implications and devotes few resources to postmarketing surveillance. ECRI and, to a lesser extent, the American Hospital Association are among the few organizations that provide comparative information on technical performance, cost, hazard reports, and other valuable information for device procurement and maintenance.

Other Private Sector Assessment Activities There is widespread and increasing interest in technology assessment among organizations in the private sector, in addition to those in the medical products industry. Private insurers, medical associations, professional and industry associations, hospital corporations and other major providers, policy institutes, and voluntary health agencies conduct and sponsor assessment activities to suit their varied needs. These include making coverage and reimbursement policies and procurement decisions, responding to practitioner inquiries, setting voluntary standards for manufacturing and practice, providing guidance to regulatory agencies and other policymakers, and improving medical practice and service delivery.

Despite this heightened interest, current private sector activity remains limited in several important ways. Other than ECRI, none of these organizations has as its primary purpose the assessment of medical technologies. Few of the evaluations undertaken in these private efforts involve original work that generates primary evaluative data. The scope of evaluations is limited—most evaluations are concerned only with matters of safety and effectiveness and do not move further to examine cost-benefit and cost-effectiveness or ethical, legal, and other broad social issues. Safety and effectiveness are addressed only indirectly in some evaluations; payers generally rely on a determination of a technology's diffusion, i.e., whether it is standard practice rather than experimental or investigative, as an indicant of a physician's judgment of its safety and effectiveness. The predominant assessment methods are literature reviews and consultation with experts. Assessments are generally conducted on a reactive, ad hoc basis rather than by systematic review and priority setting. Evaluation activity by insurers largely is to assist the insurance claims process; assessments by medical associations generally are conducted in response to inquiries by third-party payers and practitioners. The magnitude of expenditures made by providers and insurers for the extraordinarily varied array of new, emerging, accepted, and outmoded health care services makes associated efforts in technology assessment appear small.

Lags in Assessment

The total of nearly $400 billion spent in 1984 for health care tends to distract attention from the relatively small amount spent for R&D to support the health enterprise (3 percent of the total) and the nearly vanishing amount spent for technology assessment to substantiate the R&D (0.3 percent). It is difficult to determine whether that proportion of investment in medical technology assessment is in rough agreement with the spending by other sectors of industry for such assessments because estimates of expenditures for that purpose are nearly impossible to assemble with confidence. However, figures are available for R&D investment by many enterprises, and R&D expenditures in the health field are low compared with those in other technology-intensive industries.

A particular shortcoming is seen in clinical trials for medical and surgical procedures. OTA estimates that randomized clinical trials have been applied to 10 or 20 percent of medical practices. The Office of Health Technology Assessment (OHTA) has had to base its recommendations to the Health Care Financing Administration (HCFA) regarding coverage issues on evidence that is sorely lacking in rigorous experimental findings. Of the 26 full-scale assessments conducted by OHTA for HCFA in 1982, results from randomized clinical trials were available for only 2. Current NIH support for clinical trials (approximately $276 million in 1985) is provided for only a portion of those clinical trials that have been identified as being worthy of support.

Less than $50 million is spent on technology assessment devoted to the synthesis and interpretation of primary evaluation data for determining how best to apply in practice new and currently available technologies. Examples are consensus development conferences, coverage decisions by third-party payers, medical and industry association assessment programs, congressional studies, and studies by nonprofit policy institutes.

Recommendations

The descriptions in Chapter 2 of what is, and is not, being accomplished in a wide variety of medical technology assessment efforts in the United States prompted the study committee to make the following recommendations (in italics).

- *Greater commitment in medical technology assessment should be given to (1) the generation of primary data on safety and efficacy of medical and surgical procedures, (2) the determination of cost-effectiveness and public policy implications of those procedures, and (3) postmarketing surveillance of drugs and medical devices.*
- *Create a central clearinghouse to monitor, synthesize, and disseminate information about all medical technology assessment.* Several organizations already serve that function, but each only for a certain constituency, such as pharmaceutical manufacturers, hospitals, or medical device users, and there is little information flow between organizations.
- *Increase funding for medical technology assessment by $300 million in 1984 dollars primarily by instituting new contributions from payers and providers for health care.* This would be phased in over a 10-year period. The increased support should come from the health dollar because groups such as the Health Care Financing Administration and private health insurance and service plans, as well as provider groups, would see the first savings from improved technology.

METHODS OF MEDICAL TECHNOLOGY ASSESSMENT

Technology assessment offers the essential bridge between basic research and development and prudent practical application of medical technology. Fortunately, we have a substantial body of methods that can be applied to the various tasks of assessment, and their availability makes possible the acceptance, modification, or rejection of new technologies on a rational basis. That rationality, however, depends on many factors that go well beyond safety and efficacy, including economics, ethics, preferences of patients, education of physicians, and diffusion of information. The methods that have been developed can take into account most of these factors, although combining the results from examination of different factors is a major task and one that is far from settled or solved. The existence of these assessment methods provides a foundation for building a system of technology assessment for the nation.

Few people are acquainted with more than a few of the methods used for assessment. Usually investigators are acquainted only with the methods most frequently used in their own specialties. Consequently, Chapter 3 provides descriptions of the more widely used assessment methods and what they are most useful for studying.

For the purpose of evaluation through data acquisition, randomized clinical trials are highly regarded. For generating hypotheses, case studies and the series of cases have special value. Registries and data bases sometimes produce hypotheses, sometimes help to evaluate them, and sometimes aid directly in the treatment of patients. Sample surveys excel in describing collections of patients, health workers, transactions, and institutions.

Epidemiological and surveillance studies are well adapted to identifying rare events that may be caused by the adverse effects of a technology.

Quantitative synthesis and group judgment methods give us ways to summarize current states of knowledge and bridge the gaps among research findings. Similarly, cost-effectiveness and cost-benefit analyses offer ways of introducing costs and economics into these assessments. Modeling is a way to simulate the future and still include complicated features of the real life process to reveal what variables or parameters seem to produce the more substantial effects. When backed with strong empirical investigations, it may add much breadth to an evaluation.

Although randomized clinical trials offer the strongest method of assessing the efficacy of a new therapy, we recognize that it is not possible to have randomized trials for every version of every innovation. However desirable that might be, it is not feasible. Consequently, often it is necessary to depend on other methods of assessment; of course, some technologies actually require other methods. This in turn means that steps need to be taken to strengthen the other methods. These steps have two forms. First, where possible, apply the known ways of improving studies, such as observational studies (for example, have a careful protocol, use random samples, use blindness where possible, and so on). Second, many of these methods could be improved if research were carried out to find new ways to improve them. Therefore, it is often suggested that specific research be carried out that could lead to stronger results from the weaker methods of assessment.

At the same time that we recognize the need for improving the weaker methods of assessment, we also recognize that the methods we already have are not applied sufficiently often. As pointed out in Chapter 2, the Office of Health Technology Assessment evaluates the safety and effectiveness of new or as yet unestablished medical technologies and procedures that are being considered for coverage under Medicare. Requests for these evaluations come from the Health Care Financing Administration. OHTA carries out its evaluations by reviewing the literature and by getting advice from various agencies and professional organizations. The information so acquired is synthesized to reach some conclusion. OHTA does not gather primary data itself. Again and again, it turns out, and OHTA notes, that the primary data are almost nonexistent and that primary data would be required to reach a well-informed conclusion. Similarly, at the consensus conferences, speakers frequently point out the lack of primary data. Thus, the most important need is to gather more primary data.

To gather primary data, however, more primary research is needed. This effort will have to be led in part by research physicians with training in quantitative methods and will have to be supported by doctoral-level epidemiologists and biostatisticians. All three groups are in short supply. At the least the development of methods will also require epidemiologists and biostatisticians. Therefore, on the grounds of both research and methodology, funds will be needed to train research personnel.

A component of medical technology assessment is the examination of the social, ethical, and legal questions raised by the use of technology in clinical practice. Such questions do not always lend themselves to quantitative measurement and analysis, but they can be systematically identified and evaluated.

The committee's findings in reviewing research methods and myriad assessments in Chapter 3 led to the following three recommendations.

- *Increase research activity to improve and strengthen the variety of methods that are applicable to the assessment of medical technology.*

• *Increase the resources for training research workers in medical technology, both for advancing the methodology and for applying those methods to the many unevaluated technologies.*

• *Invest greater effort and resources into obtaining evaluative primary data about medical technology already in use.* (This recommendation also flowed from our analysis of the scope of technology assessment in Chapter 2.)

EFFECTS OF EVALUATION ON DIFFUSION OF TECHNOLOGY

Many forces influence the adoption or abandonment of a medical technology. Chapter 4 examines whether the method used to evaluate a technology has an effect on its diffusion. The emphasis is on physician practices and the influence of various types of clinical evaluation in changing those practices.

Diffusion and Its Determinants

Diffusion refers to the spread of an innovation over time in a social system. Built into the notion of diffusion is the expectation that social change is not instantaneous and that some difference in practice among physicians at a moment in time is therefore reasonable and likely. Of the factors that bear on the adoption and abandonment of medical technology, four (prevailing theory, attributes of the innovation, features of the clinical situation, and the presence of an advocate) are relatively insensitive to change by policymakers. Three others (practice setting, decision-making process, and characteristics of the potential adopters) may be subject over time to some policy influence. An additional three factors (environmental constraints and incentives, conduct and methods of evaluation, and channels of communication) are relatively susceptible to influence by policymakers. These are described in Chapter 4.

Types of Evaluation That Precede Accepted Medical Practice

Many studies have attempted to assess the effects of different types of evaluation in the period before general acceptance of a medical practice. Of special interest are studies that compare the influence of randomized and nonrandomized clinical trials.

In some cases the patterns of practice over time conform partially to the findings of randomized controlled trials (RCTs). For example, for coronary artery surgery, treatment of breast cancer, and the use of lipid-lowering drugs it seems highly likely that RCTs have influenced clinical practice. When multiple RCTs, and possibly other studies as well, suggest changes in practice in a similar direction, it may be difficult to discern the particular effect of a single study; yet, circumstantial evidence supporting the eventual influence of the collection of studies can be strong.

In the opinion of many oncologists and researchers involved in evaluations of cancer treatment, randomized trials have generally been more useful than nonrandomized trials in the development of cancer therapies. But, some studies that have looked quantitatively at the origins of current therapeutic practices in several types of cancer also have found nonrandomized studies to have played a dominant role in the development of therapy. For example, nonrandomized trials, more frequently than RCTs, were the source of currently accepted treatments for acute leukemia, although these were later verified by RCTs.

Clinical evaluation, being only one among many factors bearing on the diffusion of medical technology, often seems to be overwhelmed by the other nine determinants of physician behavior discussed in Chapter 4. Improving the care of patients requires both improved methods of evaluation and more effective translation of the results of evaluation into practice. Evaluations are likely to exert a greater impact on diffusion if they are buttressed by attention to other controllable factors, such as channels of communication and environmental constraints and incentives, that affect the adoption and abandonment of medical technology.

Recommendations

The discussion in Chapter 4 led the study committee to make the following recommendations (in italics).

- *Strengthen the weaker methods of evaluating medical practice and increase the use of the stronger methods.* Methods such as case studies, consensus development, and nonrandomized trials can be improved through research, and such proved mainstays as randomized controlled trials can be more widely applied. Chapter 3 also supports this recommendation.
- *Study the diffusion of medical practice concepts and procedures to understand how to speed up the adoption of good practices and discourage the use of those that are less effective or harmful.* Such research should place emphasis on factors of diffusion, e.g., channels of communication and environmental constraints or incentives, that lend themselves to some control by public policy and organizational decisions.
- *Establish lines of responsibility for making better medical practice a consequence of the evaluation of medical technology.* The connection between favorable assessment of a technology and its subsequent diffusion into practice is a wandering path among clinicians, educators, researchers, professional bodies, journal editors, hospitals, drug and device manufacturers, third-party payers, regulatory agencies, and others. Their various perspectives obscure responsibility for the diffusion of technologies. The diffuseness of the responsibility for translating the results of evaluation into improved health care is one motivation behind proposals for a public-private entity sponsored by the Institute of Medicine and for additional forms of organization discussed in this report.

REIMBURSEMENT AND TECHNOLOGY ASSESSMENT

Spending for health care in the United States rose from 6 percent of the gross national product in 1965, the year Medicare was created, to 10.8 percent in 1983. With public money being used for more than 40 percent of that spending, policymakers are searching for ways to reduce health care costs. Some analysts blame the use of new medical technologies and the overuse of existing technologies for up to 50 percent of the increases in expenditures for health care over recent years. From that perspective, one way to reduce costs would be to reduce the use of the technologies. That, however, would require that we be able to identify the technologies that are relatively ineffective, or even harmful, and discard them.

The primary purpose of medical technology assessment is to improve patient care. But it also is important to both private and public payers, receiving greater attention as its potential for cutting costs of health care has become apparent.

Chapter 5 traces the applications of medical technology assessment as they have evolved from a context of retrospective payment for health care to one of prospective payment. At first, when assessment was used largely by insurers and government to make informed decisions about coverage of health care services, its application was only partially designed to control health care costs. However, technology assessment now is seen as an aid to cost containment because it can help to determine relative cost-effectiveness of diagnostic and therapeutic procedures. The success of that application of assessment as an adjunct of economic policymaking will depend on many factors, including how to cover the costs of the assessment itself.

There are many examples of the ability and interest of private health insurers in conducting technology assessment, but there are no national or regional standards. Medicare claims recommended for payment, or subscribers' covered benefits, vary across the nation.

Despite assessment activities by the Health Care Financing Administration, insurers, and others, spending for health care has continued to rise. There are some legal reasons that technology assessment has not restrained costs. Antitrust challenges arise when insurers attempt to limit payments to certain providers. The authority to apply reimbursement sanctions to implement the findings of assessment, even if quality is at stake, must be clearly spelled out in the law. Obstacles for private insurers also lie in market forces. Buyers of private insurance policies want the widest array of benefits for the least outlay, and competition among various private insurers is fierce. Also, there are political considerations that blunt the effects of technology assessment. Public programs have not regulated physicians' fees or rationed costly services such as hemodialysis.

However, even if these constraints on the application of technology assessment were to be removed, the data bases on which insurers have to depend to make coverage decisions are inadequate. There is a growing need by payers for more information that could be used for technology assessment as well as for full analysis of the basis for differing costs for patients with different illnesses.

Assessment in the New Era of Cost Containment

Today's emphasis on cost containment is reflected in plans for altering reimbursement (payment methods) to induce and even reward cost-saving behavior. Radical changes in federal reimbursement policy have occurred through amendments related to Medicare. Until recently, most major payers such as Medicare reimbursed hospitals retrospectively on the basis of costs incurred. Under that system, the acquisition and use by hospitals of new technology and of all medical procedures (if the coverage decisions had already been made) could be fully covered regardless of their cost.

Cost-containment advocates devised a different way of calculating reimbursement. The Diagnosis-Related Group (DRG) became the product definition for hospitals. The DRG for each of hundreds of ills is the result of the distillation of patient discharge abstracts to find group characteristics that were clinically sensible and statistically clustered for cost, length of stay, and other measures of resource consumption. The Social Security Reform Act of 1983 will move Medicare payments toward a prospective reimbursement system based on an average DRG specific price.

The new reimbursement policy would appear to encourage the assessment of medical technologies for their safety, patient benefit, and costs, but the strength of demand for technology assessment will depend on many factors. These factors include (1) the dependence of a hospital on Medicare revenues, (2) the present and eventual restrictions on a hospital's capital acquisition, (3) the presence or absence of incentives for cost-efficiency in the reimbursement system, (4) how the DRG is priced and how much an institution knows about its cost variances from some norm, (5) whether and how cost performance data are used to change patterns of physician practice, and (6) incentives for assessment and appropriate use of technology.

Paying for Technology Assessment

Many authors and conferees have addressed the question of reimbursement for technology assessment. Clinical trials and similar studies have been proposed, and most of the proposals envision funds for assessment coming from the health care dollar. Chapter 5, in emphasizing the uses of technology assessment as a part of changing reimbursement policy, asks: "If the need for medical technology assessment couples so fully with the need for rational cost containment, a major policy issue is posed for lawmakers: Should reimbursement regulation be used to enforce scientific decisions about the safety, efficacy, and cost-effectiveness of technologies?"

Recommendations

In Chapter 5 it is argued convincingly that, for technology assessment to reduce the cost of medical care, the assessment process and the reimbursement system must become more congruent. Toward that end, the study committee made the following recommendations (in italics).

- *Decisions about payment for medical care should be based on more than safety, efficacy, and research status of the care.* A beginning in expanding the criteria exists in the new prospective payment system, which encourages the cost-effectiveness of care.
- *Data collected for claims purposes should be made more useful for technology assessment.* Again, the advent of prospective payment, which includes diagnosis and characteristics of care in the information needed for claims, may possibly contribute to technology assessment.
- *Payment for medical technology assessment should be made through the system that pays for medical care.* The prospective payment system already includes set-aside funding for technology, which could be earmarked for assessment. Another possibility is to pay for the use of experimental technology if the result would be the collection of data on safety, efficacy, and cost-effectiveness. Still another way is to set aside for assessment a percentage of the health care dollar, as handled by third-party payers and both public and private providers.

MEDICAL TECHNOLOGY ASSESSMENT ABROAD

Medical technology increasingly is the object of public scrutiny not only in the United States but also in other industrialized countries. A review of the current approaches and policies of different countries for assessing drugs and devices and for controlling equipment purchases shows that there is increasing concern for safety, efficacy, costs, and social and ethical issues. This has led to some new institutional mechanisms for technology assessment. However, the institutional arrangements that exist to regulate medical technology and carry out assessments vary substantially from country to country, as described in Chapter 6.

Most industrialized countries have consistent national policies and institutional arrangements for evaluating the safety and efficacy of drugs. These appear to have been strengthened in recent years, influenced to some extent by the U.S. Food and Drug Administration's example and assistance to other countries. The current World Health Organization program to assist countries that want to improve their drug regulatory systems reinforces this trend.

However, systematic regulation of devices has been established only in the United States, Sweden, Japan, and Canada; most assessment of devices elsewhere proceeds on an ad hoc basis. Even in countries that have policies for the assessment of devices, the procedures are of more recent origin and less systematic than are those for drugs.

Sweden is one of the few countries to develop a national policy or institutional arrangement for the assessment of devices, equipment, and procedures used in medical care. The Swedish Planning and Rationalization Institute of Health Services (SPRI) was established in 1968 by the Swedish government and the Federation of County Councils (which are the health care authorities in Sweden) and has been involved in the conduct of technology assessment since 1980. The organization has a mandate to solve problems confronting those who work in the health care sectors and to promote better use of existing health services resources. Additional tasks include information dissemination, establishment of standard specifications for hospital equipment, and planning.

Collaboration and exchange of information in a systematic way among countries may well provide governments with opportunities to review their policies on these matters and to draw on other countries' experiences when considering different approaches. Most countries do not yet have a coordinated coherent system for medical technology assessment. Until coordinated systems are developed within countries, it will be very difficult, if not impossible, to develop any international system of medical technology assessment.

However, most countries do appear to have a system for determining the safety and efficacy of drugs. Therefore, it is not surprising that more progress appears to have been made toward international collaboration in the assessment of drugs than in the assessment of devices or medical practices. The presence of national organizations charged with drug evaluation provides a focus for these activities and facilitates international collaboration. The presence of formal mechanisms for the assessment of drugs in developed countries is evidence of international interest in technology assessment that may be extended to devices and procedures. This shared interest may prompt standardization of methods, data exchange, and other forms of collaboration, especially if it leads to development of formal systems for such efforts. Several international organizations, most particularly the Organization of Economic Cooperation and Development and the World Health Organization, have made an important beginning to systematic approaches to the international assessment of drugs.

Recommendations

The information collected in the preparation of Chapter 6 prompted the study committee to make the following recommendations (in italics).

- *International collaboration among the industrialized nations is necessary for the fullest establishment of a comprehensive system of medical technology assessment in any one of them. A first step should be collaboration in gathering data on such technologies and on research concerning their assessment.*
- *An international clearinghouse should be established to serve as an information pool of data gathered on medical technologies and research concerning their assessment.* The World Health Organization network is a beginning. In the United States, the proposed Institute of Medicine consortium, whose initial function would be as a clearinghouse, could be part of an international union of information sources on medical technology assessment.
- *An international clearinghouse should be established for information about clinical trials.* A possible model is the British National Perinatal Epidemiology Unit at Oxford, which promotes clinical trials and conducts research on their effect on medical practice.
- *Industrialized nations with competence in medical technology assessment should work with less-developed countries to help them fill their special needs for information.*

CONCLUSIONS AND RECOMMENDATIONS

Over the years many organizations have developed assessments of medical technology in response to specific needs. Taken singly, each program fulfills a particular purpose; for example, the Food and Drug Administration's premarketing approval process protects the public from unsafe and inefficacious drugs. Taken in combination, however, these various responses do not constitute a coherent system for assessing all types of medical technologies.

The lack of a systematic approach causes some obvious problems:

- The information base for technology assessment often is inadequate; collection of primary data about medical technologies has not kept pace with their development.
- The information that has been collected is not easily available; no one office monitors, collects, indexes, and disseminates such information.
- There are no consistent and reliable procedures for identifying emerging technologies that may have major consequences.
- No one entity is responsible for setting priorities among the technologies to be assessed.
- Some technologies may be assessed too late—or never.
- New uses of established technologies may escape assessment.
- Some valuable procedures are underutilized.
- Findings of assessment can move too slowly in affecting practice.

The principal objective in assessing medical technology is the improved health of people. The primary costs of the lack of an adequate system for technology assessment are to human well-being—patients do not receive optimal care. But there also are economic costs if the most cost-effective technologies are not applied, or if ineffective technologies are.

The worth of technology assessment in medicine reaches beyond its warranty to the patient and its utility to the health professional. The results of assessment also are needed by hospitals and other facilities that buy and apply technologies; by industries that develop technologies; by the professional societies that disseminate information to health care practitioners; and by the insurance companies, government agencies, and corporate health plans that pay for the use of technologies. A strategy for assessing medical technology therefore must take into account not only the methods of assessment but also the needs, demands, and resistances of the participants and beneficiaries in the process.

The Challenge

We believe that it is possible and desirable to establish a coherent system for technology assessment. Many elements of such a system already are in place and can be built on. Numerous agencies and organizations are supporting or conducting assessments. The committee endorses this pluralism, believing that it contributes to the richness and variety of assessment activities and it serves as a system of checks and balances. Furthermore, practical methods of inquiry into medical technology exist, methods that are well developed, widely accepted, and often reliable and that have practitioners in place to apply them.

The challenge to this committee was to devise one or more strategies for medical technology assessment, built on current efforts, but in addition to strengthen and supplement them.

Key Functions for Assessment

Functions that must be well executed to ensure adequate medical technology assessment include the following:

- selecting and collecting information,
- combining information from different sources,
- disseminating information,
- identifying lacks in knowledge that require research,
- acquiring data for needed research,
- setting priorities for assessment,
- training technology assessors, and
- developing methods for assessment.

Building a System

Results of this inquiry have indicated that existing institutional arrangements, and probably existing legislative authorities, are inadequate to support an orderly system for technology assessment. Ways must be found to organize and finance the functions we have described. In addition, because some elements of an effective system already are in place, we must be alert to opportunities for building and strengthening functions that exist as well as for establishing new institutional arrangements when warranted.

In a 1982 report OTA described several possibilities for institutional arrangements: (1) congressional establishment of a private-public body, (2) re-establishment of the National Center for Health Care Technology, or (3) encouraging the secretary of DHHS to apply the existing powers of the office to develop a technology assessment system. An additional possibility would be the creation of a new federal institution. The advantages and disadvantages of the four arrangements are discussed in Chapter 7.

However, the committee acknowledges that today's most reliable health care technology assessment is being conducted as a regulatory activity—for drugs and medical devices. The success of that assessment relies on the authority of the Food and Drug Administration to demand the collection of high-quality data as a prerequisite to marketing; and, of course, the profit motive encourages fulfillment of that requirement.

The committee encourages nonregulatory approaches to technology assessment in the belief that better cooperation will be inspired by offering incentives, for instance, forms of reimbursement that encourage the needed collection of primary data.

Financing

The estimate that public and private spending on medical technology assessment totals over $1 billion yearly makes it seem like a big and costly enterprise. Yet this is a generous estimate for a broadly defined category that embraces controlled and uncontrolled clinical trials, health services research, and a wide variety of synthesis activities. Even so, it is only 0.3 percent of the money that is spent for health care. The committee believes that the importance of better assessment is sufficiently great to warrant expending on it a bigger share of the health care dollar.

Various proposals have been advanced to fund more medical technology assessment in health care and are reviewed in the full report. The committee believes that, whatever methods are chosen, there is an immediate need for $30 million to improve some of the technology assessment functions described earlier. That sum is only for "first steps," the committee states, believing that the total should grow in 10 years by about $300 million in 1984 dollars.

Recommendations

We wish to promote the development of a coordinated system for medical technology assessment that both would capitalize on the strengths and resources of the free-market economy and would meet society's needs for safe, effective medical care. The following recommendations (in italics) constitute a stepwise approach to achieve that purpose.

- *The monitoring, synthesizing, and disseminating functions of medical technology assessment should be established in some entity with a chartered mission and financing.* A private-public organization seems most appropriate.
- *The same entity should develop the research agenda for filling gaps in knowledge relevant to assessment*, as well as assign responsibility for carrying out the needed research.
- *There should be a substantial increase in the accumulation of primary data for assessment.*
- *A portion of the health care dollar should be allocated to existing Public Health Service components that already have the task of supporting research in medical technology assessment.* These components should solicit and fund research designed to fill gaps in knowledge about technologies where the profit motive does not operate to catalyze the collection of primary data, such as occurs in the drug industry.
- *Those organizations that support research in technology assessment also should engage in developing it as a scientific field, such as improving methodologies and supporting education and training of assessment personnel.*
- *Support for medical technology assessment should rise over the next 10 years to reach an annual level $300 million greater (in 1984 dollars) than at present.*

In casting its recommendations, the committee was aware that statements of generality are of little help, but that too much detail can entangle an enterprise. It recognizes that political action will be required. Building a system of medical technology assessment will require not only patient attention to improving the key functions, but also a steady emphasis on continuity and stability of effort and funding to ensure a firm foundation for its construction.

1 Introduction

Medical care has changed dramatically in recent decades; it has become more effective, more costly, and more ambitious. Changes have been impelled by new developments in biology, molecular biology, pharmacology, chemistry, physics, bioengineering, materials science, computing, and other scientific and technical fields. Medical advances have meant new medical technologies.

New technologies force changes throughout the system; old procedures are discarded, new ones replace them (perhaps too soon or too late), the definition of what is accepted medical practice shifts, third-party payers pay for medical interventions that were earlier unknown and they stop paying for some superseded ones, textbooks are revised, medical school curricula change, and old equipment is replaced with new.

The expanding gap between the health care that can be provided by the available financial resources and the health care that could be provided if there were no financial constraint makes it increasingly necessary that the health care technologies to be available and the conditions of availability be chosen knowledgeably.

One might hope that such selection processes would be guided by an orderly, well-conceived, unified system of testing and assessing the new, comparing it with the old, and moving forward as warranted by valid, reliable, evaluative information. That hope is at present only partially fulfilled.

Prompt and valid assessment of medical technology is important both to individuals and institutions. The use or nonuse of a new drug, device, or procedure directly concerns two individuals, the patient and the physician. The hospital, manufacturing firms, and insurance companies must all make and unmake various arrangements when new technology replaces old. Elucidation of medical technology assessment thus demands analysis that contemplates both the individual and the social interests.

This chapter was prepared by Lincoln E. Moses and Frederick Mosteller based on a document drafted by David Banta and Donald Young. David Banta contributed the material for the examples on electronic fetal monitoring, the computed tomography scanner, drug treatment for hypertension, and hysterectomy.

Two examples of the impact of technology assessment illustrate the contribution to be made to disease prevention and to enhancing the quality of patient care.

POLIO

Paralytic poliomyelitis used to strike many children, usually during the summer; swimming pool and other recreation facilities often would close because of a polio epidemic. The Salk vaccine was invented to prevent polio, though no one knew how effective it could be. The idea of a large public test of a vaccine on children was remarkable in itself, though having a President, Franklin D. Roosevelt, who had been afflicted with the disease lent substantial support to the trial.

To be convincing, such a trial had to be large because the annual rate of this disease was about 50 per 100,000 population but this number varied widely from year to year and from place to place. An unusual feature was that it struck well-to-do neighborhoods more often than lower-income groups. Less-hygienic living conditions are believed to lead to earlier childhood exposure to the virus while the immunity conferred by the mother still protected the child. It is also true that less educated and less well-to-do groups volunteered less often to participate in such investigations. Originally the study design proposed was to vaccinate children in grade 2 and compare them with children not vaccinated in grades 1 and 3. Some state health department officials objected that such a loose design might leave uncertainty no matter how the study results came out. They would not let their states participate without a randomized controlled study. In the end, both studies were carried out, and the results show the wisdom of having the tighter control.

The placebo controlled experiment had 201,000 children in the placebo and in the vaccinated groups and 339,000 who were not inoculated. The resulting rates of paralytic polio per 100,000 population (using laboratory determination) among the vaccinated groups was 16 and among the placebo group was 57. Those not inoculated had a rate of 36, which was considerably lower than the rate of 46 for the controls in grades 1 and 3 of the other study. The latter were not selected by their refusal to participate and thus included all groups. The reduction from 57 to 16 was substantial and led to widespread use of this and other vaccines in the United States and elsewhere and to a very diminished rate of paralytic polio (Meier, 1978).

SURGICAL PROCEDURE

A landmark assessment of a surgical technology was carried out on relatively few patients by Cobb et al. (1959) and by Dimond et al. (1958) in separate but nearly simultaneous experiments. Barsamian (1977) points out that as a treatment for angina pectoris the surgical procedure of internal mammary artery ligation was rapidly introduced by surgeons in Italy and the United States, theorizing that the operation would reduce pain by shunting blood into the coronary circulation. Early reports from operations indicated considerable success. Barsamian said that the operation was introduced rapidly because it was safe (could be done under local anesthesia), simple for the surgeon to learn and carry out, and much needed for a large population of patients with coronary artery disease. Measuring effectiveness, though important, was not a major activity for surgeons in the 1950s. An enthusiastic report in the *Reader's Digest* (Ratcliff, 1957) sent many patients to surgeons asking for the operation.

Cobb applied the operation to 17 patients; for 8 the real operation was carried out, and these patients reported a 34 percent subjective improvement in the first 6 months following surgery; 9 patients had a sham operation (which included everything in the real procedure except tying off the arteries), and these patients reported 42 percent subjective improvement. Dimond gave the real operation to 13 patients, 10 of whom showed substantial improvement, while 5 patients getting the sham operation all reported significant improvement.

Barsamian (1977) said that this test of this operation forced recognition of the possibility that surgery or medicine could have a placebo effect. From this followed the demand and acceptance of controlled studies of surgery.

Much of the nation's finest scientific and technological talent conducts research intended ultimately to improve the health of Americans. The importance of basic research for these purposes is well understood, and both the National Institutes of Health and industry invest heavily in it. The work of development also is well recognized. Less appreciated is the bridge in the road from basic research to beneficial use for human beings, namely, technology assessment. One might expect that, with all the research and development that is accomplished, any product, device, or system produced would automatically be beneficial and that the invisible hand of marketplace economics would make a new technology cost-effective. This expectation brings frequent disappointments. For example, in the area of surgery and anesthesia, Gilbert et al. (1977) found that less than half of the surgical innovations brought to careful testing in a randomized controlled trial were regarded by their assessors as successful. In addition, Gilbert et al. (1977) and Grace et al. (1966) show that weakly controlled studies tend to favor innovations more than do well-controlled studies. Gittelsohn and Wennberg (1977) find that small similar areas of a state have great variation in the frequency of performance of such surgical procedures as tonsillectomy, appendectomy, and hysterectomy. Such variation raises questions about the appropriate level of use of these operations. Thus technology assessment is necessary to verify that innovations do or do not work in practice. Cost comparisons and social consequences also require technology assessment.

It is not obvious that the step of technology assessment is required, nor are such assessments easy to make. Indeed, in some areas it is not known how to do them. Because the necessity for this step is not widely appreciated, the nation has not thoroughly developed a system for doing it, though many groups contribute to a partial effort, as will be explained in Chapter 2 and in greater detail in Appendix A. Such efforts are needed, but also costly. It is the committee's belief that additional funds are required for technology assessment and that these incremental funds should come from the health dollar. In the matter of drugs and devices that the Food and Drug Administration regulates, industry pays for testing for safety and efficacy, and the public ultimately pays when products are marketed. In other matters, such as cost-effectiveness and downstream consequences, the health system as a whole is involved with no natural agency or organization to give support to these efforts. For example, market forces like those that support assessment of drugs do not exist for surgical procedures.

The nation requires a systematic approach to technology assessment. A strategy and an organization for setting priorities is needed as well. Given the priorities, mechanisms are needed for actually making the assessments and implementing their findings. Finally a method is needed for paying for many of the needed assessments. As with any large-scale technological enterprise, it is necessary to maintain a strong body of professional personnel to carry out the assessments, and they must be encouraged to conduct work of high quality and develop new techniques as required. Although in some areas parts of this overall process are in place and contribute well to the nation's health, the system as a whole has major gaps and deficiencies, which will be described.

Simply knowing the outcomes for the health care system and their relation to the treatments and diagnoses employed might help in designing a more economical and effective system. Just now a strong link that connects outcome to care is not known. Partly this comes from not knowing how to set up such a system. A vast, sprawling monitoring system cannot be what is needed. Some keen minds should think about better indicators that relate care and outcome. Part of the trouble is that much of the current health care system contributes to quality of life rather than to morbidity and mortality. By and large, accomplishments are not assessed in these softer areas, and so medicine does not get nearly the credit due for these contributions to comfort and convenience. Part of the difficulty arises from the fact that the health delivery system is itself a dynamic process applied to a changing population. We would not have it otherwise, but it helps to explain how hard outcome studies for whole populations must be. Having mentioned this larger problem, we turn back now to the narrower ideas of technology assessment.

The questions of who should carry out assessments, how they should be done, and who should pay for them are complicated and political and have no simple answers. Consequently the study described here was conducted. This report addresses the present state of the assessment of medical technology, gives attention to processes, problems, interested parties, successes, and failures, and finally points to some needs and opportunities for improving the present system of medical technology assessment.

EXAMPLES OF TECHNOLOGY ASSESSMENT

For examples, this section begins with brief sketches of how five medical technologies have recently made their entrance into medical practice. A number of common themes recur, and these will help to shape a systematic treatment of the subject. Because medicine moves rapidly, further work will have been done on the problems treated in these examples by the time this work is published. The purpose here is not to publish the latest information but to give a feel for the varieties of technology assessment that arise.

Electronic Fetal Monitoring

Electronic fetal monitoring (EFM) is a technologic step beyond the stethoscope for monitoring the heart rate of the fetus during labor and delivery. EFM enables evaluation of fetal heart rate patterns in relation to uterine contractions and facilitates detection of certain types of abnormal patterns. Concerns about preventable perinatal mortality and brain damage led investigators to seek a more reliable and valid method of following fetal status during labor (Banta and Thacker, 1979). Advances in electronics during World War II made electronic fetal monitors feasible, as first demonstrated by a team at Yale University. Such monitors became available on the market in about 1968, and their use spread rather quickly into most of the obstetric units in the United States. By 1980 about half of the deliveries in this country were electronically monitored (Placek et al., 1983a,b).

But in the mid-1970s electronic monitoring already had become controversial because it was suspected of being associated with inappropriate cesarean sections. This question stimulated several randomized clinical trials (RCTs) (Haverkamp et al., 1976; Renou et al., 1976; Kelso et al.,

1978; Haverkamp et al., 1979; Wood et al., 1981). Although the trials consistently found no reduction in fetal or infant mortality from use of the electronic monitor as compared with auscultation, they did suggest an association with increases in cesarean delivery rates. The basic problem with these RCTs is that they were all too small. Any beneficial effects of EFM would be so slight as to require very large studies to detect them. Another shortcoming of the RCTs is that none included low-birth-weight fetuses (including prematures), who are at greatest risk of mortality and morbidity. More recently, a trial in about 13,000 low-risk women in Dublin, Ireland—a sufficient number to yield valid results—has found no benefit in terms of reduced mortality from EFM but has suggested a decrease in neurologic damage and a dramatic decrease in numbers of infant convulsions with monitoring (Ingemarsson, 1981; McDonald et al., 1983). Also the Dublin trial found no difference in cesarean rates for the monitored groups.

The risks associated with electronic monitoring are of concern. These range from infection and hemorrhage to a possible correlation with the incidence of cesarean section, which would be the greatest risk. The rate of cesarean sections in the United States was 4.5 percent of deliveries in 1965, but rose steadily to about 18 percent in 1980 (Placek et al., 1983a,b).

EFM also is expensive. Banta and Thacker (1979) estimated an annual cost of such monitoring at $411 million, including indirect costs such as those of cesarean sections and other complications. Cohen (1983), using a more thorough method of estimation, projected annual costs of from $210 million to $385 million. (These studies however do not include the possible benefits of preventing neurologic damage.) Electronic fetal monitoring is a good example of inadequate evaluation. More than 15 years after its introduction, more work is needed to define its appropriate use. One RCT is now being done in low-birth-weight infants and may answer some questions. In the meantime, a risky and costly procedure continues in widespread use.

Computed Tomography Scanning

The computed tomography (CT) scanner is a revolutionary diagnostic device that combines x-ray equipment with a computer and a cathode ray tube display to produce images of cross sections of the human body (Office of Technology Assessment, 1978). The CT scanner was the result of decades of research in such fields as mathematics, computer applications, and x-ray tomography. During the 1960s several people in the United States realized that it would be possible to develop a medical diagnostic device based on this research, but they were unable to interest either industry or government. Late in that decade, Hounsfield, working at EMI Ltd. in England, was able to convince his company to develop a prototype device (Hounsfield, 1980). The British Department of Health and Social Services also contributed some funds to the project. The first demonstrations were held at international radiology meetings in 1972, and the device was rapidly accepted by the medical community. The importance of the technological advance was recognized by the award of the Nobel Prize in medicine to some of the developers.

Plaudits notwithstanding, the CT scanner has come to symbolize the problem of high-cost medical technology (Banta, 1980). In part, this was because of the rapidity of its spread in industrialized countries. In part, it was because of its expense: the typical scanner cost $300,000 or more in 1973 and by 1984 it cost almost $1,000,000. The United States now has more than 2,000 scanners, representing a capital investment of more than $1 billion. Operation of the scanners costs the United States at least another $1 billion annually.

CT scanning is such a radical departure from conventional radiographs that it will take years of research for its proper roles to be assessed in different parts of the body and in different disorders.

Although many evaluations of CT scanning have been done, few studies have addressed a fundamental question: For what kinds of patients is application of this diagnostic technology worth its costs? (Wagner, 1980). When dealing with diagnostic technologies, answering this question requires answering another question: How does a particular technology fit into an optimal diagnostic process for a given condition? In other words, which diagnostic technologies should be used in a particular patient who needs to have a diagnosis established? The importance of this question may be illustrated by data indicating that millions of CT head scans were done each year for people with uncomplicated headaches until CT was better evaluated.

The United States now faces the emergence of nuclear magnetic resonance imaging, which is another example in the sequence of technology development. Without better evaluative studies for this and other new technologies, a great deal of money might be wasted on inappropriate diagnostic tests, and important opportunities might be missed to do diagnostic tests on people who truly need them.

Drug Treatment for Hypertension

Hypertension, or high blood pressure, is the most common chronic disease in the United States. Estimates are that about 60 million people in this country have definite or borderline hypertension (Levy, 1982). People with high blood pressure are more likely to have strokes, heart disease, and kidney failure than people with normal blood pressure.

Hypertension can be controlled by drug treatment. In the late 1960s, the Veterans Administration supported a multi-institutional RCT of treatment for men with the drugs hydrochlorothiazide, reserpine, and hydralazine. The control group was given placebos. The drug treatment was remarkably effective for men with diastolic pressures higher than 105 mm of mercury. For example, strokes were reduced by 75 percent, and congestive heart failure, renal failure, and dissecting aneurysm occurred only in the control group (Veterans Administration, 1967, 1970). The growing use of drug treatment for high blood pressure has been considered to be one of the factors that has led to a falling rate of death from heart disease in this country (Havlik and Feinleib, 1979).

However, although a growing percentage of people with high blood pressure are being treated, many still are not. Recent surveys done in Connecticut, South Carolina, Maryland, and California have shown that 18 to 28 percent of those with definite hypertension were unaware that they had the disease, and that another 21 to 34 percent were aware but were not receiving adequate therapy (National Center for Health Statistics [NCHS], 1983). Thus, very positive results of an evaluation of drug therapy have not yet been fully implemented nationally and people are still dying of cardiovascular disease at an unnecessarily high rate.

Mild hypertension is a different problem. Clinical trials have not given clear-cut evidence as to whether people with diastolic pressures under 95 mm of mercury should be treated (Hypertension Detection and Follow-up Program Cooperative Group, 1982). Yet, surveys of physicians have shown that they frequently prescribe drugs for mild hypertension (Guttmacher et al., 1981). More recent clinical trials have not resolved this scientific issue for patients under 50 years of age, which is of concern because antihypertensive drug treatment is not benign (Joint National Committee on Detection, Evaluation, and Treatment of High Blood

Pressure, 1984). Complications associated with drug treatment include dizziness, impotence, and general tiredness. Side effects can be minimized by careful medical supervision, but it is doubtful whether such care is usually available. The practice of treatment of mild hypertension has been criticized as seeking the technological rather than the social solution to disease, because the incidence of high blood pressure is often associated with stressful life situations (National Institutes of Health, 1979). The drug industry's promotion of drug treatment for mild hypertension also has been criticized. In short, drug treatment for hypertension is one of the most important medical advances of this century. However, questions remain that can be answered only by good assessments.

Hysterectomy

Surgical removal of the uterus is performed more often than any other major operation in the United States. The National Center for Health Statistics estimates that 704,800 hysterectomies were performed in the United States in 1978, compared with 678,000 in 1976. The 1978 rate is 817.3 per 100,000 women 15 years of age and older (Korenbrot et al., 1980). More recent figures for 1980 and 1981 indicate rates of 563 and 573 per 100,000 women, respectively (Easterday et al., 1983). At such a rate, more than half of American women would have their uterus removed by age 65. The high rate of hysterectomy is not peculiar to the United States (L. J. Kozak, National Center for Health Statistics, personal communication). Canada and Australia have rates approximately as high as those in the United States. It is frequently alleged that many of these hysterectomies are unnecessary.

Medical indications for hysterectomy are not standard, and this leads to variations in the rate. Wennberg and Gittelsohn (1973) have demonstrated a strong correlation between the numbers of surgical specialists and the number of operations performed in different districts in Vermont. Cross-national studies comparing the United States, the United Kingdom, and Canada have demonstrated a relationship between the number of surgeons and operations, including hysterectomy (Bunker, 1970; Vayda, 1973).

Some indications for hysterectomy, such as for cancer, are well accepted. The controversial indications are its use as a means of sterilization and its use to prevent cancer of the uterus. About 30 percent of hysterectomies done in the United States are done for these indications (Korenbrot et al., 1980).

Hysterectomy has significant risks. Death occurs in 0.1 to 0.4 percent of cases. If 30 percent of hysterectomies are elective in the United States, a 0.1 percent mortality would mean 210 deaths among this group. Much more frequent are nonfatal operative complications, including bleeding, infection, and complications of transfusion and anesthesia. In a meta-analysis of published reports carried out at Stanford University, 73 percent of women with nonemergency abdominal hysterectomy had some degree of morbidity, and more than 7 percent had moderate to life-threatening complications (Korenbrot et al., 1980).

The financial costs of hysterectomy are high. A hysterectomy was estimated in 1978 to cost from $1,700 to $2,600 in direct medical care expenses (Korenbrot et al., 1980). This figure does not include the costs of complications, nor does it include indirect costs such as lost work or psychological costs. Several cost-effectiveness studies have been done, and none found hysterectomies cost-effective for sterilization or prevention of uterine cancer. The studies have found large immediate risks and costs, with some future benefits. In a recent study, Sanberg et al. (1984) found net costs to range per year from $1,200 to

$3,700 and net increases in life expectancy were on the order of 6 to 8 months.

Thus, hysterectomy is frequently used for questionable indications. Many data that would be useful in assessing this kind of use are lacking, and available data do not strongly defend it. This raises questions of who will do the needed research and what will be done about the frequency of the procedure. Assuming that women are choosing the procedure voluntarily, it may be appropriate for society to decide that some benefits, such as the small, yet unproved likelihood of cancer prevention, are not worth the large immediate costs.

Medical Information System

El Camino Hospital, a medium-sized, nonteaching, community hospital, installed in 1971 a Technicon Medical Information System (TMIS), which processed a broad range of medical and administrative data. Two studies of it by Battelle Columbus Laboratories were funded by the National Center for Health Services Research (Coffey, 1980). The first examined the effect of TMIS on organization and administration. The second study, described here, measured the impact of TMIS on total hospital costs. This example illustrates a partial evaluation of a support system rather than of a treatment or of a diagnostic technology. A more complete evaluation might also study changes in the quality of care. (Although the study presented here discusses costs, these may actually be some form of charges.)

Costs were examined in two ways, one excluding the cost of TMIS and the other including its operational cost. The investigators used three indices: cost per patient, cost per patient day, and cost per month. Cost per patient measures the social cost, expense per patient day keys into health insurance carriers' procedures, and monthly expenses give an overall picture of the hospital budget. Expenses were broken down according to nursing care, ancillary services, and support services. The study covered a 6-year period: 2 years before TMIS, 1 year of installation, and 3 years of full operation.

Multiple regression methods and four control hospitals were used to adjust for variables that could not be controlled.

Table 1-1 shows the overall outcome of changes in costs associated with the operation of the TMIS in its third year of operation. These changes exclude the cost of the TMIS itself. The reduced cost per patient for nursing was said to be due to reduced paperwork and to a reduction in the nursing work force.

Another important impact was that faster turnaround time on tests and execution of orders led to a reduction of 4.7 percent in length of hospital stay. This was remarkable because El Camino already had a very low average length of stay.

The increase of 4.5 percent in support costs per patient was, nevertheless, unex-

TABLE 1-1 Partial Impact of TMIS (Excluding Its Cost) on Three Measures of Cost at El Camino Hospital, by Department

Department	Change in Cost per Patient	Change in Cost per Patient Day	Change in Cost per Month
Nursing	−5.0[a]	−2.0	5.3
Ancillary	−2.4	1.1	7.7[a]
Support	4.5	7.5[a]	14.3[a]
All departments	−0.6	2.3	9.2[a]

[a]Statistically significant beyond the 5 percent level.

pected. Some increase was due to increased medical records work and some to a decision unrelated to TMIS to increase nurses' training. The investigators believed that changes in support costs should not be attributed to the TMIS, and so they analyzed the data in two ways. Table 1-2 shows the results analyzed with an adjustment for these support cost charges (Method 1) and a second analysis that shows exactly what happened with adjustment for support costs (Method 2). The TMIS costs are treated separately, and the two analyses are presented in Table 1-2.

The 4.5 percent difference between the monthly costs at every level of both methods of calculation suggests that the TMIS costs 4.5 percent of the total budget. The investigators speculate that this means that the hospital may have to absorb 40 percent of the cost of the system,with 60 percent covered by improvements in productivity. Earlier studies had shown reduced error rates on orders and tests and improved completeness and accuracy of patient data. Thus, the medical benefits might justify the additional costs, but this issue was not part of the study.

The main conclusions were that (1) nursing costs per patient had been reduced by about 5 percent; (2) average length of stay was reduced by about 4.7 percent, even though El Camino started with a very low rate; (3) TMIS raised overall costs per patient by 1.7 or 3.9 percent depending on whether one ignores support department increases; (4) hospital costs rose 3.2 percent per patient day; and (5) adjusted overall monthly expenses rose 7.8 percent largely because of increased patient flow. Caution should be observed in transferring this experience because management information systems have become more fully developed since then. The outcomes might depend heavily on the patterns of work and the organizational structure of the institution installing a management information system. One would want to assess such a system to see which aspects were working well and which were not; the outcome of the assessment may be unique to the institution. Other studies assessing information systems in hospitals have been carried out by Rogers and Haring (1979) and Haring et al. (1982).

This analysis clearly shows that introducing a new system has extensive and often unexpected ramifications. Tracing the consequences is a difficult task.

SOME LESSONS FROM THE EXAMPLES

It can be seen that medical technology is a term that embraces quite a range of ac-

TABLE 1-2 Overall and Partial Impact of TMIS on Annual Expense of All Departments at El Camino Hospital During 1975, by Two Methods

Unit of Measurement	TMIS Impact Including TMIS Cost (%)	TMIS Impact Excluding TMIS Cost (%)
Method 1. Adjusted for support costs		
Per patient	1.7	−2.8
Per patient day	3.2[a]	−1.3
Per month	7.8[a]	3.3[a]
Method 2. Unadjusted Results		
Per patient	3.9	−0.6
Per patient day	6.8	2.3
Per month	13.7	9.2

[a]Statistically significant beyond the 5 percent level.

tivities. For consistency the committee follows the usage of the Office of Technology Assessment (OTA, 1982), which uses the term to refer to "techniques, drugs, equipment, and procedures used by health-care professionals in delivering medical care to individuals, and the systems within which such care is delivered."

The five examples illustrate some of the dimensions along which medical technology varies. Two examples, electronic fetal monitoring (EFM) and computed tomography (CT), are diagnostic; two, hysterectomy (Hx) and drug treatment for hypertension (DTH), are therapeutic; one, information processing, is a supporting technology; one is a drug, one is a surgical procedure, three are strongly equipment linked.

At least six issues occur in three or more of the five examples:

1. Risks—how probable and how severe are associated adverse effects? (EFM, DTH, Hx)
2. Appropriateness—are there indications for use in at least some patients? (All five)
3. Benefits—what are they? How large? How sure? (All five)
4. Insufficient evidence in the extant studies. (EFM, CT, Hx, DTH)
5. Rapidity and scope of diffusion into clinical use. (The first four suggested the possibility of too rapid and extensive acceptance; in addition, DTH suggested underutilization.)
6. Cost, both to patient and as a social investment. (All five)

Two further issues should be adduced here, although we do not undertake to measure their intensity in the examples:

7. Assessment of costs, risks, and benefits can be difficult, and requires information that is hard to get or lacks conceptual clarity about subtle matters such as quality of life.
8. Ethical questions are inherent and include equity of access to new technology, reasonableness of allocation of scarce medical resources, and mistreatment of some patients because of incorrectly established indications, etc.

These eight issues constitute problems that are addressed by technology assessment, a term that we now can treat more specifically. The term assessment of a medical technology is used here to denote any process of examining and reporting properties of a medical technology used in health care, such as safety; efficacy; feasibility; indications for use; cost and cost-effectiveness; and social, economic, and ethical consequences, intended and unintended. Comprehensive assessment examines all of these issues.

This language is chosen deliberately; it admits of an assessment that is concerned with only a portion of the full spectrum of properties. Some assessments will be only of the safety and efficacy of a technology while others may be more inclusive, adding information about costs and social and ethical impacts. This is intended, because much of assessment activity is partial in its scope. As will be seen, various participants in the health care system find different properties to be salient, focusing their studies narrowly to address the questions that interest them.

COMPREHENSIVE TECHNOLOGY ASSESSMENT

Assessment of medical technology is of course a particular instance of technology assessment as practiced by industry, government, consumers, and various agencies in other fields of applied technology such as transportation, agriculture, or housing. Technology assessment generally is an imperfect but maturing process whose consequences are exemplified in the popular press by the occasional recall of automobiles, the relatively recent redesign of bridge abutments and guard rails on highways, and the constraints imposed on nuclear energy plants.

Arnstein (1977) attributes the concept of technology assessment to Emilio Q. Daddario, former congressman and founding Director of the Office of Technology Assessment. Technology assessment has more holistic implications than such usual methods of technology evaluation as clinical trials, market research, cost-benefit analysis, or environmental impact assessment. Technology assessment ideally would be comprehensive and include evaluation not only of the immediate results of the technology but also of its long-term social, economic, and ethical consequences.

A comprehensive assessment of a medical technology—after assessment of its immediate effects—may also include an appraisal of its unintended consequences, problems of personnel training and licensure, new capital expenditures for equipment and buildings, and possible consequences for the health insurance industry and the social security system. Technology assessment provides a form of policy analysis that includes as potential components the narrower approaches to technology evaluation. Most assessments stop with a partial effort, and we include these when we speak of technology assessment.

The assessment of medical technologies presents certain qualitative and quantitative differences from technology assessment in other sectors. For example, medical technologies often can be assessed only on the basis of observing acutely ill people under conditions in which there is less than full control of important variables and with less than desirable characterization of individual circumstances.

The assessment of medical technologies often is confounded by the occurrence of large changes in the patient or process outcome due to factors outside of the study design. For example, the analysis of the effectiveness of coronary care units for the treatment of patients with myocardial infarction is complicated by the dramatic reduction in mortality from myocardial infarction over the last 15 years which is partly attributable to the change in smoking habits of the population at risk.

DIFFERENT PARTIES, DIFFERENT AIMS IN ASSESSMENTS

The Office of Technology Assessment staff, in treating this subject, wrote (OTA, 1982, p. 3):

> Medical technology assessment is, in a narrow sense, the evaluation or testing of a medical technology for safety and efficacy. In a broader sense, it is a process of policy research that examines the short and long-term consequences of individual medical technologies and thereby becomes the source of information needed by policymakers in formulating regulations and legislation, by industry in developing products, by health professionals in treating and serving patients, and by consumers in making personal health decisions.

For the purposes of this work, nearly all of health services research would be included in this definition.

According to this statement, medical technology assessment involves at least four participants: a policymaker, an administrator, a health care provider, and the patient. The provider and the patient can be seen as a dyad, concerned primarily with the safety and efficacy of particular technologies under consideration for use by that practitioner upon that patient. Although cost, equity, profit, etc., matter a great deal to the dyad, they are not primary factors in their technology assessment.

Patients should be concerned that technologies have been studied in patients similar to themselves. That aspect of equity may be up to the dyad, not in each instance, but in the sense of a general population. Those who choose not to participate in studies need not expect the findings to apply to them.

The medical scientists who test and try out new technologies may concentrate efforts mainly on one feature of the technology. The epidemiologist may study whether a particular adverse outcome is systematically related to the use of a certain treatment (e.g., thromboembolism from using high-estrogen contraceptive pills, or vaginal carcinoma in daughters of mothers who used diethylstilbestrol). The diagnostic imaging specialist may want to assess the relative or absolute information obtained with a test (e.g., echocardiography, radionuclide studies, ultrasound, etc.) because it relates to the efficacy of those technologies. Another medical scientist, evaluating diagnostic or therapeutic algorithms, may focus on a narrow question, such as "Can the algorithm be improved by introducing test Y at some stage?"

The makers of devices, drugs, or other medical equipment may have yet other interests in assessment of their technologies. The manufacturer of a drug, for instance, will seek to develop information to satisfy the requirements of the Food and Drug Administration; both the data and the manner in which they were acquired are subject to regulatory review. Manufacturers more generally will be concerned with the size of the possible market for their product, its costs as seen by the buyer, and its strengths and weaknesses in comparison with competitive products.

Various institutional components of the health profession also are involved in technology assessment, and their concerns relate to their roles. Editors of journals influence what becomes known to readers who rely upon their journals; the influence is exerted both through editorials and through decisions about which articles to publish. Medical school teachers and textbook authors must form, and then propagate, opinions that amount to assessments of safety and efficacy. Professional societies often establish standing or ad hoc panels to study questions relating to the appropriate use of technologies. It sometimes happens that different organizations reach differing conclusions on the same issue.

Third-party payers contribute substantially to medical technology assessment. Requests for payment for a new procedure are likely to trigger a review of the technology. Usually, this review is not deliberately directed at safety and efficacy, but rather it is to help in deciding whether the new procedure conforms to *accepted practice.* A negative decision about reimbursing a new technology will tend to inhibit its diffusion. But sometimes such a decision can stimulate further assessment studies, undertaken by proponents of the technology. Thus, it is reported (Cutler et al., 1973) that some of the studies concerning cost-effectiveness of routine health checkups originated in efforts to justify the provision of reimbursement for such checkups.

Large employers often are major purchasers of medical coverage for their employees. Extension of coverage benefits, perhaps as an item of union contract negotiation, raises the question of which extensions would be most worthwhile. This may quickly lead to comparison of the costs, risks, likely frequency of use, and effectiveness of several medical technologies that are alternative candidates for new coverage.

Hospitals and health maintenance organizations (HMOs) often look at new medical technologies as possible major investments, including both capital costs and costs of operation. The prospective purchaser must assess this technology from many points of view besides its costs. Its probable revenues are of equal concern. Questions of feasibility may be dominant: What are the space requirements? What training is required for personnel to operate it? Will re-education of medical professionals be called for? How about computer support? Costs from the point of view of the patient may receive little attention if reimbursement is assured, or much attention if, as in the HMO, recovery must ultimately be sought through overall increased membership fees, reserves, or other sources.

Some associations of hospitals and other institutions offer to their members assessment-like advice about new technologies. Several of these are described in Chapter 2. For example, the American Hospital Association (AHA) works to assist hospital administrators facing management and investment decisions about new and existing technologies. The AHA program evaluates diagnostic systems, therapeutic systems, computer technologies, and the like, but evaluates medical procedures only as they relate to equipment purchase or nonmedical hospital personnel. The evaluations focus on:

- cost and organizational implications;
- installation costs;
- staffing and training requirements;
- probable number of patients affected;
- effects on other hospital resources, such as the extent to which a technology will enable the replacement of existing resources, or the extent to which it will necessitate the addition of new resources;
- clinical effectiveness: not patient outcomes as such, but process outcomes such as inpatient versus outpatient application, average length of stay, etc.

Government agencies are active in medical technology assessment, often through decisions about reimbursement or about hospital investment in large equipment. Such assessments are concerned with economic efficiency, as well as with safety and efficacy, but U.S. government agencies have generally not emphasized assessments for economic efficiency and cost-effectiveness. The guidelines prepared by the federal government of Canada to assist provinces who request guidance in their hospital investments typically have 10 components (OTA, 1980). These components form a checklist of considerations to be entertained before establishing a new unit:

- patient load;
- bed requirements;
- recommended distribution;
- administrative policy, procedures, and control;
- staff establishment and coverage;
- staff training and qualifications;
- specific supporting departments and services;
- space allocation, utilization, and specific design features;
- equipment;
- relationship with other departments and services.

Concern with feasibility and coordination loom large in these governmental guidelines for assessment.

The contrast between the Canadian guidelines and the U.S. health policy statements in the 1975 health planning law and its 1979 amendments is worth noting. Title XV of the Public Health Services Act (P.L. 93-641) Section 1502 sets forth a number of National Health Priorities intended to guide national planning and investment, especially governmental, in capital facilities for health care, including expensive equipment. Among these priorities are

- provision of primary care services for medically underserved populations, with emphasis on rural and economically depressed areas;
- coordination and consolidation of institutional health services by developing multi-institutional systems (specialty services such as radiation therapy, intensive and coronary care, and emergency trauma care are singled out for special attention); development of multi-institutional systems for sharing support services;
- development of health services institu-

tions "of the capacity to provide various levels of care. . . on a geographically integrated basis."

The public policy goals also emphasize alternative health care systems to hospitals, encouraging

- the development of medical group practice;
- the training and utilization of allied health professionals such as nurse clinicians and physician assistants;
- the promotion of activities for the prevention of disease, including studies of nutritional and environmental factors affecting health and the provision of preventive health services.

Some additional priorities are consumer education so that the general public might use "proper personal health care" including prevention; cost containment and the "adoption of uniform cost accounting and simplified reimbursement"; and activities to "achieve needed improvement in the quality of health services."

Federal Medicare reimbursement for the capital portions of the hospital bill are denied to health care institutions that expand beds or certain programs without a certificate of need. The 1975 law approached cost containment primarily through institutional coordination, regionalization, the sharing of services, and nonhospital alternatives.

Technology assessment as a means of achieving these goals is not given specific mention. However, the 1979 amendments emphasized the importance of "the identification and discontinuance of duplicative or unneeded services and facilities" [P.L. 96-79, Section 102(a)(1)]. To the section of the previous law promoting uniform cost accounting and improved management procedures for institutions offering health services was added the words "and the development and use of cost-saving technology" [Section 102(a)(2)].

Finally, legislative bodies can be deeply involved in assessment of medical technology. Congress established the Office of Technology Assessment in 1972 as an advisory arm. OTA uses these words in describing its mission: "The assessment of technology calls for exploration of the physical, biological, economic, social, and political impacts which can result from applications of scientific knowledge." For medical technology this broad construction of the task reaches far beyond safety and efficacy.

The multiplicity of organizations carrying out assessments, the variety of kinds and purposes of assessments, and the amount spent on various kinds of assessments are described in Chapter 2. That inventory calls attention to the fact that no agency has the task of attending to the needed research for the nation, such as noting which medical technology assessments need to be carried out and assigning priorities and financing their execution. Appendix A supplements Chapter 2 by describing in more systematically gathered detail the work of a set of the agencies carrying out assessments of medical technologies.

To lay a foundation of methods used in medical technology assessment, Chapter 3 describes and illustrates the major methods, explains their strengths and limitations, and outlines new research in each method whose results might strengthen its use. To help us understand how medical technologies come to be adopted, dropped, or ignored, Chapter 4 examines the role of assessment, education, publications, and other stimuli to diffusion.

The role of reimbursement in encouraging and paying for the assessment of medical technologies has been much debated, and Chapter 5 discusses some of the history of these developments, both state and national. The international scene, at least in principle, is a two-way street for technology assessment, and Chapter 6 explores the current position of the United States with respect to use of international assessments. The question of what information can be usefully exchanged and what long-term policies should be instituted go beyond the purview of this report.

Chapter 7 summarizes the state of the nation's assessment of medical technologies and makes general recommendations for creating a pluralistic national system. It does not summarize the narrower recommendations scattered through the report, highlighted in the chapters, but focuses on the gaps that now prevent the United States from having a system and proposes a set of gradual steps for creating one.

REFERENCES

Arnstein, S. R. 1977. Technology assessment: Opportunities and obstacles. IEEE Trans. Systems, Man, Cybernetics, Vol. SMC-7(8):571–582.

Banta, H. D. 1980. The diffusion of the computed tomography (CT) scanner in the United States. Int. J. Health Services 10:251.

Banta, H. D., and S. B. Thacker. 1979. Assessing the costs and benefits of electronic fetal monitoring. Obstet. Gynecol. 34:627.

Barsamian, E. M. 1977. The rise and fall of internal mammary artery ligation in the treatment of angina pectoris and the lessons learned. Chapter 13, pp. 212–220 in J. P. Bunker, B. Barnes, and F. Mosteller, eds., Costs, Risks and Benefits of Surgery. New York: Oxford University Press.

Bunker, J. P. 1970. Surgical manpower: A comparison of operations and surgeons in the United States and in England and Wales. N. Engl. J. Med. 282:135.

Cobb, L. A., G. I. Thomas, D. H. Dillard, et al. 1959. An evaluation of internal mammary-artery ligation by a double-blind technic. N. Engl. J. Med. 260:1115.

Coffey, R. M. 1980. How a medical information system affects hospital costs: The El Camino Hospital experience. NCHSR Research Summary Series, DHEW Pub. No. (PHS) 80-3265. Washington, D.C.: Department of Health, Education, and Welfare.

Cohen A. 1983. Decision and Policy Analysis for Electronic Fetal Monitoring. Ph.D. dissertation. Harvard School of Public Health, Cambridge, Mass.

Cutler, J. L., S. Ramcharon, R. Feldman, et al. 1973. Multiphasic check-up evaluation study. Prev. Med. 2:197.

Dimond, E. G., C. F. Kittle, and J. E. Crockett. 1958. Evaluation of internal mammary artery ligation and sham procedure in angina pectoris. Circulation 18:712.

Easterday, C. L., D. A. Grimes, and J. A. Riggs. 1983. Hysterectomy in the United States. Ob. Gyn. Obstet. Gynecol. 62:203–212.

Francis, K., Jr., et al. 1955. An evaluation of the 1954 poliomyelitis vaccine trial-summary report. Am. J. Public Health 45(5):1–63.

Gilbert, J. P., B. McPeek, and F. Mosteller. 1977. Program in surgery and anesthesia. Pp. 124–169 in J. P. Bunker, B. A. Barnes, and F. Mosteller, eds., Costs, Risks and Benefits of Surgery. New York: Oxford University Press.

Gittelsohn, A. M., and J. A. Wennberg. 1977. On the incidence of tonsillectomy and other common surgical procedures. Pp. 91–106 in J. P. Bunker, B. A. Barnes, and F. Mosteller, eds., Costs, Risks and Benefits of Surgery. New York: Oxford University Press.

Grace, N. D., H. Muench, and T. C. Chalmers. 1966. The present status of shunts for portal hypertension in cirrhosis. Gastroenterology 50:684.

Guttmacher, S., M. Teitelman, G. Chapin, G. Garbowski, and P. Schnall. 1981. Ethics and preventive medicine: The case of borderline hypertension. Hastings Center Report 11:12.

Haring, O. M., P. M. Wortman, R. A. Watson, and N. P. Goetz. 1982. Automating the medical record: An assessment of impact on process and outcome of care in hypertension, obesity, and renal disease. Med. Care 20:63–74.

Haverkamp, A. D., M. Orleans, and S. Langedoerfer, et al. 1979. A controlled trial of the differential effects of intrapartum fetal monitoring. Am. J. Obstet. Gynecol. 134:399.

Haverkamp, A. D., H. E. Thompson, J. G. McFee, et al. 1976. The evaluation of continuous fetal heart rate monitoring in high-risk pregnancy. Am. J. Obstet. Gynecol. 125:310.

Havlik, R. J., and M. Feinleib, eds. 1979. Proceedings of the Conference on the Decline in Coronary Heart Disease Mortality. Pub. No. 79-1610. Bethesda, Maryland: National Institutes of Health.

Hounsfield, G. N. 1980. Computed medical imaging. Science 210:22.

Hypertension Detection and Follow-up Program Cooperative Group. 1982. The effect of treatment on mortality in "mild" hypertension: Results of the Hypertension Detection and Follow-up Program. N. Engl. J. Med. 307:976.

Ingemarsson, E., I. Ingemarsson, and N. W. Svenningsen. 1981. Impact of routine fetal monitoring during labor on fetal outcome with long-term follow-up. Am. J. Obstet. Gynecol. 141:29.

Joint National Committee on Detection, Evaluation, and Treatment of High Blood Pressure. 1984. The 1984 report of the Joint National Committee on

Detection, Evaluation, and Treatment of High Blood Pressure. Arch. Intern. 144:1045–1057.

Kelso, I. M., R. J. Parsons, G. F. Lawrence, et al. 1978. An assessment of continuous fetal heart rate monitoring in labor. Am. J. Obstet. Gynecol. 131:526.

Korenbrot, C., A. B. Flood, M. Higgens, et al. 1980. Elective Hysterectomy, Costs, Risks, and Benefits. Prepared for the Office of Technology Assessment, Congress of the United States, Washington, D.C.

Levy, R. I. February 1982. The National Heart, Lung, and Blood Institute Overview 1980: The director's report to the NHLBI Advisory Council. Circulation 65:217.

McDonald, D., A. Grant, M. Pereira, P. Boylan, and I. Chalmers. 1983. The Dublin Randomized Controlled Trial of Intrapartum Electronic Fetal Heart Rate Monitoring. Presented at the 23rd British Congress of Obstetrics and Gynecology, Birmingham, July 14.

Meier, P. 1978. The biggest public health experiment ever: the 1954 field trial of the Salk poliomyelitis vaccine. Pp. 3–15 in M. Tanur et al., eds., Statistics: A Guide to the Unknown, 2nd Ed. San Francisco: Holden Day.

National Center for Health Statistics, Department of Health and Human Services. 1983. Prevention Profile: Health United States. Washington, D.C.: U.S. Government Printing Office.

National Institutes of Health. 1979. Diagnosis and Management of Hypertension, A Nationwide Survey of Physicians' Knowledge, Attitudes, and Reported Behavior. DHEW Pub. No. (NIH) 79-1056. Bethesda, Maryland.

Office of Technology Assessment. 1978. Policy Implications of the Computed Tomography (CT) Scanner. Pub. No. OTA-H-56. Washington, D.C.: U.S. Government Printing Office.

Office of Technology Assessment. 1982. Strategies of Medical Technology Assessment, p. 3. Washington, D.C.: U.S. Government Printing Office.

Office of Technology Assessment. October 1980. The Implications of Cost-Effectiveness Analysis of Medical Technology; Background Paper #4: The Management of Health Care Technology in Ten Countries. Washington, D.C.: U.S. Government Printing Office.

Placek, P., K. Keppel, S. Taffel, and T. Liss. 1983a. Electronic Fetal Monitoring in Relation to Cesarean Section Delivery for Live Births and Stillbirths in the United States, 1980. Presented at the American Public Health Association Meetings, Dallas, November 16.

Placek, D., S. Taffel, and K. Keppel. 1983b. Maternal and infant characteristics associated with cesarean section delivery. Health, United States: 1983. Hyattsville, Md.: National Center for Health Statistics.

Ratcliff, J. D. 1957. New surgery for ailing hearts. Reader's Digest 71:70.

Renou, P., A. Chang, I. Anderson, and C. Wood. 1976. Controlled trial of fetal intensive care. Am. J. Obstet. Gynecol. 126:470.

Rogers, J. L., and O. M. Haring. 1979. The impact of a computerized medical summary system on incidence and length of hospital stay. Med. Care 7:618–630.

Sanberg, S. I., B. A. Barnes, M. C. Weinstein, and P. Braun. 1984. Elective Hysterectomy: Benefits, Risks, and Costs. Institute for Health Research (submitted for publication).

Vayda, E. 1973. A comparison of surgical rates in Canada and in England and Wales. N. Engl. J. Med. 289:1224.

Veterans Administration Cooperative Study Group on Anti-Hypertensive Agents. 1967 and 1970. J. Am. Med. Assoc. 202:1028 and 213:1143.

Wagner, J. L. 1980. The Feasibility of Economic Evaluation of Diagnostic Procedures: The Case of CT Scanning. Prepared for the Office of Technology Assessment, Congress of the United States, Washington, D.C.

Wennberg, J., and A. Gittelsohn. 1973. Small area variations in health care delivery. Science 182:1102.

Wood, C., P. Renou, J. Oats, E. Farrell, N. Beischer, and I. Anderson. 1981. A controlled trial of fetal heart rate monitoring in a low-risk obstetric population. Am. J. Obstet. Gynecol. 141:527.

2 The Scope of U.S. Medical Technology Assessment

The pressing need for medical technology assessment information is evident throughout the health care industry in the United States. This chapter provides a profile of medical technology assessment in the United States today. An introductory overview is followed by descriptions of the dimensions of medical technology assessment, which indicate the great diversity of current assessment activities as well as unmet assessment needs. Estimates are given for the relative magnitude of expenditures made for medical technology assessment, biomedical research and development, and national health care. Major assessment programs in the federal government, the drug industry, the medical device industry, and other sectors are described. Finally, conclusions have been drawn regarding the adequacy of our current assessment capabilities and recommendations have been made concerning investment in and conduct of medical technology assessment so as to improve those capabilities.

The detailed profiles of 20 American assessment programs in the private and public sectors, found in Appendix A, provided much of the basis for preparing this chapter. Those profiles systematically describe the purpose, technologies assessed, methods, funding, and other aspects of each program.

AN OVERVIEW

Heightened interest in medical technology assessment has prompted a wide variety of responses in recent years as one or another organization tries to meet its needs for assessment information. For instance, since late 1977, the National Institutes of Health (NIH) has conducted 50 widely reported consensus development conferences on a variety of biomedical problems and technologies. The American College of Cardiology, the American Hospital Association, and the American Medical Association are among professional and provider associations that have instituted new assessment programs. Implementation of the Medicare prospective payment system,

---

Prepared by Clifford S. Goodman.

growth in multi-institutional health care organizations, competition, and related factors have prompted health maintenance organizations, hospital corporations, and other major providers to institute new programs or expand existing ones for evaluating their delivery of health services and the cost-effectiveness of adoption and use of medical technologies. More drug companies are instituting permanent drug surveillance and cost analysis programs. The independent medical device evaluator ECRI (formerly the Emergency Care Research Institute) is responding to an expanded market for assessment information with new publications, an implant registry, a widened device-experience reporting network, and other services.

Many organizations arrange for the exchange of assessment information. Blue Cross and Blue Shield Association and other major insurers increasingly seek assistance from medical associations such as the American College of Physicians, the American College of Radiology, the American College of Surgeons, and the Council of Medical Specialty Societies in formulating coverage policies. At congressional request, the Office of Technology Assessment (OTA) has in recent years produced more than 60 reports and case studies of medical technology that have been widely circulated and cited throughout government, industry, and the public. The Department of Health and Human Services (DHHS), NIH, and the Veterans Administration (VA) are among the agencies that have recently instituted coordinating committees to enhance the exchange of information about technology assessment and to make recommendations regarding their assessment policies. The Stevenson-Wydler Technology Innovation Act of 1980 (P.L. 96-480) requires DHHS to report annually to the Department of Commerce regarding its health technology assessment and transfer activities (see Office of Medical Applications of Research [OMAR], 1984).

Several noteworthy developments recently have been made regarding establishment of new assessment entities. The Prospective Payment Assessment Commission (ProPAC) was first appointed in 1983 to make recommendations to the DHHS Secretary about adjustments in the Diagnosis-Related Groups (DRGs) used in the Medicare prospective payment system. An Institute of Medicine (IOM) report recommends the establishment of a private-public medical technology assessment consortium (IOM, 1983). In 1984, Congress set aside funds for the expansion of medical technology assessment functions of the National Center for Health Services Research and earmarked a portion of these as matching funds for a National Academy of Sciences council on health care technology similar to that proposed by the IOM (P.L. 98-551).

But the recent flurry of attention to assessment has not been accompanied by a fitting increase in new assessment information. Notwithstanding the national investment in health care and the diversity and scope of assessment needs, current assessment activities are patchy and poorly funded. Organizations are scrambling for limited available information and are relying heavily on expert opinion to fill wide gaps in the data. The bulk of all resources allocated for technology assessment is for premarketing testing of drugs for safety and efficacy. Although current premarketing assessment of drugs and devices appears adequate, insufficient attention is given to postmarketing study (Joint Commission on Prescription Drug Use, 1980; OTA, 1982b). Inadequate attention is paid to evaluating medical and surgical procedures for safety and effectiveness (Bunker et al., 1982; Eddy, 1983; OTA, 1982a, 1983b; Relman, 1980). Among all technologies, existing assessment activities are concentrated on the new and not on the widely accepted and possibly outmoded. Assessments of cost-effectiveness and cost-benefit are few; assessments for ethical, legal, and other social implications are rare.

VARIETIES OF MEDICAL TECHNOLOGY ASSESSMENT

Medical technology assessment can be described according to many attributes. As expanded in Table 2-1, these may include the type of technology assessed and its application, the stage of diffusion, the properties or concerns of assessment, the methods of assessment, and assessors. Various combinations of these attributes can be used to portray the activities of particular technology assessment programs and the great diversity among programs. Table 2-2 lists the types of technologies assessed by some of the programs discussed in this chapter. Some programs devote most of their assessment resources to one type of technology, such as ECRI for medical devices; others may address a variety of technologies, as does the congressional Office of Technology Assessment. Table 2-3 portrays 150 combinations of three attributes of assessment: technologies, concerns, and assessors. Of the 25 selected programs, 16 conduct some assessment of medical or surgical procedures for efficacy or effectiveness. However, as discussed in the remainder of this chapter, the distribution of types of assessment activity shown in Table 2-3 is indicative neither of the relative comprehensiveness of assessment nor of the relative investment made in these assessments. Figure 2-1 illustrates the relative comprehensiveness of U.S. technology assessment efforts for the various classes of technology and concerns of assessment.

It is again emphasized that a broad net is cast—broader than most—by use of the term technology assessment, as is evident from Tables 2-1 through 2-3 and Figure 2-1. Primary data gathering as well as various synthesis methods are included. Assessment concerns range from the very circumscribed, such as evaluation of safety and efficacy in support of a new drug's labeling claims, to the most comprehensive, such as a multidisciplinary effort which "systematically examines the effects on society that may occur when a technology is introduced, extended, or modified with special emphasis on those consequences that are unintended, indirect, or delayed" (Coates, 1974; see also Arnstein, 1977; U.S. Congress, 1966). In addition to drugs, medical devices, and medical and surgical procedures, we include study of support systems and organizational, delivery, and administrative systems generally known as health services research. Thus, in the discussion of various organizations engaged in

TABLE 2-1 Selected Attributes of Medical Technology Assessment

Technologies	Assessment methods
Drugs	Laboratory testing
Devices	Randomized clinical trials
Medical and surgical procedures	Epidemiologic methods
Support systems	Series
Organizational systems	Case studies
	Registries and data bases
	Sample surveys
	Surveillance
Application	Quantitative syntheses
Screening	Cost-effectiveness/cost-benefit analyses
Prevention	Mathematical modeling
Diagnosis	Group judgment methods
Treatment	Literature syntheses
Rehabilitation	
Stage of diffusion	**Assessors/sponsors**
Experimental	Biomedical and health services researchers
Investigative	Hospitals, HMOs, and other health care institutions
New to practice	Providers/provider organizations
In accepted use	Third-party payers
Outmoded	Drug and medical device manufacturers
Properties/concerns	Legislators
Technical performance	Regulators
Safety	Policy research groups
Efficacy/effectiveness	Voluntary agencies
Cost/cost-benefit/cost-effectiveness	Employers
Ethical implications	Consumers
Legal implications	
Social implications	

TABLE 2-2 Principal Technologies Assessed by 25 Programs

	Technologies				
Evaluation Programs	Drugs	Medical Devices/ Equipment/ Supplies	Medical/ Surgical Procedures	Support Systems	Organizational Systems
American College of Cardiology/American Heart Association Assessment of Cardiovascular Procedures			X		
American College of Physicians Clinical Efficacy Assessment Project			X		
American Hospital Association Hospital Technology Series		X		X	
American Medical Association Diagnostic and Therapeutic Technology Assessment	X	X	X		
Battelle Health and Population Study Center	X	X	X		
Blue Cross and Blue Shield Medical Necessity Program			X		
Blue Cross and Blue Shield Technology Evaluation and Coverage Program		X	X		
ECRI		X		X	
Food and Drug Administration Center for Devices and Radiological Health		X			
Food and Drug Administration Center for Drugs and Biologics	X				
Hastings Center Institute of Society, Ethics and the Life Sciences			X	X	X
Medtronic, Inc.		X			
National Cancer Institute (NIH)	X	X	X	X	
National Center for Health Services Research (excluding OHTA)				X	X
National Heart, Lung, and Blood Institute (NIH)	X	X	X	X	
National Library of Medicine (NIH)				X	
Office of Health Technology Assessment (National Center for Health Services Research)		X	X		
Office of Medical Applications of Research (NIH)	X	X	X	X	
Office of Technology Assessment (Congress)	X	X	X	X	X
Permanente Medical Group, Inc., Division of Health Services Research		X	X	X	X
Prospective Payment Assessment Commission	X	X	X	X	X
Prudential Insurance Co. of America			X		
Smith Kline & French Cost Benefit Studies Program	X				
University of California, San Diego, Institute for Health Policy Studies	X	X	X	X	X
Veterans Administration Cooperative Studies Program	X	X	X		

technology assessment, agencies such as the National Center for Health Services Research and Health Care Technology Assessment (NCHSRHCTA, formerly known as NCHSR) and university-based health services and policy research groups are cited that are primarily involved in health services research. This broader view recognizes the interdependence of health care technologies and that making policies to address one type of technology may have important implications for others.

TABLE 2-3 Principal Technology Assessment Concerns of Selected Organizations

	Concerns			
Technology	Safety	Efficacy/ Effectiveness	Cost/Cost-Effect/ Cost-Benefit	Ethical/Legal/ Social
Drugs	d,j,m,o,r,s,u,y	d,e,j,m,o,r,s,u, x,y	e,s,u,w,x,y	e,s,u,x
Medical Devices/Equipment/Supplies	d,e,g,h,i,l,m,o, q,r,s,u,y	c,d,e,g,h,i,l,m,o, q,r,s,t,u,x,y	c,e,h,l,s,t,u,x,y	e,h,o,s,u,x
Medical/Surgical Procedures	a,b,d,e,g,m,o, q,r,s,u,y	a,b,d,e,f,g,m,o, q,r,s,t,u,v,x,y	e,s,t,u,v,x,y	e,k,o,s,u,x
Support Systems	h,m,o,r,s,u	c,h,m,n,o,p,r,s,t, u,x,	c,h,n,p,s,t,u,x	h,k,s,u,x
Organizational/Administrative		n,s,t,u,x	n,s,t,u,x	k,s,u,x

NOTE: Letters in the body of the table correspond to the organizations listed below.

a. American College of Cardiology/American Heart Association Assessment of Cardiovascular Procedures
b. American College of Physicians Clinical Efficacy Assessment Project
c. American Hospital Association Hospital Technology Series
d. American Medical Association Diagnostic and Therapeutic Technology Assessment Service
e. Battelle Health and Population Study Center
f. Blue Cross and Blue Shield Medical Necessity Program
g. Blue Cross and Blue Shield Technology Evaluation and Coverage Program
h. ECRI
i. Food and Drug Administration Center for Devices and Radiological Health
j. Food and Drug Administration Center for Drugs and Biologics
k. Hastings Center Institute of Society, Ethics and the Life Sciences
l. Medtronic, Inc.
m. National Cancer Institute (NIH)
n. National Center for Health Services Research (other than OHTA)
o. National Heart, Lung, and Blood Institute (NIH)
p. National Library of Medicine (NIH)
q. Office of Health Technology Assessment (NCHSRHCTA)
r. Office of Medical Applications of Research (NIH)
s. Office of Technology Assessment (Congress)
t. Permanente Medical Group, Inc., Division of Health Services Research
u. Prospective Payment Assessment Commission
v. Prudential Insurance Co. of America
w. Smith Kline & French Cost Benefit Studies Program
x. University of California, San Diego, Institute for Health Policy Studies
y. Veterans Administration Cooperative Studies Program

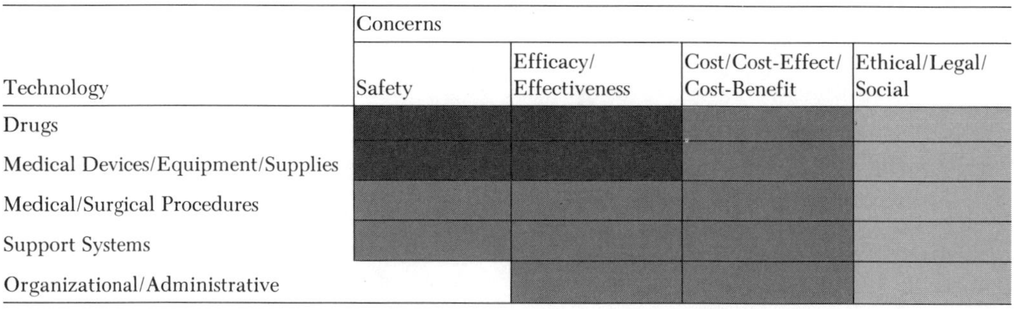

FIGURE 2-1 Comprehensiveness of U.S. technology assessment.

Most coverage ■ Inconsistent ■ Little or no coverage ■

NATIONAL EXPENDITURES FOR HEALTH RESEARCH AND DEVELOPMENT, CLINICAL TRIALS, AND TECHNOLOGY ASSESSMENT

The total dollar level of effort in technology assessment—including clinical trials, health services research, and synthesis activities such as consensus development conferences, state-of-the-art workshops, and formulation of coverage decisions—is small compared with the national effort in research and development of technologies, and can be lost in the rounding error for national health expenditures, as is evident in the relative magnitudes of the following estimates for 1984.

National health care	$384.3 billion (HCFA, 1984a)
Health R&D	11.8 billion (NIH, 1984a)
All health technology assessment	1.3 billion
Clinical trials	1.1 billion
Health services research	under 0.2 billion
Other technology assessment	under 0.05 billion

A brief look at national health research and development (R&D) expenditures will provide a context for later appreciation of expenditures for medical technology assessment. It is noted that health care products and services are of varying technological intensity requiring different levels of investment in R&D. Services include "hotel" and food services as well as microsurgery and neonatal intensive care; products include tongue depressors and bandages as well as magnetic resonance imagers and genetically engineered agents for cancer immunotherapy.

Spending for health R&D in the years since 1972 has not kept pace either with the nation's entire R&D spending or with total national health spending. In 1983, when spending for all R&D was almost $88 billion (National Science Foundation [NSF], 1984), health R&D came to $10.4 billion, or 11.8 percent, down from 12.4 percent in 1972 (NIH, 1984a).

As a proportion of the $355.4 billion in total 1983 national health expenditures (Gibson et al., 1984), health R&D amounted to 2.9 percent, down from 3.9 percent in 1972. That is a little higher than the average for all United States industry—estimated at 2.7 percent of the 1984 GNP, up from 2.3 percent in the 1970s (NSF, 1984)—but low compared with other technologically dependent industries. Those have R&D (including federal contributions) as a percentage of sales ranging from 4.2 percent for the chemical industry to 12.2 for computers and office machines to 18.3 percent for aircraft and missiles (NSF, 1984). Even the defense establishment pegs R&D at 11 percent of estimated fiscal year (FY) 1984 outlays ($231 billion), which include pay and pensions, housing, maintenance, and other items of little technological content (U.S. Office of Management and Budget, 1984). The pharmaceutical industry, separately from the rest of health, spends nearly 12 percent of sales on R&D.

When we come to expenditures for medical technology assessment, the estimates indeed become rough. At the outside they amounted to $1.3 billion in 1984. By far the biggest item is $1.1 billion for clinical trials. Health services research expenditures hardly amount to $200 million. Spending for all the rest of medical technology assessment will not reach $50 million for 1985. Some of the details in these categories are explained below.

The $1.1 billion figure for clinical trial expenditures represents 0.3 percent of 1984 national health expenditures. The drug industry is the largest spender for clinical trials—perhaps $750 million in 1984—constituting over one-fifth of that industry's R&D expenditures (using Pharmaceutical Manufacturers Association estimates of allocation of pharmaceutical R&D expenditures; see section below on the drug industry). The next largest contributor is NIH with $235 million in FY 1984 obligations (NIH, 1985), or 5 percent of its budget. The third largest contributor may be the medical device industry, with approximately $35 million in 1984 (4 percent of that industry's R&D expenditures). Other contributors are the VA (approximately $20 million); the Alcohol, Drug Abuse, and Mental Health Administration (ADAMHA) ($12 million; OMAR, 1983); and the Department of Defense (DOD) (under $10 million; H. Dangerfield, U.S. Army Medical Research and Development Command, personal communication, 1984). Clearly, the roles of the drug industry and NIH are dominant; a 5 percent error in the drug industry estimate would likely exceed the contributions of any of the others except NIH.

Research and evaluation of organizational and support systems technologies (e.g., health services delivery modes, payment systems, data bases, and manpower) are generally grouped under health services research. Total annual expenditures for health services research are probably under $200 million, including some expenditures for demonstration projects. The bulk of health services research support comes from the Health Care Financing Administration (HCFA), the National Institutes of Health (NIH), the National Center for Health Services Research and Health Care Technology Assessment (NCHSRHCTA), and private foundations.[1] Other sources include ADAMHA, the Office of the Secretary, DHHS, the Health Resources and Services Administration (HRSA), the VA, Agency for International Development, and major private providers such as hospital corporations and health maintenance organizations (HMOs).

Total estimated expenditures in 1984 for medical technology assessment activities other than clinical trials and health services research are well under $50 million. This includes assessment expenditures* for HCFA ($3 million, FY 1984) and NCHSRHCTA (under $4 million, including the $0.7 million Office of Health Technology Assessment budget, FY 1985) and medical technology assessment activities of the Food and Drug Administration (FDA) ($5 million) and the Centers for Disease Control (CDC) ($4 million, FY 1982). Also included are the entire budgets of such prominent technology assessment activities as the NIH Office of Medical Applications of Research, coordinator of the NIH Consensus Development Program ($1.8 million, FY 1985); the Prospective Payment Assessment Commission ($3.1 million, FY 1985); the congressional Office of Technology Assessment (OTA) Health Program ($1.6 million, FY 1985); the larger medical and industry association programs for technology assessment such as the American College of Physicians Clinical Efficacy Assessment Project ($0.16 million, 1985), the American Medical Association Diagnostic and Therapeutic Technology Assessment program ($0.38 million, 1985), and the American Hospital Association Hospital Technology Series program ($0.25 million, 1985); nonprofit research groups such as the independent medical device evaluator ECRI ($5 million, 1985) and the Hastings Center Institute of Society, Ethics, and the Life Sciences ($0.25 million, 1985); and the investment in coverage and reimbursement assessment activities by major third-party payers such as the Blue Cross and Blue Shield Association ($0.35 million, 1984) in support of its plans.

The following four sections of this chapter describe technology assessment activities in the federal government, the drug industry, the medical device industry, and

* Estimates of recent program expenditures and applicable year are shown in parentheses. Rough estimates are used where budget line items are unavailable. Sources for these estimates are cited later in the text, with the discussions of assessment programs.

other types of organizations in the private sector. Where available, estimates of program expenditures for R&D and for clinical trials and other assessment activities are provided. Estimates are subject to variations in terminology and budgeting practices and are necessarily rough in certain cases. Expenditures for technology assessment activities usually are included in R&D budgets but may not be identifiable as separate line items. Among organizations that do not generally conduct R&D, such as insurers and medical associations, technology assessment expenditures may be included in administrative budgets but not identified as such. For certain organizations, it is difficult to make estimates of the cost (or value) of personnel time devoted to technology assessment. Examples are the value of unpaid participants in medical association assessment programs and the cost of personnel time devoted by NIH and FDA personnel in response to inquiries made by the NCHSRHCTA Office of Health Technology Assessment (OHTA) in assessments conducted for HCFA. Available figures for clinical trial expenditures may include all costs of patient care (hospitalization, physician services, etc.), or, as is the case for the VA, they may be confined to the additional costs of conducting a trial over routine patient care costs. By reimbursing for hospital and physician services, private and public third-party payers provide an indeterminate amount of indirect support for some clinical trials, series, case studies, and other observations.

FEDERAL GOVERNMENT

The federal government conducts and supports medical technology assessment to serve its roles in medical research; health services research; health care delivery, payment, regulation, and legislation; and defense. Federal government expenditures for medical technology assessment were approximately $450 million in 1984. This included $280 million for clinical trials (primarily NIH support), roughly $100 million to $150 million for health services research,[1] and $30 million for other assessment activities including consensus development conferences and other syntheses and special studies by NIH, HCFA, NCHSRHCTA, FDA, CDC, OTA, and other agencies as described below. Federal expenditures for medical technology assessment—including health services research expenditures—constitute about 7 percent of federal health R&D expenditures and 0.4 percent of federal health care expenditures.

Federal government emphasis on the various types of medical technologies and the properties for which they are assessed (safety, efficacy, etc.) are uneven. Consistent with FDA requirements, the assessment of new drugs and certain medical devices (new class III devices; see discussion below) for safety and efficacy prior to marketing for use as specified in their labeling is comprehensive. However, as described later in this chapter, FDA assessments do not adequately address the broader scope of evaluations beyond safety and efficacy and deal only minimally with these technologies once they are marketed. The bulk of the nation's efforts in evaluating medical and surgical procedures is supplied by the federal government in the form of certain clinical trials and synthesis activities supported by NIH, the VA, ADAMHA, HCFA, and NCHSRHCTA. These are not overseen or otherwise coordinated by any one agency. The Health Care Financing Administration, the nation's single largest payer for medical and surgical procedures, relies heavily for its coverage decisions on the NCHSRHCTA Office of Health Technology Assessment (OHTA)—a $0.7 million per year program—and less formal linkages with other federal agencies and private sector sources.

Recognizing the need for improved coordination, several federal agencies have formed technology assessment coordinating bodies. For instance, the DHHS Technology Coordinating Committee serves as a forum for information exchange and coordination of assessment activities. Chaired by the Director of OHTA, the committee includes representatives of DHHS agencies such as NIH, FDA, CDC, ADAMHA, NCHSRHCTA, National Center for Health Statistics (NCHS), Health Resources and Services Administration (HRSA), and HCFA; OTA, ProPAC, DOD, and others of the legislative and executive branches; and nongovernmental organizations such as Blue Cross and Blue Shield and medical and industry associations.

The following are brief descriptions of selected major technology assessment activities in the federal government, including those of NIH, FDA, OTA, ProPAC, HCFA, NCHSRHCTA, OHTA, NCHS, VA, CDC, and DOD. Other federal agencies that conduct and support evaluations of health care technology include other agencies in the Office of the Assistant Secretary for Health (OASH), ADAMHA, HRSA, and the Office of the Secretary, DHHS.

National Institutes of Health

The National Institutes of Health is the principal biomedical research agency of the federal government. Consistent with its mission of improving the health of the people of the United States by increasing our understanding of processes underlying human health and acquisition of new knowledge (NIH, 1982), R&D activities take 94 percent of the entire NIH budget and are weighted to basic research, which accounts for nearly 60 percent of the R&D budget. Another 32 percent goes to applied research and 9 percent goes to development (NSF, 1984). As the nation's main engine for basic and applied biomedical research, NIH does not particularly set its priorities to address current issues of medical practice.

Resources devoted by NIH to clinical trials and other technology assessment comprise a small portion of its total budget. Even so, NIH is the nation's largest supporter of clinical trials outside the combined efforts of the drug industry. NIH currently obligates about 5 percent of its total budget to clinical trials—$235.4 million in FY 1984 and $275.7 million in FY 1985 (NIH, 1985). The institutes' investment in clinical trials varies; the National Cancer Institute (NCI) alone accounts for 59 percent of 1985 NIH clinical trial obligations. NCI clinical trial expenditures account for about 13 percent of that institute's budget; clinical trial expenditures average 3 percent of other institutes' budgets. NIH is considering the reinstatement in 1985 of a detailed inventory of clinical trials, using standardized information categories across the institutes, bureaus, and divisions of NIH.

At NIH, technology assessment refers to assessing the results of clinical trials and creating state-of-the-art reports on medical technologies.

> [T]echnology assessment. . . consists of synthesizing complex scientific information in such a way that the reports are useful for decision-making by practitioners or policy makers (NIH, 1983).

NIH "synthesis" activity includes workshops, symposia, and conferences, notably the NIH Consensus Development conferences coordinated by the Office of Medical Applications of Research and responding to Public Health Service (PHS) requests for expert opinions regarding the safety and efficacy/effectiveness of drugs, devices, and procedures. Including the OMAR budget, NIH expenditures for such synthesis activities probably are less than $10 million annually, about 0.2 percent of the $4.5 billion 1984 NIH budget. Precise figures for NIH technology assessment expenditures are unavailable, largely because of differences among NIH bureaus, institutes, and divisions in drawing up budget categories and defining terms.[2] NIH reports that it devotes $40 million to health services research, however, this may be a high estimate.[1]

Office of Medical Applications of Research The Office of Medical Applications of Research is the NIH focal point for coordinating, improving, and promoting NIH technology assessment and transfer activities. The FY 1985 OMAR budget was approximately $1.8 million (I. Jacoby, OMAR, personal communication, 1985). OMAR jointly sponsors and administers with the NIH bureaus, institutes, and divisions (BIDs) the NIH Consensus Development conferences, over 50 of which will have been held by the end of 1985. The cost of conducting a Consensus Development conference in 1985 was $145,000, including contractor costs, NIH staff time, and information dissemination (I. Jacoby, OMAR, personal communication, 1985). OMAR also acts as a clearinghouse for NIH patent-related activities, coordinates NIH medical and scientific review of HCFA Medicare coverage issues referred to NIH by the Office of Health Technology Assessment, and supports studies to evaluate and improve assessment efforts. The OMAR director serves as chairman of the NIH Coordinating Committee on Assessment and Transfer of Technology. The committee includes representatives from the NIH BIDs and liaison representatives from ADAMHA, FDA, CDC, OHTA, NCHSRHCTA, and the Occupational Safety and Health Administration (OSHA).

Food and Drug Administration

The Food and Drug Administration is primarily a scientific regulatory agency for the development of regulations and product standards; development of methodologies and protocols for evaluation of product safety and efficacy; and approval of drugs, medical devices, and other products prior to marketing. Although the FDA reviews evidence accumulated in assessments directed by product sponsors, the agency does not conduct clinical trials of medical products. FDA assessment requirements address safety and efficacy but not cost, cost-effectiveness, or broader social issues. Sponsors must show that their products are safe and efficacious as claimed in their labeling, but they are not required to show safety and efficacy relative to similar products. Thus, FDA-required assessments do not generally produce comparative safety, efficacy, or cost-effectiveness information that may be useful to providers for choosing among alternative products, e.g., different drug treatments, or alternative technologies, e.g., treatment with drugs versus surgical treatment.

In 1984 the FDA spent about $2 million to conduct and support postmarketing surveillance of drugs and roughly $1 million to support its network for reporting problems with medical devices. The FDA participates in OHTA assessments of medical devices and drugs conducted for HCFA. The agency does conduct applied R&D, e.g., the development of methods and devices for measuring the quality of diagnostic devices and emissions of radiological products and the storage and transmittal of radiographic information. In FY 1984 the FDA spent an estimated $79.3 million on applied R&D and $3.9 million on technology transfer (OMAR, 1984). The agency's regulatory role in drug and device assessment is described in the sections of this chapter on the drug and device industries.

Office of Technology Assessment

The Office of Technology Assessment is an analytical support agency of Congress. The Health Program of the Health and Life Sciences Division of OTA has conducted many health care technology assessments and has issued other reports directly related to health care technology assessment issues. OTA staff integrates information from the literature with the help of expert advisers from industry, academia, public interest groups, and other government agencies. OTA focuses its evaluation efforts either on generic technological issues or on case studies from which further research questions or generalizable lessons can be gained. Subjects of case studies have included drugs, devices, procedures, and organizational and support technologies. In order to identify the policy implications of technologies, OTA assessments consider economic implications, cost, and cost-effectiveness of technologies, as well as evidence of safety, effectiveness, and efficacy. OTA is one of a few assessment organizations that addresses social, legal, and ethical aspects of technologies when they are relevant issues. By 1985 the OTA Health Program had generated 24 main reports on technology assessment issues, 34 case studies, and other related technical memoranda and background papers. The 1985 OTA Health Program budget is approximately $1.6 million (C. J. Behney, Office of Technology Assessment, personal communication, 1985). Other agencies of the legislative branch such as the General Accounting Office (GAO), the Congressional Budget Office, and the Congressional Research Service have issued reports regarding technology assessment issues. Under its auditing authority, the GAO has made recommendations to Congress for greater economy, efficiency, and effectiveness of federal health programs (see, e.g., U.S. Congress GAO, 1982, 1983, 1985).

Prospective Payment Assessment Commission

The Prospective Payment Assessment Commission was established by Congress under the Social Security Act Amendments of 1983 (P.L. 98-21), when the new Medicare prospective payment system was enacted. ProPAC was established as an independent commission to advise and assist Congress and the DHHS secretary in maintaining and updating the Medicare prospective payment system administered by HCFA. ProPAC will address itself initially to two primary responsibilities: (1) recommending annually to the DHHS secretary the appropriate percentage change in the payments made under Medicare for inpatient hospital care and (2) consulting with and recommending to the secretary and reporting to Congress necessary changes in the Diagnosis-Related Groups (DRGs) used in the prospective payment system and their relative weights. The first report of ProPAC on these subjects was submitted April 1, 1985. ProPAC has the authority to assess safety, efficacy, and cost-effectiveness of new and accepted medical and surgical procedures. In collecting and assessing information, ProPAC must use existing information when possible. If existing information is inadequate, the commission may support original research and experimentation, including clinical research. However, in order to carry out such activities, ProPAC will require substantially more money than was budgeted in each of its first 2 years: approximately $1.5 million for FY 1984 and $2.4 million in FY 1985. (ProPAC operated on $3.1 million in FY 1985, using funds carried over from FY 1984.) Support of ProPAC, both financial and in the form of close cooperation with other public and private health organizations, is especially important to the viability of prospective payment. The use of DRGs has yet to be adequately evaluated for its validity as an indicator of patient resource needs or for its impact on medical technology under prospective per-case payment. Furthermore, the periodic DRG adjustment process requires sufficient supporting mechanisms for identifying and assessing new hospital cost-raising technologies and will rely on accurate and timely data collection (OTA, 1983a).

Health Care Financing Administration

The Health Care Financing Administration is responsible for the Medicare program and federal participation in the Medicaid program and is the nation's largest third-party payer. Estimated federal outlays for health care services and supplies by Medicare ($68.1 billion) and Medicaid ($20.2 billion) totaled an estimated $88.3 billion in FY 1984 (HCFA Bureau of Data Management and Strategy, unpublished data, 1984). HCFA has two major types of assessment efforts: the process it uses to make coverage decisions and research, evaluation, and demonstration projects directed by the HCFA Office of Research and Demonstrations.

HCFA coverage decisions are especially far-reaching, because they apply not only to Medicare coverage but often are followed by other third-party payers. HCFA coverage questions generally arise when a Medicare carrier or intermediary receives a claim for a new or unfamiliar service or when there is some other reason to question whether a procedure is *reasonable and necessary*. When these questions are of national importance and cannot be resolved locally or by the HCFA regional offices, HCFA's central office is asked to make a decision, with the assistance of HCFA's physician panel where medical judgment is needed. If HCFA does not have sufficient information on which to base a decision, it refers the question to the Public Health Service, where the Office of Health Technology Assessment conducts an assessment, as described below. In a few cases, such as heart transplantation and treatment of end-stage renal disease, the HCFA Office of Research and Demonstrations will sponsor a special study to assist the agency in making a coverage decision. (See DHHS Office of the Assistant Secretary for Planning and Evaluation [OASPE; 1984] for a detailed description of the HCFA coverage decision process.)

The HCFA Office of Research and Demonstrations (ORD) directs over 200 intramural and extramural research, evaluation, and demonstration projects to improve the effectiveness of the Medicare and Medicaid programs (HCFA, 1983). The FY 1984 budget of HCFA ORD was about $31 million. With the decrease in funding for NCHSRHCTA, HCFA has become the federal leader in supporting health services research. But HCFA seldom provides direct support of assessments of clinical technologies. Only about $3 million of the 1984 HCFA ORD budget was devoted to assessments of cost, safety, efficacy/effectiveness, and other concerns regarding medical technologies such as heart transplantation, kidney dialysis and transplantation, magnetic resonance imaging, and implantable devices (HCFA ORD, unpublished data, 1984).

Given the magnitude of Medicare's contribution to U.S. health care and the numerous requests for coverage determinations made to HCFA, the agency's investment in technology assessment is miniscule. Expenditures for HCFA technology assessment activities, including the $31 million ORD budget (devoted largely to health services research and demonstrations rather than clinical technologies) and the indeterminate but certainly minor cost of the HCFA coverage decision process, are imperceptible in the estimated $88.3 billion paid by HCFA for health care in 1984. This is the case even if we take into account the additional investment in assessment activities made not by but on behalf of HCFA—primarily the $0.7 million for OHTA and related advice from other agencies, and the few million dollars for ProPAC, which evaluates and makes recommendations regarding the Medicare prospective payment system administered by HCFA.

National Center for Health Services Research and Health Care Technology Assessment

The National Center for Health Services Research and Health Care Technology Assessment (formerly the National Center for Health Services Research) has extramural and intramural programs primarily devoted to health services research topics such as health services financing, organization, quality, and utilization; health information systems; the role of market forces in health care delivery; and health promotion and disease prevention. Whereas HCFA R&D activities are addressed to improving the Medicare and Medicaid programs, NCHSRHCTA efforts reach more widely and are intended to add to a broader understanding of health services delivery in all sectors. The agency's budget has decreased steadily from the 1972 high of $65 million to approximately $17.5 million in FY 1985 (current dollars not corrected for inflation), including about $1 million from the Medicare Trust Fund. This drop limits investigator-initiated health services research and may erode the basis for making national policy changes in health care delivery.

Office of Health Technology Assessment The NCHSRHCTA Office of Health Technology Assessment has the responsibility for preparing assessments and recommendations regarding Medicare coverage issues referred to the Public Health Service by HCFA. OHTA assumed these responsibilities following the dissolution of the National Center for Health Care Technology in 1981. OHTA assessments are concerned with the safety and effectiveness of diagnostic and therapeutic procedures or techniques and normally address a procedure's acceptability and appropriateness and requisite facilities and support systems. OHTA assessments currently do not entail the generation of primary evaluative data but are based on literature searches and consultation with medical specialty societies and federal agencies such as NIH and FDA. (See Finkelstein et al. [1984] for analysis and comparison of coverage decision processes of OHTA and a Blue Shield plan.) Since 1981, OHTA has prepared over 100 assessments for HCFA. Virtually all of the HCFA coverage decisions made on issues referred to OHTA have been consistent with OHTA recommendations. OHTA activities, supported primarily by the Medicare Trust Fund, were budgeted for $0.7 million in FY 1984 and again in FY 1985. Most of the FY 1985 NCHSRHCTA research budget of $15.5 million is for intramural and extramural health services research, with perhaps a few million dollars for other technology assessment activities, including the OHTA budget.

In the Health Promotion and Disease Prevention Amendments of 1984 (P.L. 98-551), Congress renamed the agency the National Center for Health Services Research and Health Care Technology Assessment and set aside $3 million of its FY 1985 budget (and $3.5 million in FY 1986 and $4 million in FY 1987) specifically for technology assessment. This increased support is intended primarily to strengthen the agency's ability to make recommendations regarding Medicare coverage of medical technologies and to undertake and support studies of technology diffusion, assessment methods, and specific technologies. Congress earmarked a portion of these set-aside funds ($0.5 million in FY 1985, $0.75 million in FY 1986, and $0.75 million in FY 1987) as matching funds for the planning, development, establishment, and operation of a council on health care technology at the Institute of Medicine, National Academy of Sciences.

National Center for Health Statistics

The National Center for Health Statistics is the federal agency established to collect, analyze, and disseminate data on the nation's health. NCHS provides data on the health status of the population (e.g., through its "Vital and Health Statistics" reports); the nature and use of health resources, costs, and expenditures for health services; and other areas of national concern. NCHS supports and helps to coordinate statistical programs of other organizations such as the Duke University Cardiovascular Data Bank and the American Rheumatism Association Medical Information System. NCHS also conducts research in data collection methods and statistical methodology. As discussed in Chapter 3, NCHS routinely produces data that can be used in technology assessment efforts of other federal agencies, health researchers, industry, and the public. NCHS data are useful for monitoring changes in health services utilization and practice behavior. Furthermore, they may provide a national yardstick for indicating the effect of medical and public health interventions and call attention to health services research and other technology assessment needs. NCHS devoted approximately $2 million of its $46 million 1984 budget to R&D (OMAR, 1984).

Veterans Administration

The Veterans Administration devoted about $192 million in FY 1985 to R&D activities conducted or sponsored by the Medical Research Service ($171 million), Rehabilitation Research and Development Service ($15 million), and the Health Services Research and Development Service ($6 million; VA Central Office figures for FY 1985). Total 1985 VA health care costs were approximately $9 billion. The VA Cooperative Studies Program of the Medical Research Service coordinates multihospital studies conducted by investigators at different VA medical centers under common protocols. In FY 1985, the VA spent approximately $20 million on clinical trials, including $12 million by the Cooperative Studies Program (P. Huang, VA, personal communication, 1985). The VA Health Services Research and Development Service supports and conducts evaluations of alternative policies and interventions of care (P. Goldschmidt, VA, personal communication, 1984). The VA Supply Service evaluates (including bench testing) new equipment for safety and effectiveness for procurement by VA facilities. In 1984, the VA instituted a Technology Assessment Committee to make recommendations to the chief medical director of the VA regarding priority technologies for assessment and appropriate assessment methods and purchasing and deployment of technologies, to track assessment activities of other agencies, and to coordinate these and other agency-wide assessment activities (P. Goldschmidt, VA, personal communication, 1984). In 1982, the VA initiated a Prosthetics Technology Evaluation Committee to coordinate the evaluation of VA prosthetic products and devices.

Centers for Disease Control

The Centers for Disease Control medical technology assessment activities consist primarily of improving the performance of clinical laboratories, including setting standards for laboratory practices and research and evaluation of laboratory materials (e.g., reagents) and procedures, and developing and testing disease prevention, control, and health promotion programs. The CDC provides laboratory support to other agencies, e.g., to the National Heart, Lung, and Blood Institute for its cardiovascular intervention trials, and to the FDA for investigating medical devices (especially laboratory test kits) and assistance in developing FDA guidelines and performance standards for these products. In 1982, the CDC devoted approximately $4 million[3] to medical technology assessment activities (C. Blank, CDC, personal communication, 1984). CDC spent an estimated $76.1 million of its $378 million 1984 budget on R&D (OMAR, 1984).

Department of Defense

The Department of Defense conducts medical and life sciences R&D under the Navy Medical R&D Command, Army Medical R&D Command, and the Air Force Aeromedical Division. Total defense health care expenditures, including care for retirees and military dependents, were $6.6 billion in 1983 (Gibson et al., 1984). The total medical and life sciences R&D budget is $446 million for 1985. These R&D activities are primarily addressed to military needs not met in the civilian sector. Included are infectious and parasitic disease research; combat casualty research; medical defense against biological and chemical weapons; effects of electromagnetic radiation; and diving, submarine, and aviation medicine. Among the medical technologies under development and evaluation are field-operated imaging systems, noncontact monitoring systems, and combat information systems. Expenditures for clinical trials are probably under $10 million annually (Vorosmarti, 1985; H. Dangerfield, personal communication, 1984).

DRUG INDUSTRY

The U.S. drug industry is one of the nation's most profitable in terms of returns on sales and investments (Standard & Poor's Corporation, 1983a,b). The industry has three major components as classified by the U.S. Department of Commerce (USDOC): biological products, medicinals and botanicals, and pharmaceutical preparations. Pharmaceutical preparations, including ethical (prescription) and proprietary (nonprescription, over-the-counter) products, accounted for 75 percent of the estimated $27.9 billion in 1984 U.S. drug product shipments (USDOC, 1985). When adjusted for inflation, annual growth in dollar shipments of drugs over the 10-year period from 1972 to 1982 was 3.8 percent (Standard & Poor's Corporation, 1983a). Drug industry after-tax profits were an estimated 13.5 percent of sales in 1984 (USDOC, 1985). The industry places great emphasis on research and development, which produce many successful product innovations. The number of prescriptions filled in the United States was 1.5 billion in 1983 (USDOC, 1985).

Drug Industry Research and Development

Drug industry R&D and successful product innovation provide the impetus for the industry's profitability. Individual drug firms depend on a handful of successful innovations. Failure to produce new products—to replace those that lose market share to imitators or for which patents expire—would be devastating to many drug firms. Of the 30 top-selling products in 1965, only four remained in the top 30 by 1980. Some 95 unique prescription drug products (i.e., different, new chemical entities) were introduced into the U.S. market in the 5-year period 1980–1984 (USDOC, 1985; Pharmaceutical Manufacturer's Association [PMA], PMA Statistical Factbook, unpublished, 1984). In 1984, nearly 400 new drug products were in various stages of development (USDOC, 1984). Taking a new chemical entity from discovery through FDA approval for marketing currently requires from 7 to 10 years and over $90 million,[4] according to the Pharmaceutical Manufacturers Association (PMA Statistical Factbook, unpublished, 1984).

The importance of new product R&D and competition in the drug industry is exemplified by the antiulcer drug Tagamet (active ingredient cimetidine), a product of the SmithKline Beckman Corporation. Between 1977, when Tagamet was approved for the U.S. market, and 1982, the company's total annual sales quadrupled. In 1984, Tagamet was the world's largest-selling drug; its worldwide sales (including chemical sales of cimetidine), approached $1 billion, half of which was accounted for by U.S. sales. This single drug accounted for 60 percent of SmithKline Beckman's ethical pharmaceutical sales in 1983 and 30 percent of corporate sales (SmithKline

Beckman, 1983; M. L. Paterson, Smith Kline & French, personal communication, 1984). However, a new, similar antiulcer drug, Zantac, a product of the British-based firm Glaxo, Inc., challenged Tagamet in 1984. Popular in the United Kingdom and Europe, in 1984 it was accounting for 25 percent of all new antiulcer drug prescriptions, following its introduction to the U.S. market by mid-1983 (Kleinfield, 1984; Koenig, 1983).

Drug companies invest high proportions of sales and profits in R&D and spend relatively high amounts on basic research. Ethical pharmaceuticals account for the bulk of drug industry R&D. Drug industry expenditures for R&D have been increasing at a rate of about 15 percent a year since 1978, compared with about 11 percent for all industries (Standard & Poor's Corporation, 1983a; USDOC, 1985). Drug R&D expenditures were an estimated $3.5 billion in 1984 (including 5 percent for veterinary use) and is projected to be $4.0 billion in 1985 (USDOC, 1985). This amounts to 12 percent of drug product shipments. The Pharmaceutical Manufacturers Association (1984) estimates that its member firms devote over 14 percent of sales to R&D and that 80 percent of pharmaceutical firm R&D expenditures is devoted to new product development, and the remaining 20 percent is devoted to improvement and modification of existing products. (PMA members number about 130 of the well over 1,000 U.S. drug companies and primarily are the larger, brand name pharmaceutical firms, accounting for over 90 percent of total U.S. drug sales.) There is little (less than 1 percent) direct government financing of drug industry R&D, although much of the basic research that precedes the development of new drugs is federally supported, primarily by NIH, and is performed in universities and medical centers.

Assessment of Drugs

Following basic research and discovery, drug evaluation largely is guided by the regulatory process administered by the FDA. FDA involvement begins when a sponsor seeks to investigate a drug's safety and efficacy using clinical testing in humans. The FDA has established a two-part process for premarketing drug evaluation: (1) the investigational new drug (IND) application process and (2) the new drug application (NDA) process (FDA, 1977). In an IND application, a drug sponsor describes the proposed clinical studies, the qualifications of the investigators, the chemical description of the drug, and available data on its pharmacology and toxicity gained from studies in animals (and humans when available, usually from foreign studies). If the IND application is approved by the FDA, the sponsor may proceed with a three-phase clinical investigation of the drug. Following completion of testing under the approved IND application, a sponsor may file an NDA, which is a request for FDA permission to market the drug. About 1 in 10 drugs for which INDs are issued complete all phases of clinical investigation and receive NDA approval by the FDA (FDA, 1983c).

Premarketing clinical studies do not provide an adequate picture of a drug's potential adverse effects or indications. The total drug-exposed populations in such studies are relatively small (usually 700–3,000 patients) and do not permit detection of uncommon effects, such as those occurring less often than in 1 in 1,000 patients. Many types of patients who ultimately will use the drug are excluded from the premarketing study (e.g., certain age groups, pregnant women, patients with diseases other than the one being studied, patients taking concomitant medications, specific degrees of severity of disease), which may preclude identification of effects that occur only in other types of patients or effects that result from drug-drug interactions. The duration of premarketing studies is limited, usually 1 to 2 years, and thus may not enable identification of long-term effects. The conduct of premarketing studies often is limited to specialists affiliated with major medical centers and so may not permit assessment of effects of a drug as used by the average physician engaged in clinical practice. New indications for a drug may be found after marketing, raising efficacy issues not previously addressed (FDA, 1983a; Joint Commission on Prescription Drug Use, 1980; OTA, 1982b).

Although the FDA closely regulates the introduction and labeling of new drugs, the use of legally marketed drugs in practice is not regulated. The agency approves of what the manufacturer may recommend about uses in its labeling and advertising, but it cannot approve or disapprove of how a legally marketed drug is used by a physician in practice (Archer, 1984). Industry and the FDA conduct postmarketing studies of drugs which address some of the needs left unfilled by the premarketing study. However, compared with the volume of data that is collected prior to marketing, far fewer data are collected in the United States on drugs after they are approved for marketing (Altman, 1983; Borden and Lee, 1982; Joint Commission on Prescription Drug Use, 1980; OTA, 1982b). This reflects differences both in level of effort and types of study.

Postmarketing studies include so-called phase IV studies and a variety of surveillance activities. Phase IV studies are not mandated in FDA regulations but are discussed in FDA guidelines. A phase IV study may be a condition of FDA marketing approval if the uncertainty over a drug's safety or efficacy does not warrant delaying its release on the market, or it may be initiated by companies to further substantiate drug safety and efficacy and to support marketing efforts. Phase IV studies may be experimental or nonexperimental. Although a number of drug manufacturers have periodically conducted postmarketing studies of adverse and beneficial drug reactions and drug-drug interactions for specific drugs, only a few have established permanent units for these activities (Blue Sheet, 1983), e.g., those of Burroughs Wellcome, Hoffman-La Roche (E. Roberson, Hoffman-La Roche, personal communication, 1984), and Upjohn (Borden and Lee, 1982). A few companies are venturing into studies beyond safety and efficacy; Smith Kline & French Laboratories initiated a cost-benefit studies program in response to the increased emphasis on cost containment and to justify the prices of its leading products (M. L. Paterson, personal communication, 1984).

The FDA conducts, coordinates, or sponsors a number of surveillance programs, including spontaneous reaction reporting programs, adverse reaction registries, and research programs. Other agencies such as the CDC, the National Institute on Drug Abuse, and the World Health Organization share drug surveillance information with the FDA (Jones, 1985; OTA, 1982b).

Expenditures for Drug Assessment

Data for making direct estimates of drug industry expenditures devoted to technology assessment activities such as clinical trials and postmarketing surveillance are not available, as company budgets do not generally show line items for such activities. However, indirect estimates can be made from survey data.

Based on a recent survey of its members, the Pharmaceutical Manufacturers Association estimates that clinical evaluation (including controlled and uncontrolled trials in phases I, II, and III and in postmarketing phase IV) accounts for 23.1 percent of R&D expenditures for ethical pharmaceuticals in 1982 (PMA, 1984). Assuming that clinical evaluation accounts for a smaller proportion of R&D costs for other drug product makers than it does for PMA-member ethical pharmaceutical makers, we estimate that roughly $700 million to $750 million of the $3.3 billion in 1984 human-use drug R&D expenditures was devoted to clinical evaluation, including postmarketing studies. A rough estimate of 1984 expenditures for postmarketing studies is $100 million, most of which was spent by industry.[5]

Despite its shortcomings, premarketing assessment of drugs for safety and efficacy in the United States is the most comprehensive and well-funded area of medical technology assessment in the world. The federal government and the drug industry have had sufficient opportunity since the 1962 amendments to the Food, Drug, and Cosmetic Act to clarify, improve, standardize, and adapt to drug assessment procedures. The industry's vitality evinces little sign of deleterious effects of the regulatory process, which may have enhanced overall provider and consumer confidence in drug products, both in the United States and worldwide. Adjustments in the regulatory process are being made to address the role of generic drugs, patent restoration, orphan drugs (notably the Drug Price Competition and Patent Restoration Act of 1984 and the Orphan Drug Act of 1983), and other issues related to industry innovation and competition.

Improvement is needed in gathering data for identifying drugs' adverse and beneficial effects, their rates of use, and indications for use. Methodological shortcomings in the current premarket approval process are not adequately compensated by existing provisions for postmarketing surveillance. These efforts are scattered, relatively uncoordinated, and rely heavily upon voluntary participation (Blue Sheet, 1984; Joint Commission on Prescription Drug Use, 1980; OTA, 1982b).

Increased cost-consciousness of physicians, hospitals, and consumers; increased availability of alternative therapies; and expanded capabilities in diagnosis and treatment posed by new biotechnologies are among the factors that press for widening of drug assessment beyond safety and efficacy, to include greater study of cost, cost-effectiveness, and certain public policy implications.

MEDICAL DEVICE INDUSTRY

The medical device industry generates a great diversity of products. More than 8,500 device establishments currently registered with the FDA have listed some 42,000 makes and models in 1,740 generic categories of medical devices (FDA Center for Devices and Radiological Health [CDRH], unpublished data, 1985). These include diagnostic and therapeutic equipment, prostheses, surgical and medical instruments and supplies, dental equipment and supplies, ophthalmic goods, and in vitro diagnostic products—reagents, instruments, and systems used in the collection, preparation, and examination of specimens taken from the human body to determine the state of a patient's health. The FDA definition of medical devices excludes drugs, which achieve their effects through chemical action within or on the body. The great majority of medical device manufacturers are classified by the U.S. Department of Commerce in five industries: x-ray and electromedical equipment, surgical and medical instruments, surgical appliances and supplies, dental equipment, and ophthalmic goods. The value of medical device product shipments in these industries exceeded $20 billion in 1984 (USDOC, 1985).[6]

Medical Device Industry Research and Development

Because of the limited availability of medical device industry R&D data, direct estimates of industry-wide R&D are not available. The range of R&D spending by device manufacturers is wide; makers of such devices as heart pacemakers, intraocular lenses, and certain diagnostic technologies spend greater amounts on R&D. For example, Medtronic, Inc., the world's leading producer of implantable devices, devoted about 9 percent of sales to R&D in 1983 (R. Flink, Medtronic, personal communication, 1984). For most dental products firms, R&D expenditures average less than 2 percent of sales; even the larger firms invest only about 3 to 4 percent of sales in R&D (USDOC, 1985).

A rough estimate of R&D expenditures across the medical device industry, including federal contributions, is 5 percent of sales.[7] Applying the 5 percent estimate to an estimated $20 billion in 1985 sales, total annual medical device industry R&D expenditures would be on the order of $1 billion.

Principal federal participants in medical device research and development include NIH, the VA, CDC, and the National Institute for Handicapped Research (NIHR) in the Department of Education. The VA is a leader both in the R&D and the use of rehabilitative technologies and devices. The VA Rehabilitation Research and Development Service does extensive work in amputation prosthetics, spinal cord injury, and sensory aids; the Prosthetic and Sensory Aids Service provided $81 million in appliances and services to one million disabled veterans in 1982 (VA, 1983). NIHR has the largest federal budget (estimated at $36 million in FY 1984; American Association for the Advancement of Science [AAAS], 1984) specifically directed toward disability-related research. The National Aeronautics and Space Administration (NASA, 1982), National Bureau of Standards, and the Department of Energy also contribute to medical device R&D.

Assessment of Medical Devices

Assessment of medical devices is influenced by and may be described in terms of the device classification and premarket notification and approval processes stipulated in the Medical Device Amendments of 1976. This legislation gave the FDA significant authority to regulate the testing and marketing of medical devices to ensure their safety and efficacy. Congress required classification of all devices into one of three regulatory classes differentiated according to the extent of control necessary to ensure their safety and efficacy: class I, general controls; class II, performance standards; and class III, premarket approval. The amendments instituted systematic premarket notification and screening procedures rather than continued reliance on postmarket regulatory actions on a case-by-case basis. The FDA does not regulate the use of approved medical devices in clinical practice, but has the power to ban devices of any classification that present substantial deception or unreasonable and substantial risk of illness or injury that is not correctable by labeling (FDA, 1980, 1983b).

All post-1976 devices require premarket approval unless exempted by the FDA as being *substantially equivalent* to one already in use before the 1976 amendments or unless the sponsor successfully petitions the FDA for reclassification into class I or II. By 1985, nearly 29,000 premarket notifications for new post-Amendment devices had been received—including over 5,000 in 1984 alone. Over 98 percent of these have been found to be substantially equivalent to pre-Amendment devices; the others—405 devices by 1985—have been placed in class III (FDA CDRH, unpublished data, 1985). For a class III device not substantially equivalent to a pre-1976 device, the sponsor must provide information to the FDA concerning all investigations about safety and efficacy. (Pending final classification by the FDA and after a designated grace period, the agency may require the filing of evidence of safety and efficacy for pre-Amendment devices and their post-Amendment substantial equivalents in order to allow for continued marketing.) This information normally is provided through the premarket approval process, involving an investigational device exemption (IDE) and submission of a premarket approval application (PMAA). The IDE, which is analogous to the investigational new drug process in FDA drug regulation, permits limited use of an unapproved device in controlled settings for the purpose of collecting safety and efficacy data.

In a PMAA, the sponsor submits to the FDA the results of clinical investigations made under the IDE together with manufacturing data. The FDA will approve a PMAA if the results demonstrate the device to be safe and efficacious. As is the case for new drugs, FDA may require specified postmarketing study of a new medical device as a condition of marketing approval. FDA approval of a PMAA authorizes a sponsor to distribute commercially a device for the purposes for which it is labeled subject to any FDA-imposed restrictions. Sponsors may be required by the FDA to file "supplemental" PMAAs with clinical data to support new labeling claims for previously approved devices.

PMAAs remain a comparatively new and infrequently implemented regulatory requirement, although they account for a significant portion of the FDA's device-related workload, and the median time for processing them is about 10 months (FDA CDRH, unpublished data, 1985). Through 1983, only one medical device firm in 25 had any direct experience with PMAAs (Blozan and Tucker, 1984). Of the 358 PMAAs submitted through 1983, 46 percent were for ophthalmic devices (intraocular lenses, contact lenses, and related products); the rest were mostly alpha-fetoprotein test kits, pacemakers/pulse generators, plasma exchange systems, transcutaneous carbon dioxide (CO_2) monitors, antimicrobial test systems, and heart valves. Based on an FDA survey of 20 manufacturers of various types of medical devices, the cost of bringing a new device to market through the PMAA process—including device development, clinical trials, manufacturing and controls, application preparation, and other activities conducted during review—ranges from \$370,000 to \$1,025,000 (Blozan and Tucker, 1984).

Pursuant to the 1976 Amendments, FDA published in 1984 final rules on medical device reporting (MDR), which require manufacturers and importers of medical devices to report adverse experiences suggesting that a device may have caused or contributed to a death or serious injury or has malfunctioned and would be likely to cause or contribute to a death or serious injury if the malfunction were to recur (Federal Register, 1984a). In addition, the FDA will maintain its voluntary, and less than comprehensive, Device Evaluation Network (DEN). As part of DEN, the FDA supports the Medical Device and Laboratory Product Reporting Program (PRP) administered by the United States Pharmacopeial Convention, Inc. (\$250,000 1984 budget; D. M. McGinnis, U.S. Pharmacopeial Convention, personal communication, 1984). PRP receives approximately 2,000 device problems reports annually. The agency also has a contract (\$50,000 in 1984) with the Consumer Product Safety Commission for similar data. Other sources for DEN are FDA field offices, the VA, the Department of Defense, and the independent medical device and equipment evaluator ECRI (C. Reynolds, FDA, personal communication, 1984).

Expenditures for Medical Device Assessment

The range of resources devoted to clinical trials of medical devices varies widely by type of product. Many devices (e.g., many of the 1,600 types of class I and class II devices which are remote from the body or otherwise pose minimal hazard) require little investment in clinical evaluation; others, such as implantable devices, require a great deal. Medtronic, Inc., spent approximately 7 percent of its 1983 heart pacing products R&D budget on clinical trials (R. Flink, personal communication, 1984); IOLAB, Inc., and other manufacturers of intraocular lenses may spend 20–25 percent of their intraocular lens R&D budgets on clinical trials (M. Nimoy, IOLAB, personal communication, 1984). (A company's expenditures for clinical trials in a given year depend on the stage of development of its new products.)

Medical device industry expenditures for clinical evaluation were probably on the order of $35 million in 1984, or about 4 percent of medical device industry R&D expenditures. At least half of this amount may be accounted for by clinical trial expenditures associated with devices submitted for FDA approval under PMAAs.[8] Clinical evaluation costs other than those for devices submitted under PMAAs include costs for devices tested under investigational device exemptions (IDEs), but not carried through the entire premarket approval process, and for the several thousand devices annually that bypass the PMAA process as being substantially equivalent to marketed devices. However, few of these entail costly, if any, clinical evaluations.

Medical device assessment has yet to emerge from a shakedown period, partly because the relative newness of the 1976 Medical Device Amendments (as compared with the 1962 Amendments to the Food, Drug, and Cosmetic Act) and the great diversity of devices subject to regulation. Many thousands of devices—from implantable, programmable dual chamber cardiac pacemakers and diagnostic reagents using monoclonal antibodies to porcine heart valves, injectable silicone, snakebite kits, ice bags, and bed boards—must be properly classified and regulated to protect consumers and to be responsive to provider needs and manufacturers' concerns. Congress has reproved the FDA for being slow to implement certain major provisions of the 1976 Amendments (U.S. Congress, House, 1983; U.S. Congress GAO, 1983). In 1984, the FDA required for the first time premarket approval data for a pre-Amendment device (an implanted cerebellar stimulator, the first of 13 such devices identified in 1983) and its post-Amendment substantial equivalents (Federal Register, 1984b). As noted above, the FDA did not establish final mandatory medical device reporting rules until 1984. The agency has not set performance standards for the 1,100 generic types of class II devices as specified by the law, although Congress set no time limit for doing so.

The FDA is faced with making decisions regarding priorities in device regulation, and these will have implications for industry and the public. The workload for handling premarket approval of class III devices, already substantial given current technological advances, may increase, depending on the emphasis placed on requiring premarket approval applications for pre-Amendment devices and their substantial equivalents. Greater resources should also be devoted to expanded postmarketing surveillance of devices, addressed only in part by the new mandatory medical device reporting requirements, and perhaps to work in classifying devices and setting performance standards for class II devices. This type of work will require additional properly trained people, both in the FDA and in industry.

As is the case for drugs, resources for device assessment are limited and too narrowly focused. Device assessment rarely extends beyond safety and efficacy to matters of cost-effectiveness and broader social implications and devotes few resources to postmarketing surveillance. ECRI and, to a lesser extent, the American Hospital Association are among the few programs that make available comparative information on technical performance, cost, hazard reports, and other valuable information for device procurement and maintenance.

OTHER PRIVATE SECTOR ASSESSMENT ACTIVITIES

There is widespread and increasing interest in technology assessment among organizations in the private sector in addition to those in medical product industries. Private insurers, medical associations, professional and industry associations, hospital corporations and other major providers, policy institutes, and voluntary health agencies conduct and sponsor assessment activities to suit their varied needs. These include making coverage and reimbursement policies and procurement decisions, responding to practitioner inquiries, setting voluntary standards for manufacturing and practice, providing guidance to regulatory agencies and other policymakers, and improving medical practice and services delivery.

Despite this heightened interest, current private sector activity remains limited in several important ways. Except for the private, independent health devices-testing organization ECRI, few of the evaluations undertaken in these private sector efforts involve the generation of primary data, and no other organization has as its primary purpose the assessment of medical technologies. The scope of evaluations is limited—most evaluations do not extend beyond matters of safety and effectiveness to cost-benefit and cost-effectiveness and ethical, legal, and other broader social issues. Safety and efficacy/effectiveness are addressed only indirectly in some evaluations; third-party payers generally rely on medical providers' acceptance of a technology as standard practice—rather than experimental or investigative—as an indicant of its safety and effectiveness. The predominant assessment methods are literature reviews and consultation of experts. Assessments are generally conducted on a reactive, ad hoc basis rather than by systematic review and priority setting. Evaluation activity of insurers largely is driven by the insurance claims process; assessments by medical associations generally are conducted in response to inquiries by third-party payers and practitioners. The magnitude of expenditures made by providers and insurers for the extraordinarily varied array of new, emerging, accepted, and outmoded health care services merits a much more serious commitment to technology assessment.

Insurers

Blue Cross and Blue Shield Plans, commercial insurance companies, and prepaid and self-insured plans paid an estimated $100 billion in medical benefits in 1983, or 32 percent of total U.S. personal health care expenditures (Gibson et al., 1984). The purpose of assessment efforts by private insurers is to fulfill equitably the contractual responsibility to pay for care of good quality at a reasonable cost. Insurance contracts generally cover only technologies that are "medically necessary" and reimburse for covered procedures in amounts that are "usual, customary, and reasonable." Most contracts exclude investigational and experimental procedures or those done for educational purposes.

Technology reviews by insurers generally arise through the claims process; in very few instances do providers inquire before providing a service as to whether it will be reimbursed. For the most part, burden of proof for payment decisions rests on the payer rather than the provider. Claims reviewers may question procedures that are new, unorthodox, outmoded, or applied in an unconventional manner. Few third-party payers explicitly evaluate safety, effectiveness, appropriate use, or cost-effectiveness of medical technologies. Payers generally rely on a determination of a technology's diffusion, i.e., whether it is standard practice rather than experimental or investigative, as an indicant of physicians' judgment of its safety and effectiveness. Because assessments are triggered by the claims process, they can be bypassed by concealing new technologies under old coding and nomenclature.

Insurers increasingly rely on claims review committees and assistance from medical associations such as the American College of Radiology, the American College of Physicians, and the American College of Cardiology for making coverage and reimbursement decisions. Very few insurers are able to assign dollar amounts to their assessment activities, because these generally are not budget line items and involve the efforts of a variety of personnel having additional responsibilities.

The Blue Cross and Blue Shield (BCBS) Association has a number of activities in technology review. The Technology Evaluation and Coverage Program develops medical policies for the Association's *Uniform Medical Policy Manual*, which is used by plans in administering certain national account contracts. These policies are formulated by the BCBS Medical Advisory Panel, which determines the status, i.e., experimental, investigative, or standard, of new and emerging technologies, and if appropriate any special indications for coverage or noncoverage. The purpose of the BCBS Medical Necessity Program is to identify outmoded, duplicative, and unproved technologies, as well as procedures, that are standard practice but that are utilized more often than warranted by good medical practice. Medical Necessity Program guidelines are distributed to the BCBS Plans to assist them in determining their subscriber contractual obligations. Including these two programs, the Blue Cross and Blue Shield Association spends approximately $350,000 annually on medical policy and coding activities (L. Morris, Blue Cross and Blue Shield Association, personal communication, 1984). In addition to the activities of the association, the 87 local Blue Cross and Blue Shield Plans have medical departments and engage in various levels of technology review activities. The California Blue Shield Medical Policy Committee ($100,000 1985 budget) assesses for coverage purposes new diagnostic and therapeutic technologies and initiated the review of obsolete procedures that grew into the Medical Necessity Program of the Blue Cross and Blue Shield Association. Beginning with percutaneous transluminal coronary angioplasty in 1982, California Blue Shield became the first private third-party payer to institute selective reimbursement—i.e., payment for certain procedures at designated institutions only—and currently reimburses selectively for heart transplants and liver transplants.

Direct private payer support of medical R&D and technology assessment is negligible (Gibson et al., 1984; Kahn, 1984). A few private payers provide funds for research and technology assessment activities. For example, since 1982, Blue Cross of Massachusetts has obligated over $5 million in matching funds to the Massachusetts Fund for Cooperative Innovation, a grant program for hospital cost-containment experiments administered jointly with the Massachusetts Hospital Association (MHA) (Blue Cross/MHA, 1985).

Medical Associations

Many of the major national medical associations and societies conduct assessments in response to inquiries from their members and from government and third-party payers. Some associations establish panels to set voluntary guidelines for practice. Evaluations often are undertaken in response to requests made by government and private payers trying to determine whether technologies are standard practice as opposed to investigational or experimental. Some associations set voluntary guidelines for practice, e.g., American Academy of Pediatrics recommendations for immunization practice. For the most part, medical association assessment activities are confined to matters of safety and efficacy and do not involve original studies. Methods generally consist of literature searches by staff and informal polling and review of association committees and other experts. Studies that collect primary data are the exception; probably the foremost example is the ongoing American College of Radiology's Patterns of Care Study of cancer treatment supported by the National Cancer Institute, currently funded at approximately $500,000 annually (J. Diamond, American College of Radiology, personal communication, 1984). Medical associations generally are unable to provide budget figures for their assessment efforts. A few of the larger assessment programs do have their own budgets; e.g., the American College of Physicians (ACP) Clinical Efficacy Assessment Project has a $160,000 1985 budget (L. J. White, American College of Physicians, personal communication, 1985), and the American Medical Association's new Diagnostic and Therapeutic Technology Assessment program has a $380,000 1985 budget (N. E. Cahill, American Medical Association, personal communication, 1985).

Policy Research Groups

A number of independent assessment and policy research groups undertake technology assessment studies and analyses of related issues. These are generally supported by government contracts, contributions of philanthropic foundations, corporations, and private individuals; membership and conference fees; and publication sales. Examples are the American Enterprise Institute for Public Policy Research; the Battelle Memorial Institute; the Brookings Institution; the Hastings Center Institute of Society, Ethics and Life Sciences; Project HOPE Center for Health Affairs; InterStudy; and the Rand Corporation. Although some nonprofit institutes have health divisions that conduct medical technology assessments on request under contract, few have ongoing technology assessment programs. The Hastings Center ($250,000 1985 health-related budget; A. L. Caplan, Hastings Center, personal communication, 1985) is one of very few organizations that deals consistently and explicitly with ethical and legal issues of medical technologies. Assessments usually consist of findings drawn from reviews of the literature. A notable exception is ECRI (formerly the Emergency Care Research Institute), a self-sufficient organization that provides a number of assessment services, including published reports of comparative laboratory testing of medical devices and equipment and information on device alerts and related developments ($5.0 million 1985 budget; M. VanAntwerp, ECRI, personal communication, 1985). Examples of assessments that generate primary data are the Battelle heart transplantation and kidney transplantation and hemodialysis studies conducted for DHHS and the Rand health insurance experiment (Brook et al., 1983) funded by DHHS.

Industry Associations

Many industry and professional associations have strong interests in medical technology issues and often are particularly concerned with effects of government regulation on industry innovation and marketing. Although a few of these organizations conduct technology assessments on a contractual basis, most of their technology assessment-related activities consist of setting voluntary standards, monitoring and responding to legislation, and conducting conferences and educational programs for members.

Particularly active with regard to FDA regulation of drugs and medical devices and related congressional activity are the Pharmaceutical Manufacturers Association and the Health Industry Manufacturers Association. The American Hospital Association (AHA) has helped to formulate hospital industry positions with regard to Medicare prospective payment and related issues. The Group Health Association of America recently established a medical technology panel to examine policies for inclusion of technologies in benefits plans; of particular interest is the effect on competitive status among health maintenance organizations (HMOs) and other third-party payers of mandatory coverage by federally qualified HMOs of expensive new technologies such as liver transplantation (Group Health Association of America, 1984).

The AHA Hospital Technology Series Program provides medical equipment procurement guidelines, alerts, and related evaluative information to its hospital subscribers for medical equipment ($225,000 1985 budget; M. Goodhart, AHA, personal communication, 1985). Other associations active in medical technology issues include the Alliance for Engineering in Medicine and Biology, American Public Health Association, American Society for Testing and Materials, Association for the Advancement of Medical Instrumentation, Health Insurance Association of America, Institute of Electrical and Electronics Engineers, National Electrical Manufacturers Association, and Rehabilitation Engineering Society of North America.

Provider Institutions

Major medical centers, hospitals, hospital corporations, health maintenance organizations, private clinics, and other provider institutions have played important roles in the development, application, and evaluation of medical technologies.

Although it is not possible to account for even a substantial fraction of the assessment work conducted by provider organizations, we can cite a few examples that illustrate the evolution and variety of these activities, even within single institutions. The Cleveland and Mayo Clinics were particularly active in the early evaluation of the computed tomography (CT) scanner. The Cleveland Clinic has conducted major research and assessment programs in cardiovascular diseases, including an artificial heart program. The Mayo Clinic has done important work in many areas of biomedical research and has conducted surveillance studies of Guillain-Barré syndrome, leukemia, vaginal cancer associated with diethylstilbestrol (DES), hip arthroplasty, and other conditions and procedures (Kurland and Molgaard, 1981; Melton et al., 1982). The Mayo Clinic also has a health care studies unit examining corporate health care cost-containment, measures of illness severity, cost-effectiveness of liver transplantation, cost studies comparing coronary bypass grafting and percutaneous transluminal coronary angioplasty, and issues in rural health services delivery (F. Nobrega, Mayo Clinic Health Care Studies Unit, personal communication, 1985).

Health maintenance organizations have made important contributions in health services research, cost-effectiveness of new technologies, and other aspects of technology assessment. Group Health Cooperative of Puget Sound, Harvard Community Health Plan, Health Insurance Plan of Greater New York, and Kaiser-Permanente Medical Care Program are examples of some of the larger HMOs that have significant and evolving assessment activities.

The Harvard Community Health Plan has conducted noteworthy evaluations in such areas as psychotherapy and quality assurance. It recently merged its research department with the Harvard Center for Analysis of Health Practice to form the Institute for Health Research, which examines cost-benefit of health care practices, resource allocations, system response to patients' needs, and methods of measuring performance in health care (Harvard Community Health Plan, 1984). Among numerous evaluation activities, Group Health of Puget Sound (GHC) has been involved in the Rand Health Insurance Experiment (Brook et al., 1983) and the Boston Collaborative Drug Surveillance Program, a joint effort with Boston University. GHC has consolidated and expanded its research and evaluation activities under the Center for Health Studies ($1.8 million 1985 budget) which, in addition to serving GHC internal evaluation needs, conducts studies of wider interest in preventive care, reproductive health, primary care, mental health, geriatrics, cancer control, and accidents and injuries (GHC, 1984; M. Durham, GHC, personal communication, 1985).

The implementation of the Medicare prospective payment system and the growth of multi-institutional providers able to pool information resources and take advantage of purchasing power are two major factors expanding the interests of provider organizations in technology assessment. The Medicare prospective payment system has increased the stakes for cost-containment measures in provider institutions and has broadened the market for assessment information. Prospective payment provides incentives for hospitals to shift their behavior regarding adoption and use of medical technologies. Because Medicare accounts for such a large portion of hospital revenues, these may be strong incentives. Hospitals are rewarded for technology use that attracts admissions of profitable DRGs, reduces patient length of stay, and controls the use of ancillary services. (See, e.g., Anderson and Steinberg [1984], OTA [1984, 1983a], and Roe and Schneider [1984] for projected effects of Medicare prospective payment on technology adoption and use.)

Traditionally, providers have gathered procurement information from vendors and trade shows, medical specialty societies, and other providers. Currently, providers seek concise comparative purchasing information regarding product price and value, useful life, operating costs, and service support, as well as product updates, alerts, and corrective actions such as are provided by ECRI and the American Hospital Association. In addition, more hospital corporations, HMOs, and other large provider organizations are undertaking their own assessment of medical devices, equipment, supplies, and facilities. Hospital Corporation of America (HCA), Humana, Inc., and Kaiser-Permanente Health Care Program are examples of organizations with units for examining effectiveness, regulatory and reimbursement status, cost, service requirements, and other attributes of medical devices and equipment and for assisting member hospitals in capital equipment selection and purchasing (Collen, 1985; T. Dwyer, Humana, personal communication, 1985; D. Foutch, HCA, personal communication, 1984). Major provider organizations are especially likely to use group purchasing and sole source supply for volume discounts and competitive bidding for equipment and supplies. The increased market for assessment information and the leverage afforded by economies of scale should make provider institutions into more discerning buyers of medical technologies.

Similar to the manner in which the VA Cooperative Studies Program facilitates the conduct of multicenter clinical trials sharing common protocols, the networks of hospitals managed and owned by hospital corporations may provide resources for multicenter clinical trials of medical technologies. HCA Medical Research Services, an affiliate of HCA, has begun contracting with pharmaceutical firms to conduct and manage clinical trials of new drugs, using common protocols in selected HCA hospitals (J. Butler, HCA Medical Research Services, personal communication, 1985). HCA Capital Corporation, the venture capital arm of HCA, has invested in and provided other forms of support for applied R&D and assessment of emerging technologies such as cochlear implants, the artificial heart, lithotripters, microwave heat treatment for cancer, and reusable imaging media for x-ray systems. In exchange for its support, HCA receives certain licensing rights for some of these technologies, in addition to the benefits of involving its providers, patients, and facilities in these projects (HCA, 1984; L. Coleman, HCA Capital Corporation, personal communication, 1985). These activities may increase the facilities and other resources available for clinical research beyond university teaching hospitals and other traditional settings. Another HCA affiliate, the Center for Health Studies, coordinates corporate studies and services implementation in management development and medical education, strategic planning and services, and telecommunications (K. Hoot, HCA, personal communication, 1985). Such efforts among multi-institutional providers may widen the bridge of technology transfer.

Academic Institutions

Academic institutions performed about $3.6 billion in health R&D in 1983 (NIH, 1984). Most of this is basic and applied biomedical research supported by NIH; amounts for technology assessment are relatively small. Universities perform health services research, clinical trials, and other technology assessment activities supported by federal (especially NIH, HCFA, and NCHSRHCTA) and state agencies; foundations and other private, nonprofit sources; and industry. These activities often are carried out at centers for health services and policy research in schools of public health and medicine. A directory compiled by the Association for Health Services Research (1983) lists 37 centers, based in or affiliated with academic institutions, whose primary (although not necessarily sole) mission is the conduct of health services and policy research. Annual budgets of the 35 centers providing budget data range from $0.12 million to $5.5 million, average $1.1 million, and total $38.3 million. Of that total, 39 percent was provided by the federal government; 34 percent by private foundations; 7 percent by corporate sources; 7 percent by universities; and 13 percent by other sources such as state and local governments, individual gifts, and endowments. Examples of centers associated with academic institutions are the Boston University Health Policy Institute, Brandeis University Center for Health Policy Research and Analysis, Duke University Center for Health Policy Research and Education, Georgetown University Institute for Health Policy Analysis, Harvard University Division of Health Policy Research and Education, Johns Hopkins Health Services Research and Development Center, Northwestern University Center for Health Services and Policy Research, University of California at San Francisco Institute for Health Policy Studies, and Yale University Health Systems Management Group.

Employers

Employer contributions for employee health insurance benefits were an estimated $70.7 billion in 1983 (Federation of American Hospitals Review, 1984). The portion of production and service costs attributable to health benefits has increased with the expansion of employee and retiree health care benefits. Across all U.S. industries, employer-paid benefits for hospital, surgical, medical, and dental care averaged nearly $1,400 per employee in 1983, accounting for approximately 7 percent of the total payroll (U.S. Chamber of Commerce, 1985). Although a few companies are taking harder looks at proposed additions of technological innovations to health benefits plan coverage, many employers are taking other measures to decrease their health care costs. These include sponsoring HMOs, increasing employee health plan copayments and deductibles, requiring second opinions for certain types of surgery, providing incentives for outpatient instead of inpatient care, providing reimbursement for the cost of generic drugs only, and instituting wellness and fitness programs.

CONCLUSIONS

The estimate that public and private spending on technology assessment totals over $1 billion yearly makes it seem like a big and costly enterprise. Yet this is a generous estimate for a broadly defined category embracing controlled and uncontrolled clinical trials, epidemiologic and other observational studies, health services research, and a wide variety of synthesis activities. Even so, it is a nearly vanishing 0.3 percent of the money that is spent for health care.

Whether that proportion of investment in medical technology assessment is in rough agreement with the spending by other sectors of industry for technology assessment is difficult to tell, because estimates of expenditures for that purpose are nearly impossible to assemble with confidence. However, figures are available for R&D investments by many enterprises. Health R&D takes 3 percent of total health spending, which is low compared with other technology-intensive or -dependent industries, such as the chemical industry, information industries, and the defense establishment. Another indication that health R&D is lagging comes from figures that show a decline in the proportion of spending for R&D since 1972.

A particular shortcoming is seen in clinical trials for medical and surgical procedures. OTA (1983b) estimates that randomized clinical trials have been applied to 10 or 20 percent of medical practices. The NCHSRHCTA Office of Health Technology Assessment has had to base its recommendations to HCFA regarding coverage issues on evidence sorely lacking in rigorous experimental findings. Of the 26 assessments conducted by OHTA for HCFA in 1982, results from randomized clinical trials were available for only two (OTA, 1983b; see NCHSR, 1984a). NIH support for clinical trials (an estimated $276 million in FY 1985 obligations) is provided for only a portion of the clinical trials that have been identified as worthy of support. Due to uncertainties in future funding and competing priorities, the National Heart, Lung, and Blood Institute (NHLBI) has had difficulty in initiating any new large-scale clinical trials since 1978; its support of clinical trials overall has dropped from the $40 million to $60 million range of the mid- to late 1970s to an estimated $25 million in FY 1985 (current dollars not adjusted for inflation; NIH, 1985).

Less than $50 million is spent on technology assessment devoted to synthesis and interpretation of primary evaluation data for determining how best to apply in practice new and currently available technologies. Examples are consensus development conferences, coverage decisions by third-party payers, medical and industry association assessment programs, congressional studies, and policy institute studies.

Despite its oft-cited shortcomings—including the absence of comparative studies of medical products—the premarket approval processes for drugs and medical devices regulated by the FDA is the only coherent, coordinated systems for medical technology assessment. Premarketing notification requirements for these products are sufficient for identifying and classifying new technologies for assessment according to levels of risk posed to the public. Current provisions for drug and device assessments are less concerned with post-marketing assessment and with matters beyond safety and efficacy. Whereas premarketing reporting of drug safety and efficacy is mandatory, most of the available data on postmarketing adverse reactions to drugs is derived from voluntary reporting. Funding for drug assessment accounts for the bulk of all medical technology assessment funding. In 1984, roughly $700 million to $750 million of $3.3 billion in human use drug industry R&D expenditures was devoted to clinical evaluation of drugs, including an estimated $100 million for postmarketing study. Although the amount devoted to premarketing drug assessment may be adequate, greater attention needs to be devoted to postmarketing study of drugs.

Because of their more standard treatment under FDA assessment requirements and the time since passage of the 1962 amendments to the Food, Drug, and Cosmetic Act, assessment procedures for drugs are more widely understood and consistently carried out by industry and government than are those for medical devices. Certain important aspects of medical device assessment are still being clarified pursuant to the 1976 Medical Device Amendments, which address many thousands of diverse products. Most medical devices do not require rigorous clinical evaluation; roughly $35 million was spent in 1984 on clinical evaluation of medical devices, much of which was devoted to the relatively few class III devices subject to FDA premarketing approval requirements. Resources for postmarketing study of medical devices are limited, as are those for getting information about comparative technical performance, cost, and other information useful in the procurement and maintenance of devices. The demand for such information will continue to increase.

Much less formal than premarketing drug and device assessment is the loose network of relationships among public and private third-party payers, medical associations, private physicians, and the biomedical research community that characterize the assessment of medical and surgical procedures. Although the FDA is the gatekeeper to the marketing of new drugs and medical devices and has the authority to recall products presenting "imminent hazard to the public health," the agency holds little sway in the application of drugs and devices in medical practice. It is left to the loose network to determine whether medical and surgical procedures meet the subjective criterion of "standard and accepted practice."

Other nodes and strands of the network arise ad hoc; e.g., an NIH consensus development conference on liver transplantation; publication of results of an NHLBI study on coronary artery bypass surgery; a special HCFA study on end-stage renal disease; the issuance of voluntary mammography guidelines by the American College of Radiology; or OHTA's pulling together of literature, opinions, and other resources from medical associations, NIH, and the FDA to synthesize recommendations for a HCFA coverage decision. Assessments of new, accepted, or possibly outmoded medical and surgical procedures are not undertaken systematically. Rather, they are often prompted by new or unusual insurance claims, by inquiries made to medical associations, and occasionally by political pressure. The rigor of assessment methods varies widely, from a landmark NHLBI randomized controlled clinical trial to a medical association staff literature search informally reviewed and approved by a small committee of physicians. Where assessments require group judgments, methods may be used which are methodologically unsound, and decision rationale and literature sources may go undocumented. The NIH Consensus Development Program is one of few ongoing group judgment efforts that has been subject to serious evaluation.

RECOMMENDATIONS

Five interrelated recommendations are offered covering assessment concerns, coordination of assessment information, responsibility for conduct of assessments, evaluation of assessment programs, and increased financial support for medical technology assessment.

Assessment Concerns

We recommend increased commitment to technology assessment, especially for the following:

- *generation of primary data on the safety and efficacy of new, accepted, and possibly outmoded medical and surgical procedures, with emphasis on information useful in making medical practice decisions and coverage decisions, especially comparative data on the safety and efficacy of alternative technologies*;
- *determination of cost-effectiveness and public policy implications of adopting selected drugs, medical devices, and medical and surgical procedures*; and
- *postmarketing surveillance of drugs and medical devices.*

Coordination of Assessment Information

We recommend the implementation of a coordinative capacity for monitoring, synthesizing, and disseminating technology assessment information. To some extent, a number of organizations already serve certain constituencies in this way. Examples are ECRI for medical device users; the Health Industry Manufacturers Association, the Pharmaceutical Manufacturers Association, and the American Hospital Association for their respective and somewhat overlapping constituencies; and the NIH Office of Medical Applications of Research for the PHS and NIH in particular. Clearly, much new assessment information is of interest to wide constituencies; for example, within 1 year the American Medical Association (AMA; 1983), ECRI (1982), and OHTA (NCHSR, 1984b) each assessed automatic implantable infusion pumps. The effects of instituting prospective payment and developments in such technologies as magnetic resonance imaging, monoclonal antibodies, and computer-aided decision support systems sweep across much of the health care community. A coordinative capacity placed in one or more clearinghouses would serve as a central directory and source for current assessment information. To be responsive to both government and the private sector, yet not directed by either, this capacity should be vested in one or more jointly supported private-public organization. Once it has firmly established this capacity, such an organization may be a logical agent for coordinating the development of an agenda to address unmet assessment needs.

Responsibility for Conduct of Assessments

The committee is in favor of vesting expanded assessment activity in multiple organizations, to best serve the diverse needs for assessment. Increased federal commitment should be devoted especially to greater NIH clinical trial support, consensus development activities, PHS advisory capacity to HCFA, fulfilling ProPAC responsibilities, and FDA-coordinated postmarketing surveillance of drugs and medical devices. Designation of increased private funds for assessment should be made by private sources; funds should be devoted to support clinical trials, medical association assessment programs, and private payers' own assessment activities. Both federal and private support should be made available to independent assessors such as ECRI and various policy research institutes. An independent, private-public assessment entity such as was proposed by the Institute of Medicine (1983) and Bunker et al. (1982) could be supported by balanced federal and private contributions.

Evaluation of Assessment Programs

We recommend that assessment programs make formal provisions for their own evaluation and improvement, with special emphasis on the effectiveness of assessments used (e.g., clinical trials, epidemiological methods, consensus development) and the dissemination of results. Examples of programs that have undertaken such evaluation are the NIH Consensus Development Program and the American College of Physicians Clinical Efficacy Assessment Project.

Financial Support for Medical Technology Assessment

Amount of Support The committee recommends a prompt increase in medical technology assessment activities and the resources devoted to them. We believe that support for medical technology assessment should rise over an appropriate period to reach an annual level $300 million greater (in 1984 dollars) than at present. This represents a modest increase, perhaps 25 percent more than the estimate cited herein, of current assessment expenditures. The bulk of this new funding would be devoted to generating primary data for assessing medical and surgical procedures, with remaining funds allocated to assessments for assisting payers in administering plans and making coverage and reimbursement decisions, postmarketing study of drugs and medical devices, health services research, medical information system assessments, group judgment efforts, training, and clearinghouse activity. A substantial effort is needed to find the costs of various kinds of research in efficacy and effectiveness. These costs probably vary considerably from one kind of technology to another. Finding out about these costs would be an appropriate task for a priority-setting agency.

The increased support might be allocated somewhat as follows. The amounts cited are not meant to be prescriptive, but are intended to illustrate approximate magnitudes of investments that can be effectively allocated.

- $150 million to $250 million for clinical trials. $200 million per year would pay for 30 ongoing large-scale clinical trials requiring an average of $5 million in annual support, plus 200 smaller-scale trials requiring an average of $0.25 million in annual support.[9]
- $30 million to $50 million in increased support for health services research. In the face of accelerating changes in the organization, delivery, and financing of health services, funding for health services research is at a low ebb following years of budget cuts. This report projects that 1984 national expenditures for health services research will be less than $200 million. The total NCHSR budget dropped from $65 million in 1972 to $17.5 million in 1985 (current dollars).
- $10 million to $20 million in increased

support for assessment activities intended to assist HCFA in administering the Medicare prospective payment system and making coverage and reimbursement policy, including support for assistance from the Public Health Service (OHTA, NIH, ADAMHA, FDA, etc.); special HCFA ORD assessments of drugs, devices, and procedures; and increased support for ProPAC.

- $10 million to $20 million in increased support for assessment activities intended to assist private payers in administering plans and making coverage and reimbursement policy, including, e.g., studies of alternative benefits plans, determining appropriate reimbursement levels for technologies, and support of medical association group judgment efforts.
- $5 million to $15 million in increased support for postmarketing study and surveillance of drugs and medical devices, to be coordinated by the FDA.
- $5 million to $10 million in increased support for assessments of medical information technologies. Included are technologies for medical information processing, storage, retrieval, and transfer, which provide the foundation of technology assessment efforts as well as other biomedical endeavors. Also included are such emerging technologies as computer-assisted diagnosis and treatment and research on and evaluation of the dissemination and diffusion of medical technology assessment findings.
- $2 million to $5 million in increased support for group judgment and other synthesis efforts and workshops, symposia, and conferences conducted by federal agencies and medical, professional, and industry associations. A portion of these funds should be allocated to consensus development conferences such as those cosponsored by OMAR at NIH. Currently, OMAR cosponsors about seven NIH consensus development conferences annually at a cost of $145,000 each. Ten additional such conferences would amount to less than $1.5 million. Over the 3-year period 1981–1983 with a total budget of approximately $650,000, the Clinical Efficacy Assessment Project of the American College of Physicians generated recommendations regarding some 50 technologies. Programs such as these can be most useful in focusing interest on assessment issues, establishing the extent of available information on technologies, calling attention to further needs, and broad dissemination of findings.
- $2 million to $5 million per year in medical technology assessment training fellowships to provide for academic training and on-site participation in assessment activities undertaken by a sponsoring organization. It is important that leaders in health care appreciate and understand the role of assessment in health care. Candidates for these fellowships would include persons with backgrounds in such fields as medicine, epidemiology, biostatistics, allied health, engineering (e.g., electronic, materials, mechanical, and bioengineering), hospital administration, policy analysis, economics, law, risk management, and information management. Fellows would be supported by both private and public sources. Government sponsors might include NIH, FDA, NCHSRHCTA, HCFA, OTA, VA, CDC, and NLM (the National Library of Medicine); private sector sponsors might include drug and medical device manufacturers, insurers, and independent assessment organizations such as ECRI, Battelle, and Hastings Center. These might be 2-year fellowships, for example, in which the first year would be spent at an academic institution and the second on site. In a given year, 50 fellowships at an average cost of $50,000 each (including stipend, tuition, expenses, indirect costs, varying according to source of support, sponsor, and fellows' previous training) would amount to $2.5 million. These could be apportioned, for instance, in 6-year training grants of $1.5 million

each, to 10 academic institutions, each providing for 15 2-year fellowships.

- $2 million to $5 million for a medical technology assessment clearinghouse.[10]

Sources of Support Support for increased technology assessment should come from the health care dollar. A number of mechanisms have been proposed, including percentage-of-payment (or premium) set-asides by payers, per capita levies from provider organizations, grants and contracts from payers and providers, and charges for membership in and subscription to research findings of assessment institutes. (Third-party set-asides for technology assessment and biomedical research based on percentages of expenditures have been suggested by, e.g., Relman [1980, 1982] and Kahn [1984].) Further work is needed to formulate alternatives for tapping the health care dollar, and prompt political action will be required to implement one or more of them.

One alternative would be for all private and public third-party payers to set aside a fraction of a percent of their benefit payments, e.g., 0.2 percent [Relman (1980)]. In 1984, this would have amounted to about $490 million—$200 million from federal payers, primarily HCFA; $70 million from state and local payers; and $220 million from the private health insurance industry and other private third-party payers. To generate $300 million under such a plan would require a lesser investment. Across-the-board participation by private third-party payers, including self-insured plans, would deflect the "free-rider" problem.[11] A portion of these contributions could take the form of selective coverage for experimental technologies in exchange for evaluation data. (Blue Shield of California is using selective coverage for a few technologies [Schaffarzick, California Blue Shield, personal communication, 1985]. See, e.g., Bunker et al. [1982] for discussion of selective coverage.)

A Worthy Investment Expenditures for unproven or unnecessarily used medical technologies are certainly in the tens of billions of dollars annually. Although inconsequential as a percentage of health care expenditures, a $300 million annual investment would pay for itself many times over if it resulted in justified nonreimbursement for even a handful of unnecessary technologies, aside from gains made in quality of care. Savings from nonreimbursement of only several of the technologies recommended for nonreimbursement by the National Center for Health Care Technology (NCHCT) (which operated on a $4 million budget in its final year) have been estimated to be in the hundreds of millions of dollars annually.[12] The results of the NHLBI coronary artery surgery study, a large-scale clinical trial, are also instructive. It is estimated that 159,000 patients in the United States had bypass surgery in 1981 at a cost to the nation of $2.5 billion to $3 billion. Results of the NHLBI coronary artery surgery study, a large-scale randomized clinical trial, suggest that 25,000 potential bypass patients per year should not have the surgery (Kolata, 1983). The study was conducted over a 14-year period at a cost of $26.3 million (current dollars), or approximately $37 million in 1984 dollars. It will have paid for itself if it results in decreasing unnecessary surgery for only 2,000 patients.

NOTES

[1] HCFA spent approximately $28 million of its $31 million 1984 Office of Research and Demonstrations budget on health services research (HCFA, 1983, 1984b). The bulk of NCHSR's $15 million FY 1984 research budget was for health services research; some was for assessment activities involving other medical technologies (J. E. Marshall, National Center for Health Services Research, personal communication, 1984). The FY 1984 budget of the VA Health Services Research and Development Service was $5 million (VA, 1985). Expenditures by foundations in 1980 for health services research were estimated at $25 million by Dooley et al. (1983). A review of Foundation Cen-

ter (1984) data indicates that a total of approximately $20 million was contributed for health services research in 1-year budget periods spanning 1982–1983 by the following major contributors (listed alphabetically): Commonwealth Fund, John A. Hartford Foundation, Robert Wood Johnson Foundation, Henry J. Kaiser Family Foundation, W.K. Kellogg Foundation, John D. and Catherine T. MacArthur Foundation, and the Pew Memorial Trust.

An NIH estimate for total 1983 federal obligations for health services research is $169.9 million (NIH, Analysis Branch, Department of Planning and Evaluation, Office of Program Planning and Evaluation, Biannual Report of Federal Obligations for Health Research and Development, unpublished, 1984). However, this may be a high estimate, including certain expenditures made for biomedical research and other activities outside health services research as the term is used in this report. Included in that estimate is $39.7 million for NIH health services research, nearly half of which is devoted to NIH health promotion and disease prevention activities which may be more oriented to biomedical research than to health services research. Also included is the entire $29.3 million R&D budget of the National Institute for Handicapped Research (in the Department of Education), which conducts a wide range of rehabilitation-related activities, including services delivery, training, and R&D of rehabilitative devices. The estimate by NIH includes amounts for the following agencies: NIH ($39.7 million), ADAMHA ($17.3 million), HRSA ($12.5 million), Office of the Assistant Secretary for Health ($16.6 million, primarily NCHSRHCTA), HCFA ($30.2 million), Office of the Secretary (DHHS) ($12.4 million), Department of Education ($29.3 million), and other agencies ($12 million).

[2] OMAR (1983) indicates that NIH budgeted $560 million for technology assessment and technology transfer in 1982. Taken alone, however, this may be misleading. First, OMAR was unable to get consistent itemizations of expenditures from the NIH bureaus, institutes, and divisions (BIDs). Second, estimates for technology assessment encompassed support for (1) clinical trials, (2) specialized centers, (3) state-of-the-art workshops and conferences, (4) various clearinghouses, (5) development and dissemination of publications, and (6) evaluation of biomedical inventions and monitoring of patent and licensing activities. Of these six activities, the latter three are technology transfer activities, amounting to approximately $148 million in 1982, according to the report. Another $230 million of the $560 million is for specialized centers. Although the use of specialized centers support varies among NIH BIDs, most of it is for resource development; virtually all of the over $75 million provided to specialized centers by the National Cancer Institute (the largest supporter among the BIDs of specialized centers) was for resource development (salaries of professional and administrative personnel, equipment, facilities, renovations, etc.). Specialized centers do get funds for basic research, clinical trials, and related activities, but these funds are for the most part listed under other categories. Approximately $176 million of the 1982 technology assessment and transfer budget was for clinical trials. This leaves $7 million for technology assessment activities such as consensus development conferences, workshops, seminars, and related activities, including the $2 million OMAR budget and nearly $4 million for National Eye Institute technology assessment research grants. Using similar categories of activities, the OMAR report estimated that ADAMHA expenditures for technology assessment and transfer amounted to $38.44 million.

[3] This figure excludes expenditures for environmental health and occupational safety and health assessment activities.

[4] This figure is based on an estimate made by Hansen (1979) and has been updated by the Pharmaceutical Manufacturers Association in cooperation with Dr. Hansen to account for inflation in R&D costs. The figure includes the cost of new chemical entities (NCEs) that enter clinical testing but are not carried to the point of FDA approval for marketing. Thus, the figure—$91 million in 1983—should be interpreted as the average expected cost of discovering and developing a marketable NCE (Grabowski, 1982). Others have made similar types of estimates; see Hutt (1982) for further discussion.

[5] According to the PMA survey data for 1982, 3.2 percent of U.S. R&D expenditures for pharmaceuticals were allocated to phase IV studies. Applied to a total 1984 human use drug R&D budget of $3.3 billion, this would amount to more than $100 million (included in the estimate of clinical evaluation expenditures). However, this is probably an overestimate, as the larger ethical pharmaceutical makers surveyed by PMA may be more likely than other drug makers to invest in nonrequired, expensive postmarketing trials. In 1984, FDA spent under $1 million on intramural postmarketing surveillance activities and another $1.1 million in support of extramural programs such as the Boston Collaborative Drug Surveillance Program, the Drug Epidemiology Unit of Boston University, the Medicaid postmarketing surveillance programs in Michigan and Minnesota, and the Drug Product Problem Reporting Program administered by the United States Pharmacopeial Convention, Inc. (J. K. Jones, FDA National Center for Drugs and Biologics, personal communication, 1984).

[6] Product shipments in 1984 for x-ray and electromedical equipment, surgical and medical instruments, surgical appliances and supplies, and dental equipment totaled an estimated $18.6 billion (USDOC, 1985). In 1977, the last year for which data

are available, ophthalmic goods product shipments were $0.84 billion (USDOC, 1981).

[7] One reasonable approximation of industry-wide R&D commitment may be made using the figures for the USDOC optical, surgical, photographic, and other instruments industry group, which includes surgical and medical instruments, surgical appliances and supplies, dental equipment and supplies, and ophthalmic goods. Including federal contributions, total R&D for that industry group was 6.9 percent in 1980 (NSF, 1984). According to a 1981 poll of more than 500 medical device manufacturers, one-quarter of them reported R&D expenditures of less than 1 percent of sales, one-third reported 1 to 5 percent, and one-third reported spending 6 percent or more. (Others did not know or did not respond.) Thirteen percent spent fifteen percent or more (Louis Harris, 1982). This distribution is not inconsistent with the 5 percent estimate. Finally, a recent OTA report cites a special survey of limited available USDOC data that indicates industry R&D expenditures were 3 percent of medical device shipments in 1980, but the report concedes that this is probably an underestimate (OTA, 1984). As is the case in the drug industry, many medical device concerns are part of large, multiproduct firms which manufacture low R&D-intensive products in addition to medical devices.

[8] According to an FDA survey of 20 medical device manufacturers (Blozan and Tucker, 1984), the cost of clinical evaluation reported in PMAAs differs greatly for implantable and other devices. Reported costs for clinical trials (including protocol development, conduct of studies, payments for physician time, equipment, evaluation, printing costs, etc.) of ophthalmic devices range from $5,000 to $270,000 (averaging $144,000), implantable nonophthalmic devices range from $100,000 to $1,440,000 (averaging $813,000), and other nonophthalmic devices range from $40,000 to $200,000 (averaging $109,000). (These figures should be considered approximations in light of the survey's small sample size.) If we apply these cost estimates for PMAA clinical trials to a group of 88 PMAAs (the number submitted in 1982, the most in any year thus far) having characteristics of PMAAs submitted thus far (50 percent ophthalmic, 18 percent implantable nonophthalmic, 32 percent other nonophthalmic), then associated clinical trial costs would be on the order of $20 million annually.

[9] Large-scale trials referred to here might be comparable to the eight large-scale NHLBI trials, conducted primarily in the 1970s, for prevention and treatment of heart and vascular diseases. These trials ranged from $17 million to $150 million in total costs over periods ranging from 6 to 18 years (including intervention and follow-up), with average annual costs ranging from $2 million to $10 million per trial. The overall average cost of these eight trials was $5 million per trial per year. The average cost for all 20 NHLBI clinical trials ongoing in 1979 was $2.8 million. The average cost for all trials supported by NIH in 1979 was $0.16 million.

[10] The formation of a clearinghouse for information on medical technology assessment has been recommended by the Institute of Medicine (1983). Annual budgets for other types of clearinghouses in NIH, CDC, and ADAMHA range from $0.15 million to $6 million. Examples (with FY 1982 budgets) are the High Blood Pressure Information Center ($0.150 million), National Diabetes Information Clearinghouse ($0.208 million), Clearinghouse for Occupational Safety and Health ($1.03 million), National Clearinghouse for Alcohol Information ($3.41 million), and International Cancer Research Data Bank Program ($6 million) (OMAR, 1983).

[11] The free-rider problem here refers to the ability of nonparticipating, private, third-party payers to take advantage, at no cost and with potential for competitive advantage, of evaluative information gained through the investment of others.

[12] A Harvard School of Public Health (1981; Braun, 1981) study gave low, middle, and high estimates for 10-year savings expected from nonreimbursement of four medical procedures. Estimates were given for the savings to Medicare (for the population 65 and over) and to the nation (for all ages). Middle estimates of 10-year national savings for the four technologies were as follows (in 1980 dollars): endothelial cell photography, $130 million; dialysis for schizophrenia, $146 million; hyperthermia for cancer, $272 million; and radial keratotomy for myopia, $477 million. Among the assumptions used in arriving at the savings estimates is that two of the procedures (radial keratotomy and hyperthermia for cancer) would eventually be reimbursed.

A UCLA School of Public Health (1981) study gave low and high estimates for annual savings to Medicare from restricted reimbursement of three procedures (in 1980 dollars): home use of oxygen, $6 million to $20 million; telephonic monitoring of cardiac pacemakers, $87 million to $97 million; and plasmapheresis for rheumatoid arthritis, $10,000 million to $15,000 million.

REFERENCES

Altman, L. K. March 22, 1983. How safe are prescription drugs? New York Times.

American Association for the Advancement of Science Intersociety Working Group. 1984. AAAS Report IX: Research & Development, FY 1985. Washington, D.C.

American Medical Association. 1983. Diagnostic and therapeutic technology assessment (DATTA):

Implantable infusion pump. Journal of the American Medical Association 250:1906.

Anderson, G., and E. Steinberg. 1984. To buy or not to buy: Technology acquisition under prospective payment. New England Journal of Medicine 311:182–185.

Archer, J. D. 1984. The FDA does not approve uses of drugs. Journal of the American Medical Association 252:1054–1055.

Arnstein, S. R. 1977. Technology assessment: Opportunities and obstacles. IEEE Transactions on Systems, Man, and Cybernetics SMC-7(8):571–582.

Association for Health Services Research. 1983 (and June 1984 addendum). Health Services and Policy Research Centers Directory. Washington, D.C.: Association for Health Services Research.

Blozan, C. F., and S. A. Tucker. 1984. A Profile of Premarket Approval Applications and Their Costs: A Background Paper. Washington, D.C.: Office of Planning and Evaluation, Food and Drug Administration.

Blue Cross of Massachusetts/Massachusetts Hospital Association Fund. 1985. Blue Cross/MHA Fund for Cooperative Innovation: Report for 1984. Boston.

Blue Sheet. 1984. Adverse Reaction Reporting: FDA System Must Permit "Early Triage" (Interview of FDA Commissioner Hayes). 27(35):P&R-4.

Blue Sheet. 1983. Drug companies are establishing post-marketing surveillance systems as a way to avoid unpredictable outbreaks of adverse reactions. 17(26):7–8.

Borden, E. K., and J. G. Lee. 1982. A methodologic study of post-marketing drug evaluation using a pharmacy-based approach. Journal of Chronic Diseases 35:803–816.

Braun, P. 1981. Need for timely information justifies NCHCT. Medical Instrumentation 15:302–304.

Brook, R. H., J. E. Ware, W. H. Rogers, E. B. Keeler, A. R. Davies, C. A. Donald, G. A. Goldberg, K. N. Lohr, P. C. Masthay, and J. P. Newhouse. 1983. Does free care improve adults' health? New England Journal of Medicine 309:1426–1434.

Bunker, J. P., J. Fowles, and R. Schaffarzick. 1982. Evaluation of medical-technology strategies: Proposal for an institute for health-care evaluation. New England Journal of Medicine 306:687–692.

Coates, J. 1974. Some methods and techniques for comprehensive impact assessments. Technological Forecasting and Social Change 6:341–357.

Department of Health and Human Services, Office of the Assistant Secretary for Planning and Evaluation. 1984. Technology Assessment and Coverage Decisionmaking in the Department of Health and Human Services. Washington, D.C.

Dooley, B., C. Jackson, J. Merrill, J. Reuter, and K. Tyson. 1983. How do private foundations spend their money? A description of health giving. Health Affairs 2(3):104–114.

ECRI. 1982. Implantable Drug Infusion Pumps. Issues in Health Care Technology 5.I.4.:1–3. Plymouth Meeting, Pa.

Eddy, D. M. 1983. Flying without instruments: Analyzing medical policies by consensus and expert opinion. The John Hartford Foundation Bulletin. Winter:1–4.

Federal Register. 1984a. Department of Health and Human Services, Food and Drug Administration: Medical Device Reporting: Final Rule. 21 CFR Parts 600, 803, 1002, and 1003:36326–36351. Washington, D.C.: U.S. Government Printing Office.

Federal Register. 1984b. Department of Health and Human Services, Food and Drug Administration: Neurological Devices; Premarket Approval of the Implanted Cerebellar Stimulator: Final Rule. 21 CFR Part 882:26573. Washington, D.C.: U.S. Government Printing Office.

Federation of American Hospitals Review. 1984. Business and the health marketplace: testing grounds for competition, cost containment. 17:26–35.

Finkelstein, S. N., K. A. Isaacson, and J. J. Frishkopf. 1984. The process of evaluating medical technologies for third-party coverage. Journal of Health Care Technology 1(2):89–102.

Food and Drug Administration, U.S. Department of Health and Human Services. 1977. General Considerations for the Clinical Evaluation of Drugs. Washington, D.C.: U.S. Government Printing Office.

Food and Drug Administration, U.S. Department of Health and Human Services. 1980. Guideline for the Arrangement and Content of a Premarket Approval Application. Silver Spring, Md.: FDA Bureau of Medical Devices.

Food and Drug Administration, U.S. Department of Health and Human Services. 1983a. A Review of Safety Information Obtained from Phases I-II and Phase III Clinical Investigations of Sixteen Selected Drugs. Rockville, Md.: National Center for Drugs and Biologics.

Food and Drug Administration, U.S. Department of Health and Human Services. 1983b. Regulatory Requirements for Medical Devices. Washington, D.C.: U.S. Government Printing Office.

Food and Drug Administration, U.S. Department of Health and Human Services. 1983c. New Drug Evaluation Project, Briefing Book. Rockville, Md.: FDA Office of New Drug Evaluation.

Foundation Center. 1984. The Foundation Center Grants Index, 13th Edition. New York: Foundation Center.

Gibson, R. M., K. R. Levit, H. Lazenby, and D. R. Waldo. 1984. National Health Expenditures, 1983. Health Care Financing Review 6:1–29.

Grabowski, H. 1982. Public policy and innovation: The case of pharmaceuticals. Technovation 1:157–189.

Group Health Association of America. 1984. GHAA establishes medical technology panel. Group Health News 24(7)1–3.

Group Health Cooperative of Puget Sound. 1984. 1983 Annual Report. Seattle.

Hansen, R. W. 1979. The pharmaceutical development process: Estimates of current development costs and times and the effects of regulatory changes. Issues in Pharmaceutical Economics, in R. I. Chien, ed. Cambridge, Mass.: Lexington Books.

Harvard Community Health Plan. 1984. 1983 Annual Report. Cambridge, Mass.

Harvard School of Public Health Center for the Analysis of Health Practices. 1981. Impact on Health Costs of NCHCT Recommendations for Nonreimbursement for Medical Procedures. National Center for Health Care Technology Monograph Series. Rockville, Md.: National Center for Health Care Technology.

Health Care Financing Administration, U.S. Department of Health and Human Services. 1983. Health Care Financing Status Report: Research and Demonstrations in Health Care Financing. Office of Research and Demonstrations. Baltimore.

Hospital Corporation of America. 1984. Getting to Know HCA. Nashville, Tenn.: Hospital Corporation of America.

Hutt, P. B. 1982. The importance of patent term restoration to pharmaceutical innovation. Health Affairs 1(2):6–24.

Institute of Medicine. 1983. Planning Study Report: A Consortium for Assessing Medical Technology. Washington, D.C.: National Academy Press.

Joint Commission on Prescription Drug Use. 1980. Final Report. Washington, D.C.: U.S. Government Printing Office.

Jones, J. K. 1985. Post-Marketing Surveillance: A Description of the U.S. Approach and Some Considerations for a General Program of Post-Marketing Surveillance. In J. L. Alloza (ed.), Clinical and Social Pharmacology: Post-Marketing Period. Aulendorf, Germany: Editio Cantor.

Kahn, C. R. 1984. A proposed new role for the insurance industry in biomedical research funding. New England Journal of Medicine 310:257–258.

Kleinfield, N. R. May 29, 1984. SmithKline: One drug image. New York Times.

Koenig, R. December 22, 1983. SmithKline's Beckman unit gets slow start. Wall Street Journal.

Kolata, G. 1983. Some bypass surgery unnecessary. Science 222:605.

Kurland, L. T., and C. A. Molgaard. 1981. The patient record in epidemiology. Scientific American 245:54–63.

Louis Harris and Associates, Inc. 1982. A Survey of Medical Device Manufacturers. Study No. 80205, report submitted to the Bureau of Medical Devices, Food and Drug Administration, Washington, D.C.: Louis Harris and Associates.

Melton, L. J., R. N. Stauffer, E. Y. S. Chao, and D. M. Ilistrup. 1982. Rates of total hip arthroplasty. New England Journal of Medicine 307:1242–1245.

National Aeronautics and Space Administration. 1982. Spinoff 1982. Washington, D.C.

National Center for Health Services Research. 1984a. Health Technology Assessment Series: Health Technology Assessment Reports, 1982. DHHS Publication No. (PHS) 84-3371. Rockville, Md.: Department of Health and Human Services.

National Center for Health Services Research. 1984b. Health Technology Assessment Series: Health Technology Assessment Reports, 1983. DHHS Publication No. (PHS) 84-3372. Rockville, Md.: Department of Health and Human Services.

National Institutes of Health. 1982. Orientation Handbook for Members of Scientific Review Groups. Bethesda, Md.: National Institutes of Health.

National Institutes of Health. 1983. Draft Research Plan: FY: 1985. p. 60. Bethesda, Md.: National Institutes of Health.

National Institutes of Health. 1984a. NIH Data Book. Bethesda, Md.: National Institutes of Health.

National Institutes of Health. 1985. Office of the Director. Report on the Patterns of Funding Clinical Research. Bethesda, Md.

National Science Foundation. 1984. National Patterns of Science and Technology Resources 1984. Washington, D.C.: National Science Foundation.

Office of Medical Applications of Research, National Institutes of Health. 1983. Technology Assessment and Technology Transfer in DHHS: A Report Submitted to the Department of Commerce in Compliance with the Stevenson-Wydler Technology Innovation Act of 1980 (P.L. 96-480). Bethesda, Md.: National Institutes of Health.

Office of Medical Applications of Research, National Institutes of Health. 1984. Technology Assessment and Technology Transfer in DHHS: A Report Submitted to the Department of Commerce in Compliance with the Stevenson-Wydler Technology Innovation Act of 1980 (P.L. 96-480). Bethesda, Md.: National Institutes of Health.

Office of Technology Assessment. 1982a. Strategies for Medical Technology Assessment. Washington, D.C.: U.S. Government Printing Office.

Office of Technology Assessment. 1982b. Postmarketing Surveillance of Prescription Drugs. Washington, D.C.: U.S. Government Printing Office.

Office of Technology Assessment, U.S. Congress. 1983a. Diagnosis Related Groups (DRGs) and the Medicare Programs: Implications for Medical Technology. Washington, D.C.: U.S. Government Printing Office.

Office of Technology Assessment, U.S. Congress.

1983b. The Impact of Randomized Clinical Trials on Health Policy and Medical Practice. Washington, D.C.: U.S. Government Printing Office.

Office of Technology Assessment, U.S. Congress. 1984. Federal Policies and the Medical Devices Industry. Washington, D.C.: U.S. Government Printing Office.

Pharmaceutical Manufacturers Association. 1984. 1980–1983 Annual Survey Report. Washington, D.C.

Relman, A. S. 1980. Assessment of medical practices: A simple proposal. New England Journal of Medicine 303:153–154.

Relman, A. S. 1982. An institute for health care evaluation. New England Journal of Medicine 306:669–670.

Roe, W. I., and G. S. Schneider. 1984. Technology in a changing environment. Business and Health July/August:33–35.

SmithKline Beckman. 1983. Annual Report 1982. Philadelphia.

Standard & Poor's Corporation. 1983a. Industry surveys, health care: basic analysis 151:H13–H35.

Standard & Poor's Corporation. 1983b. Industry surveys, health care: current analysis 151:H1–H5.

U.S. Chamber of Commerce. 1985. Employee Benefits 1983. Washington, D.C.: U.S. Chamber of Commerce.

U.S. Congress, General Accounting Office. 1982. Medicare payments for durable medical equipment are higher than necessary. Comptroller General's Report to Congress. GAO/HRD-82-61. Washington, D.C.: U.S. Government Printing Office.

U.S. Congress, General Accounting Office. 1983. Federal regulation of medical devices—problems still to be overcome. GAO/HRD-83-53. Washington, D.C.: U.S. Government Printing Office.

U.S. Congress, General Accounting Office. 1985. Information requirements for evaluating impacts of Medicare prospective payment on post-hospital long-term services: Preliminary report. PEMD-85-8. Washington, D.C.: U.S. Government Printing Office.

U.S. Congress, House, Committee on Science and Astronautics. 1966. Inquiries, legislation, policy studies re: science and technology: Review and forecast. Second Progress Report. Washington, D.C.: U.S. Government Printing Office.

U.S. Congress, House, Committee on Energy and Commerce. 1983. Medical device regulation: The FDA's neglected child. Committee Print 98-F. Washington, D.C.: U.S. Government Printing Office.

U.S. Department of Commerce. 1981. Census of manufactures, industry series. Washington, D.C.: U.S. Department of Commerce.

U.S. Department of Commerce, Bureau of Industrial Economics. 1984. 1984 U.S. Industrial Outlook. Washington, D.C.

U.S. Department of Commerce, Bureau of Industrial Economics. 1985. 1985 U.S. Industrial Outlook. Washington, D.C.

U.S. Office of Management and Budget. 1984. Budget of the United States Government, FY 1985. Washington, D.C.: U.S. Government Printing Office.

University of California at Los Angeles School of Public Health. 1981. The effect of third party reimbursement on expenditures for medical care. Monograph prepared for the National Center for Health Care Technology Monograph Series. Rockville, Md.: National Center for Health Care Technology.

Veterans Administration. 1983. Administrator of Veterans Affairs Annual Report 1982. Washington, D.C.: Veteran's Administration.

Vorosmarti, J. 1985. Office of the Undersecretary of Defense for Research and Engineering. Interview in HIMAFOCUS. January 21. Washington, D.C.: Health Industry Manufacturers Association.

3 Methods of Technology Assessment

As Chapter 1 indicates, technology assessment offers the essential bridge between basic research and development and prudent practical application of medical technology. We have a substantial body of methods that can be applied to the various tasks of assessment, and their availability makes possible the acceptance, modification, or rejection of new technologies on a largely rational basis. That rationality, however, depends on many factors that go well beyond safety and efficacy, including, among other components, economics, ethics, preferences of patients, education of physicians, and diffusion of information. The methods that have been developed can take some account of most of these components, although combining the results for the components is a major task and one that is far from settled or solved. The existence of these assessment methods provides a foundation for building a system of technology assessment for the nation.

Most innovations in health care technology rest on some theoretical ideas held by the innovators. These ideas inevitably range in strength from very well informed to hopeful speculation. Beyond this, a few innovations are purely empirical in the sense that someone has noticed that the technology seemed to work, even though no underlying mechanism was proposed or understood. In considering medical technologies, no matter how strong or weak the theoretical justification, experience must be decisive. If *in practice* the innovation is clearly better or clearly worse than existing technologies, then the innovation deserves adoption or rejection. It is known from much experience that merely having a good idea, a good theory, or a constructive observation is not enough because there are so many unexpected interfering variables that may thwart the innovation and the innovator. Learning from controlled experience is central to progress in health care.

Learning from experience itself without formal planning often presents great difficulties and sometimes leads to long-main-

The outline, introduction, and conclusions of this chapter were developed by Frederick Mosteller. The various sections of the chapter were drafted primarily by other authors identified at the opening of each section.

tained fallacies, partly because of the lack of control of variables. This method is slow and expensive unless the effects are huge. Planning and analysis and scientific testing provide ways to strengthen the learning process. This chapter describes a number of techniques or methodologies that help to systematize learning from experience in health care technology.

Few people are acquainted with more than a few of the methods used for assessment. Usually investigators are acquainted with the few methods most frequently used in their own specialties. Consequently, it seems worthwhile to give a brief description of the more widely used methods and what they are most useful for studying.

For direct attack on evaluation through data acquisition, clinical trials are highly regarded. For generating hypotheses, the case study and the series of cases have special value. Registries and data bases sometimes produce hypotheses, sometimes they help evaluate hypotheses, and sometimes they aid directly in the treatment of patients. Sample surveys excel in describing collections of patients, health workers, transactions, and institutions.

Epidemiological and surveillance studies, although not synonymous, are well adapted to identifying rare events that may be caused by adverse effects of a technology.

Quantitative synthesis (meta-analysis) and group judgment methods give us ways to summarize current states of knowledge and sometimes to predict the future. Similarly, cost-effectiveness analysis (CEA) and cost-benefit analysis (CBA) offer ways of introducing costs and economics into these assessments. Modeling provides a way to simulate the future and still include complicated features of the real life process and to see what variables or parameters seem to produce the more substantial effects. When backed with strong, although limited, empirical investigation, it may add much breadth to an evaluation.

Sometimes what is learned to be true in a scientific laboratory may not, at first, be successfully applied in practical circumstances. Myriad reasons can explain this: the new technique is not correctly applied, or to the right kinds of cases, or it is not applied assiduously enough, or too assiduously, etc. This idea in medical contexts is captured in the terms *efficacy* and *effectiveness*. Efficacy refers to what a method can accomplish in expert hands when correctly applied to an appropriate patient; effectiveness refers to its performance in more general routine applications. The relevance of these ideas here is that some of the methods presented below are more naturally adaptable to assessing one of these or the other. The reader will probably appreciate, for example, that surveillance and data banks point toward assessing effectiveness, and most randomized clinical trials point toward assessing efficacy.

Although randomized clinical trials offer the strongest method of assessing the efficacy of a new therapy, it is recognized that it is not possible to have randomized trials for every version of every innovation. However desirable that might be, it is not feasible. Consequently, other methods of assessment are often going to be depended on; of course, some technologies actually require other methods. This in turn means that steps need to be taken to strengthen the other methods. These steps have two forms. First, where possible, apply the known ways of improving studies, such as observational studies (for example, have a careful protocol, use random samples, use blindness where possible, and so on). Second, many of these methods could be improved if research were carried out to find new ways to improve them. Therefore, specific research that could lead to getting stronger results from the weaker methods is often suggested.

Possibly, research will find that particular methodologies are best when applied to special classes of treatments. For example, perhaps noninvasive drugs and devices could be handled in one way and invasive methods in another. Perhaps data banks and registries could offer good results from some class of problems. Answers to such questions are not now available.

At the same time that the need for improving the weaker methods is recognized, it is also recognized that the methods already in existence are not sufficiently often applied. The Office of Health Technology Assessment (OHTA) evaluates the safety and effectiveness of new or as yet unestablished medical technologies and procedures that are being considered for coverage under Medicare. Requests for these evaluations come from the Health Care Financing Administration (HCFA). OHTA carries out its evaluations by reviewing the literature and by getting advice from various agencies and professional organizations. The information so acquired is synthesized to reach some conclusion. OHTA does not gather primary data itself. Again and again, it turns out, and OHTA notes, that the primary data are almost nonexistent and that primary data would be required to reach a well-informed conclusion. In advising HCFA about coverage for various medical technologies, OHTA prepared 65 reports in the years 1982, 1983, and 1984. Lasch (1985) reviewed these reports to see what the state of the informational base on safety and efficacy seemed to be (K. E. Lasch, Synthesizing in HRST Reports, unpublished report, Harvard School of Public Health, 1985). Lasch sorted the reports into four categories, as follows:

1. The technology enjoyed widespread use and was considered an established technology.
2. The data base for the technology was insufficient; there was a call for more studies and better research designs, or accuracy was questioned for diagnostic tests.
3. The data base was sufficient; the technology was not recommended.
4. The technology was outmoded, not routinely used, and not an established therapy.

After the studies were categorized for the 3 years, Lasch found the results shown in Table 3-1. The percentage values of the results are similar from year to year. The category of insufficient data stands out.

In noting that 69 percent of these assessments have insufficient data to reach a satisfactory conclusion, it should not be assumed that the technologies in the other categories have always been evaluated on the basis of strong data. The categories were chosen to generate a clear set when the evidence was inadequate. The first category of widespread use may also include poorly evaluated technologies. This study, then, offers a clear message that many technologies that physicians wish to use have not been adequately evaluated. Similarly, at the consensus conferences, speakers frequently point out the lack of primary data (National Institutes of Health [NIH], 1983, 1984). Thus, the most important need is to gather more primary data.

As we report later in this chapter, the Office of Technology Assessment (OTA; 1980a) polled data analysts who conduct cost-effectiveness and cost-benefit analyses of health care technologies and found lack of information to be a uniformly significant problem.

More primary research is needed, and this will have to be led in part by research physicians with training in quantitative methods and supported by doctoral-level epidemiologists and biostatisticians. All three groups are in short supply (National Academy of Sciences, 1978, 1981, 1983). At the least the development of methods will also require epidemiologists and biostatisticians. Therefore, on both grounds, we will need funds for training research personnel.

Many assessment methods are described in some detail in the sections that consti-

TABLE 3-1 Distribution of Technologies for Years 1982, 1983, and 1984 into Four Types[a] when Reviewed by OHTA for HCFA

	Percentages for Each Year[b]			
Category	1982	1983	1984	Total
Widespread use	16 (4)	19 (4)	21 (4)	18 (12)
Insufficient data	68 (17)	76 (16)	63 (12)	69 (45)
Data sufficient; technology not effective	4 (1)	0 (0)	0 (0)	2 (1)
Technology not used or outmoded	12 (3)	5 (1)	16 (3)	11 (7)
Totals	100 (25)	100 (21)	100 (19)	100 (65)

[a]Each of the 65 reports was assigned to one of the above categories based on a reading of the summary and discussion sections. Coding of the 65 reports revealed that the four categories were mutually exclusive; each report fell neatly into one of the categories.
[b]Numbers of studies shown in parentheses.

tute the main body of this chapter. Unless explicitly interested in research methods, some readers may wish to scan cursorily through the chapter.

Most sections follow a pattern that opens with a brief description of the method, followed by typical purposes and uses and by a subsection addressing capabilities and limitations, including some remarks on ways of strengthening the method in practical use. Sometimes a final subsection discusses research that could be done that might lead to improvements in the method.

RANDOMIZED CLINICAL TRIALS*

The randomized clinical trial (RCT) is a method of comparing the relative merits (and shortcomings) of two or more treatments tested in human subjects. A well-designed and -executed RCT is widely regarded as the most powerful and sensitive tool for the comparison of therapies, diagnostic procedures, and regimens of care.

More broadly, the RCT can be regarded as an unusually reliable method for learning from experience; its success lies in structuring that experience so as to foreclose many sources of ambiguity. In the health sciences the method is applied not only in comparing therapies but also diagnostic methodologies, ways of imparting information to patients, and regimens of care (e.g., home care versus critical care units for certain heart patients). In general, if alternative ways of accomplishing an aim are in competition, the RCT may be the best technique for resolving their relative merits.

Notice that *comparison* is at the heart of the method. A clinical trial is not a device for ascertaining the health consequences of a toxic substance in food or for elucidating the etiology of a disease. It is a method for comparing interventions that are applied and controlled by the investigator. The clinical trial becomes an RCT if there is a deliberate introduction of randomness into the assignment of patients (eligible for both, or all, of the treatments) to treatment A, treatment B, etc. The reasons for such a method of assignment are discussed below.

Hereafter, when referring to an RCT, it is contemplated that it satisfies these two conditions:

1. No subject is admitted without having been judged to be equally suitable to

*This section was drafted by Lincoln E. Moses.

receive any one of the treatments being offered to the subject's class of patients.

2. No subject is admitted without having volunteered to receive either treatment, as may be assigned.

Practical Problems of Comparing Treatments

Two factors make it intrinsically difficult to compare different treatments. First, the subjects receiving the treatments usually are different people, so differences found between the treatments could be due to differences among the subjects in the groups. If the groups differ in any systematic way (whether recognized or not), the treatment comparison may be biased; bias can exaggerate, nullify, or reverse true differences. Second, even if the treatments could be compared in the same patients (as sometimes happens), the contrast between the treatments will vary from one patient to another, producing uncertainty in the overall assessment. This is the problem of variability. Large samples can reduce the disturbance of variability but do not help with bias.

If two treatment groups are differently constituted, then bias in the treatment comparison must be regarded as likely. The phrase "differently constituted" applies, for example, where the treatment groups are (1) admitted to the study by different means; (2) treated in different places, at different times, or by different sets of practitioners; (3) assessed by different groups; or (4) analyzed and reported by different teams.

Randomization in a clinical trial is aimed at preventing bias. Two characteristic features are essential to realizing that aim.

First, the study is conducted under a *protocol* that makes explicit exactly what questions are to be studied, what treatments are to be applied; and how, to what kind of patients, when, and where. It also specifies how assessment of outcomes will be done and how statistical analyses will be conducted.

Second, the RCT calls for assignment of the respective treatments to each eligible patient admitted to the study by means of a *random* choice. The effect of this is to ensure that the two treatment groups are not "differently constituted"; indeed, they are brought into being as random subsets of a singly constituted group which is operationally defined by the protocol.

The protocol-controlled RCT is even stronger whenever knowledge of which treatment a patient has received is screened from participants (patients, treating physicians, outcome assessors). A result of such "blinding" is to ensure that placebo effects remain randomly assorted to the treatments. Another result is to prevent differential decisions about care during the study. It is especially important that those assessing outcomes be blind to the type of treatment—unless the outcome is entirely objective, e.g., length of survival. In some cases, blinding of physicians may not be possible, such as when a medical modality is being compared with a surgical one.

The Protocol

The protocol is a written prescriptive document that spells out the purposes and rationale of the trial and how it will be conducted. Specifics include the criteria of eligibility for inclusion of patients in the trial—and criteria for exclusion—and description of treatments, adjuvant therapy, outcome measurements, patient follow-up, and statistical analyses to be performed. The protocol also specifies the numbers of patients to be entered and the mechanics of randomization. The protocol is both a planning document and a procedures manual. The aim is to provide trustworthy answers at the end of the study to the following questions: What treatments were applied, to what kinds of patients, with what results? What do the results mean?

Provisions for blindness and for the order in which processes are to be performed can be central to the validity of a study and to the value of the protocol that governs it. If the decision to enter each patient into the trial is made in the knowledge of which treatment the next patient will receive, then ample opportunity for building up noncomparable treatment groups is at hand, so the protocol should not use alternate-patient assignment to the treatments. If a rather subjective diagnostic test W assesses a condition thought to be related to another test V, then W measured after V is not the same as W measured before V; it may be important that the protocol specify the order in which they are to be done. The careful protocol attempts to specify in advance all procedural steps that may materially affect execution of the trial and interpretation of its results.

A well-conducted RCT requires not only a good protocol but also that the trial be carried out in accordance with it. The protocol may call for specific steps to check on (and promote) protocol adherence. Staging and laboratory analyses may be checked by introducing (blindly) occasional standard specimens. Samples of study records may be checked back to more basic clinical records. Visits by monitors, combined with audit, may be routinely conducted in multicenter studies.

The protocol also has the character of a compact among the participating investigators, relevant human subjects committees, and funding sponsors. This contractual character lends stability to a study over its lifetime, helping to supply definite answers to the questions concerning what was done, to what kinds of patients, and with what results.

Random Assignment to Treatment

The primary reason for random assignment is to prevent bias by breaking any possible systematic connection of one treatment or the other with favorable values of interfering variables (whether recognized or not). A fuller appreciation of this principle may be gained by considering two alternative modes of treatment comparison that are sometimes advocated. The first is the use of historical controls, the second is the use of statistical procedures to adjust for treatment group differences in the important interfering variables.

The historically controlled trial (HCT) compares outcomes on a new treatment to outcomes in previous (historical) cases *from the same setting*. The motivation is to arrive at decisions sooner by assigning all eligible patients rather than only half of them to the new treatment. But because the treatment and control groups come from different time periods, they are "differently constituted groups." This raises the spectre of bias—and sometimes the actuality. The drop in cardiovascular deaths and the decrease in perinatal mortality over the last decade are both not really understood, and both exemplify temporal shifts in control levels of the sort that vitiate historical controls. Time changes all things, including the patients' characteristics at a hospital, the effectiveness of adjuvant treatments not under study, the skill of surgeons with a new operation, and the skill of physicians with a new drug. Thus, it is hard to know when an HCT does reach a valid conclusion. There are successes and there are failures.

An example of what seems to be a successful HCT is that of a changing policy by an institution toward stab wounds. Originally, the policy had been to perform an exploratory laparotomy on all patients presenting with abdominal stab wounds. On the basis of advances in handling wounds and some data from refusals to give consent, the institution decided to change to a policy allowing surgical judgment to be exercised. This reduced considerably the number of laparotomies performed (92 to 40 percent) and also the numbers of infections (Nance and Cohn, 1969). The overall complication rate dropped from 27 to 12 percent, and no complications occurred in 72 unexplored patients.

Byar et al. (1976) call attention to an RCT comparing placebo and estrogen therapy for prostate cancer in which the survival of placebo controls admitted in the first 2.5 years was significantly shorter ($p = .01$) than the survival of those admitted in the second 2.5 years, although admission criteria, in a fixed setting, were unchanged. They point out that the use of the early placebo group (as historical controls) would have falsely led to the conclusion that estrogen therapy (in the second period) was effective.

It is possible to consider the use of historical controls whenever the variation in successive control levels is statistically taken into account. However, it may be difficult or impossible to estimate that variation; that is a practical difficulty. Furthermore, there is a theoretical principle that applies. The work of Meier (1975), and later Pocock (1976), show that for a given standard deviation in batch-to-batch random bias, there is a minimum study size number (the number of experimental subjects) beyond which relying on historical controls, no matter how numerous they are, is inferior to dividing the sample into two equal groups, half experimental and half control. In summary, historical control trials are inferior to RCTs because (1) differently constituted groups are inherently likely to produce bias; (2) if the historical controls *were* comparable and if the random bias of successive batches of controls had variability that was exactly known, then reliance on the historical control data would be preferable to randomization only for studies below a certain threshhold size; and (3) knowledge of variability of the random bias is often not available.

One often sees the argument that the need for randomization can be circumvented by making statistical adjustments for differently constituted subgroups, correcting for differences in the influential variables that affect outcomes, and rendering the subgroups comparable. It is easy to find statisticians who place little credence in this trust of statistical adjustment, and for cogent reasons. First, some of the most influential variables may not even be recognized as important. Second, the ones that are recognized as important may not have been measured, or they may not have been measured comparably. Third, just how to make the adjustment can be very unclear; mutually influential variables can be interrelated in ways that both are important and poorly understood. Randomization avoids these difficulties by ensuring that whatever the critical variables may be and however they may conspire together to affect the outcomes, they cannot systematically benefit one treatment over the other, beyond those vagaries of chance for which the significance test specifically makes allowances. This approach avoids the effort of trying to unravel the Gordian knot of causation and cuts through it at one stroke, by random assignment.

Before leaving the subject of random assignment, the idea of randomization within strata should be addressed. If some pretreatment variable, say stage of disease, is known to be strongly related to outcome, then it can be wise to design the study so that (nearly) equal numbers of both treatments occur at each level of that pretreatment variable. This kind of design is quite natural for multi-institutional studies, when each institution is treated as a stratum. Refining the randomization to be done separately within strata does not give added protection against bias, but it may increase the efficiency of a study, i.e., increase its effective sample size (usually only moderately).

Limitations of RCTs

The method, powerful as it is, is hard to apply under certain circumstances. If outcomes mature after decades, then completion of the RCT requires long-term maintenance of protocol-controlled follow-up, which is difficult and expensive.

If a sufficiently rare outcome is the endpoint of interest, then detection of treatment differences may call for unworkably large sample sizes. One example was concern about the safety of the anesthetic, halothane. Detection of differences in surgical death rates (about 2 percent overall) that might relate to anesthetic choice would amount to trying to distinguish between death rates such as 1.9 percent and 2.1 percent—a task calling at least for hundreds of thousands of patients. The retrospective study that was done did arrive at conclusions, but they were expressed with diffidence made necessary by the possible existence of unrecognized biases.

Sometimes it is objected that an RCT is not applicable because treatments are too variable to be controlled with the specificity that an RCT demands. This objection is sometimes false; for example, a treatment may be defined to allow modification as indications arise in the course of therapy. In other cases, the objection is simply specious, for it asserts the impossibility of answering the question "What is the treatment?" That impossibility would block any kind of objective assessment of it.

A rather more difficult limitation to deal with grows out of the possibility that a new procedure started in an RCT may, outside that trial, evolve into a superior modified version of the treatment. Then, continuation of the RCT is at risk of being irrelevant or unethical. **There is a real problem here, and it deserves more study; the question is how the use of protocol and randomization can help to speed sound evolution of new therapies.** One proposal has been to "randomize the first patient." (See, for instance, Chalmers, 1975, 1981.) Inherent in the concept of randomizing the first patient is a fluid protocol that allows a change in the details of a new treatment as the investigators improve their performance (the "learning curve") or as other information appears. It has not found wide agreement. The definitive treatment of these issues is not yet at hand.

The sample size of an RCT may have been planned to resolve differences of a stated size, but when it is completed, questions about treatment comparisons in certain subclasses of patients cannot be resolved. This is not a limitation of the RCT per se, for more questions always can be asked of a body of data than can be answered by it, but one should be warned to think at the planning stage about choosing sample sizes large enough to support adequate treatment comparisons in particularly salient subgroups.

It is sometimes argued that RCTs are too costly. The cost of disciplined, careful, checked medical work is of course high; the advantages of the protocol are not cheaply bought. But in many medical centers with already high standards of recordkeeping, diagnosis, etc., the incremental cost of the protocol might not be great. The incremental cost of randomization is negligible. Costs can be high when the base costs of bed, drugs, tests, and care are all loaded onto the RCT budget. Most of these costs would have been incurred anyway, regardless of how the patients were treated.

Failure to distinguish between total costs, which include those that would be incurred anyway, from *incremental costs* of RCTs is inherently misleading and could lead to grievous policy errors. Good measurements of incremental costs of RCTs are needed. This will involve both conceptual effort and data gathering. **Better information concerning actual incremental costs of RCTs is a topic that should receive systematic research attention.**

Two other limitations of RCTs also are drawbacks to any investigational method. The first is that dispute may grow around unwelcome conclusions and hinder adoption of the findings. The second is that the

RCT may give a clear verdict in patients of the kind used in the trial, but leave unanswered the question of efficacy in different kinds of subjects. This issue, dubbed external validity sometimes is readily dealt with; thus, the Salk vaccine trials showed the vaccine to be effective in first-, second-, and third-grade children. No difficulty was found in generalizing the conclusion to both older and younger children. Sometimes things are harder—they may even demand further RCTs. External validity is of course a problem *whenever* we undertake to learn from one body of experience and then apply the results to other experience; it is not a peculiar difficulty of RCTs. **We do not know as much as we could afford to about designing studies with an eye on external validity. This is another area that deserves further research effort.**

Strengthening RCTs

The primary paths to good quality lie in designing a strong protocol and executing it faithfully. The paper by Goodman in Appendix 3-B of this committee's report gives a systematic treatment of most of the key features of a strong protocol. Extensive accounts of RCT protocol are given in works by Friedman et al. (1981) and Shapiro and Louis (1983). Some additional ideas on pre- and post-protocol execution deserve comment here.

First, the study should be large enough; if it is too small to have a good chance of establishing the existence of a plausibly sized actual improvement, then it needs to be made larger or to be abandoned. Otherwise, work, money, and time will be devoted to an effort that lacks a good chance of producing a useful finding. Statistical methods for assessing adequacy of planned study size (power calculations) are well established and should be used. (Sometimes, however, the opportunity to do a study is too good to be missed even if it is too small to be definitive. This should be reported with the study in hope that results of other studies can be combined with these and together they may reach firm conclusions.)

Second, the participating investigators should fully understand and be fully supportive of the investigation. Persons with initial convictions about relative merits of the treatments may prove to be encumbrances to successful execution of the protocol.

Third, in planning for the time and number of cooperating centers that will be needed to carry the study through, be realistically guarded about the flow of eligible patients that can be anticipated. Seasoned RCT veterans recommend safety factors of two, five, even ten.

The foregoing suggestions all relate to the planning phase. A final way of strengthening the RCT applies to the completion phase.

Write about and report it well. In particular, the operational definitions of all terms should be clear. Thus, the reader should not be left with doubts about how the subjects were defined and selected, how they were assigned to treatments, what treatments were applied, or how outcomes were measured. In addition, the report should specify whether study staff were blind to treatment allocation at key steps like enrollment in study, determination of eligibility, interpretation of diagnostic tests, measurement of outcome, etc. These issues were prominent among those that DerSimonian et al. (1982) checked in reviewing reports of clinical trials in four leading medical journals and that Emerson et al. (1984) checked in reviewing reports in six leading surgical journals. Both studies answered five questions: (1) What were the eligibility criteria for admission to the study? (2) Was admission to the study done prior to allocation of treatment? (3) Was allocation to treatment done at random? (4) What was the method of randomization? (5) Were outcomes assessed by persons who were blind to treatment?

Good reporting will also explain the quality control measures that were applied, methods of follow-up used, and audit checks employed.

Not only should the reader be told what was done, and how, but also what happened. Summary statistics should have the aim of revealing information to the reader.

The methods of statistical analysis should be explained. The best way to do this is topic by topic. The analysis was actually *done* in such a pattern; it should be reported that way: for understanding, for specificity, and, incidentally, for ease of writing. Sometimes one finds a published paper which lists statistical procedures in the methods section. "We used chi-squared, the t-test, the F-test, and Jonckheere's test." The use of this style of reporting for banquet recipes would list all the ingredients in all the dishes together and report the use of stove, mixer, oven, meat grinder, egg beater, and double boiler.

In addition to showing the data, or generously detailed summaries of them, the statistical analysis should state each of the principal questions that motivated the study and what light the data shed on those questions. (Note that this is not the same thing at all as reporting just those results that are statistically significant.) To lend understanding both to significant and non-significant results, it is wise to use confidence intervals whenever feasible and to report the power of statistical tests that are applied (Freiman et al., 1978). Interesting statistical results that arise out of studying the data (rather than from studying the principal questions that motivated the study) are necessarily on a different, and somewhat ambiguous, logical footing. It is usually wise to regard such outcomes with considerable reserve, more as hypotheses turned up than as facts established. It is especially important to be candid about the nature and amount of "data dredging" that has accompanied the analysis.

A Final Remark

The protocol has been described as a compact; its construction is typically a collegial exercise. This entails some advantages. Of course, deliberation and consultation give opportunities for better planning. Sometimes a sequence of RCTs leads to cumulative expertise and strategizing. But, some of the greatest advantages may lie in the ethical domain.

The use in human beings of a new treatment with only partially understood properties raises certain problems of ethical portent. (This is true whether that new treatment is tried in an RCT or in any other way.) Among these questions are the following: How strong is the evidence that this new treatment may be at least as good as the best available current therapy? How shall we know when we should stop using both treatments and prefer only one of them? Who shall be able to receive this new treatment, and who shall not? Each of these questions is likely to be better answered when decided by a group of professionals, acting explicitly and consultatively, in a process open to review. Wishful thinking blooms wherever *Homo sapiens* is found, but group consultation tends more often than not to restrain it.

Another advantage of the collegial building of the protocol is that investigators who already believe they know which treatment is superior have the opportunity to drop out, leaving to the trial's execution investigators able to proceed in good conscience to participate themselves and to invite their patients to participate.

EVALUATING DIAGNOSTIC TECHNOLOGIES*

Accurate diagnosis is central to good medical practice. Diagnostic technology provides the physician with diagnostic information. However, all diagnostic tests and procedures have associated costs and risks. Thus, persons involved with medical care must determine whether an individual test or procedure provides significant new diagnostic information and whether the information provided and its impact on subsequent medical care offset the costs and risks of the technology. For each diagnostic test, these and related questions require assessment of (1) the diagnostic information provided and (2) the impact of the resulting therapy on patient outcome. Such assessments of diagnostic technology rarely are performed. Most diagnostic technology undergoes only narrow and limited evaluation. The lack of more comprehensive assessment severely limits the efficient and optimal use of diagnostic tests and procedures.

Fineberg et al. (1977) has formulated a hierarchy of evaluation of diagnostic technologies:

1. *Technical capacity*—Does the device or procedure perform reliably and deliver accurate information?
2. *Diagnostic accuracy*—Does the test contribute to making an accurate diagnosis?
3. *Diagnostic impact*—Does the test result influence the pattern of subsequent diagnostic testing? Does it replace other diagnostic tests or procedures?
4. *Therapeutic impact*—Does the test result influence the selection and delivery of therapy? Is more appropriate therapy used after application of the diagnostic test than would be used if the test was not available?
5. *Patient outcome*—Does performance of the test contribute to improved health of the patient?

Clearly, if diagnostic technology fails utterly at any step in this chain, then it cannot be successful at any later stage. If it succeeds at some stage, this implies success in the prior stages (even if they have not been explicitly tested) but does not tell what success may be attached to later stages. Thus, an accurate test may or may not lead to more accurate diagnosis, which in turn may or may not lead to better therapy, and that in turn may or may not eventuate in better health of the patient. Because many tests may be involved, it can require carefully designed studies to gauge success or failure of any particular one at stages 2 through 5.

Present Evaluation Methods

The first step in the hierarchy of evaluating diagnostic tests and procedures is determination of the technical performance of the test. Several factors are involved in this evaluation. The first deals with the ability of the test actually to measure what it claims to measure. Replicability and bias of test results are important measures of test performance. Replicability (i.e., precision) reflects the variance in a test result that occurs when the test is repeated on the same specimen. A highly precise test exhibits little variance among repeated measurements, an imprecise test exhibits great variance. The greater this variation, the less faith one may have in a single test's results. However, a precise test is not necessarily a good test. A test may exhibit a high level of replicability yet be in error. A good test must be reliable (i.e., unbiased); that is, it must exhibit agreement between the mean test result and the true value of the biologic variable being measured in the

*This section was contributed by J. Sanford Schwartz.

sample being tested. Evaluations of clinical tests should consider both the replicability and reliability of the technology. Finally, the safety of a diagnostic technology should be determined. Performance of the test should involve no unusual, unacceptable, or unexpected hazard. FDA regulations require some minimal level of safety and technical performance to be demonstrated for many diagnostic tests before marketing approval is granted (OTA, 1978a).

The purpose of a diagnostic test or procedure is to discriminate between patients with a particular disease and those who do not have the disease. However, most diagnostic tests measure some disease marker or surrogate (e.g., a metabolic abnormality that is variably associated with the disease) rather than the presence or absence of the disease itself. The performance level of a diagnostic test depends on the distribution of the marker being measured in diseased and nondiseased patients and on the technical performance characteristics of the test itself (its precision and reliability).

Each disease marker has a distribution in populations of diseased and nondiseased patients. Unfortunately, these distributions frequently overlap so that measurement of the markers does not permit complete separation of the diseased and nondiseased populations (Figure 3-1). In these circumstances no matter what cutoff value, k, is chosen it is not possible to ensure that all patients on one side have the disease and all those on the other are free of the disease. We are instead left with some false positives and some false negatives, as indicated in Figure 3-1. By moving k to a larger or smaller value the relative probabilities of these two kinds of error will be altered. These probabilities can be tabulated in a format like that in Table 3-2.

It should be borne in mind that the numerical values of these probabilities will change if the cutoff value of k is changed.

The two most commonly used measures of diagnostic test performance are sensitivity and specificity (Table 3-3). These test characteristics deal with the ability of the diagnostic test to identify correctly subjects

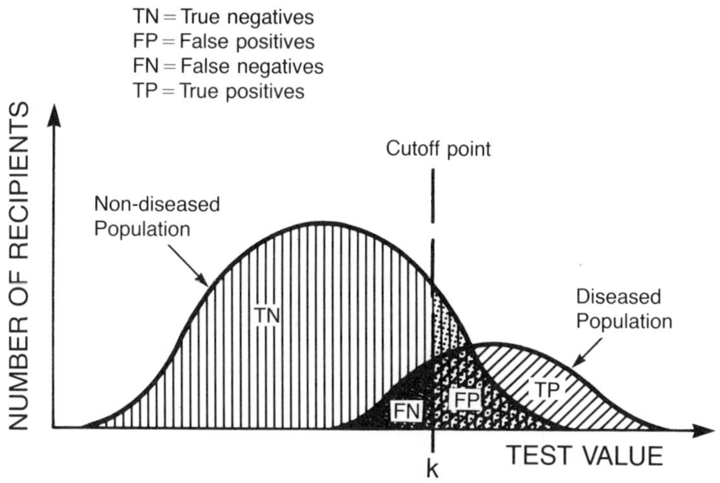

FIGURE 3-1. Relationship of test value to diseased and nondiseased populations for a hypothetical diagnostic test.

TABLE 3-2 Outcomes of Diagnostic Test Use

TEST RESULT	DISEASE STATUS	
	Disease Present	Disease Absent
Positive	True positives	False positives
Negative	False negatives	True negatives

with and without the condition of interest. Sensitivity measures the ability of a test to detect disease when it is present. It measures the proportion of diseased patients with a positive test. This can be expressed by the ratio,

$$\frac{\text{True positives}}{\text{True positives} + \text{False negatives}}.$$

Specificity measures the ability of a test to correctly exclude disease in nondiseased patients. It measures the proportion of nondiseased patients with a negative test. This can be expressed as

$$\frac{\text{True negatives}}{\text{True negatives} + \text{False positives}}.$$

Sensitivity and specificity have been adopted widely because they are considered to be stable properties of diagnostic tests when properly derived on a broad spectrum of diseased and nondiseased patients. That is, under such circumstances their values are thought not to change significantly when applied in populations with different prevalence, presentation, or severity of disease. However, if diagnostic tests are not derived on an appropriately broad spectrum of subjects their values will change as the prevalence and severity of disease are varied in the populations tested (Ransahoff and Feinstein, 1978).

Test sensitivity and specificity as measures of diagnostic test performance taken alone do not reveal how likely it is that a given patient really has the condition in question if the test is positive, or the probability that a given patient does not have the disease if the test is negative. The fraction of those patients with a positive test result who actually have the disease is called the predictive value positive of a test. It is calculated by the ratio of

$$\frac{\text{True positives}}{\text{True positives} + \text{False positives}}.$$

The fraction of patients with a negative test result who are actually free of the disease is called the predictive value negative and is determined by the ratio of

$$\frac{\text{True negatives}}{\text{True negatives} + \text{False negatives}}.$$

TABLE 3-3 Operating Characteristics of Diagnostic Tests

Measure of Performance	Characteristic
Sensitivity =	$\frac{\text{True positives}}{\text{True positives} + \text{False negatives}}$
Specificity =	$\frac{\text{True negatives}}{\text{True negatives} + \text{False positives}}$
Predictive values positive =	$\frac{\text{True positives}}{\text{True positives} + \text{False positives}}$
Predictive values negative =	$\frac{\text{True negatives}}{\text{True negatives} + \text{False negatives}}$

The predictive value positive and predictive value negative of a diagnostic test measure respectively how likely it is that a positive or negative test result actually represents the presence or absence of disease in a given population of patients with a given prevalence of disease. The positive and negative predictive values of a diagnostic test, however, are not stable characteristics of that test. Rather, they depend strongly on the prevalence of the condition being examined in the population being tested. As the disease prevalence (pretest likelihood of disease) decreases, the proportion of individuals with a positive test result who actually are diseased falls and the proportion of nondiseased patients falsely identified as being diseased rises. Conversely, as the prevalence of disease increases, the proportion of patients with a positive test result who are in fact diseased increases, while the proportion of patients with a negative test result who are not suffering from the disease falls. This fact has enormous implications for diagnostic tests, particularly when they are used in populations with a low prevalence of disease, such as when a test is used to screen for the presence of an uncommon disease.

The receiver operating characteristic (ROC) curve (Lusted, 1969; Metz, 1978; Metz et al., 1973; Robertson and Zweig, 1981; Swets, 1979; Swets and Pickett, 1982) provides an economical display of the information in the two-by-two table *for various values of k*. Figure 3-2 is an example showing for each of five values of k the sensitivity and specificity information. Consider the point marked B; we see that using the cutoff value of k = 1.0 mm in the exercise stress test yields sensitivity of about 0.65 and specificity of about 0.85 (since

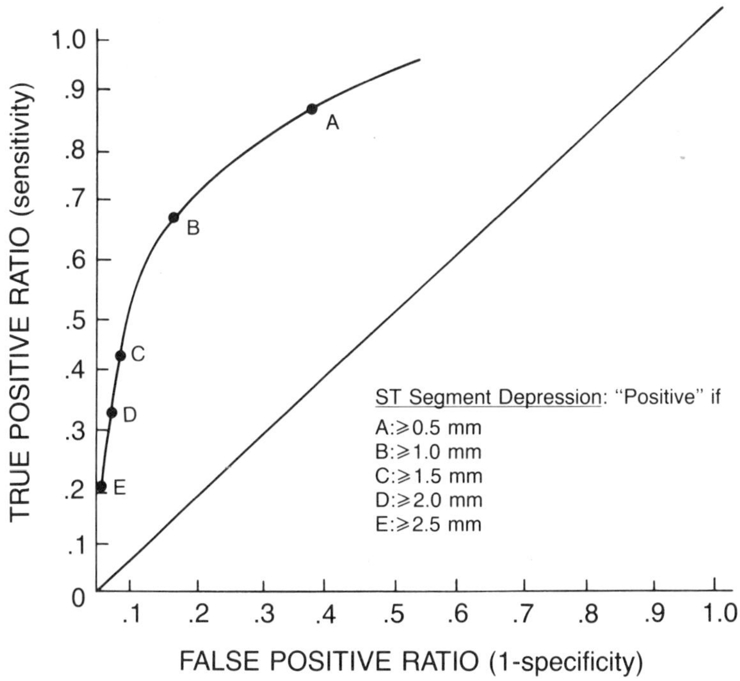

FIGURE 3-2 Receiver operating characteristic curve for the exercise stress test for the diagnosis of coronary artery disease as the criterion for a positive test is varied.

1 − specificity is about 0.15). From the curve, it is easy to see how lowering the cutoff value increases the sensitivity at the cost of also increasing the false-positive ratio.

Figure 3-3 shows another use of ROC curves. The curves of tests A and B make it evident that test A is the better of the two, because at every false-positive ratio it has higher specificity than does test B (or equivalently, at every specificity, test A has a lower false-positive ratio than does test B). The more closely an ROC curve can fit into the upper left-hand corner, the better its performance. The diagonal curve C represents a test based on pure chance; if the test called every patient positive with a probability of one-fourth (for example, if cutting a deck of cards produced a spade), the point P would result, showing specificity and a false-positive ratio both to equal 0.25.

So, an important use of the ROC curve is *to compare* alternative tests; an ROC curve that lies above and to the left of another corresponds to the better of the two tests. Then, the choice of a particular k value for that test amounts to choosing the sensitivity and specificity that will be employed. The particular choice of k may depend on the purpose for which the test is being used. One might require more stringent criteria to confirm (rule in) a suspected clinical diagnosis than to screen for or exclude (rule out) disease. A cutoff criterion with high specificity (to the left on a ROC curve) is desired when confirming a disease. A cutoff point with high sensitivity is desired when screening for a disease, although such a point is accompanied by lower test specificity. Such a cutoff point corresponds to a point upward and to the right on a ROC curve.

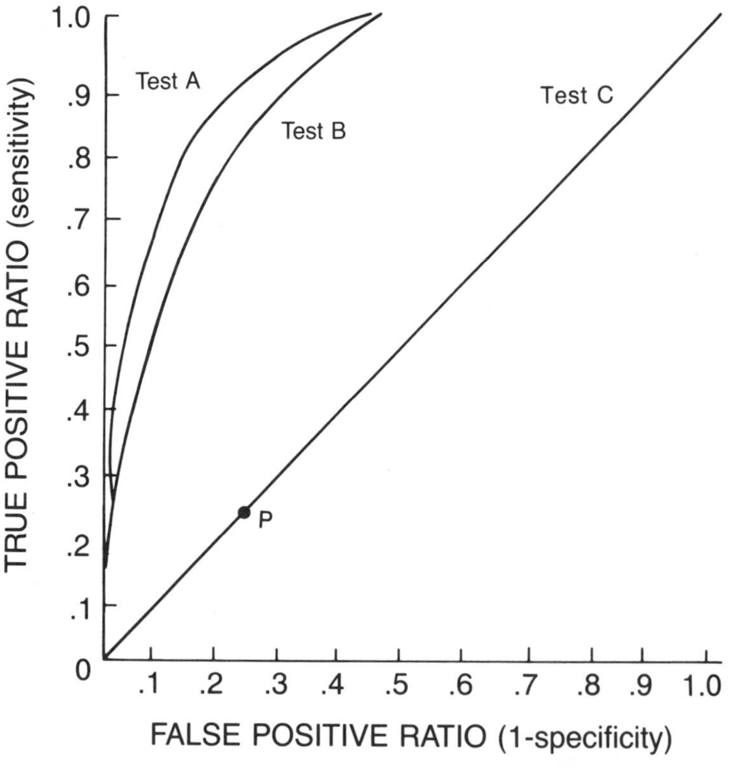

FIGURE 3-3 Three hypothetical ROC curves: for tests A and B and for the chance test C.

Comparison of two tests by means of their ROCs is far better than attempting to do so from the two-by-two tables, as can be seen by the following argument.

If one test (A) has a higher sensitivity but a lower specificity than the other test (B), one cannot be sure which test performs better. Three alternative possibilities exist: test A may perform better than test B (Figure 3-4a), test B may perform better than test A (Figure 3-4b), or they may represent the same or equivalent tests with different cutoff values used (Figure 3-4c). But ROC curve analysis can differentiate among these possibilities by empirically determining test performance and comparisons over a range of cutoff points (Lusted, 1969; Metz, 1978; Metz et al., 1973; Robertson and Zweig, 1981; Swets, 1979).

When one test performs better than a second test at some levels of use (e.g., with high specificity) but worse at other levels of use (e.g., with high sensitivity), the ROC curves cross and comparison is then more complicated (Schwartz et al., 1983).

Limitations of Present Evaluation Methods

Diagnostic technologies usually are evaluated adequately with respect to technical performance. However, issues of test replicability and reliability commonly receive less consideration.

Evaluations of diagnostic tests are hampered by the common practice of excluding indeterminate or uninterpretable results from published reports of test performance. Some patients cannot cooperate with a diagnostic test or procedure. In other patients, the test is uninterpretable because of technical factors. Few investigators evaluating diagnostic tests identify such patients in their published evaluations. Usually these patients are deleted from evaluations of test performance because they do not fit neatly into a two-by-two table or ROC. However, such patients may constitute a considerable portion of patients for whom a test is advocated. Inclusion only of those patients with definitive test results represents reporting of a selected sample. In these cases published results of test performance overstate the diagnostic test's actual performance in clinical application.

The range of patients on whom diagnostic tests are evaluated often is inadequate. Commonly, a test first is evaluated on patients with advanced disease and on young, very healthy controls. Such a strategy may be appropriate at a preliminary stage of test evaluation, because if a diagnostic test cannot separate patients with extremes of disease presentation, it is unlikely to perform well when the diagnosis is less obvious. However, many tests perform well in patients with extreme cases of disease but

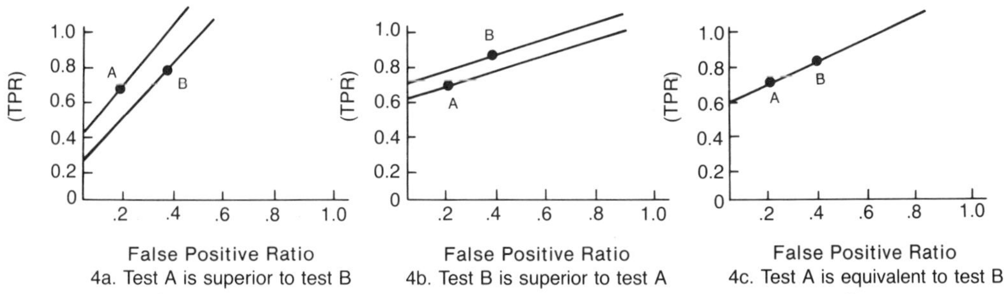

FIGURE 3-4 Comparison of two hypothetical tests (A and B) illustrating the need for receiver operating characteristic curve analysis to compare their performance over a range of cutoff points.

perform poorly in those patients with intermediate probabilities of disease. The performance estimates of diagnostic tests that are derived from extremes of populations (patients with severe disease and healthy controls) will deteriorate as the test is performed on a broader spectrum of patients. Feinstein (1977) has identified several groups of patients on whom a diagnostic test should be evaluated: (1) patients with the disease who are asymptomatic, (2) patients with symptoms and signs representative of the spectrum of the disease of interest, (3) patients without the disease of interest who have other diseases which produce similar signs and symptoms, and (4) patients without the disease of interest who have other diseases which affect the same organ(s) as the disease of interest or which occur in a similar anatomical location(s). Most important for the clinician are those patients in whom they will apply the test. Generally this group is composed of those patients suspected of the disease by virtue of their symptoms or clinical findings, but in whom disease presentation is not obvious or is somewhat atypical. The irony is that while it is in such patients that the diagnostic test is most needed, it is in this population that its performance may be poorest and least predictable and in which it is least likely to be evaluated. The lack of a proper spectrum of patients in diagnostic test evaluations has been shown to lead to overstated performance of diagnostic tests (Ransahoff and Feinstein, 1978).

A very large percentage of new evaluations in diagnostic radiology are currently based on ROC curves, whose use also is increasing in other areas of investigation. Although ROC curve analysis represents the state-of-the-art method to evaluate diagnostic tests, it has several limitations. Unless used to analyze data in a timely fashion it usually is impossible to construct such curves at a later time. Second, as with other procedures adequate methods are not available at present to determine the importance of differences among the ROC curves. As with other methods to evaluate diagnostic technologies, statistically significant differences among several ROC curves (Centor and Schwartz, in press; Hanley and McNeil, 1982; Swets and Pickett, 1982) do not necessarily imply clinically important differences.

Many diagnostic tests require some degree of interpretation to arrive at a test result. Thus, diagnostic test performance commonly depends on a combination of the technical performance of the test and how it is interpreted (the test-interpreter unit). For example, the diagnostic performance of a chest radiograph depends both on the technical quality of the film image and the expertise of the radiologist or other physician interpreting the film. ROC curves evaluate the complete test-interpreter unit. However, when evaluating a technology it may be important to differentiate between deficiencies in the performance of the technology and deficiencies in the performance of the technology interpreter, as one or the other may be more easily improvable.

A major problem in determining the performance characteristics of diagnostic tests is the lack of an appropriate reference standard (gold standard) against which to judge the test. The true state of nature generally is not known in clinical medicine. For most diseases even the best available diagnostic test has some associated error rate. In practice one is forced to accept the best available, albeit imperfect, diagnostic test as a pseudo-reference standard. Evaluating a diagnostic test against an imperfect reference standard obviously results in an inaccurate measurement of test performance.

The clinical use of a reference standard often presents a number of other problems, many of which are avoidable. A true reference standard should be a means of determining the correct diagnosis independent of the measures of the diagnostic technology being evaluated. In some circumstances a reference standard is adopted that depends on the subjective judgment of an observer whose judgment in turn might be based, in part, on the technology in question. Another common reference standard is the degree of concordance between its results and those found by subsequent tissue examination. This is a partial and inadequate solution. The problems here involve case selection bias and work-up bias so that the results may not be generalizable to many cases. A third method is to use clinical follow-up as a reference standard. Such an outcome measure provides some inferential data regarding reference standard performance. However, outcome measures may be confounded by the effects of time or intervening therapy. A low correlation between a positive test and a bad outcome might be consistent with a correct diagnosis and an appropriate, successful intervention. A high correlation might arise with ineffective diagnoses that result in deleterious treatment.

The dynamic evolution of many diagnostic technologies complicates the timely evaluation of many tests and procedures. Diagnostic technologies must be evaluated before they are adopted widely. This requires early evaluation. However, the results of early evaluations often are questioned or rejected in light of improvements in the technology which occurs subsequent to the evaluation. The problem of technological creep and how to identify optimal times to assess diagnostic technologies is important, unsolved, and vexing.

Strengthening the Method

Assessments of a diagnostic technology typically are confined to evaluation of the diagnostic performance of the test and do not often measure clinically important impacts of diagnostic tests, such as the therapy chosen or the clinical outcome following therapy. The scope of evaluations of diagnostic technologies should be broadened more often to include consideration of the diagnostic decisions, therapeutic choices, and health outcomes. When appropriate, financial and social impacts of a test (e.g., a screening test) may call for careful evaluation.

Diagnostic tests often are used in combination, and it can require carefully designed studies to disentangle separate contributions of individual tests to clinical decisions and outcomes.

Although one diagnostic procedure may be superior to a second as judged from their ROC curves, the choice between them may have to take account of other information such as the comparative invasiveness of the two tests, patient acceptance, or the time scale on which results are available.

ROC curve analysis can measure the differences in diagnostic performance of various combinations of diagnostic tests, but only rarely has it been used for this purpose (Feinstein, 1977).

Diagnostic technology often is evaluated on patient populations that are small in size, limited in disease spectrum, and highly dependent on expert interpretation, limiting the adequacy of the evaluation of the test or procedure. Pooling of data from different studies and different sites may help resolve many of these methodologic problems, particularly when studies consist of small numbers of observations or have conflicting results. **Thus, data pooling should be explored further as a mechanism to improve the quality and timeliness of evaluations of diagnostic technology.** However, several methodologic issues must be investigated before it can be determined that data pooling is both possible and appropriate. Data pooling requires studies with similar clinical situations, study design (randomization, selection criteria), diagnostic methods and techniques, observer interpretations and skills, and outcome measures. It is possible that studying diagnostic tests in collaborative studies at several institutions, as therapies are often studied in clinical trials, would be a constructive move. **Unresolved methodologic issues include questions of weighing in various studies (by size, quality), selection of appropriate methods of statistical analysis and hypothesis testing, and specification of criteria for inclusion of studies in pooled analysis.**

Summary

Although assessing diagnostic technologies unquestionably is difficult, a conceptual base has been laid. The most important problems remaining to be addressed are practical ones. One of the important problems for those researchers engaged in the evaluation of diagnostic technologies is to appreciate and acknowledge the uncertainty involved in test performance and interpretation and to consider the many factors that confound the results of such evaluations. Awareness of these problems must be coupled with improved evaluation methodologies. In particular, adoption of better experimental design standards and use of ROC curve analysis will improve the results of such evaluations. Diagnostic tests should be evaluated in terms of their use with and contribution to other diagnostic tests and not merely as to the absolute accuracy of a test in isolation of already known clinical information.

Even if these problems are addressed, other important factors remain unresolved. **One of the most important of these includes the definition and measurement of appropriate clinical endpoints for evaluation.** Up to the present most research has dealt with the validity of tests, and few studies have evaluated the outcome of testing through clinical trials. For example, what is the impact of a test on the diagnostic process or on therapy? How is performance of a test related to ultimate health outcome? How does one evaluate a diagnostic test when there is no adequate reference standard? How do patients and physicians value positive test results when there is no effective treatment for the disease of interest? How do patients and physicians value the reassurance inherent in an expensive technological examination as compared with that of a careful physical examination? How much are patients consulted about their desires for immediate diagnosis?

Investment in medical research has led to major advances in physiology, pathophysiology, biochemistry, genetics, and other basic sciences. These in turn have led to the development of many technological advances in diagnosis. However, knowledge of how best to apply such information clinically has lagged significantly. A major reason is underinvestment in this kind of research. Thus, we have the ironic situation in which important and painstakingly developed knowledge often is applied haphazardly and anecdotally. Such a situation, which is not acceptable in the basic sciences or in drug therapy, also should not be acceptable in clinical applications of diagnostic technology.

It is clear that existing research does not provide a firm basis for comprehensively assessing the usefulness of diagnostic tests. Diagnostic testing in the setting of patient care is expensive and has been the subject of increasing scrutiny and concern. Diagnosis is one of the most rapidly expanding activities of medical practice, with estimated annual growth rates of 15 to 20 percent. Concern for health care costs has led to moves to limit expenditures for medical care. Programs that employ such categories as Diagnosis-Related Groups (DRGs) for provider reimbursement certainly will affect the use of diagnostic testing. Present limitations of knowledge, however, will continue to hamper the physician's ability to arrive at appropriate decisions regarding the utilization of diagnostic tests and procedures, regardless of the reimbursement and planning systems in place. Substantial progress in the measurement of test performance and more appropriate utilization of tests and procedures requires more comprehensive technology evaluation that focuses on the clinical impact of the technology on the patient and the patient's health.

THE SERIES OF CONSECUTIVE CASES AS A DEVICE FOR ASSESSING OUTCOMES OF INTERVENTION*

An air of serving the common good clings to the process of publishing for general information the results of one's own extensive experience. Medicine enjoys a long tradition of such publication; valuable results sometimes ensue. Moreover, a large share of medical knowledge has been accumulated in just this way, through the publication of series of cases. This paper examines the usefulness and limitations of series for assessing safety and efficacy of medical interventions. Two historical examples initiate the discussion; the first *demonstrates* results with a new technique; the second *compares* outcomes between two differently treated subsets of a single series of patients.

In 1847 John Snow published an epochal work, *On the Inhalation of the Vapor of Ether in Surgical Operations* (Snow, 1847). In it he described the equipment he had devised, his procedure, and a description of the 52 operations at St. George's Hospital and the 23 operations at University College Hospital in which he had delivered ether anesthesia by September 16, 1847.

These two series (with four and two deaths, respectively) doubtless were, in the eyes of the author and his readers, harbingers of the future. For a modern reader they are, as well, a window on the past; in all 75 operations, neither the thorax nor the abdomen was ever entered. The two series showed the effectiveness of Snow's apparatus for vaporizing the ether for patient inhalation and that with the new apparatus and procedure (1) anesthesia was induced in all patients, (2) they all revived from the anesthesia, and (3) the surgery went forward more easily. All this helped to dispel the mistrust of ether anesthesia that had grown up around earlier, inept applications of ether in England during 1846.

In 1835 Pierre Louis published, from his practice over the years, an account of 77 patients who had had pneumonia, uncomplicated by other disease (Louis, 1836). He classified them by whether or not they had survived the disease and by the day in the course of their illness on which he had begun bleeding them. Early bleeding turned out to be associated with reduced survival. That series of observations was an important part of his attack on bleeding as a panacea.

These accounts, although much abbreviated, allow us to see some of the issues relating to series as an information source in medicine. First, a series typically contains information acquired over a period of time. Second, the patients in the series are all similar in some essential way; with Snow they had all received ether, although with various operations; with Louis they all had the same disease (and physician), but varied in how they were treated. Third, *all* the patients of a defined class are reported; with Snow, all ether administrations on or before September 16, 1847, were reported; with Louis, all the pneumonia patients for whom he had records indicating no other disease, and whom he had bled, were reported. Fourth, comparison is involved either directly, as with Louis, or indirectly, as with Snow; fairness of comparison becomes a crucial issue. (Louis

*This section is adapted from an article written by Lincoln E. Moses for the New England Journal Project in the Department of Biostatistics, Harvard University.

assured his readers that the two groups, survivors and decedents, were as alike in initial severity of disease as he could arrange by including and excluding cases from his files. Fifth, the series, whatever its value as evidence, may be influential or it may not. Louis was a member of the faculty at Paris; that lent weight to his series. (This contrasts notably to the low impact of James Lind's beautifully controlled experiment demonstrating the curative power of lemons in treating scurvy; he was a naval surgeon without high standing, and his study's effect on the policy of the Royal Navy was delayed by some 40 years.)

Description of a Series

The term series will be applied to studies of the results of an intervention if the study has certain characteristics:

1. It is longitudinal, not cross-sectional; postintervention outcomes are reported for a group of subjects known to the investigator before the intervention.
2. All eligible patients in some stated setting, over a stated period of time, are reported. These eligible patients are *alike*; they have a common disease, they have received the same intervention, or they share some other essential characteristic.

Series may have other important design characteristics, such as (1) the presence or absence of comparison groups and (2) whether the research was planned before or after the data were acquired.

Thus a series, as the term shall be used, studies the outcomes of an intervention applied to all eligible subjects, chosen by criteria that depend only on pretreatment status. The actual data collection may go forward in time according to a research plan, or it may be undertaken after all cases are complete. (Intermediate cases can occur.) The data are regarded as if the subjects were first identified as to eligibility, and then given the intervention, and then observed as to outcome.

A significant fraction of current medical literature consists of articles that meet this description. Feinstein (1978) reviewed all issues of the *Lancet* and the *New England Journal of Medicine* (*NEJM*) appearing between October 1, 1977, and March 31, 1978. Of the 324 structured research papers that he identified, 47 (transition cohort and outcome cohort) contained reports of series, as the term is used here. This 15 percent of articles was approximately equaled by 16 percent (53 papers) which reported clinical trials. Bailar et al. (1984) reviewed all Original Articles published in *NEJM* during 1978 and 1979. Among the 332 articles studied, there were 80 that apparently met the description of series used here.

Needed Information

At a minimum, to interpret a series' findings securely, it is necessary to know answers to the cub reporter's legendary questions: *Who* were the subjects (i.e., what were their relevant characteristics?)? *What* was done? (This calls for defining the treatment, diagnosis, staging, adjuvant care, follow-up, etc.) By *whom* was it done? (By world-class experts? By teaching hospital staff? By community hospital staff?) *When* was it done? (Over a time span long enough to permit the existence of large trends of various sorts within the series?) We may even need to know *why* a treatment was done. (Because other treatments had already failed? Because the patients were not strong enough to tolerate other treatment? For palliation? For cure?)

Adjustment for Interfering Variables

Recent series from the United Kingdom of 5,174 births at home and 11,156 births in hospitals show perinatal mortality of 5.4/1,000 in the home births and 27.8/1,000 in the hospital births (Health and Social Service Journal, 1980). What use can be made of these numbers? A moment's thought fills the mind with questions about the comparability of the two series of mothers: How did they differ in age, parity, prenatal care, prenatal complications, home circumstances, general health, and disease status? Without answers to these questions, we must hold back from any firm interpretation whatsoever. With information on all these variables—and doubtless some others—we are better off. But with such information in hand, we would still face the hard question of how to adjust the raw results for differences in these other variables: their relevance to perinatal mortality is likely, but we do not know how to adjust numerically for these factors, even if we had the information.

The complexities that are attached to adjustment are nicely exemplified in a study of more than 15,000 consecutive (eligible) deliveries at Beth Israel Hospital in Boston, about half of which involved electronic fetal monitoring, which was the intervention being studied (Neutra et al., 1978). The authors identified many variables as risk factors; among them were gestational age, hydramnios, placental, and cord abnormalities; multiple birth; breech delivery; and prolonged rupture of membranes. Their primary analysis used 18 variables in a multiple-regression-derived risk index scored for each delivery. Then, each case was assigned to one of five (ordered) strata, depending on its risk score. In addition to the primary analysis just sketched, the authors applied risk stratification in two other ways, and they also independently analyzed the data in terms of log-linear models. Clearly, how to adjust is not always a straightforward question. The authors qualify their results with this observation: "Since we are applying our risk score to the set of data from which the weights for the score were computed, we may be overstating the concentration of benefit in the high-risk categories." This candid caveat further attests to the intrinsic difficulty of adjusting for relevant variables in the effort to interpret series results.

The message here is that the interpretation of even an apparently crisp series-based difference may make heavy demands for additional information about the data in the series, and even with such additional information the meaning of the series' result may remain ambiguous.

Capabilities and Limitations

Just as a series can advance correct understanding, so can a series promote the pursuit of bad leads. It is probable that nearly every discarded, once-popular therapy was supported by a series of favorable cases. This is known to be true, even in recent times, with portacaval shunt for the treatment of esophageal varices and with gastric freezing for the treatment of ulcers.

The strengths and weaknesses of series as information sources deserve analysis. Perhaps there are straightforward ways to identify trustworthy information conveyed by series and to recognize spurious, misleading information from them. We turn now to these matters.

The publication of a series of successive cases provides readers with vicarious experience. The reader acquires this new "experience" with little outlay of effort. Often the writer also has expended relatively little effort in collating and writing up the experience to report the series. Thus, in terms of effort, the series may be regarded as an efficient information source.

The useful interpretation of this vicarious information is likely to involve considerable difficulty. Good knowledge of surrounding circumstances is ordinarily necessary; the series may not adequately report these. Even if the needed supplementary information is reported, correct methods for taking quantitative account of it may be hard, or even impossible, to devise.

Face value acceptance of the result of a series is almost never justified. Any statistic is simply the reported outcome of some process; until the process is known, one cannot know what the statistic means, however it may be named or labeled. Thus, the use and interpretation of a series result is typically a task calling for analysis—analysis which in some instances will prove to be feasible and in others infeasible.

A series is a record of experience, and as such it has prima facie value; it may give very useful information about how to apply a new technique and what kinds of difficulties and complications may be encountered. The reader of Snow's (1847) book will see this. Postmarketing surveillance produces what might be called partial series (where total numbers under observation can only be estimated). It is a method of study that has its just role in medical investigation.

The series is most liable to infirmity as an arbiter of treatment effectiveness. The two principal threats to validity are vagueness and bias.

Interpretation of Series

A number of factors bear on the interpretation of a report of a series.

Integrity of Counting The definition of a series used here has included the word all, and that word is essential. Conclusions based on selected cases are notoriously treacherous because selection can grossly affect the data; in the extreme, only the successes or only the failures might be reported. Presumably, the limitations of selected cases underlie the skepticism sometimes voiced about the usefulness of voluntary disease registries.

At a minimum the reader needs to know what criteria were used to determine inclusion and exclusion, how many subjects were included, and what happened to each of them. There lurk here two kinds of problems. The first is operational; it may be difficult or impossible to learn some of the essential information in retrospect. The outcomes for some who belong in the series may be unknown. Patients who cannot be followed up often differ on average from ones who can; more of them may be dead; more of them may be cured. Without complete follow-up, the available figures lose much of their meaning.

The second counting problem is definitional. The series report, to avoid being a recital of selected cases, needs to describe what was done to (all) eligible patients and how things turned out for each of them. Who is (was) eligible? This may depend on diagnostic criteria that require making judgment calls. What was done to the patients? Judgment calls may be involved here as well; if the intervention is a new surgical procedure that has changed somewhat with time, the designation of patients who did and did not receive the new operation requires a decision by the investigator. Even identifying the outcome for a patient may demand a judgment call. If the surgical patient dies on the operating table, there may be a question (and a decision) as to whether it was an anesthetic death, a treatment failure, or a result of the patient's disease.

The definitional and operational problems of counting are likely to loom larger when the series study is planned after the data are already in existence.

Consequences of No Protocol The absence of a protocol, prepared before data are acquired, may allow certain kinds of defects to arise in a series-based study. Exactly what interventions were performed on what kinds of patients for what indications may be unclear in hindsight. Who was counted eligible and so included and who was omitted may have been based on judgment calls. Withdrawals may be ill-documented or entirely tacit, with possibly a great effect on the results. The reader may be left to wonder whether the results reported were searched out from among many possible endpoints and thus less likely to be reproducible than significance tests indicate. There are indications of an increasing number of studies in which the research is planned after the data have been collected. Fletcher and Fletcher (1979), studying articles in the *Lancet* and the *Journal of the American Medical Association*, found that in 1946, 24 percent of the articles were post hoc in this sense; in 1976 the corresponding figure was 56 percent. Of course difficulties can be mitigated by careful reporting, but they can be eliminated only if the data are gathered so systematically as to conform to an invisible protocol in all important respects.

Consequences of No Randomization
The series-based study stands vulnerable to the many dangers that randomization forestalls. The key considerations are comparability of cases receiving different interventions and equivalence of outcome evaluation. Were the patients who got the new treatment chosen because they were strong enough to be able to tolerate it or so sick that there was no other possible therapy? In either case, they are not likely to be comparable to the controls. Was any judgment needed in assessing the outcomes? If so, then evaluation biases can easily masquerade as treatment differences—i.e., as treatment effects.

Thus, in the absence of randomization, doubts about interpretation can, and should, nag the reader. Crossing over illustrates the difficulty. Suppose that a serious disease can be treated effectively by surgery, but operative mortality and post-surgical sequelae are drawbacks, so a medical therapy is an attractive alternative. If there is a class of patients for whom the two treatments appear to be equally reasonable, then a suitably designed and executed RCT should tell which treatment is actually superior in that class of patients. Now, it may happen that some medically treated patients do not respond, and the gravity of the disease requires that they receive the surgical treatment, after having begun therapy in the medically treated group. This is crossing over.

The effect of this in an RCT is simply to change the research question from its original form to this one: "Which is the superior policy, for patients of the class originally defined, (1) apply surgery immediately or (2) treat medically and defer surgery until it may become indicated?" This question is very likely to be a better, i.e., more realistic and practical, question to answer than was the original one, so no harm is done.

It is in nonrandomized studies in which crossing over is more likely to be a serious problem. Now the two policies, surgery immediately and medical therapy until surgery may be necessary, can be very difficult to compare because the patients receiving surgery may not be identifiable in retrospect as to which policy had been applied to them.

A summary of this point would suggest that series-based studies are liable to grave difficulties, although of course not every study comes to a false conclusion. The problem lies in checking out the value of the individual study under consideration. This amounts to ascertaining whether selection biases have operated, whether assessment of treatment outcomes have differed with treatment, and whether withdrawal of patients has biased the results. The reader may recognize the questions but be powerless to answer them from the information published. The investigator may be unable to answer them from the records. These difficulties are larger when the research plan comes after the data have already been recorded.

Advance planning is not the only way in which timing enters as a strategic variable in reporting a series; there is a second way. The cases can be defined as all those present at one of several temporally ordered stages. Thus, the series study might look at all cases of a certain disease that are present in a given setting. It might look at the subset of those who (after presenting) receive treatment A or B. It might study all those who received treatment A or B more than 6 months ago. In general, the later the stage in terms of which the series is defined, the greater the need for retrospective inference (judgment calls) and the larger the difficulties with ambiguous or unobtainable information.

What About the Clear-Cut Series?

The reader may think that the picture has been presented too negatively. One may reason, "If a small series is done, clear differences may be observed at once, and the complexities referred to may not need to be unraveled. If a new approach is so good that it has an explosive impact, then an acceptable study can be devised readily enough." This objection raises fair questions. Isn't a large fraction of medical practice based on series results? Aren't there many examples, like penicillin and ether anesthesia, in which the series unambiguously asserts the truth? It is true that the bulk of medical practice has evolved largely from series-based information. We know also that much of the accepted doctrine will be discarded when more and more careful evaluations are done. The problem is to ascertain which series (which uncontrolled studies) have right answers and which do not.

What about penicillin for syphilis, sulfa against pneumococcus, and other examples? These have been called "slam-bang" effects. When they occur, they are dramatic. The very fact that these are so dramatic should remind us that they are also rare. An effort to enumerate them will bring us to vitamin B_{12} against pernicious anemia, penicillin for subacute bacterial endocarditis, x rays to guide setting of fractures, cortisone for adrenal insufficiency, insulin for severe diabetes, propranolol for hypertrophic aortic stenosis, methotrexate for choriocarcinoma, indomethacin for patent ductus arteriosus, and perhaps as many again, or twice or thrice as many, or possibly even more. But more than one or two per year in the last half-century? Perhaps not.

Slam-bang effects are uncommon. They result from only a tiny part of the thousands of studies published each year. Furthermore, they are not always open and shut cases. In 1847, the year that Snow published his ether series, J. Y. Simpson published his results lauding chloroform anesthesia. Controversy about comparative merits of the two anesthetics extended at least until the Lancet Commission (1893) examined the matter more than four decades later. At that time 64,693 administrations of chloroform and only 9,380 administrations of ether were identified, both since 1848. The commission (1893) recommended ether as safer than chloroform in general surgery "in temperate climes." Similarly, x rays in fractures clearly work, but how long did it take to discard x rays for the treatment of acne? Prefrontal lobotomy as a treatment for schizophrenia stands as a reminder that a treatment may come into wide use and prominence on the basis of inadequate evidence—only to be discarded later. The occasional slam-bang effect, confidently detectable from an uncontrolled study, is at the favorable end of the spectrum; at the other lies the sequence of series-based studies that defy interpretation. The Office of Health Research Statistics and Technology, in its assessment report concerning transsexual surgery (1981), reviewed the nine published series that reported at least 10 cases, and then declared:

> These studies represent the major clinical reports thus far published on the outcome of transsexual surgery. None of these studies meets the ideal criteria of a valid scientific assessment of a clinical procedure, and they share many of the following deficiencies:
>
> a. There is often a lack of clearly specified goals and objectives of the intervention making it difficult to evaluate the outcomes;
>
> b. The patients represent heterogeneous groups because diagnostic criteria have varied from center to center and over time;
>
> c. The therapeutic techniques are not standardized with varying surgical techniques being combined with various other therapies;
>
> d. None has had adequate (if any) control groups (perhaps this is impossible);
>
> e. There is no blinding with the observers usually being part of the therapeutic team;
>
> f. Systematically collected baseline data are usually missing making comparison of pre- and postsurgery status difficult;
>
> g. There is a lack of valid and reliable instruments for assessing pre- and postsurgery status and the selection and scoring of outcome criteria usually involve arbitrary value judgments;
>
> h. A large number of patients are lost to followup, apparently due in great part to the desire of transsexuals to leave their past behind; and,
>
> i. None of the studies are presented in sufficient detail to permit replication.

Although the procedure under consideration is quite unusual, most of the difficulties listed are general threats to assessments using series of patients receiving a new treatment or procedures. They also amount to a list of most of the problems that the protocol of an RCT is intended to forestall.

Some Additional Issues

Subgroups The difficulties of directly relying on data in the whole series worsen if one attempts to pick out subclasses marked by strikingly good or bad results. The idea seems reasonable enough but ignores a somewhat subtle, inescapable fact: there are *always* to be expected some good-looking and some bad-looking subsets in any body of data, even when no preferential influences have operated on any part of it. Furthermore, such subset differences can easily be large enough to look quite convincing to the unsophisticated analyst. Numerical statistics can be used to elucidate the point.

Suppose that n subjects, a random sample from some population with standard deviation s, are further divided at random into k equal-sized subgroups. Then the standard error (SE) for the mean of the undivided sample is $s/\sqrt{n} = SE$. Now, of course, the largest of the subgroup means *must* exceed the whole-group mean, but it can be surprising how large the excess must be. The average excess of the largest subgroup mean over the whole-group mean to be expected from random division, if $k = 4$, is 2.06 SE; if $k = 7$, then 3.56 SE; if $k = 10$, then 4.75 SE. The comparison of the best and the worst of subgroup means can produce even more vivid-looking (but meaningless) differences. The following rule of thumb shows this well; if a group of n subjects are divided at random into k equal-sized subgroups, then the difference between the largest subgroup mean and the smallest one has an expected value that is approximately k times the standard error of the whole group. (This rule applies for a k value of not more than 15.)

With such large subgroup differences to be expected by random division, we must temper our enthusiasm when we search out a series subset that looks better than the whole group; we should face the question:

"Is this large enough to believe, considering what chance alone would produce?" There are methods for answering this question, which also arises with RCTs (Ingelfinger et al., 1983).

Temporal Drift If a series has accumulated over a long time (as happened with Louis, but not Snow) additional problems are likely. Over a long enough time period, shifts can occur—indeed, they are to be expected. The patient population may change as referral patterns do; demographic composition may drift. Supportive care, diagnostic criteria, and exposure to pathogenic agents may change over time. Even treatments may change. It follows that information about the sequence and timing of the cases in the series may be essential to a realistic analysis. The issue here is not hypothetical; Schneiderman (1966) gives examples of clinical trials in which, because treatments were modified part way through a trial, a second control group was initiated. Analysis then showed that the two successive control groups in the same setting, meeting the same criteria, differed importantly in their survival experience.

Grab Samples Statistical inference is a powerful tool for learning from experience. It is at its best if data are obtained in ways in which probability theory can be correctly applied, e.g., with random sampling from a population or with data from a randomized clinical trial. Where probabilistic structure is unknown, the data constitute what is often called a grab sample. Inference from such a sample is necessarily treacherous, whether by application of formal statistical methods or otherwise. The personal experience of a single physician is in some sense a grab sample; so is the case study; so is the series of successive cases. The fact that we can learn from experience shows that it is not impossible to reach valid conclusions from grab samples; but the process is fraught with difficulty, uncertainty, and error.

Grab sample data may be especially useful where the following two conditions are obtained: First, the data come from a well-identified setup that is relatively stable over time. Second, the data are taken from this setup at regular intervals over a protracted period.

Two examples help explain. First, statistical reports from the Metropolitan Life Insurance Company have long given useful indication of *trends* in longevity and disease attack rates, despite the fact that their statistics could not wisely be used to estimate U.S. population *averages* of longevity and attack rates (because of selective factors that apply to insurance policyholders.) Similarly, cross-sectional information from particular health care populations such as Kaiser, Mayo Clinic, and Veterans Administration (VA) hospitals would not be expected to apply directly to larger or different groups, but temporal changes in such series might so apply.

Second, air pollutants are monitored at stations situated in particular locations; the relation of pollutant levels at such stations to levels experienced by persons in the schools, homes, roads, and factories near the monitoring stations are, in general, poorly known. Nonetheless, when those monitored levels rise or fall, we feel justified in thinking that the pollution levels experienced by the nearby population rise or fall as well. The monitored pollutant levels would serve less well, or even not at all, as measures of absolute dose to nearby persons.

Even such restricted use for trends depends strongly on the assumption of stability in the system. For example, a change in membership, fees, reporting methods, etc., can affect the interpretation of trends observed in the statistics of a health plan. Similarly, seasonal changes in prevailing wind direction might cause some areas to receive higher levels of pollution, even though every monitoring station shows lower levels. To see this, consider a location, near a major pollution source, which is upwind of that source during the region's high-pollution season but is downwind from it during the region's low-pollution season.

Epidemiology is largely devoted to methodically—and often imaginatively—identifying, estimating, and correcting for interfacing variables that obscure direct interpretation of grab samples, natural experiments, and series.

So the message here again is that the interpretation and reliance that can be placed on the data in a series are generally obscure until resolved by detailed study. It is possible that detailed study will reveal essential flaws that bar trustworthy interpretation of a kind that one might have initially hoped would have been available.

Strengthening the Method

The author can do much to mitigate problems of interpretation by advanced planning and full, careful reporting. The planning should be done while contemplating the way he or she would investigate the problem by an RCT. The author can identify probable disturbing variables—and measure them and report them. It is impossible to reliably make two differently constituted groups comparable by doing statistical adjustments, so doubts about selection bias and assessment bias cannot ordinarily be entirely removed. But more complete information helps with the difficult task of interpretation.

The series of consecutive cases is a device much used in the cumulation of experience concerning medical technology. In general, trustworthy interpretation of series-based data demands clear and complete information about (at least) (1) the defining characteristics of the cases in the series, (2) the intervention(s) applied, and (3) the outcomes and how they were assessed. When one or more of these is ambiguous, then the meaning of the series becomes correspondingly obscured. Typically, the reliable interpretation of a series requires an analytic effort, which may or may not be crowned with success.

THE CASE STUDY AS A TOOL FOR MEDICAL TECHNOLOGY ASSESSMENT*

Case studies can be useful tools for medical technology assessment. Although limited in important ways, case studies can reveal some of the implications of medical technology that are not readily exposed by other methods of evaluation. Case studies also can provide insight into decision making about a new technology in a vivid and memorable way. The contribution of case studies may be enhanced when they incorporate the findings of other forms of evaluation (controlled clinical trials, epidemiologic surveys, simulation studies, cost-effectiveness analysis, etc.) and when they are prepared as part of a series of related case studies. The example of El Camino management information system given in Chapter 1 could be regarded as a case study. The book by Yin (1984) is useful in pointing to the case study as a research strategy.

In this paper we describe the features that characterize case studies of medical technology and then review some recent efforts by the U.S. Congress Office of Technology Assessment to conduct case studies of medical technology, discuss the strengths and weaknesses of the method, and end with a summary.

What Is a Case Study?

In the most general sense, any coherent discussion of events related to a topic might

*This section was drafted by Harvey V. Fineberg and Ann Lawthers-Higgins.

be considered a kind of case study. For the purpose of evaluating a medical technology, a case study is a detailed account of selected aspects of the technology. These aspects include issues, events, processes, decisions, consequences, and programs occurring over time and affecting individuals, institutions, and policies. A case study is particularistic in its detail and may also be holistic in the scope of its coverage of a medical technology (Wilson, 1979b). The form and content of case studies reflect the values and points of view of the writers, their intended audiences, and the purposes of the evaluation.

In sorting out the variety of documents described as case studies, it is helpful to distinguish several types of cases, as indicated in Figure 3-5.

Case studies of medical technology tend to take one of two forms. The first type of case study attempts to reveal causes, to explain the basis for decisions about a medical technology. The second type of case study attempts to reveal consequences, to describe the direct and indirect effects of medical technology. Some case studies of medical technology are concerned both with causes and consequences.

The kinds of case study concerned with causes include studies of policymaking about medical technology, studies of the development of new technology, and studies of the diffusion of medical technology. This type of case study typically spans a particular time horizon and may be aptly characterized as a narrative history of a process. A case study of this type usually portrays the interests, motivations; and opportunities of different players, describes the institutional environment in which they work; and characterizes the external forces acting on the decision makers. The elements in such case studies may be related in complex ways, and even those closely involved in decisions about a medical technology may have only a dim perception of the interests and actions of others. The aim of such a case study is to describe what happened in a vivid way and, more importantly, to provide insight into why certain decisions were made at certain times and produced certain reactions and responses.

The second type of case study is an effort to enumerate the consequences of a medical technology. This type of evaluative case study organizes and presents diverse information on the impact of a medical technology. This information may be derived in part from clinical trials, epidemiologic studies, and other forms of evaluation as well as from data banks, insurance records, vital statistics, and other sources of

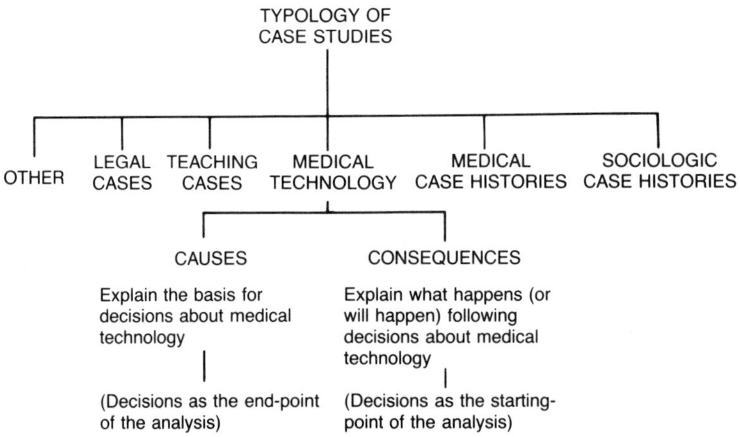

FIGURE 3-5.

primary data. There is a continuum between review papers that synthesize evidence from such primary evaluations as controlled clinical trials and case studies that characterize the manifold consequences of a medical technology. Compared with a typical clinical review paper, a case study of medical technology highlights a wider array of consequences, such as ethical issues, effects on the organization of medical care; and economic, social, and political consequences. A case study typically contains qualitative as well as quantitative assessments of a medical technology. Instead of measuring experienced effects of technology, a case study of an emerging medical technology may aim at anticipating expected consequences. The values and judgment of a case writer are likely to be prominent parts of such an evaluative case study.

Both case studies aimed at causes and case studies aimed at consequences draw upon eclectic sources of information. These range across personal interviews, historical documents, news accounts, company and institutional records, data banks, epidemiologic studies, clinical trials, and more. Any source of information bearing on the subject properly is grist for the case writer's mill. A case writer may employ a similarly varied array of analytic methods in developing a case study, including, for example, historical and journalistic research, survey methods, cost accounting, and statistical analysis.

The challenge in writing a useful case study is to create an accurate and coherent picture of the subject. Stylistically, a case study may be written in academic prose for an academic audience or, to engage a busy policymaker, in the form of a vivid narrative, complete with dialogue.

Closely related to case studies of particular medical technologies are case studies whose subjects are diseases, medical institutions, or health care policies, because these all bear directly on medical technology. The kinds of case studies considered here are quite different from case reports of individual patients or of unusual clusters of patients that may be reported in the medical literature.

A case study developed for technology assessment also differs from cases developed for teaching purposes. A teaching case study in a school of management, government, or public health typically presents a cast of characters and a chronology of events. The case may describe the values and attitudes of the characters, and it may discuss outside factors affecting the situation. The cases used in teaching may or may not adhere to all the facts of a real-life situation. The aim of the case study is to project the student into a decision-making role and to stimulate discussion about the best way to deal with the situation. Through vicarious experience with a number of cases, the student is expected to become better prepared to face real situations that resemble the cases. In this sense of aiming to produce lessons that will apply to new situations, teaching case studies are like case studies of medical technology.

Case Studies from the Office of Technology Assessment

The U.S. Congress Office of Technology Assessment (OTA) has sponsored a series of case studies of medical technology. As of the spring of 1984, two dozen had been published (OTA, 1983a). These cases cover a range of technologies (drugs, devices, equipment, procedures) at different stages of diffusion; the technologies are used by diverse medical specialists for a variety of clinical purposes (prevention, diagnosis, therapy, rehabilitation); they involve high costs and raise a variety of ethical and policy issues.

The first 19 of these studies were undertaken as part of OTA's assessment of cost-effectiveness analysis of medical technology. As such, a principal emphasis in most of the studies was to synthesize available information on the costs and clinical effects of the subject technology. Some of the cases represent new areas of application of cost-effectiveness analysis, and several develop new methods for assessing the costs and benefits of particular types of medical technology, such as diagnostic equipment. Some of the case studies describe events and decisions about the subject technology and discuss the reasons behind some of the decisions.

The OTA relied on the collection of studies to identify common problems and advantages of cost-effectiveness and cost-benefit analysis in health care. The cases also illustrated numerous observations and conclusions in the OTA report on the implications of cost-effectiveness analysis of medical technology (OTA, 1980a).

The remaining case studies in the OTA series cover sundry health technologies and topics: passive restraint systems in automobiles, telecommunications devices for hearing-impaired persons, alcoholism treatment, therapeutic apheresis, and the relation between hospital length of stay and health outcome. The issue of cost-effectiveness arises in some of these cases, and they also deal with questions of technical feasibility, variation in medical practices, political decision making, and ethical consequences.

Weaknesses of Case Studies

The accuracy and completeness of a case study depend on the skill and insights of the case analyst. If the case writer is biased, careless, or misguided, the case study will be similarly misleading. Similar comments might be made about the analyst in any type of evaluation. However, oversights and analytic errors in a case study may be more difficult to detect than similar problems in other forms of evaluation, such as reports of a clinical trial.

A central problem in the use of case studies for technology assessment is the derivation of generalities from particular instances. The main interest in a case study is usually less what it says about the subject itself than what it implies about a class of technologies (decisions, institutions, issues, etc.) that are like the subject of the case study in some ways. This kind of implication is prone to error, because the case study omits important considerations or misrepresents causes and consequences, because the reader misinterprets the case study, or because the new situation differs from the case study in unrecognized ways.

Campbell and Stanley (1963) regarded case studies as useless tools for evaluating the benefits and risks of a program or treatment because individual case studies lack controls. In making this judgment, they did not take account of case studies as methods for revealing the process of decision making, nor did they consider the role of case studies in assessing the ethical and social consequences of medical technology.

Strengths of Case Studies

In some instances of major policy decisions about medical technology, case studies may be the only practical means of investigating the causes and consequences of those decisions. Case studies can provide some leads and suggest more detailed and structured studies. Cases like the artificial heart (OTA, 1983a) and the swine flu immunization program (Neustadt and Fineberg, 1983) are complex and singular events. Case studies of each may help decision makers prepare to deal with similar situations that are likely to arise in the future.

Case studies can convey the complexity involved in decisions about many medical technologies. The open form of a case study makes it suitable for raising some of the ethical, social, legal, and political consequences of technology. A case study allows these issues to be presented from different points of view and can juxtapose these issues against evaluations of the safety and efficacy of a medical technology.

The vividness and concreteness of a case study may carry a powerful intellectual and emotional impact on the reader. A single case, properly presented, may motivate a decision maker to act more surely than a scientifically sounder abstract analysis. A case study can provide the kind of memorable paradigm that people use to interpret other experiences. This feature is, of course, a hazard as well as a benefit.

Strengthening Case Studies

Some analysts have suggested that sets of case studies may overcome some limitations of generalizability that apply to individual cases (Kennedy, 1979; Hoaglin et al., 1982). When case studies are grouped with an eye toward using them as sample surveys, data collected for the cases should reflect a range of attributes that relate to the specific purposes of the case analysis. Even if it is not possible to assemble a sample that permits estimates of the fraction of instances in which an attribute occurs, it still may be possible to represent the bulk of pertinent attributes in the sample. Kruskal and Mosteller (1980) use the term coverage to describe the idea of such a broadly representative sample.

Including both examples and counterexamples (successes and failures) in the set of cases may help reduce the chances of drawing misleading conclusions. For example, one set of case studies of medical innovations examined only instances of clinically valuable innovations (Globe et al., 1967). This study found that enthusiastic advocates appeared to accelerate the acceptance of good medical innovations, not recognizing that strong advocates can be equally effective in promoting what turn out in retrospect to have been medical mistakes (Fineberg, 1979).

Conclusions

Case studies of the causes and consequences of decisions about medical technology can be useful forms of technology assessment. Case studies provide the most practical means of investigating some complex and exceptional medical technologies. Case studies also provide a mechanism for discussing some of the ethical, social, and political consequences of medical technology that are not readily assessed in other ways. Case studies can link assessments of the development and diffusion of medical technology with evaluations of the impact of the technology.

Among the principal weaknesses of case studies are their dependence on the perceptions and judgments of the case analyst and the hazards of generalization from uncontrolled observations. The vividness and memorability of a case study can produce unwarranted convictions as well as helpful lessons. **These shortcomings may be at least partially overcome by integrating the results of stronger methods of analysis into case studies and by undertaking a series of related case studies to investigate a class of medical technologies or a set of issues about medical technology.**

REGISTERS AND DATA BASES*

In this section we distinguish between registers (lists of patients, usually with limited clinical and demographic descriptors about each patient) and data bases (with more detailed and comprehensive data about each patient). Except in names of organizations, we reserve the term registry for an organizational structure that develops and maintains a register.

The distinction between registers or series and data bases is not sharp, and many sources of data have some characteristics of

*Contributors to this section were John Laszlo, John C. Bailar III, and Frederick Mosteller.

each. Table 3-4 lists additional features that tend to distinguish between registers and data bases but that may occur in either. Registers generally cover larger numbers of cases, and they often are suitable for use by numerous cooperating institutions, whereas data bases usually serve more restricted uses. Registers are better adapted for general, multiuse, and multiuser public resources and may be used for measuring trends in disease incidence or in the use of medical facilities, for tracking patients, or sometimes as indexes to more detailed patient records for special studies. Data bases are more often developed to answer research questions dealing with clinical epidemiology, such as questions about prognostic factors or the natural history of disease. Registers generally are file-oriented and readily searchable by patient name or key word identifiers. Data bases generally have a hierarchical structure, and they contain and can generate multiple files. Many registers and most data bases are stored in computers, and data bases are maintained and used with the help of a data base management system.

Research investigators develop disease-oriented registers of many descriptions largely to identify patients for epidemiologic studies and to track identified patients for data on the outcome of the disease and for treatment. Such registers have often been misunderstood by persons not directly involved. One might expect that health professionals would want and need an accurate filing and tracking system to identify numbers and types of patients and treatments given, to quantify and evaluate the usage of expensive and sometimes hazardous resources, and to ascertain treatment results and survival. However, there is no recognized consensus on the value of existing registers, nor even a well-accepted definition of their functions. Furthermore, the services that registers provide are diffi-

TABLE 3-4 Comparison of Health Registers and Data Bases

Features	Health Registers	Data Bases
Data source	Single institutions, regional, or nationwide	Limited number of institutions. Often uni-institutional
Job characteristics	Epidemiology of disease categories for large populations. Large-scale follow-up. Large numbers of patients	Specifically oriented to a particular disease, therapy, and/or procedure. Smaller numbers of patients
Detail required	Minimal	Comprehensive
File structure	Single-file oriented; can be manually stored	Multiple file capabilities Generally computer stored by a data base management system
Types of benefits	Assessment of public health programs. Influence on distribution of health resources. Regional variations in diseases, treatments.	Clinical applications
Time scale of major benefits	Long-term	Short-term to long-term

cult to evaluate quantitatively, leaving only intuitive or global impressions.

These difficulties reflect, and ultimately contribute to, several problems that often affect disease registers: unstable funding, weak local support (especially from persons asked to provide the raw data), and uncertain long-term continuity.

Some of these issues about registers and data bases will be examined. Bailar (1970a,b) has expanded on some of the points below. Many of the examples refer to cancer registers, which, taken together, are both the oldest and the largest of these enterprises. Approximately 1,000 hospital-based cancer registries are included in the cancer programs approved by the American College of Surgeon's Commission on Cancer (Commission on Cancer, 1974); these cover 55 to 60 percent of all patients found to have cancer in the United States, exclusive of superficial skin cancers that are not treated in hospitals and present very little threat to life and health. Numerous other registries are not yet approved or are seeking approval. A rough estimate is that the total cost of approved cancer registries in the United States is at least $20 million per year.

Medical accrediting agencies consider that registers are crucial to cancer programs, presumably because registers have important functions in patient follow-up, education, and research. Oncologists consider them useful as an index for case finding at best and woefully incomplete at worst. Hospital administrators consider them costly and often fail to understand their need, and most physicians have never used a register or been inside of a cancer registry office.

Data bases tend to be of two types. One type covers specified diseases or populations, the other covers procedures or therapies. Either type may also collect information about a control group. For example, the Coronary Artery Disease (CAD) data bank at Duke University Medical Center includes all patients with chest pain, regardless of cause. This data base originally was limited to patients who had cardiac catheterization but has been expanded to collect information from additional patient groups regarding noninvasive tests and coronary care unit (CCU) admissions (Rosati, 1973). The Duke data base is used to evaluate various technologies that may be used for patients with stable chest pain. Data from coronary care units, such as arrhythmia monitoring, hemodynamic monitoring, rehabilitation programs, and electrophysiology studies, contribute to knowledge about the management of patients with myocardial infarction.

In contrast, the National Heart, Lung, and Blood Institute (NHLBI) data base of angioplasty candidates remains procedure oriented, because it covers only patients undergoing percutaneous transluminal coronary angioplasty (PTCA) (NHLBI, 1982). Unlike the Duke CAD data base, the NHLBI data base does not collect data about patients who are considered candidates for the procedure but do not receive it.

Some other clinical data bases are those of the Seattle Heart Watch (Bruce, 1974, 1981), the Coronary Artery Surgery Study (Principal investigators of CASS and their associates, 1981; Chaitman, 1981) the Maryland Institute of Emergency Medicine (MIEM) (Cowley, 1974), and patients seen at the Mayo Clinic (Kurland and Molgaard, 1981). Other disease-oriented data bases focus on rheumatology (Dannenberg et al., 1979; Fries et al., 1974; McShane et al., 1978), gastrointestinal diseases (Graham and Wyllie, 1979; Hovrocks et al., 1976; Wilson, 1979a), radiology (Jeans and Morris, 1976), mental health (Evenson et al., 1975), head injuries (Braakman, 1978; Galbraith, 1978; Jennett, 1976; Knill-Jones, 1978; Teasdale, 1978), and cerebral ischemia (Heyman et al., 1979).

Uses of Registers and Data Bases

The largest cancer registry system in the United States (really a consortium of regional registries) is the Survival, Epidemiology, and End-Results (SEER) program of the National Cancer Institute, which gathers data on cancer incidence and mortality rates in several widely dispersed areas of the United States (five states, five additional metropolitan areas, and Puerto Rico) with about 10 percent of the U.S. population. The SEER data file includes all known invasive cancers (excluding superficial skin cancers) diagnosed in residents of these areas since 1973. Data elements include demographic factors, disease site, type of cancer, and whether or not surgery was done (Pollack, 1982a). National estimates of cancer incidence rates are largely based on these data. Quality control procedures include a regular program of workshop training for medical record abstractors. The currently available 5-year base of data (1973–1977) contains about 350,000 cases (Young et al., 1981). More recent data are to be published soon.

Regional registers with a direct and immediate role in patient care have been developed to support programs of organ transplantation, by the timely matching and transport of donor kidneys to potential recipients. The present 32 regional hemodialysis registries may in time be coordinated, perhaps along the lines of the European Dialysis Transplant Association (Groot, 1982).

The National Implant Registry, a private organization, contracts with hospitals to track patients with mechanical and prosthetic implants, such as heart valves and vascular grafts, to preserve accountability between the manufacturer of a device and its recipient and to alert hospitals and physicians to defects and deficiencies. The National Implant Registry has a research component that permits plain language inquiries of its computer records for such things as the frequency and location of use of a specific brand, model, or generic class of a device. If a device is replaced and a second implant is registered for the same patient, the system flags the episode for further investigation.

Because registers tend to be large and complex, the kinds of data to be collected must be carefully thought out. This often is in terms of a minimal data set of items to be submitted for each patient, with or without optional supplementary items. Settling on the minimal data base for a register requires careful thought and agreement by the sponsors of such matters as the general problems to be attacked, data items the registry will collect, what can profitably be analyzed, what will be the cost, and who will pay which costs at various steps from the initial collection of data through the analysis and dissemination of results. For example, if a cancer register is to be used for more than studies of crude counts of patients, it should contain demographic descriptors, information about the type and severity or extent of the disease, and considerable follow-up and survival data.

Very strict requirements for completeness of documentation can have the effect of restricting the coverage of the registry by excluding otherwise appropriate cases that fail to meet those requirements. On the other hand, lax standards of documentation can result in the mistaken inclusion of patients whose disease status is not actually appropriate to the registry. Balancing these opposed considerations is a challenge that should not be shirked or ignored.

Disease registers that have nearly complete coverage of a defined population, such as residents of a given state, are especially useful. They can avoid or measure certain biases from factors that cause different kinds of patients to go to different hospitals, and they can be used for important classes of studies that require the computation of incidence rates.

Additional functions of a disease registry, such as deriving statistics on patient survival for each hospital, comparing modes of treatment, and finding clues regarding predisposing occupational, environmental, or genetic risk factors, are highly desirable when they can be obtained in a cost-effective manner. Administrative uses of registers are important in resource allocations. Questions of patient access to the hospital, travel distance, and availability of a local physician are easily answered from demographic data. Such data have some value to medical investigators and health administrators and offer the potential for substantial cost-effective use.

Despite the attractiveness of using registers to answer questions about the effectiveness of treatments, experience shows that retrospective analysis of hospital charts often is imprecise. The necessary data about diagnostic evaluations and the nuances that affect therapeutic decisions and outcomes seem to be unobtainable with a basic registry system. The same considerations apply to certain kinds of epidemiologic analyses in which only a detailed prospective search for occupational, environmental, or genetic factors can be given serious attention. A cancer registry in the Netherlands is specifically oriented to look for genetic predisposition (Lips et al., 1982). Older cancer staging systems are based solely on anatomic and pathologic factors, whereas functional tests, hormonal status, and the like are now recognized as important in describing disease biology and prognosis.

Opportunities to use large registers or specialized data bases for clinical research and for exchange of information among various centers were mentioned above; see also Laszlo (submitted for publication). Previous publications (Blum, 1982; Cox and Stanley, 1979a; Cox et al., 1979b) have illustrated the kinds of information that can be obtained and have offered recommendations on how to modernize cancer staging systems. For example, Blum (1982) has developed a computer program that searches a substantial data base for causal hypotheses.

The numbers of drugs on the U.S. market is huge, but the number of combinations of drugs is astronomical. If there were only 1,000 drugs in common use, there would be essentially 500,000 pairs of such drugs and a far greater number of combinations when three or more drugs are used. Some patients take many drugs simultaneously (Blum, 1982). Physicians cannot hope to keep track of the consequences for patients of each possible combination. Both Stanford University and Massachusetts General Hospital have computer systems that track and warn of adverse drug reactions. In the Stanford system, each prescription for a hospital inpatient triggers a literature-based listing of potential drug interactions between the prescribed drug and other previously prescribed drugs. The program automatically notifies pharmacists, nursing staff, and physicians of these potential interactions (Cohen et al., 1974; Tatro et al., 1979).

The Kaiser-Permanente organization developed and used a Drug Reaction Monitoring System (DRMS) which the Food and Drug Administration (FDA) and the National Center for Health Services Research (NCHSR) supported for 5 years as a demonstration project. The DRMS followed both inpatients and outpatients to assess the frequency of drug and event association, to assist in determining causality, to assess the size of the public health problem, and to support other scientific investigations (Friedman, 1972). One long-range goal of such studies is to build up evidence of safety and risk for many drugs. Using the DRMS, Friedman (1983a) was able to review earlier concerns that long-term use of rauwolfia predisposes to breast cancer after age 50. He found no statistically significant relation and estimated that for this population the risk ratio is less than twofold, if in fact there is any excess risk at all.

An extension of this approach can screen drugs for carcinogenicity, as Friedman and Ury (1983b) have done. They reported on 143,574 patients followed from 1969 through 1978. The 95 most commonly used drugs or drug groups and 120 selected drugs used less commonly were screened. Because many drugs and many cancer sites lead to many statistical tests, the authors point out that results can be no more than preliminary and suggestive. As an example, concern had been expressed about an association between amphetamines and Hodgkin's disease. The authors found only one case of Hodgkin's disease among 506 users of phenmetrazine hydrochloride and 880 users of diethylpropion hydrochloride.

Capabilities and Limitations of Registers and Data Bases

The strengths and weaknesses of disease registers will be reviewed in this section, again using cancer registers as a model (Bailar, 1970a,b; Commission on Cancer, 1974; Cutler et al., 1974; Demographic Analysis Section, 1976; Feigl et al., 1981; Gershman et al., 1976; Maclennan et al., 1978; Queram, 1977; WHO, 1976a,b, Young et al., 1976). The old-style registry is characteristically in or near a medical record room, often at a site remote from physicians' offices. This separation creates two related problems: It is unnecessarily difficult for registrars to consult physicians about questions (i.e., what did the surgical staging reveal?; was this a primary pancreatic cancer?), and distance and the lack of frequent contact inhibit the use of registry data. A register that is used little is largely useless, doomed to mediocrity, and likely to contribute to the poor reputation of disease registries in general. Registries work best when they are not separate and distant appendages but rather an integral part of both the clinical program (as some cancer registries are integral to cancer consultation, treatment, and follow-up) and the patient data program (Laszlo et al., 1976) Such an approach has been successfully employed in many cancer centers.

A surprising number of problems and concerns arise even in a basic registry system (Bailar, 1970a,b; Laszlo et al., 1976). Completeness of case findings is difficult to document but may be a major problem at many institutions that code only the records of inpatients. Furthermore, uniformity of approaches at different centers can be assured only by an extensive and costly set of quality control procedures.

As an example of the efforts required to maintain data quality at even the most basic level, the Centralized Cancer Patient Data System (CCPDS) worked for several years to develop a 36-item minimal data set. These items require the inclusion of an entire volume of definitions. Even so, reabstracting studies performed by CCPDS showed that coding disagreements at comprehensive cancer centers were primary site, 6 percent; histology, 14 percent; and stage, 23 percent (Feigl et al., 1981). It seems likely that less thoroughly supervised registry systems have error rates that are at least as large.

Timeliness of record completion is often a problem. Medical record libraries or other organizational units that house registries may be pressed to meet other business, office, and professional review functions, so that records often are not abstracted until many months after patients have been discharged from the hospital. Thus data are not current, and to the extent that they rely on fading memories they even may not be accurate. Some record libraries are also so large or so inefficient that a return clinic visit note fails to find its way back to the chart promptly, thereby giving an inappropriate signal that the patient has not kept a return appointment. Reminder letters under such circumstances may reflect adversely on the competence of the institution.

Registry organizers may ask questions

that are too numerous or too complex to be collected quickly by clerks, or require a level of detail that cannot be found in charts or cannot be used for analysis. Such pitfalls are well known in cancer registries; for example, many cancer registries once asked for extensive staging information as well as detailed information about treatment, including the drugs and doses used. Individual hospital and state tumor registries invested many years of work to abstract hundreds of thousands of cases of cancer with classifications of tumor stage that have never been carefully studied and classifications of treatment that have never been subjected to critical analysis. This was a matter of fundamental purposes, objectives, and methods, not a quality control problem; even if the abstracting could have been done to perfection, it would still have been of limited value. A system which has such encumbrances cannot be monitored for its quality, cannot be operated by clerks, and cannot be justified in terms of its cost.

The process of organizing cancer registries as part of hospital cancer programs does serve a cohesive function that is important but difficult to quantitate. These benefits have only recently been recognized and are being addressed by the network of hospitals served by the registry program of the Joint Committee on Accreditation of Hospitals and its agent in this matter, the American College of Surgeons, and by the Surveillance, Epidemiology, and End Results Program (Demographic Analysis Section, 1976; Feigl et al., 1981; Young et al., 1976).

Roos (1979) illustrates the thoughtfulness and multiplicity of methods that good analyses of nonexperimental data require, although each situation may require special approaches not transferable to other studies or other data bases. Roos found that 75 to 95 percent of ordinary tonsillectomy patients could not meet the criteria for a current randomized trial of this operation. Several different analyses, including a simulation, led to different answers because some analyses tended, on their face, to give less credit to the operation than others. The overall effect of the several analyses was to suggest that during the year following surgery, the average patient experiences between 0.1 and 0.8 fewer episodes of respiratory disease than if the operation had not been performed. Because the operation has some hazards and offers modest gains, Roos concluded that physicians should take a very conservative approach to tonsillectomy.

The costs of operating a registry may be calculated in widely different ways: with or without the costs of lifetime follow-up of registered patients; with or without the salaries of staff (who also have other duties); with or without the costs of using registry data for various purposes (such as computer costs of data analysis); with or without overhead and fringe benefits, etc. This explains in part the very wide divergence in quoted costs, ranging from a few dollars to perhaps $150 per registered case. **There would be much value in a study that would assess, on a uniform basis and in a variety of settings, the real costs of specific registry activities, including extra chart handling, abstracting, follow-up, and data analysis (manual or computerized).** Despite the uncertainties, real marginal costs might be estimated at about $65 per case for a registry recording 300 new cases per year, as indicated in Table 3-5.

Total costs for the SEER program, which include costs of analysis, lifetime follow-up, coordination of many diverse registries, and intensive quality control, probably exceed $100 per case entered (Pollack, 1982b).

The capabilities and limitations of data bases are similar to those of registers except that data bases offer richer possibilities for detailed study, generally at greater real cost. Perhaps the greatest challenge in organizing a data base system is to gain

TABLE 3-5 Approximate Costs of Registry for 300 New Cases per Year

Budget Item	Cost (1982 dollars)
Salary and Benefits	$15,000[a]
Space and Equipment	1,000
Printing and Postage	1,500
Telephone	1,200
Miscellaneous	500
Total	$19,200

[a]Varies with experience and geographic location.
SOURCE: Kindly provided by the American College of Surgeons (1974).

agreement as to its elements. Many persons naively think that a broad-based data set on all patients, with records for each interesting event over time, could be quite usefully browsed and queried. Such an approach is not practical for large-scale studies that depend on retrospective searches through data bases, particularly when the data records have been compiled and entered by a variety of observers from hospital records that were not regularly and consistently collected for each patient of the type being studied.

Each data base should have extensive input from persons with a variety of interests, beginning with the initial organization phase and continuing through the life of the data base. These persons should represent the data users; the persons who will supervise data collection and analysis; and the administrators who are responsible for providing space, money, and other resources. These individuals should be authorized to speak for their colleagues in the case of an institutional venture, particularly because registries require long-term commitments. Legal advice also is needed when questions of data access are discussed, for the system must be designed to protect patient and doctor confidentiality, with access governed by established guidelines. There should be an executive committee that set policy for the use of data, as has been described for the CCPDS (Feigl et al., 1981). In the case of federally sponsored programs, particularly those funded by contract, special (although simple) systems are needed to protect the confidentiality of data that might be misused by persons who request access thereto through the Freedom of Information Act. (The Act includes special provision for the protection of individual privacy, but not for statistical summaries.) This seems not to be a problem for grant-funded research data, which remain the property of the investigator.

Registries are most likely to survive if they are attached to other successful programs (such as tumor clinics) and if the leaders of those programs are willing to help in acquiring the needed financial and other resources. The chances of success are improved for registries that are part of more extensive data bases that become an accepted part of the hospital and clinic environment, that are used often by physicians, that can be used to evaluate systems of health care or new technologies, and that are reimbursable as part of the medical care system. Stand-alone registries and data bases can exist for research purposes, but their future as permanent parts of the medical scene is no more secure than that of the research grants that support them (Laszlo, 1984).

The recruitment, training, and supervision of registry staff depend on the type, size, and scope of the register; but general requirements include (1) meaningful physician supervision for education and morale of staff as well as to enlist the necessary cooperation of other physicians, (2) able and motivated clerical staff as registrars, (3) locally designed as well as regional or national training programs for initial and continuing training, (4) membership of the chief registrar on the hospital cancer committee, (5) hospital by-laws that specify the functions of the registry, and (6) a close functional relationship (but not necessarily physical proximity) with the medical record library, which must provide and later refile charts as needed. Hospital administrators need to understand and support the registry, and the support of the chief record librarian can be invaluable.

The simpler registry file systems are being supplemented and/or supplanted by more extensive data bases with multiple file capabilities. These are of many varieties and represent major new trends as physicians discover their capability to manipulate medical information in computers. The next decade may see a large increase in the number of such systems, and those that survive will be those used to improve patient care, to assess medical technology, or both.

Strengthening Uses of Registers and Data Bases

Roos (1979) states: "So many different types of analyses are possible given these data bases that some dialogue with reviewers and readers is necessary. Researchers obviously have their own emphases, priorities, and biases. Without suggestions from others at each stage of the research process, significant opportunities for improving both our methodology and our substantive understanding will be lost." **Clearly some education about possible analyses will help the medical community to make more appropriate use of data bases for the comparison of therapies. Research on ways to improve such usage might be helpful.**

Aspects of patient confidentiality sometimes constrain the sharing of data among institutions. Thus a patient may be followed by two or more hospital registries that do not communicate with each other, especially if the patient has not given permission to share data and there is no centralized (state or regional) registry. **Although considerable effort has been devoted to examining data sharing problems on multi-institutional research (Boruch and Cecil, 1979; National Academy of Sciences, 1985), action and research on ways to reduce these problems is needed.**

Because data bases ordinarily contain information from patients whose treatment was chosen in an uncontrolled manner and delivered in an uncontrolled and poorly monitored fashion, groups receiving different treatments cannot be expected to be similar in prognosis. Attempts to use data to compare the effects of different treatments must therefore use analytical devices to attempt to remove the effects of biases. **Such devices are not entirely satisfactory, and both new methods and a better understanding of old methods are needed.**

SAMPLE SURVEYS*

Sample surveys (of, for example, medical records, health care providers, or the population) are useful for evaluating medical technologies in clinical use. Surveys can estimate disease incidence and prevalence rates; quantify the use of medical care services and procedures; and estimate costs and benefits of drugs, procedures, and other technologies. Population-based health surveys collect information on health status, functional capacity, medical care utilization, and costs or charges. The information may be obtained in person, by telephone, or by mail.

Surveys of health care providers capture information about patients' demographic and medical characteristics, the medical diagnoses associated with contacts in the health care delivery system, the tests and procedures carried out, and charges for the services provided.

Sample surveys of vital records—birth, death, and stillbirth certificates—can also

* This section was drafted by Dorothy Rice with assistance from John C. Bailar III.

yield information useful for technology assessment. Files of registered births and deaths, for example, provide lists of events for which considerable additional information may be obtained from various sources (perhaps on a sample basis), including hospitals and physicians who provided care to the individual whose record is selected for the study.

The focus in this section is on national sample surveys that are designed to provide accurate representation of the universe that provided the samples. Such surveys are very large undertakings that must serve many diverse and sometimes competing purposes, not only that of technology assessment. They may therefore not exactly suit the needs of the technology assessor with a specific question, but they have many other important strengths such as ready availability of past as well as current data, large sample sizes, and the immense but unquantifiable advantages of data quality that come from having a large, full-time, experienced staff capable of state-of-the-art methods.

Uses of Sample Surveys

A few of the ways in which sample survey data have been used in relation to technology assessment are shown below; many others could be cited.

- Scitovsky (1979) used data from the National Health Interview Survey (NHIS) conducted by the National Center for Health Statistics to develop national estimates of visits to physicians' offices and then combined these results with data from the National Ambulatory Medical Care Survey (NAMCS) to estimate the percentage of physician visits that had a laboratory procedure ordered or provided.
- A report from the National Center for Health Care Technology (NCHCT) (1981) estimated from NAMCS data that there are in the United States 80,000 to 110,000 new candidates each year for surgical treatment of coronary artery disease.
- The Office of Technology Assessment (OTA) report (1982c) "Technology and Handicapped People" used NHIS data to estimate the number of persons with selected impairments.
- Much of the data for OTA's report (1983b), "Variations in Hospital Length of Stay: Their Relationship to Health Outcomes," came from the National Hospital Discharge Survey.

NCHS Surveys

Under the National Health Survey Act of 1956, the National Center for Health Statistics (NCHS) has developed a model set of population-based sample surveys for government and private uses. The purpose is to present a broad picture of the nation's health status and of the use of health resources, and to show various aspects of health and health resources in relation to each other. The surveys draw their information from the people, the institutions and professions that provide health services, and from vital records. These cross-sectional surveys assess the health status of the population at specific points in time and allow examination of changes over time. They encompass and produce statistics on the extent and nature of illness and disability in the United States; the determinants of health; environmental, social, and other health hazards; and health care costs and financing.

Several national sample surveys conducted by NCHS have special functions concerned with health care technology; these are briefly described below.

The National Hospital Discharge Survey (NHDS) has collected data about discharges from nonfederal short-stay hospitals continuously since it began in 1964 (NCHS, 1980b). NHDS can provide a wide range of data on both trends in diagnoses associated with hospitalization and the treatments received by patients in hospitals. While the survey is designed primarily to produce national estimates it can also produce some estimates for the four major geographic regions of the country, as well as data by characteristics of hospitals such as type of ownership or number of beds.

Technology diffusion in hospitals has been rapid and extensive over the past few decades. New equipment and techniques are introduced, and old techniques are used differently or discarded (Russell, 1979). The NHDS is an excellent source of data for monitoring such trends.

NHDS data on deliveries by cesarean section show how surveys can detect and illuminate trends in certain procedures and diagnoses over the past decade (NCHS, 1980e). In 1970 cesareans were 5.5 percent of all deliveries; by 1978 the percentage was 15.2; in 1981 the NHDS reported 17.9 percent of all deliveries were by cesarean section (NCHS, 1983e). A report on hospital discharge diagnoses showed that in 1977 the discharge rate for sterlization of healthy females age 15–44 was over five times as great as in 1970. Most were for tubal sterilizations, usually by laparoscopy (NCHS, 1981a).

There also have been rapid changes in diagnostic tools and surgery for heart disease, including steady increases in cardiac catheterization, the use of angiograms, and bypass surgery (Grossman, 1981). Between 1979 and 1981 cardiac catheterization increased 97 percent for men 65 years of age and over and 34 percent for men 45 to 64 years of age. During the same period, coronary bypass surgery increased 27 percent for men 45 to 64 years of age (from 3.0 to 3.8 per 1,000) and 89 percent for older men (from 1.8 to 3.4 per 1,000) (NCHS, 1983c).

The NHDS has documented increases in lens extraction (cataract surgery) and in lens implantation following cataract surgery. Lens extraction among the elderly increased about 30 percent between 1979 and 1982; 57 percent of these procedures were accompanied by the insertion of a prosthetic lens in 1981, compared with 36 percent in 1979 (NCHS, 1980d).

The use of computerized axial tomography (CT scan) among hospitalized persons increased from 0.8 to 1.8 per 1,000 population between 1979 and 1981 (NCHS, 1983c).

The National Ambulatory Medical Care Survey, a survey of physicians in private office-based practice, began in 1973. Physicians selected into the NAMCS sample are asked to complete a patient record for each sampled patient seen during a 1-week survey period. That form includes information on the physician's diagnosis and on diagnostic services ordered or provided during the visit. Prior to this reporting period physicians are inducted into the survey by a brief interview that obtains information about their training and about characteristics of their practice (NCHS, 1980b). The survey does not, but could, include queries about the physician's knowledge, attitudes, accessibility, and use of specified types of technologies. In 1980 and 1981, a special supplement on drug therapy was added to the NAMCS patient record after several feasibility tests and pretests. The drug data were coded using a system of therapeutic categories based on the Pharmacologic-Therapeutic Classification of the American Society of Hospital Pharmacists (NCHS, 1980d). A national estimate of 679,593,000 drug mentions (a physician's record of a pharmaceutical agent ordered or provided for the purpose of prevention, diagnosis, or treatment) resulted from the 1980 survey.

The survey also produces a listing of the 100 agents most frequently utilized by physicians in office practice (NCHS, 1983b). Periodic supplements of this type would permit study of changes in the use of certain types of medication. Followback surveys of NCHS also contribute to the measurement of technology diffusion. For a sample of registered births and deaths, considerable additional information is sought from various sources, including hospitals where care was received and physicians who gave care to the sampled person. The first National Mortality Survey covered a sample of deaths in 1961 (NCHS, 1983a). Since that time NCHS had conducted several mortality and natality surveys and an infant mortality survey.

The National Natality Survey of events occurring in calendar year 1980 includes an oversampling of low-birth-weight infants and a sample of fetal deaths. This survey shows how the followback mechanism can provide a range of data relevant to the use of health care technology. For sampled infants, information was requested from both the mothers and the providers of medical care (primarily the physician who delivered the baby) about prenatal care, delivery, and postpartum care. Emphasis was given to whether, during the 12-month period prior to the delivery, the mother had received x rays; ultrasound; thyroid tests; scans or uptakes (nuclear medicine); sonograms or deep heat diathermy; or microwave, short-wave, or radio-frequency treatments. Mothers were asked to identify the providers of each of these examinations or treatments, and the providers were asked for more specific information about the exact type of procedure, why it was performed, and the date and place where it was performed. Information is available about the delivery, including drugs or surgical procedures used to induce or maintain labor, type of delivery, anesthetics, and condition of the infant at birth such as the Apgar score at 1 and 5 minutes for live births. These data, in conjunction with demographic and socioeconomic information from the mother's questionnaire, her health habits during pregnancy, and information on many aspects of pre- and postnatal care make this survey uniquely valuable for study of the ways that health care technology is used and how it affects the outcome of pregnancy and delivery.

Data from the survey show that in 1980 about 13 percent of mothers received an x ray during pregnancy; nearly one-third of all pregnant women received at least one ultrasound examination; 29 percent of mothers 35 years of age and over received amniocentesis; and almost one-half of mothers in the survey received fetal monitoring (NCHS, 1983f).

Similar surveys of deaths are in the early planning stages, including development of sample design specifications that deal with specific diagnoses listed on the death certificate. The samples for past National Mortality Surveys conducted by NCHS have been straightforward, without focus on any particular cause of death, but a future survey could be designed from a different perspective.

None of the surveys previously mentioned collect data on costs or charges needed to measure the cost and impact of medical technology. Two recent surveys were specifically designed to obtain information on health care utilization, the expenditures associated with medical care, and the sources of payment for the care received. The first of these—the National Medical Care Expenditure Survey (NMCES)—was conducted in 1977 by the National Center for Health Services (NCHSR) in collaboration with NCHS (NCHS, 1981b). A somewhat modified version—the National Medical Care Utilization and Expenditure Survey (NMCUES)—was conducted in 1980 by NCHS in collaboration with the Health Care Financing Administration (HCFA) (NCHS, 1983d).

The National Medical Care Utilization and Expenditure Survey (NMCUES) was a longitudinal panel study, having five contacts with each household in the initial sample. The contacts were spread over a period of about 15 months in order to obtain information for the entire calendar year. Each interview asked about health care received in a variety of locations, including dentists' offices, emergency rooms, hospital outpatient departments, and physicians' offices. Information was obtained about the type of provider, the reason for the visit, the specific condition—if any—for which the visit was made, whether certain kinds of tests were done, the total charge for the visit, and expected sources of payment for the bill. Information not available at the time of the first report about the health care encounter was sought at subsequent interviews.

Analyses of specific conditions or groups of conditions will examine the total range of services received and the expenses associated with those services. The NMCES and NMCUES data should go a long way toward answering questions about charges for various types of services and how those charges are paid.

Other NCHS surveys produce data that can be used to assess medical technology, or they could be modified to enable such use. A guiding tenet of the NCHS is that the statistical data it gathers should be available to all interested users as promptly as resources permit. The principal forms used are published reports, special and unpublished tabulations, and public use data tapes. NCHS policy is to release public use data tapes from all its surveys in a manner that will not in any way compromise the confidentiality guaranteed to the respondents who supplied the original data (NCHS, 1980a). These public use data tapes are a major resource for analyses by health services researchers, including those involved in technology assessment.

The potential uses for technology assessments of NCHS sample surveys and the associated data collection methodologies are great despite the limitations outlined above and the lack of any systematic effort to assess needs and capabilities. **There is considerable interest in making connections between sample surveys and controlled experiments in an attempt to combine the generalizability that surveys offer with the accuracy that experiments offer. This suggestion seems especially pertinent to longitudinal surveys (Boruch, 1985).**

Health Care Financing Administration Data

Through its administration of the Medicare and Medicaid programs, the Health Care Financing Administration routinely receives data on such items as its beneficiary population, providers certified to deliver care to the beneficiaries, the use of services, and reimbursements to providers. These materials can be studied by either census (100 percent) methods or sample methods. While HCFA generally uses census methods, these files are described here because we believe that many nongovernment investigators will prefer to use samples.

The Medicare Statistical System (MSS) was designed to provide data to measure and evaluate the operation and effectiveness of the Medicare program. The statistical system is a by-product of three centrally maintained administrative record systems:

Health Insurance Master File contains a record on each person who is enrolled in Medicare. Data elements for each individual include the Medicare claim number, age, sex, race, place of residence, and reason for entitlement. This file provides enrollment statistics and denominators for calculating all Medicare utilization rates.

Provider of Service File contains information on each hospital, skilled nursing facility home health agency, independent laboratory, or other institutional provider that has been certified to participate in the program.

Utilization File contains Medicare billing information, including such data elements as copayments, deductibles, and spells of illness. For a sample of bills the MSS obtains more extensive information, for example, the nature of the hospital episode (diagnostic and surgical procedures), for approximately 20 percent of the hospital bills.

Because each record in the utilization file contains the beneficiary's claim number and the provider's identification number, utilization records can be matched to enrollment and provider records to determine population-based statistics or provider-based statistics. These record systems are extremely large: about 12 million inpatient hospital bills, 30 million outpatient hospital bills, and 150 million physician payment records were received and processed in 1981 (Lave, 1983).

HCFA data bases have not been widely disseminated, but they have been utilized by HCFA grantees and contractors. An example of an innovative use of Medicare data for assessing variations in health outcomes is Wennberg's analysis of small area variations in health care delivery in Vermont (Wennberg and Gittelsohn, 1973). The use of HCFA data undoubtedly will grow and may be bolstered by the development of general purpose public use tapes that provide summary information on Medicare enrollment and utilization.

Capabilities and Limitations of Sample Surveys

Sample surveys have many potential advantages over studies based on complete enumeration. If the universe surveyed is large or geographically widespread, sampling can be economical. Nonresponses can usually be handled more effectively, the data can be processed more quickly, and the quality of responses can almost always be improved because of the greater opportunity for individual handling of problems in smaller data sets. These advantages are not always realized, however; and each reported survey must be studied in detail by prospective users to determine whether the data really will serve their needs. The national sample survey data collected and produced by the NCHS and HCFA are useful and reliable sources for some aspects of technology assessment, provided their scope and limitations are understood. For example, NHDS data are abstracted from the face sheets of medical records; any diagnostic or therapeutic information in the medical record that is not cited on the face sheet is lost to analysis.

NCHS national sample survey data are designed to measure the rate of diffusion, cost, and medical impact of medical technologies when they are reasonably well established and in general use. When new, experimental, or emerging technologies are first introduced there is little impact that these data programs can measure, but as they become established they are incorporated into various classification and coding schemes, and there is a chance to quantify their effects.

The capacity to characterize the recipients of a given procedure in terms of additional variables is perhaps the major advantage of surveys over routine record sources. For instance, it was possible on the basis of NCHS's 1980 National Natality Survey to compare the characteristics of pregnant women on whom amniocentesis, ultrasound, and electronic fetal monitoring were performed (NCHS, 1983c). It is also possible in principle to examine combinations of procedures. This could potentially increase our understanding of the diffusion process and affect policy regarding technology transfer.

Data now are limited by the coding schemes used. Current Procedures Terminology (CPT) is generally used in the United States to code procedures for reimbursement purposes. Diagnoses, surgical operations, and procedures may be coded to the most recent revision of the International Classification of Diseases (ICD), which permits comparison with similar data from other countries. The approximately decennial revision in the ICD may damage the comparability of data over time, although periodic changes in code systems are essential to permit introduction of new terms and procedures that reflect changes in the delivery of medical care. Efforts are made to preserve the same code designations, but special problems are associated with the recent change from coding procedures according to surgical speciality to coding based on the various body systems. When the NHDS made the conversion to ICD-9-CM beginning with the 1979 data year, NCHS increased the maximum number of diagnoses carried on its data tapes from five to seven; similarly, the maximum number of procedures and surgical operation codes assigned was increased from three to four.

The type and character of respondents profoundly affect the design of and instructions for survey questionnaires. Thus, survey of members of the general population must be limited to the level of medical detail that most lay persons can provide in response to survey questionnaires. Lay respondents may in some instances provide information of little value for the assessment of medical technologies.

The Office of Technology Assessment (1980a) recently polled data analysts who conduct cost-effectiveness and cost-benefit analyses of various health care technologies and found that unmet data and information needs were considered a significant problem by all respondents. Information needs more often were reported to affect the cost of a given study than such factors as complexity of the problem being studied or the stage of development of the technology (NCHCT, 1981). Thus, investigators need to rely on primary data collected for other purposes as well as on secondary data analyses.

Strengthening Uses of Sample Surveys

The scarcity of resources for the design of new specialized surveys is likely to require that established national sample surveys continue to be a major resource for monitoring trends in the incidence, prevalence, diffusion, cost, and medical impact of technologies in clinical use. Several changes could strengthen the use of these surveys for technology assessment.

Sample surveys are conducted by many public and private organizations for a variety of uses (Mullner et al., 1983). Standardization of data elements across programs would facilitate cross-survey comparisons. The National Committee on Vital and Health Statistics sponsored the development of three minimum data sets dealing with hospital discharges, ambulatory medical care, and long-term health care (NCHS, 1980c,f; 1981c). These may form a useful beginning for development of a broader collection of minimum data sets for the multiple data collection systems needed in technology assessment.

Data systems in the public and private sectors could be utilized more fully. Analysis of existing data, if adequate for technology assessment, is generally less expensive than collection of new data. Existing national sample surveys might be expanded, where feasible, to assist in monitoring trends in health status, medical care utilization, and health outcomes. Questions could be added to existing continuing surveys; information can sometimes be inexpensively "piggy-backed" onto ongoing sample surveys. Sample surveys can often be used for follow-up studies, in which a specific population group is studied again, and for followback surveys, in which the past experience of a group is analyzed.

A major problem in monitoring the diffusion of new technologies is the fixed character of most classifications and coding schemes. It takes several years for classifications to be modified so that new procedures can be distinguished from older procedures. **A mechanism needs to be developed to make classification more responsive to emerging technologies.**

Health data are collected by a variety of organizations. These data could be shared more widely among agencies, often without introducing problems of confidentiality, if other problems of data compatability and record linkage can be solved. **To encourage sharing of data, methods should be developed that will increase the capacity to integrate data sets.** Linkage of data files should be encouraged when there is a good reason to believe that the results of a specific linkage program will be sufficiently complete for the purpose and that biases and other limitations of linkage studies will not be so severe as to vitiate results.

Longitudinal surveys, in which a sample of the population is followed through time, can record systematically changes in health status and can be useful for technology assessment. Careful evaluation of the health of persons in these samples and their use of drugs, surgical procedures, and other medical technologies could be useful for technology assessment.

EPIDEMIOLOGIC METHODS*

In this section will be discussed several kinds of data sources, including registers and data bases, surveillance systems, and sample surveys. Data from these sources are rarely usable in their original form to assess technologies. Analytic methods, often designated collectively as epidemiology, may be applied to data from these and other sources.

Epidemiologic methods, narrowly defined, deal with diseases as they are observed in defined populations. An extended definition of epidemiologic methods might take in the entire range of observational studies of such things as rates of disease incidence or mortality, causes and risk factors for specific conditions, characteristics of screening and diagnostic tools (including sensitivity and specificity), the efficacy of preventive measures, follow-up, and outcome. Epidemiology is essentially an observational science; intervention by an investigator is uncommon, and controlled intervention is rare. Thus in most instances in which these methods apply, bias in data is a greater threat to interpretation than is random error. Epidemiology (in contrast to clinical medicine) is not ordinarily concerned with identified individuals except as the identification is needed to match records or assign persons to the right population group.

Clinical studies of the effects of treatment share much with epidemiologic methods in the overlap of problems, methods of attack, analytic tools, and problems of interpretation. However, epidemiology itself is not ordinarily concerned with the responses of a disease to treatment, although more general responses of the host (e.g., increased susceptibility to other diseases) may be included.

Epidemiologic investigations of acute illness (infections, trauma, or acute chemical toxicity) are quite different from those of chronic or long-delayed illness (e.g., cancer, chronic obstructive lung disease, or schizophrenia). The differences are not only in the problems studied but include the methods of research study, the nature of various impediments to sound conclusions, the kinds of risk factors including past applications of technologies, and the means for evaluating those technologies. Examples can be found in the range of differences between studies of acute organ damage by some chemical substance and studies of the carcinogenicity of the same substance.

Another important dichotomy separates input variables from output variables. In-

* This section was drafted by John C. Bailar III.

put variables, somewhat loosely defined, are those observed prior to some effect, event, or use of a technology to be studied and might be more roughly labeled *causes and correlates of causes*. Output variables are those observed after the use of a technology or other intervention or event and include at least all those features that are *effects*. Thus the definitions of input and output variables are somewhat broader than the usual concepts of independent and dependent variables.

To illustrate, consider a study of a new treatment for hypertension. Input variables include such things as the nature, causes, severity, and pretreatment complications of the disease; age, race, occupation, and other demographic variables; concomitant illnesses and family history; and, of course, the treatment itself. Output variables include such things as vital status and survival time, change in the disease process, and complications of treatment.

Three very broad categories of epidemiologic methods will be discussed: cohort studies, case-control studies, and cross-sectional studies.

Both cohort studies and case-control studies focus on relations between input and output variables, but differ in a critical aspect of the way subjects are selected for investigation: in cohort studies, selection of subjects is based on input variables, while in case-control studies, selection is based on output variables (White and Bailar, 1956). Thus one might examine the relation between polio immunization and the later incidence of polio by:

- comparing a sample or series of persons immunized with a similar sample not immunized, to see how many in each group develop polio (a cohort study, because the groups are defined on the basis of treatment—an input variable);
- comparing a sample or series of new polio patients with a control series free of such infection to see how many in each group had been immunized (a case-control study, because the two groups are defined by the presence or absence of polio—an output variable).

Critical to both approaches is the concept of cause and effect, which implies the observation of or reporting of change over time—change in the patient, in a disease, in physiologic or biochemical features, or even in features of whole populations or social milieus.

Cross-sectional studies are rather different and not as precisely defined. Their characteristic feature is the search for *correlations* from which inferences (including cause-effect inferences) can be made, rather than the search for change over time. Studies of many familial diseases are cross-sectional; so are many population-based studies of disease screening.

Some epidemiologic studies are strictly cross-sectional and do not involve change, but do permit strong inferences about change (i.e., cause and effect) and may be treated as if they were ordinary cohort or case-control studies (Bailar et al., 1984). An example is the reported correlation (Needleman, 1979, 1985) between behavioral changes in school children and the lead content of deciduous teeth, which are presumed to reflect lead levels some years earlier when the teeth were formed.

Uses of Epidemiologic Methods

Cohort Studies Cohort-based epidemiologic studies can play a substantial role in technology evaluation. Consider the following example:

Sherins et al. (1978) reported an unexpectedly high incidence of gonadal dysfunction in African boys who had received cytotoxic drugs as treatment for Burkitt's lymphoma. The study was strictly observational; there was no treatment protocol, no parallel control group, no prior hypothesis, not even a well-defined population from which the subjects were a describable sample. Various features of the report, however, suggested that the observation was quite solidly based and established a previously unrecognized complication of an important drug technology that is used, with variations, for many other neoplastic diseases. This is considered a cohort study because subjects were selected on the basis of input variable (age, sex, and geographic location as well as disease and treatment) rather than because they did or did not have known gonadal dysfunction. The study had no internal controls, but the authors cited results in untreated, well North American boys (presumably supported by the author's own knowledge of physiology in adolescent Africans) to establish that there was indeed a high risk.

Case-Control Studies Case-control studies of medical technologies are often an outgrowth of the unstructured observation of something odd. If the oddity is sufficiently striking, there may be little need for an explicit control group in the initial report on some possible technologic effect. The function of controls at this initial stage of identifying and reporting a possible problem may be filled by earlier case series, reports in the literature, or even common knowledge. However, more definitive work, including quantitative estimates of such things as the frequency or degree of effect, will nearly always demand careful attention to controls.

For example, Herbst et al. (1971) reported a remarkable cluster of cases of a very rare disease (adenocarcinoma of the vagina in adolescents). They also reported data for a control group and established that the occurrence of the disease was closely linked to maternal use of diethylstilbestrol (DES) before the offspring were born. This initial identification of a technologic effect was based on sampling an output variable (all subjects had cancer; the controls did not), not the relevant input variable (DES exposure). Later, more tightly designed studies confirmed the association and left little doubt that it was cause and effect. Fortunately, only a very small proportion of "DES daughters" developed the cancer—a quantitative result that could not have been established by Herbst's original approach and was in fact unexpectedly reassuring.

Cross-Sectional Studies The object of cross-sectional studies is to understand some state of nature rather than to study changes in state. Examples of cross-sectional studies include the identification and description of new (or newly recognized) diseases, determinations of disease severity or extent, establishing normal ranges for laboratory tests, and investigation of pathophysiologic mechanisms. Although data over time may be collected in such studies, change is used only as a tool of investigation; it is only when change itself is the object of study that the work is classified as cohort or case-control.

Cross-sectional studies are commonly used in the evaluation of medical technologies. For example, new techniques for the diagnosis and staging of disease are nearly all of this type. Re et al. (1978) provide an illustration. Narrowing of a renal artery is sometimes a cause of hypertension; this cause is likely when plasma renin activity (PRA) is at least 1.5 times as high in blood from one renal vein as in blood from the other. Re et al. (1978) proposed a modification in technology (administration of a substance called CEI) to increase the sensitivity of the test. They found that the mean PRA ratio was 2.94 before and 8.36 after the administration of CEI in seven unselected patients with known renal artery disease, while in patients without that condition CEI changed the mean PRA from 1.99 to 1.17. The authors conclude that CEI increases the diagnostic accuracy of the PRA test, but they are careful not to imply that their study is definitive.

Capabilities and Limitations of Epidemiologic Methods

Epidemiologic methods have many uses in technology assessment besides the identification and characterization of health outcomes. These include studies of:

- the prevalence of use of technologies, such as surgery, in various types of communities;
- the prevalence of various health outcomes that may be technologically related, such as the Reye Syndrome, or complications of elective abortion;
- the prevalence of disease (e.g., patient load), risk factors, or other input variables, without study of output variables, such as a survey to determine potential demand for an artificial heart;
- the distribution of availability of a technology or of its actual use and rate of diffusion;
- data on technology-related costs or charges.

Although these items may have some evaluative uses in themselves, results are more likely to be passed on to other evaluation methods discussed elsewhere in this book (e.g., cost-effective analysis/cost-benefit analysis).

Epidemiologic studies of health technologies rarely are planned before a specific need is noted, usually in relation to concerns about some undesirable effect. Most are attempts to gather information after astute clinical observation, or other methods discussed elsewhere in this book, have shown that there may be a problem.

Epidemiologic assessments are done most often in academia, sometimes in government, but rarely by manufacturers, providers, or third-party payers—health maintenance organizations (HMOs) being a strong exception. This may introduce bias in selection of topics and specific methods, types of patients available, etc.

Epidemiology used for technology assessment can have the capability of: (1) exploiting populations that come to hand; (2) derivation and testing of inferences (see, e.g., U.S. Public Health Service, [1964] for a thoughtful discussion); and (3) providing more satisfactory modes of post-marketing surveillance.

On the other hand, epidemiologic findings are often straitened because (1) data often are limited, biased, and in inappropriate forms, sometimes because the data are a by-product of a process that is conducted largely for other purposes (such as death certification); (2) study performance may be damaged by problems of access to data (concerns about confidentiality, etc.), the chronic shortage of trained epidemiologists, and perhaps other structural problems not related to particular diseases, particular patient groups, or particular technologies; (3) good epidemiology is almost always expensive and time consuming.

Strengthening Uses of Epidemiologic Methods

The greatest opportunity may lie simply in extending the application of epidemiologic methods to what are called outcome studies. The aim of such studies is to learn about patient status after considerable time has elapsed following treatment. Topics include matters like 1-year survivorship after a certain operation or after discharge from intensive care or coronary care units. Such data are valuable in making individual decisions and in designing health care policy. Surprising findings can arise when such studies are done (Garber et al., 1984; Wennberg, 1984). More outcome studies are needed. The methodology for outcome studies is at a relatively early stage of development and more research will be needed. **There is a need for faster, easier, less expensive, and more accurate measurement of many kinds of outcomes (e.g., the carcinogenic effects of drugs or**

the outcome of treatment for many kinds of chronic diseases).

Problems and gaps both in present data and present applications should be better identified, and ways to improve the techniques and uses of epidemiologic evaluation for purposes of health technology assessment (new knowledge, new organization, etc.) should be developed.

Epidemiologists have been in critically short supply for at least 30 years; the supply of those trained for (and interested in) technology assessment may be even tighter (National Academy of Sciences, 1978, 1981). Efforts to increase the supply of epidemiologists should be expanded.

SURVEILLANCE*

Surveillance was widely used by health departments in the nineteenth century,† but modern nationwide surveillance was substantially strengthened some 30 years ago when the Centers for Disease Control (CDC) began its efforts to monitor and control outbreaks of infectious disease (American Public Health Association [APHA], 1981; Bell and Smith, 1982; CDC, 1982a; White and Axnick, 1975). A national morbidity reporting system is based on data forwarded from the states to CDC for aggregation. There are detailed surveillance procedures and report forms of some 30 diseases using a variety of sources. Some of these efforts are laboratory based, such as identification of strains of salmonella. Some are hospital acquired infections. Some are practitioner-based, such as the reporting by neurologists of Guillain-Barré neuropathy following swine flu immunization. No direct information is available on the costs and benefits of such programs; indeed it would be difficult to approach such issues in this manner (see below). However, certain benefits of the surveillance system have recently been summarized (Kimball, 1980).

Reports of morbidity and mortality are generated weekly, monthly, and annually by the CDC. Their weekly reports have worldwide distribution as the Morbidity and Mortality Weekly Report (MMWR).

Surveillance is the continuing scrutiny of the occurrence, spread, and course of a disease for aspects that may be pertinent to its effective control (APHA, 1981). Surveillance traditionally has been associated with communicable disease epidemiology, but now it is applied to noncommunicable diseases, health indicators, environmental and occupational hazards, and other health problems and conditions. Included in disease surveillance are the systematic collection and evaluation of a broad range of epidemiologic data, such as (1) morbidity and mortality reports; (2) results of special field investigations; (3) laboratory reports; and (4) data concerning the availability, use, and untoward effects of a variety of substances and devices used in disease control, such as vaccines, drugs, and surgical procedures. The concept and practice of surveillance can be extended from standard features of health and disease to medical practices, such as surveillance of surgical procedures or vaccine use, of adverse reactions to drugs, and of health risk factors such as smoking or environmental hazards.

Surveillance may be passive or active. Passive, voluntary surveillance puts the burden of reporting on health care providers or institutions, who, as cases occur, respond by mail or telephone to a health department or other central repository of surveillance data. Such voluntary reporting may be useful but provides incomplete data biased by the individual reporter's experience.

Active surveillance, which might apply to the same disease or practice, supple-

* This section is based on material prepared by Jeffrey Koplan and John C. Bailar III.

† John Garunt reported surveillance using the bills of mortality in the seventeenth century.

ments or replaces passive reporting with systematic, specific inquiries directed to persons or institutions that may be able to supply data. For example, passive surveillance of adverse reactions to rabies vaccine might involve a periodic flyer to practicing physicians, along with a package insert asking them to report such information to the manufacturer, state health department, or a federal health agency. Active surveillance might involve tracking by state health officials of all doses of rabies vaccine distributed and periodic telephone calls to physicians and/or patients asking for specific information on circumstances of use and adverse reactions. Systematic reporting is likely to be more comprehensive, better standardized, and better able to detect previously unknown effects (good or bad), but it requires a more expensive and complex system.

Under the postmarketing surveillance program of the Food and Drug Administration (FDA) for drugs approved for general use, the sponsor is required to forward to FDA any reports of adverse effects of the drug. Additional information about adverse drug reactions comes to the FDA from several sources. These sources include reports from physicians, pharmacists, and hospitals; a monthly literature review; studies in special populations (largely, but not entirely, passive surveillance); registries and data bases; and the World Health Organization (WHO).

Uses of Surveillance

Evaluation of technologies such as vaccines has always relied considerably on surveillance methods. Even when the technique has been evaluated independently, as by a randomized controlled trial (RCT), surveillance provides for continued assessment of the vaccine and the disease it prevents. The reporting of measles, combined with reports on the use of measles vaccine and possible adverse reactions, permits a quantitative assessment of vaccine efficacy and safety (CDC, 1982a; White and Axnick, 1975).

Surveillance has an important role in supplementing clinical studies of rare events that may not be observed in studies with modest sample sizes. For example, if a drug therapy causes blurred vision in 1 person per 1,000 persons treated, a clinical trial including 200 treated patients has only a .18 probability of observing one or more such events. Increasing the sample to 2,000 raises this probability to .86 and a sample of 5,000 to .993. Thus one argument for postmarketing surveillance is that comparative premarketing trials of modest size may not detect rare but important adverse reactions, whereas continued study after the drug is released for general use increases the probability of detection (OTA, 1982a).

Reporting may not be as rigorous as during a clinical trial, so that an adverse event that occurs to 1 individual in 1,000 might be properly reported less than half the time. A factor of one-half would affect the numbers given above as follows:

	Probability of Observing at Least One Adverse Drug Reaction		
Sample size	200	2,000	5,000
Full reporting	.18	.86	.993
Fifty percent reporting	.10	.63	.918

Whether omissions are more or less frequent than 50 percent seems not to be known. Furthermore, the incomplete and perhaps inaccurate reporting of adverse events, while unlikely to establish a causal link to the therapy, can increase the vigilance of the medical community and initiate more extensive and more reliable studies (Finney, 1965, 1966).

Postmarketing surveillance information may lead the FDA to remove a drug from the market or constrain its advertising or labeling. In recent years FDA received an average of about 11,500 reports of adverse events per year, with 71 percent reported through manufacturers.

When adverse drug effects are long delayed, some form of postmarketing study may be required, because few randomized clinical trials can be continued for many years. More generally, methods other than clinical trials are used to detect many kinds of adverse outcomes (Bell and Smith, 1982).

Surveillance, even in the crude form of national incidence figures, can offer insight into changes in the epidemiology of a disease, including changes caused by effective disease control measures and programs.

Assessment of a vaccine, drug, or device requires data on frequency of use, characteristics of persons treated, frequency and types of adverse sequelae, etc., all of which are amenable to collection by surveillance methods. Thus, disease surveillance monitored the progress of the World Health Organization's successful smallpox eradication program at the same time that it identified where cases were occurring and improved the targeting of control activities (Foege, 1971).

Surveillance can provide data useful for decision analysis, including cost-benefit and cost-effectiveness analysis (CBA/CEA). Benefit-risk studies of smallpox vaccination based on surveillance of vaccine use and reactions and worldwide disease occurrence led to the conclusion and subsequent federal government recommendation that routine smallpox vaccination was no longer warranted (Lane, 1969). Recent studies of CBA/CEA of vaccination programs for measles (White and Axnick, 1975), pertussis (Koplan et al., 1979), mumps (Koplan and Preblud, 1982), and hepatitis (Mulley et al., 1982) have used surveillance data for disease incidence, disease complication rates, rates of vaccine usage, and rates of adverse vaccine reactions.

Evaluations of screening procedures also require estimates of disease prevalence. For example, routine surveillance has provided data crucial for assessments of prenatal cytogenetic screening (Hook et al., 1981), maternal serum alpha-fetoprotein screening for neural tube defects (Layde et al., 1979), screening for rubella immunity (Farber and Finkelstein, 1979), and lead screening (Berwick and Komaroff, 1982).

As the scope of epidemiology has broadened, so has the subject matter found suitable for surveillance. The Boston Collaborative Drug Project collects data on the uses and adverse effects of various pharmaceuticals for use in epidemiologic studies of benefits and risks (Boston Collaborative Drug Surveillance Program, 1973). Surveillance of techniques for contraception and pregnancy termination has led to increased information about their benefits and risks (CDC, 1979), such as recognition of the association between a particular intrauterine device (the Dalkon shield) and pelvic inflammatory disease. Programs designed to identify and modify medical procedures associated with high rates of nosocomial (hospital-fostered) infections have relied on surveillance methodologies (Dixon, 1978; Haley et al., 1980). Surveillance of environmental and occupational hazards and disease, including injuries, is helpful in the assessment of technologies, including those aimed at controlling environmental hazards and reducing illness and injuries in the workplace (U.S. Consumer Product Safety Commission, 1982).

The surveillance of local and regional trends in the use of surgical procedures, such as surgical sterilizations, can raise questions to be answered by more directed analytic studies. Data from the National Survey of Family Growth and from the Centers for Disease Control (1982b) have been used to estimate the cumulative prevalence of hysterectomy and tubal sterilization among women of reproductive age in the United States. The cumulative prevalence of tubal sterilization for women aged

15–44 years more than doubled from 1971 to 1978, and the rate at least tripled for woman under 30 years old. Proportionate increases in the cumulative prevalence of hysterectomy were not as great, but by 1978, 19 percent of women 40–44 years old had undergone hysterectomy.

Although the main methods for post-marketing surveillance are cohort studies, case-control studies, and voluntary reporting by physicians, Wennberg has proposed some additional types of population studies that use insurance claims and hospital discharges. He and his colleagues use such data to study per capita use of procedures, hospital expenditures, use of beds and personnel, and outcomes of care in various subpopulations of a state or region (Wennberg and Gittelsohn, 1973; Wennberg et al., 1980; Wennberg, 1981; Vermont Health Utilization Survey, unpublished report, 1973). They used surveillance methods to show that rates of tonsillectomy and adenoidectomy varied across 32 hospital areas in Rhode Island, Maine, and Vermont by a factor of 6, while hysterectomy varied by 3.6, prostatectomy by 4, and herniorrhaphy by about 1.5. The point is not that reductions are required, because a comparison of rates does not in itself tell whether the high rates provide corresponding health benefits, but rather that such large variations in usage deserve study and explanation. When physicians become aware of such variations their practice may change. Gittlesohn and Wennberg (1977) found that in the highest-rate area of Vermont, the cumulated rate of tonsillectomy during childhood dropped from 65 percent to 8 percent when the Vermont Medical Society provided a new information program for local physicians. Earlier studies by Lembcke (1956) and Dyke et al. (1974) showed similar effects from surveillance on the number of hysterectomies in Canada.

Such methods also can be applied to study the costs, health benefits, and mortality associated with various policies about the use of procedures. For example, in the United States a strategy of low use of prostatectomy has been projected to lead to 1,900 deaths annually while a high use strategy would lead to 6,800, a ratio of about 3.6 (Wennberg, 1981).

Surveillance also can be used to study longer-term survival and thus to contribute information about the risks of various medical procedures. Wennberg proposes using insurance claims data as a kind of surveillance mechanism to study rates of complications. For example, Schaffarzick et al. (1973) found that various types of complications following intraocular lens transplant were resolved in 42 percent by lens removal alone, in 9 percent by lens removal and replacement, and 50 percent without lens removal.

Some new and existing technologies might be usefully evaluated in a surveillance system. Although maternal serum alpha-fetoprotein appears to be a valuable screening test for neural tube defects, its performance in the field could be better assessed by developing a surveillance system in which laboratory accuracy and standards (including false positives and false negatives), distribution of services, patient follow-up, interpretation of results, and actions taken are all monitored in a regular and systematic manner. The recently available hepatitis B virus vaccine is being evaluated by surveillance directed toward determining both its efficacy and any adverse effects (Wennberg, 1981).

Capabilities and Limitations of Surveillance

Surveillance mechanisms may be as carefully designed and controlled as, for example, the RCT, but surveillance is intended to serve different functions, including a role in disease control. Skilled staff can institute surveillance on a routine basis relatively quickly, and surveillance can provide data useful for technology assessment from diverse geographical areas and over long periods of time.

Jick et al. (1979) and Remington (1976) believe that more general mechanisms are both needed and feasible. Finney (1965) has outlined many aspects of a good monitoring system.

Although surveillance data often are incomplete, they can be used to evaluate disease trends if the manner of data collection is consistent and variations in the completeness of reporting are small. When the reporting fraction varies over time, conclusions drawn from reported trends can be erroneous. During the World Health Organization's Smallpox Eradication Program, graphs of smallpox incidence revealed peaks that reflected improved surveillance and the reporting of cases that previously went unreported rather than an increase in incidence (Foege et al., 1971). Similarly, changes in disease definitions, professional interest and activity (reporting physicians, clinics, etc.), and incentives (economic, political, social) can influence disease reporting to create spurious trends in disease incidence. A map showing the incidence of syphilis by state could reflect differences in such matters as case-finding activity, availability of public clinic facilities, program priorities, and reporting practices, as well as actual differences in incidence (CDC, 1982a).

Passive surveillance systems usually provide information at little cost, but they may be neither timely nor accurate and have problems of underreporting and ascertainment bias. A passive surveillance system in Washington, D.C., failed to detect an epidemic of diarrheal disease caused by a drug-resistant strain of *Shigella sonnei* (Kimball et al., 1980).

Strengthening Uses of Surveillance

Various ways to improve postmarketing surveillance have been suggested (IMS America Ltd., 1978). For example, the Joint Commission on Prescription Drug Use recommended that comprehensive postmarketing drug surveillance be developed for the United States to detect serious adverse events that occur more often than 1 in 1,000 patients and that methods be developed to detect rarer adverse events and delayed events as well as to evaluate benefits. It proposed a private, nonprofit center to aid in these developments.

One possibility is to divide the nation into geographic regions and to release new drugs and other technologies to some regions and not others, recognizing in the analysis the possibility of region-to-region variations in frequency of use for various purposes (OTA, 1978a). This approach would fit well with some aspects of decentralized decision making (e.g., to states or to third-party carriers) but would have to be developed carefully to avoid problems of both practicality and ethics. The regions should be selected on logical grounds after careful study, rather than by simple contiguity (such as northeast, south, midwest, and west). The use of population samples in comparable regions could avoid having the whole country be the guinea pig for all drugs, and a means for rotating first marketing regions would assure that no one region would always bear the burden—or reap the benefits—of first marketing.

Postmarketing surveillance mechanisms for drugs are now extensive and rather well developed, and surveillance of major infectious disease appears adequate, but other areas lag behind. Substantial well-targeted surveillance systems might be quite helpful in such areas as iatrogenic illness, environmental health hazards, and long-term occupational risks. **Research is needed on ways to develop surveillance programs for such health problems in the context of budget restraints, growing concerns for individual privacy, and a general lack of incentives to develop and preserve the necessary records (e.g., of occupational exposure to potentially toxic chemicals).**

QUANTITATIVE SYNTHESIS METHODS—META-ANALYSIS*

Meta-analysis is a statistical method for obtaining quantitative answers to specific questions from collections of primary articles dealing with the same subject. From information obtained from each article, a synthesis is made which may produce a much stronger conclusion than any of the separate articles can provide.

There are many methods of combining information from several sources, and some of these are discussed here. Louis et al. (1985) give a large collection of examples of meta-analyses in public health.

Uses of quantitative synthesis methodology, especially for obtaining overall significance levels from groups of studies, have expanded steadily since the 1930s (e.g., Fisher, 1938, 1948; Mosteller, 1954; Pearson, 1938, 1950). Although applications of synthetic methods have been most prominent in the social sciences, the utility of these methods has been demonstrated in applications to data from medical trials. Certain of these applications are described as examples in this section.

Two models are often applied. The first supposes that each study measures the same true quantity, although with differing precision for the different studies. The second, usually more realistic, model assumes that each study estimates a somewhat different quantity, and that we want to assess the properties of the distribution of these different quantities. For example, the gains from a treatment might be different in different institutions, not just because of sampling errors, but because the characteristics of the patients and procedures at institutions differ. In spite of these differences, we want to know how well a treatment works when we aggregate across institutions, perhaps by averaging. The methods of Cochran (1954), Gilbert et al. (1977), and DerSimonian and Laird (1982) offer ways to estimate the means and the variability of the true effects.

There are several major benefits to quantitative synthesis of groups of trials. One is the increase in power, the ability to detect significant differences between treatment and control groups. The larger the sample size of patients (or other subjects) assumed to be drawn from a common distribution, the more likely that a certain effect will be detected as statistically significant.

A second benefit of quantitative synthesis is in obtaining improved estimates of effect size (usually defined as the difference in means divided by the standard deviation of single observations in the control group). Where effect sizes from each of a group of studies are assumed to be estimates of a single true effect size, averaging (or otherwise cumulating) effect sizes may provide a better estimate. A third benefit is in describing the form of a relationship. Combining studies provides more data or a greater range of data with which to describe relationships among variables. A fourth benefit is in detecting contradictions or discrepancies among groups of studies. Faced with a collection of studies in a particular area of research, a reviewer may analyze and compare subgroups of studies with, for instance, divergent findings to detect mediating factors of study design, treatment, context, measurement, or analysis that otherwise may not have appeared noteworthy (Pillemer and Light, 1980).

A prevalent criticism of quantitative synthesis of findings across trials is that there may exist unpublished negative (or zero-effect) trials that are not available for pooling, thus biasing the sample of trials included in the synthesis. In their quantitative synthesis of 345 studies on interpersonal effects (discussed below, under

* Clifford Goodman contributed this section.

"Cumulation of Significance Levels"), Rosenthal and Rubin (1978b) address this "file drawer" problem, demonstrating that the number of studies averaging a zero effect that would be required to reduce significant findings of that synthesis to insignificance ($p \geq 0.05$) is in the tens of thousands. Of course, the "file drawer" could have negative results as well.

Devine and Cooke (1983) compared results in journals and books with those of unpublished dissertations. They were studying reductions in length of hospital stay associated with patient education. They found the reductions in the published articles to be 17 percent while those in the unpublished articles were 14 percent. These published effects are a little larger than unpublished ones, as many critics expect.

Of course, studies should not be indiscriminately grouped for achieving the benefits of synthesis. As discussed throughout this section, the utility of these quantitative synthesis procedures requires making certain assumptions about similarities among grouped studies.

As is the case in any synthesis, the reviewer should specify the criteria for selection of studies included in the calculation of average effect size. The notion of scope of studies selected for synthesis is most important. If a wide-scope synthesis shows small differences among treatments designed to achieve the same effect, then hypotheses about differences among these treatments may be of minor importance. If the wide-scope synthesis shows large differences among treatments, then the synthesis can be applied on a smaller scope, so as to identify important differences among treatments.

Deciding which studies should be included in synthesis is a controversial topic. Glass (1976) and Hunter (1982) suggest that restriction of scope of studies considered for synthesis should be more topical than methodological. They suggest that when a reviewer excludes studies because of methodological deficiencies, valuable information may be wasted based on an assertion (of deficiency) which is not tested. Glass proposes grouping studies on some measure of quality as an alternative to dropping studies thought to be poorly done. If no relationship is found between quality and outcome, there is no reason to drop the studies with low measures of quality. If a relationship is found, then the reviewer and those agreeing with the definition of quality should weight the better studies more heavily (Glass, 1976; Rosenthal and Rubin, 1978b). For studies of psychotherapy, Glass notes that the "mass of 'good, bad, and indifferent' reports" show almost exactly the same results.

Glass's procedure for study selection has been met with criticism by those who favor rejection of studies which utilize insufficient methodological controls (Eysenck, 1978). Pillemer and Light (1980) note that agreement on what constitutes a good study, or which of two measurement procedures provides better information, may be difficult to attain. They suggest that, although it seems sensible to exclude studies that do not meet basic methodological standards, variation in study designs may be an asset, as follows.

> An analyst actually may want to insure that several major types of designs are represented, not to combine them blindly, but so that the outcomes can be compared. He or she may choose to stratify by type of design and/or general type of outcome measure, and then randomly select a number of studies from each stratum. This would build diversity.

Voting Methods

Several voting methods use tests to determine whether the result of a voting method is statistically significant (Hunter, 1982). One set of methods rests on the assumption that if a null hypothesis is true, then the correlation between treatment and effect is zero (or if significance levels are used, half would be expected to be larger than 0.50 and half smaller than 0.50). Statistical tests are used to determine whether the observed frequency of findings is significantly different from the 50/50 split of positive and negative correlations expected if the null hypothesis were true. Thus, if 12 of 15 results are consistent in either direction, the sign test indicates that results so rare as this occur by chance only 3.6 percent of the time (Rosenthal, 1978a). In another approach to vote testing, the proportion of positive significant findings can be tested against the proportion expected under the null hypothesis (typically, $p < 0.05$ or $p < 0.01$). These methods do not take magnitude of effect into account.

Another set of voting methods estimates effect sizes across studies, given the sample sizes of the studies used and the relative proportion of studies showing positive and negative effects (Hedges and Olkin, 1980). Confidence intervals may also be constructed around the overall effect sizes. These methods rest on the assumption that there is one true effect size for the treatment and that each study represents a sample of a distribution of measurements taken of the true effect size. (This assumption, and pooling effect sizes, is discussed below.) Because these voting methods for estimating effect size do not use information about effect-size magnitudes from individual studies, their estimates of overall effect size are not as good as certain methods that do make use of such information when it is available (Hunter, 1982).

Cumulation of Significance Levels (*p*-Values)

Several methods may be used to cumulate significance levels across studies to produce an overall significance level for the set of studies as a whole. This enables an overall test of a common null hypothesis, which is generally that the compared groups have for outcomes the same population mean. Where this overall significance level is small enough, it is concluded that the treatment effect exists. A primary reason for cumulating significance levels is to increase power. The increased sample size of combined studies may detect differences which could not be detected by individual studies.

Rosenthal (1978a) has summarized and provided guidelines for using nine methods for cumulating significance levels across studies. The major advantages of these techniques are their computational simplicity, low informational requirements, and few formal assumptions. The general caution offered by Rosenthal is that the studies should have tested the same directional hypothesis. In general, these methods are helpful when the individual studies can be considered independent and random samples. Where the studies exhibit a split of significantly positive and significantly negative study outcomes, there may be systematic differences between some studies and others. In the case of a conflict, combining these studies might lead to a false conclusion, e.g., of no effect when there are different true effects. When conflicts arise, an explanation should be sought, and other more sensitive methods should be used (Pillemer and Light, 1980).

Other Statistical Synthesis Procedures

A variety of other methods exist for statistically combining the results of studies.

Pillemer and Light (1980) summarize approaches for investigating interactions and comparing similarly labeled treatments that are more analytic than synthetic in that they pull together studies to search for variation and discrepancies. Rosenthal and Rubin (1978b) present a blocking technique involving comparisons of study outcomes using analysis of variance techniques. Light and Smith (1971) present a cluster approach where similarly labeled subgroups of studies must be screened before they are combined. The screening involves determining that the means, variances, relationships between dependent variables and covariates, subject-by-treatment interactions, and contextual effects are similar across subgroups. Once it is determined that subgroups are similar, or that proper statistical adjustments have been made to correct for explained differences, subgroups may be combined for overall tests (e.g., of significance). In addition to increasing confidence in overall findings, the major benefit of such approaches may be in identifying conflicts and discrepancies among studies which can provide clues to previously unknown variables moderating effects.

For summaries and reviews of the quantitative methods discussed in this section, see especially the collection in Light (1983) as well as Cook and Leviton (1980), Glass (1976), Glass et al. (1981), Hunter (1982), Jackson (1980), Light and Smith (1971), Pillemer and Light (1980), Rosenthal (1978a), Wortman (1983), and Wortman and Saxe (1982a). The review of validity considerations for the synthesis of medical evidence in these last two references is especially instructive.

The following example of synthesizing groups of studies by Baum et al. (1981) pools similar pairs of treatment and control groups progressively through time. This pooling has the effect of increasing overall sample size so that statistically significant differences between the pooled treatment and control groups are observed, where such differences had been observed in only a minority of the nonpooled groups.

Example of Synthesis A synthesis was performed on 26 randomized control trials, published between 1965 and 1980, comparing the effects of antibiotic prophylaxis and no-treatment controls on postoperative wound infection and mortality following colon surgery. The synthesis cumulated treatment and control groups, respectively, year by year. (Using a technique described in Gilbert et al. [1977], the authors found that the pooled estimate of the within-trial variance of the difference between infection rates was larger than the estimate among trials, and likewise for the estimates of the variance of the difference in death rates. Given these findings, the authors judged the degree of homogeneity among trials sufficient for pooling.) For each additional year, cumulative effect sizes (i.e., differences between treatment and control groups) were calculated, and confidence intervals were determined around each. As early as 1975, pooled data indicate a noteworthy and significant difference in effect size between antibiotic prophylaxis and no-treatment controls for both infection and mortality rates.

The authors used the Mantel-Haenszel (1959) procedure to test the difference in infection rate and in mortality rate between treated patients and untreated controls. The difference between both cumulative infection and mortality rates was analyzed by the Z-test for the difference between proportions, and 95 percent confidence intervals for the true difference were calculated. The 95 percent confidence intervals were a 14 ± 6 percent difference for infection (36 percent for the control group versus 22 percent for the treatment group) and a 6.7 ± 4.4 percent difference for mortality (11.2 percent for the control group versus 4.5 percent for the treatment group). By 1970, the significance level of the difference between treatment and control groups had reached $p < 0.01$, even though only one of the six studies conducted through 1970 was statistically significant.

Among the 14 RCTs conducted after 1975 (11 of which were significant), the 95 percent confidence intervals for the difference between treatment and control groups was 26 $\pm$ 6 percent for infection and 5.3 $\pm$ 3.4 percent for mortality. The synthesis made significant findings for mortality possible, since no single study had enough data to demonstrate a significant difference between treatment and control for mortality.

The authors conclude that continued use of no-treatment control groups is inappropriate and that future studies should compare various prophylaxes for the surgery, using a previously proven standard of comparison. The authors note that this poses a "scientific dilemma" of diminishing returns, because it would take a RCT with more than 1,000 patients to demonstrate a reduction in infection rate from 10 to 5 percent. Nevertheless, 1,019 patients were involved in the 12 trials studied for 1965–1975, and 1,033 were involved in the 14 trials studied for 1978–1980.

GROUP JUDGMENT METHODS*

Group judgment efforts for evaluating medical technologies reflect interests in bridging gaps and resolving disparity among research findings, defining state of the art, and establishing medical and payment policies. Since 1977, the National Institutes of Health Consensus Development Program has conducted 50 conferences on a wide variety of biomedical technologies. The Clinical Efficacy Assessment Project of the American College of Physicians has evaluated more than 60 medical procedures and tests since 1981. The Diagnostic and Therapeutic Technology Assessment Program of the American Medical Association was initiated in 1982 to answer questions regarding the safety and effectiveness of medical technologies. The Health Care Financing Administration, Blue Cross and Blue Shield Association and member plans, and other third-party payers have expert panels for resolving coverage issues.

Evidence from well-designed clinical studies is unavailable for certain drugs (some of those first used prior to 1962), medical devices, and most medical and surgical procedures. The scope even of the best clinical studies rarely touches upon matters of cost, cost-effectiveness, and social and other issues relevant to policymaking of health care delivery and payment. Most clinical and payment policies rely on the implicit consensus of standard and accepted practice. However, clinicians, payers, and others increasingly seek a more explicit consensus. Thus, for many new technologies, and some others that have questionable utility, they establish panels of experts to distill available evidence, add informed opinion, and render findings that will guide policy. These panels weigh, integrate, and interpret evidence, experiences, beliefs, and values and then formulate guidelines, recommendations, or other findings. The evidence may consist of a sparse patchwork of contradictory research results of varying quality. The technologies being assessed may be rapidly evolving. Panelists are subject to biases and errors of reasoning; experts and nonexperts alike are subject to oversimplification, empiricism, case-selection biases, incentives, and advocacy (Eddy, 1982).

The better group judgment efforts spell out their assumptions and identify inconsistencies, contradictions, and gaps in research. They provide participants the opportunity to learn from the perspectives and insights of others and have the means to disseminate their findings effectively. But they do not generate new scientific findings. (As discussed earlier in this chapter, some quantitative methods are available that, under specified conditions, may be used to combine research results to add precision to and strengthen significance of findings.) The finding of an expert panel that a procedure is "standard and accepted

* Clifford Goodman contributed this section.

practice" does not constitute new evidence of safety, efficacy, or cost-effectiveness.

This section describes two categories of group judgment methods. The first category includes two formal methods that have been applied in many fields, including health, and for which a considerable amount of literature describes methodology and applicability: the Delphi process and nominal group technique. The second category includes newer group methods designed specifically to develop documents for use by health practitioners and policymakers, e.g., NIH Consensus Development, Glaser's state-of-the-art process, and computerized knowledge bases.

Formal Group Methods

Delphi Technique The Delphi technique is an interactive survey process that uses controlled feedback to isolated, anonymous (to each other) participants. The process normally includes (1) obtaining anonymous opinions from members of an expert group by formal questionnaire or individual interview; (2) obtaining several rounds of systematic modifications/criticisms of the summarized anonymous feedback provided to the groups; (3) obtaining a group response by aggregation (often statistical) of individual opinions on the final round.

The Delphi technique was developed by the Rand Corporation to integrate expert opinion in making predictions for national defense needs (Dalkey, 1969). It is currently used in many fields to obtain predictions of events and estimates where empirical data are unavailable or uncertain. It is also used to generate forecasts, plans, problem definitions, programs and policies, summaries of current knowledge, and selections from alternatives (Olsen, 1982).

For health issues, the Delphi technique has been used to obtain estimates, where empirical data are insufficient, of influenza epidemic parameters (Schoenbaum et al., 1976b) and of incidence of disease and rates of adverse drug reactions in preventive treatment of tuberculosis (Koplan and Farer, 1980). The method has been used to develop national drug abuse policy (Jillson, 1975; Policy Research Incorporated, 1975a,b), the identification of statewide health problems (Moscovice et al., 1977), the design of a statewide health policy research and development system (Gustafson et al., 1975), consensus on physician practice criteria (Romm and Hulka, 1979), and the implications of advances in biomedical technology (Policy Research Incorporated, 1977).

The primary advantages attributed to the technique are that participants generally have no direct contact with each other, so that variables of professional status and personality have little chance to influence opinions as they might in face-to-face meetings, the process can obtain opinions at low cost from geographically isolated participants, and panelists may complete their questionnaires within their own time constraints (Delbecq et al., 1975; Olsen, 1982).

The Delphi technique does not provide the opportunity for clarification of ideas and other benefits of face-to-face interaction. Insights to be gained by considering conflicting or minority viewpoints may be obscured or lost through pooling of responses and ranking procedures (Delbecq et al., 1975; Linstone and Turoff, 1975). Although the method's reliability may increase with the numbers of participants and iterations, so does its cost. Participation also drops off with more iterations. Considerable concern has been voiced that the consensus achieved in some applications has been "forced," or is "artificial" (Sackman, 1975). Although advantages and disadvantages of the Delphi technique have been cited by many, few of these are substantiated by rigorous study. Their relevance likely depends on the type of problem under consideration (Herbert and Yost, 1979).

Nominal Group Technique The nominal group technique (NGT) is a group decision process developed by Delbecq et al. (1975). The product of an NGT is a list of ideas or statements rank-ordered according to importance. The process usually involves the following.

1. Participants generate silently, in writing, responses (opinions, rankings, views) to a given problem.
2. The responses are collected and posted, but not identified by the author, for all to see.
3. Responses are clarified by participants; a round-robin format may be used.
4. Further iterations of silent, written response, posting, and clarification may follow.
5. A final set of responses is established by voting/ranking.

Like the Delphi technique, NGT benefits from pooling opinion and certain group interactions, while postponing evaluation and criticism and minimizing certain effects of individual status and personality that may skew individual participation in less structured group interactions. Unlike the Delphi technique, NGT allows for immediate clarification of responses. Because it requires bringing participants together, NGT may be costly in certain situations.

NGT has been used to formulate priorities for quality assurance activity in multispecialty group clinics and their associated hospitals (Horn and Williamson, 1977; Williamson, 1978). Policy Research Incorporated (1975b) used an NGT to develop ranked national objectives and strategies against drug abuse. NGT was compared to a Delphi process for developing procedures for handling emergency medical services cases. Physician participants were assigned randomly to the NGT and Delphi groups to develop the procedures. Six months later, they were surveyed for their opinions regarding their respective groups' conclusions. Although the degree of consensus reached by the nominal and Delphi groups was comparable, the NGT participants changed their opinions to a significantly greater extent than did the Delphi group participants (Thornell, 1981).

Group Methods Designed for Health Issues

NIH Consensus Development Conferences The primary purpose of the National Institutes of Health Consensus Development Conferences is to evaluate the available scientific information on biomedical technologies and to produce consensus statements for use by health professionals and the public. Examples of technologies assessed are breast cancer screening, intraocular lens implantation, coronary bypass surgery, the Reye Syndrome, liver transplantation, and diagnostic ultrasound imaging in pregnancy.

Conference panels of 8 to 16 members usually address five or six predetermined questions. Panelists include research investigators in the relevant field; health professionals who use the technology; methodologists or evaluators such as epidemiologists and biostatisticians; and public representatives such as ethicists, lawyers, theologians, economists, public interest group representatives, and patients.

Consensus conferences are open meetings that usually last 2 1/2 days. The first 1 1/2 days are devoted to a plenary session in which experts or representatives of task forces present information on the state of the science and the safety and efficacy of the technology. These presentations are followed by an open discussion involving speakers, panelists, and members of the audience. Following the plenary session, the panel drafts consensus answers to the predetermined questions. This draft document is read to the audience on the morning of the third day for further comment and discussion among the panel and audience. The panel may incorporate comments received during this session for inclusion in the final consensus statement. The process concludes with a press conference. Consensus statements may reflect opposing or alternative opinions if these exist; however, few statements thus far have reflected lack of consensus.

The NIH consensus format is not designed to limit problems associated with face-to-face interaction (e.g., relative dominance of viewpoints due to social or hierarchical factors) in group settings, as are Delphi, nominal group, or other group processes. The program has been exploring the use of decision analysis models as a reference framework to assist panelists in formulating consensus (S. G. Pauker, Tufts-New England Medical Center, personal communication, 1985).

The NIH Consensus Development program is one of few medical technology assessment programs that has undergone formal evaluation. An impact study of the 1978 consensus conference on supportive therapy in burn care indicated high clinician awareness of the conference's recommendations (Burke et al., 1981). The Office of Medical Applications of Research (OMAR) conducted a survey to measure physician awareness of two consensus conferences (computed tomography [CT] scan of the brain, 1981; and hip joint replacement, 1982) and their results, how that awareness was obtained, and the relative effectiveness of various means of information dissemination. Among the samples of five physician specialties targeted for the CT scan conference, awareness that the conference was being held ranged between 11 and 37 percent, and awareness of its conclusions ranged from 1 to 15 percent. Among the samples of six physician specialties targeted for the hip joint conference, awareness that the conference was being held ranged between 7 and 21 percent, and awareness of its conclusions ranged from 0 to 10 percent. The study concluded that there is significant room for improvement in conveying information about the program, the individual conferences, and their results (Jacoby, 1983). The NIH program has implemented a number of recommendations made in a study conducted by the University of Michigan of the NIH consensus development process (Wortman and Vinokur, 1982b). The Rand Corporation is conducting a study, to be completed by 1985, of how consensus conferences have affected the knowledge, attitudes, and practices of health care professionals (Rand Corporation, 1983).

The NIH program has successfully established its role as provider of information, rather than as government regulator dictating methods of clinical practice. The issuance of consensus statements has not precipitated a flurry of malpractice actions based on consensus panel findings, and there is no evidence that the program has stifled innovation (Perry and Kalberer, 1980). Currently, at least one conference question solicits the panelists' opinion on directions for future research.

Other concerns have been at least partially alleviated by modifications in conference preparations and format. The earlier absence of biostatisticians, epidemiologists, and other methodologists who could speak on the validity of scant and/or controversial scientific evidence has been addressed by current panel representation requirements. Concern has been voiced that consensus statements are prone to consist of generalities representing the lowest common denominator of discussion, i.e, the only points on which panel members can fully agree (e.g., Rennie, 1981).

Group judgment efforts such as the NIH

program often seek to bridge gaps in and otherwise make sense of available research, so as to provide guidance for clinical practice. In so doing, expert panels may render recommendations relying to some extent on suggestive but not rigorously founded clinical evidence, e.g., derived from weaker epidemiologic studies as opposed to randomized clinical trials. One recommendation of the NIH consensus panel on lowering blood cholesterol—to lower dietary cholesterol for all Americans age two onward—may have been such an instance. (See Kolata [1985], Lenfant et al. [1985], and Steinberg [1985] for discussion.) This is a methodological concern of any group judgment effort and is best addressed with documentation of group judgment methodology and the characteristics of the research considered and assumptions made by the panelists.

A number of consensus statements have fallen short of directly addressing certain prominent issues. In the 1981 Reye Syndrome consensus statement, none of the 15 conference questions addressed the controversial role of aspirin, although limitations of studies indicating its association with the Reye Syndrome were cited.

Consensus development conferences usually examine only the safety and effectiveness of medical technology. By not addressing such matters as cost and availability of other resources, many consensus statements may be of limited value in suggesting guidelines for use of technologies. The consensus statement on liver transplantation does not address the reimbursement of this very expensive procedure; the existing and potential demand for the procedure; or how such demand could be met in terms of available transplant teams, facilities, and donor organs. At issue is the conflict between the intent to avoid conference topics for which insufficient data are available for reaching scientifically valid conclusions and pressure to hold conferences on controversial issues, as was the case with the liver transplantation conference.

State-of-the-Art Diagnosis and Care of COPD Glaser (1980) coordinated a broad-based consensus development effort to compose a state-of-the-art journal article on the diagnosis and care of chronic obstructive pulmonary disease (COPD). This project, which took approximately 2 years from initiation to publication, involved a project team of 11 physician researcher-practitioners in the COPD field, a project facilitator, and a large network of reviewers in the field. The project consisted of the writing, review, and revision of 13 drafts. The first 5 drafts were composed and revised by a single project team author, incorporating the detailed review and critique of each draft by the other team members. Drafts 6 through 13 were reviewed by groups of reviewers chosen out of a lot of 120 experts. The product, published in the *Journal of the American Medical Association* (Hodgkin et al., 1975), invited further critique for use in a revised and expanded state-of-the-art monograph. This monograph, which was also composed by the project team using outside reviewers, was published in 1979 by the American College of Chest Physicians (Hodgkin, 1979).

Medical Practice Information Project The Medical Practice Information Demonstration Project conducted by Policy Research Incorporated (1979a,b) used expert teams to reach consensus on four aspects (epidemiology, diagnostic validity, therapeutic efficacy, and economics) of three health problems: bipolar disorder (characterized by manic and depressive states), malignant melanoma, and rheumatic heart disease.

The process involved health problem expert teams and research validation teams. For each health problem, expert teams completed two instruments. In the first, expert team members provided certain health problem data (e.g., incidence) and cited the sources of that data (e.g., empirical study, extrapolation from empirical study, or assumption). An independent research validation team assessed the documentary literature cited by the expert teams to determine how well the research design and statistical work of the sources supported the data.

Using the first instrument summary and the report of the research validation team, the four expert teams completed second iteration surveys of health problem data and sources and rated the probable validity of the cited data, i.e., the degree of certainty with which they held the data to be valid. The final report included narrative summaries for each of the four aspects of the health problem, best sources of information, documentation and rated validity of information, and policy implications.

Rand-UCLA Health Services Utilization The Rand-University of California, Los Angeles (UCLA), study of health services utilization, scheduled for completion in 1985, uses consensus panels to (1) compile indications for performing selected medical and surgical procedures (e.g., coronary artery bypass surgery and upper gastrointestinal endoscopy), (2) select the indications that account for the majority of procedures, and (3) evaluate the relationship between frequently used reasons for performing the procedure and patients' health. Panelists participate both independently and as a convened group and have tasks of reviewing the literature, amending lists of indications for the use of a procedure, rating, and estimation. The panels have nine members, including specialists and internists, family practitioners, or other generalists. Prior to a 1-day meeting, panelists review staff-prepared literature reviews and sets of indications for a procedure. Panelists may amend the list of indications and then rate the clinical appropriateness of each and select the most frequently used of the lot. At the consensus meeting, panelists discuss and rate in at least two rounds those indications that showed high disagreement in their initial ratings of clinical appropriateness and that account for the majority of the procedures. Panelists estimate the proportion of procedures for which each of the frequently used indications is responsible in a high- and low-use area of the country. Finally, panelists will rate each indication in terms of the improvement to be expected by use of the procedure (A. Fink and J. Kosecoff, Fink and Kosecoff, Inc., personal communication, 1983).

Computer Knowledge Bases The National Library of Medicine (NLM) Lister Hill National Center for Biomedical Communications developed a computerized synthesis of information about a specific disease: viral hepatitis (Bernstein et al., 1980). This was a process for establishing and updating a state-of-the-knowledge base for viral hepatitis. The project was active from 1977 through 1983, when the NLM Knowledge Base Program was discontinued.

Because of the infeasibility of sifting through the massive amount of literature (16,000 publications on hepatitis in English over a 10-year period, drawn from 3,000 serials indexed by the NLM), the project's initial information sources were limited to 40 current review articles recommended by a few authorities in the field.

The initial knowledge base was formulated by consensus of a panel of 10 experts who reviewed a draft synthesis of the 40 selected review articles prepared by one person. Each expert reviewed the entire initial draft and reviewed in detail one-tenth of the draft. The experts identified weaknesses, inaccuracies, and missing information and made suggestions for changes. Decisions on inclusion or modification of content were made by vote of the expert group, and areas of unresolved conflict were noted. Generally, when there were two or more (out of the 10-person panel) dissenting views, the paragraph under consideration was modified or reconsidered by the entire group. Developers of the Hepatitis Knowledge Base have initiated a new, similar project to develop and update a gastroenterology data base (L. M. Bernstein, Knowledge Systems, Inc., personal communication, 1983).

One of the noteworthy aspects of the Hepatitis Knowledge Base project was the use of a computer conferencing network as the principal medium of communication linking the geographically dispersed experts and project staff. This was the electronic information exchange system (EIES) under development and study by the National Science Foundation and operated by the New Jersey Institute of Technology (see e.g., Hiltz and Turoff, 1978, and Siegel, 1980). EIES and other forms of computer support are under further development and application for group judgments in a number of fields (Turoff and Hiltz, 1982). The advantages of computer conferencing—participants' independence of space and time constraints and automatic recording of data, communications, and other transactions—may be quite suitable for engaging group judgment efforts in medical technology assessment and for documenting, evaluating, and improving the group deliberative process.

Strengthening Group Judgment Efforts

The current level of group judgment efforts to determine how best to put medical technologies to use is not commensurate with the effort and care devoted to developing these technologies. Although we do quite well at assembling experts, we often provide them with inadequate, largely untested means for drawing upon their expertise and for organizing and weighing the evidence. Group judgment methods currently used are difficult to validate, because they do not adequately document evidence and provide rationale for findings or provide estimates of the effects of adopting their recommendations. The following are guidelines that may be helpful in implementing and evaluating a successful group judgment effort.

1. The procedures and criteria for selecting topics and panel members should be documented.
2. Sponsors and panelists should agree on the nature and technical understanding of the intended users and the means used in disseminating findings.
3. A chair/facilitator should be selected who is a skillful moderator and working-group coordinator, with standing in the relevant field but not necessarily expert on the particular topic, and having no particular position on the topic.
4. Panelists should be chosen whose interests can be served by working on and using the findings of the process. They should represent the relevant medical specialties, general practitioners, methodologists such as epidemiologists and biostatisticians, economists, administrators, and others who can provide important perspectives.
5. The questions to be addressed by the panel should be specific and manageable, i.e., commensurate with the available data, the time available for the process, and other resources. Panelists should be able to participate in specifying the questions to be addressed, responsibilities for tasks, and project format.
6. An operational definition of consensus should be specified (e.g., full agreement, majority agreement, etc.), as well as how to present less than full agreement in the panel's findings (e.g., cite minority opinions).
7. Panelists should be provided with the most comprehensive scientific data possible. A summary description of the avail-

able studies (topic, study design, findings) should be provided and cited in the final panel statement.

8. Process methodology, facts, assumptions, estimates, criteria for findings, and rationale should be documented. Findings should include estimates of outcomes expected if the panel's recommendations are followed. This documentation should enhance internal consistency, allow others to check reasoning, and provide the basis for reassessment in light of new developments.

9. The panel should recommend research needed to resolve those issues concerning which it could not reach full agreement and to otherwise advance understanding of the topic.

10. The dissemination and effects of panel findings should be evaluated to enable improvement of the process. Panel members and other participants should be apprised of the evaluation findings.

Group judgment processes could be improved by answering several types of research questions.

- **What conditions inhibit and enhance panelists' participation in group judgment?**
- **Do group judgment processes achieve increased understanding and convergence of opinion or lowest common denominator views of panelists?**
- **Are some processes better than others at achieving consensus?**
- **How effective are group judgment processes in modifying policies and practices concerning medical technology?**
- **What factors (scientific findings, ethical considerations, stature of other panelists, personal experience, etc.) are most important in influencing panelists' decisions?**
- **What factors (stature of panelists, identity of sponsoring organization, documentation of groups' reasoning, media used to disseminate findings, etc.) are most important in influencing the adoption of group judgment findings?**

COST-EFFECTIVENESS AND COST-BENEFIT ANALYSES*

The Office of Technology Assessment defined the terms cost-effectiveness analysis (CEA) and cost-benefit analysis (CBA) as normal analytic techniques for comparing the negative and positive consequences from the use of alternative technologies (OTA, 1980a,b). There is thus possible a continuum of such analyses involving measurements of the costs of using a technology, the effectiveness of the technology in achieving its intended objectives, and determination of the positive and negative benefits from both intended and unintended consequences (Arnstein, 1977).

The principal distinction between a CEA and a CBA is in the valuation of the effects/benefits of using the technologies. In measuring benefits, a CBA requires that all important effects and benefits be expressed in monetary (dollar) terms. Thus some estimates are required of the monetary value of all benefits gained so that they can be compared with all dollar costs expended (Cooper and Rice, 1976). CEA avoids the requirement of attributing a monetary value to life by simply counting the lives (or years of life) saved or lost. An attempt to assess the quality of life of the years saved usually weighs differences in health status (e.g., from a value of "O" for the state of death up a positive scale of values for decreasing disability and increasing health status).

The burgeoning interest in health care CEA/CBA is a phenomenon that began budding in the late 1970s. This interest is derived largely from provider, payer, and consumer concern over increasing health care costs and governmental spending for health care services. (For an overview of the history of CEA/CBA and health care

* This section was contributed by Morris Collen and Clifford Goodman.

CEA/CBA concepts, methods, uses, applications, and relevant references, see OTA, 1980a,b.)

OTA (1980b) reported on a study of health care CEA/CBAs conducted by medical function and year (1966–1978). This report (Table 3-6) shows not only the accelerating increase in the use of CEA/CBA but the change from the early emphasis on prevention studies to the current dominance of studies on diagnostic and treatment technologies.

An extensive survey and classification of the growth and composition of the CEA/CBA literature for the same period 1966–1978 is also reported by Warner and Luce (1982) and in abbreviated form by Warner and Hutton (1980). This survey found over 500 references addressing CEA/CBA for health services. It identified a number of significant trends in the literature (Table 3-7). It reported that the considerable growth in the CEA/CBA literature over the period surveyed was more rapid in medical than in nonmedical journals and that a preference appeared to be emerging for CEA over CBA. This study also found that while the number of all types of CEA/CBA studies increased, those related to diagnosis and treatment technologies showed considerable increases in prominence relative to those on preventive health. The decision orientation of the studies shifted away from organizational and societal decision makers to those of individual practitioners. The authors observed that the rapid growth of the CEA/CBA literature over the period was not matched by adequate skill in methodology, noting a higher proportion of technically low-quality analyses in the later years than in the earlier years of the period surveyed.

In conducting a CEA/CBA, OTA (1978a, 1980b) recommended a series of steps to follow:

1. Define the problem for which the technology is used. The problem, which should be stated as clearly and explicitly as possible, may be in clinical disease or treatment, preventive medicine, or in a health care process or service.

2. State the intended objectives for using the technology. These objectives may

TABLE 3-6 Numbers of Health Care CEA/CBAs by Medical Function and Year (1966–1978).

Year	Prevention	Diagnosis	Treatment	Other[a]
1966	0.0	0.0	0.0	5
1967	0.0	0.3	1.7	3
1968	2.5	3.0	3.5	6
1969	1.5	0.5	2.0	2
1970	3.0	2.0	3.0	8
1971	6.5	3.5	4.0	11
1972	7.0	2.0	4.0	14
1973	14.5	4.0	10.5	15
1974	2.5	5.0	14.0	22
1975	5.0	10.0	14.5	22
1976	15.0	16.0	28.0	33
1977	12.5	17.0	37.5	35
1978	18.0	25.5	18.5	31
Total	88.0	88.8	141.2	207

[a]Includes mixes of all three functions (prevention, diagnosis, and treatment), administration, general, and unknown.

SOURCE: Office of Technology Assessment (OTA, 1980b).

TABLE 3-7 Trends in Health Care CBA/CEA, 1966–1973 and 1974–1978[a].

Trend	1966–1973	1974–1978
Average annual number of publications	17.0	73.0
Publications in medical journals as percent of total journal publications	40.2	62.7
CEAs as percent CEAs + CBAs	42.1	63.2
Percent articles on:		
Prevention	44.7	22.0
Diagnosis	18.8	30.9
Treatment	36.5	47.2
Percent articles with orientation of:		
Individual	8.3	15.8
Organization	21.3	10.8
Society	70.4	73.4

[a]All differences significant at $p = 0.05$.
SOURCE: Warner and Luce (1982).

be expressed in terms of patient outcomes (e.g.,decreasing mortality) or in terms of health care processes (e.g., decreasing costs).

3. Identify any alternative technology that can be used to achieve the stated objectives. Usually the analysis compares a new or modified technology with old or currently used technologies.

4. Analyze the effects and benefits resulting from the use of the technology. "Effectiveness" is generally expressed as the extent to which intended objectives are actually achieved in ordinary practice and is distinguished from "efficacy" which is usually defined as the probability or extent of achieving the objectives under ideal conditions (OTA, 1978a).

A wide variety of evaluative approaches, including randomized clinical trials and epidemiological studies, form the basis for assessing effectiveness of medical technology. Effects of a diagnostic technology may be expressed in terms such as the percentage of correct diagnoses achieved, time and cost to complete the diagnostic process, or cost per true-positive test. Effects of a treatment technology may be expressed in terms of disability, mortality, patient well-being or reassurance, or time and cost to complete the treatment process. Effects of a supporting/coordinating technology such as an information system may be expressed in terms of data error rates, response times to queries, or cost for retrieval per information unit.

All intended consequences (effects/benefits) should be studied, and all important unintended consequences should be identified and assessed (OTA, 1980b). Some effects/benefits will be positive (i.e., desirable), some will be negative (i.e., undesirable), and some may be indeterminate. Generally in CEA/CBA, all important effects/benefits should be considered to whomsoever they accrue (Klarman, 1973). Included are those affecting the individual patients, effects upon other health care resources/services, and effects on the family/society/employer. For some technologies it is not possible to ascertain final patient outcomes so that as a compromise one measures intermediate outcomes, such as the diagnostic accuracy of clinical testing procedures or the resultant changes in patients' smoking habits from a smoking cessation program.

5. Analyze costs associated with the use of the technology. Costs of the health care process should include all expenses to all participants resulting from the use of required resources (personnel, facilities, equipment, supplies), including the direct controllable costs and overhead uncontrol-

lable costs (Klarman, 1973). Patient-consumer costs should be identified, including charges for services received, time and earnings lost from work, transportation costs, and any other expenses. For a technology system or program, opportunity cost should be considered as an estimate of the value of other opportunities that are forgone because of the investment in the specific technology selected. In CEA/CBA all negative-costs, i.e., savings attributed to the use of the technology, are considered to be effects or benefits.

All future costs and monetary values of future benefits should be discounted to their present value in order for them to be compared appropriately with one another. The discount rate attempts to adjust for what a dollar invested today would earn in interest. For long-term projections, low discount rates tend to favor projects whose benefits accrue in the distant future (OTA, 1980a,b); accordingly, selection of appropriate discount rates are often controversial and usually are subjected to sensitivity analysis (redoing the calculations with different rates). OTA (1980b) provides an example of how the particular discount rate chosen can have a substantial impact on the outcome of the analysis, because investment in health programs often means spending present money (which is not discounted) for future benefits (which are). In such programs, the higher the discount rate, the less attractive the program appears. As an example, suppose one spends $1,000 today, expecting to save $2,000 in medical costs 10 years later. In order to compare the expected benefit ($2,000 savings) with the costs of program ($1,000), one must discount the benefit to its estimated "present value." Consider the varied results using different annual discount rates with a cost of $1,000 (in present dollars) and a benefit of $2,000 (in year 10).

Discount rate (%)	Present Value of benefit	Present Value of net benefit (B − C)
0	$2,000	$1,000
5	1,228	228
7	1,017	17
10	771	−228

And, if the benefit were not related for 20 years, the results would be:

Discount rate (%)	Present Value of benefit	Present Value of net benefit (B − C)
0	$2,000	$1,000
5	754	−246
7	517	−483
10	297	−709

This example shows the power of discounting and the resultant importance of the choice of the discount rate.

6. Differentiate the perspective of the analysis. Since the explicit objectives sought may vary somewhat from the viewpoint of the patient, the physician, the administrator, and the policymaker, a comprehensive CEA/CBA may be very complex if the aim is to satisfy all participants. Objectives, benefits, and costs differ for each of these participants. Public societal benefits and costs often differ substantially from private benefits and costs. For the public policymaker, societal benefits sought may be primarily in cost reduction of improved accessibility of health care services. From the viewpoint of the private hospital administrator, the cost-effective capital-intensive technology may be that with the highest financial return on investment. The health care provider will seek the technology that minimizes his costs or maximizes the desired patient outcomes. From the viewpoint of the patient-consumer, the primary benefits desired are improved health outcome at an affordable cost, yet other important considerations are length of time to complete the care process and satisfaction with the process.

7. Analyze uncertainties. Relevant retrospective data for a CEA/CBA are often uncertain as to their accuracy, and some-

times they are entirely unavailable. Timely prospective data for predicting future events is rarely available. In such instances of uncertainty, a sensitivity analysis for important variables should be performed to test the sensitivity of the analytic results to potentially important variations in the data used. By a variety of techniques, such as by consensus development of experts who are selected appropriately to attempt to minimize bias, estimates can be derived that can be used as substitutes (valid or not) for valid primary data. Usually a series of scenarios are tested in which various assumptions are specified for critical uncertain variables.

8. Interpret results. The results of the analysis should be discussed in terms of validity, sensitivity to changes in assumptions, likely variations in benefits and effects over time (e.g., by discounting), and implications for policymaking. If it is not possible to arrive at a single decision or recommendation, the important consequences from using the alternative technologies studied should be presented in order to decrease the uncertainty of decision making.

Important ethical, legal, or societal issues should be identified and their implications discussed. Strictly on the ground of efficiency for a CEA, the alternative with the lowest cost-effectiveness ratio would be preferable because it could achieve the desired objectives at the lowest cost. Similarly for a CBA, the alternative with the greatest net of benefits minus costs should be preferred, except that the monetary values attributed to years of life may make the results controversial. In any actual decision, however, policymakers should consider also social effects such as equity and political importance (Banta et al., 1981). Social and ethical consequences of medical technology are increasingly being questioned in such applications as support systems for prolonging life in incurable terminal patients, organ transplants (e.g., heart, liver, and kidney) for which the demand exceeds the supplies, and artificial organs (e.g., heart and kidney) where equity of funding and distribution will always be an issue.

An example of a CBA is given in Appendix 3-A of this chapter to illustrate the analytic process.

Uses of CEA/CBA

The uses of CEA/CBA for technology assessment can be categorized by (1) the type of technology (i.e., drugs, devices, procedures, instruments, equipment, or a group of these components into a system) and (2) the application of the technology (i.e., for medical diagnosis, medical treatment, preventive medicine, or for supporting/coordinating functions of medical services).

Drugs, chemicals, vaccines, and similar agents have been studied using CEA/CBA, with special consideration of their efficacy and safety (OTA, 1978a). OTA (1980a) proposed a hypothetical CEA model for assessing a drug's cost-effectiveness if the efficacy and safety of the drug could be quantified in measurable units of "net health effect." Then the "net cost of achieving a desired net health effect" (e.g., specified reduction in morbidity and mortality) could be derived by determining the cost of the drugs and of the treatment of any of its side effects and subtracting the savings from the use of the drug. A cost-effectiveness ratio for the drug would be the net cost divided by units of net health effect. Similarly, the cost-effectiveness ratios could be derived and compared for alternative drugs or existing treatment modalities. CEA/CBA have been applied to immunizations, such as for pneumococcal pneumonia (Patrick and Woolley, 1981; Willems et al., 1980), influenza (OTA, 1981a), and rubella (Schoenbaum et al., 1976a).

CEA/CBA have been used for a variety of devices, instruments, machines, and equipment. Such assessments require detailed analysis of the process, technical procedures, and personnel using the devices; and they employ different analytic methods for diagnostic, therapeutic, or coordinating/supporting applications.

A notable example is the case of computed tomographic scanning (OTA, 1978b, 1981b). This study generally followed the traditional model for the economic evaluation of diagnostic procedures, and it considered outcomes, benefits, and effects. Usually the assessment of diagnostic technology separates the evaluation of the cost-effectiveness of the process in achieving its diagnostic objectives from the cost-effectiveness of subsequent treatment technologies which have a different set of specific objectives (McNeil, 1979). A variety of diagnostic and screening tests have been studied, including hypertensive renovascular disease (McNeil et al., 1975), cancer (Eddy, 1980), multiphasic screening (Collen et al., 1970, 1973, 1977; Collen, 1979b,d), lead screening (Berwick and Komaroff, 1982), mammography (Collen, 1979a), diagnostic x-rays (Collen, 1983), and endoscopy (Showstack et al., 1981).

CEA/CBA for treatment technologies have been reported for a wide variety of therapeutic devices and procedures, such as surgery (Bunker et al., 1977), psychotherapy (OTA, 1980c), hemodialysis for end-stage renal disease (Stange and Summer, 1978; OTA, 1981c), preoperative antimicrobial prophylaxis (Shapiro et al., 1983), and for therapeutic decision making in general (Pauker and Kassirer, 1975).

CEA/CBA have been used for assessment of multiple devices aggregated into complex systems (Collen, 1979c), such as medical information systems (Drazen and Metzger, 1981; Richart, 1974), and alternative health care programs such as ambulatory versus inpatient care (Berk and Chalmers, 1981). See Appendix 3-A of this chapter for a more detailed example.

Capabilities and Limitations

OTA (1980a) has emphasized that CEA/CBA should not serve as the sole or primary determinant of a health care decision, but the CEA/CBA process could improve decision making by considering not only whether the technology is effective but also whether it is worth the cost.

In general, a CEA is most useful for making a choice as to the lowest cost technology to achieve a specified objective, benefit, or effect; and CBA is most useful for making a choice between technologies producing various objectives, benefits, or effects as to which could produce the highest value for the costs expended.

A CEA is especially useful for assessing the past performance of a technology when specific limited objectives are defined and reliable data are available to achieve these same defined objectives. Such retrospective analysis can be relatively simple and inexpensive and can be used to support rational decision making to the extent that the CEA does permit comparison of costs per unit of effectiveness among competing alternatives for achieving the same objectives. Still, the accurate determination of actual costs of resources used, or of appropriate associated incremental costs, is not always readily obtainable, and charges or fees for services are often substituted that may not be directly related to true costs (Finkler, 1982).

When a CEA extends the analysis to study unintended consequences from using alternative technologies, the analysis becomes more complex and expensive. Uncertain or missing data is then an important problem and a sensitivity analysis becomes necessary. CEA does not permit comparison of complex technologies having different or multiple objectives associated with different process or outcome measures unless uniform composite indexes of outcome measures are used.

A CBA is capable of assessing the values of technologies that have differing objectives by converting all of their effects/benefits to dollar values. Thus, as has been emphasized, a CBA requires a dollar determination of added years of life, quality of life, etc., so that costs expended can be compared to the dollar value of benefits gained. The dilemma for a CBA of valuing life and death in monetary terms can be avoided by a CEA; however, a CEA is not as useful for setting policy priorities among different types of technologies because expressing all of the effects/benefits in equivalent units is usually possible only with dollars.

OTA (1980b) emphasizes that there are certain technical considerations that can significantly alter how a CBA is interpreted, as, for example, the use of net benefit (that is, benefit minus cost) rather than the cost-benefit ratio as a criterion to compare programs. The former (net benefit) approach is usually preferred, especially when the alternative programs are widely variant in scope. As an illustration, OTA (1980b) considered two programs.

Program A costs $2,000 and reaps gross benefits of $4,000; program B costs $2 million and reaps gross benefits of $3 million. A net benefit approach yields the following results.

Program A

$$\$4{,}000 - \$2{,}000 = \$2{,}000$$

Program B

$$\$3 \text{ million} - \$2 \text{ million} = \$1 \text{ million}$$

Clearly, program B is preferred, given the ability to finance the project and setting aside for the example all considerations of equity and distributional effects.

However, a benefit-cost ratio (B/C) would yield the following results:

Program A $\qquad$ Program B

$$\frac{\$4{,}000}{\$2{,}000} = 2 \qquad \frac{\$3 \text{ million}}{\$2 \text{ million}} = 1.5$$

Now, program A is clearly preferred. Notice that the ratio gives the reader no indication of the size of the expected benefits, nor the size of the program. Also, although program A gives a better rate of return for the money invested, there is no reason to believe that it can be increased in scale and still maintain the high rate of return.

Sometimes a marginal analysis (i.e., the additional benefit derived from adding one more unit of expense) may help determine the optimal size of a program and the point at which a given technology is no longer cost-effective.

Because CEA/CBA are primarily economic types of analysis and most useful for cost-containment decisions, they are limited in their ability to help with policy decisions that affect primarily the quality of care. Valid quantitative measures of effects and benefits of quality of care are not available, and the validity of the estimates of any such variables used are controversial. Similarly, social values, ethical considerations, and political realities may well take precedence over analytical economic results (Banta et al., 1981). OTA (1980a) has noted the conflict between equity and efficiency as an important issue in the use of CEA/CBA and cites the difficulties of measuring a person's worth; of rating better or worse welfare states; of assigning values to equity, fairness, and justice; and of valuing lives.

Although significant advances have been made in rational clinical decision making (Weinstein and Feinberg, 1980), OTA (1980a) has pointed out that CEA/CBA has had little relevance to decision making in practice because the primary focus of CEA/CBA is cost-effectiveness from a societal or policymaking viewpoint. In addition since the physician's major responsibility is to the patient-consumer, the perspective of the physician is often very different from that of the policymaker.

The stage of development of the technology is an important factor affecting the validity of the analysis. Often, for a new technology when an assessment might be especially useful, insufficient time has elapsed to permit adequate reliable evaluative data to have accumulated.

CEA/CBA can be a useful tool for planning for the future, and prospective analytic simulation models can attempt to predict costs and effects/benefits of competing alternative programs. OTA (1980a) emphasizes the importance of sensitivity analysis to cope with the problem of missing data and the uncertainties about the future by testing a range of discount rates, varying the weights used to compute quality-adjusted life expectancy, and testing all important variables over a range from best to worst cases.

OTA (1980a) emphasized the infinite number of unintended consequences (also called externalities, second-order effects, side effects, spillovers, or unintentional effects from using the technology), such as the effects on technical manpower and the training programs needed for a new technology. The costs of such important effects should be estimated and included in the CEA/CBA.

Strengthening Use of CEA/CBA

It is an important question as to what extent CBA/CEA are actually used by policy decision makers. Certainly, the usefulness of CEA/CBA will depend upon the importance of the technology in affecting medical care costs and patient outcomes. Accordingly, the criteria for selecting medical technology for CEA/CBA should recognize that approximate analyses of timely technology can be more useful than certain analysis for unimportant technology.

Also, the usefulness of CEA/CBA for decreasing the uncertainty of policy decision making for cost-containment or budgetary planning can be enhanced by judicious application of sensitivity analysis. For missing or uncertain data, an appropriate group of experts, selected carefully to minimize bias, can use consensus development techniques to provide credible estimates of missing data. Then by studying a variety of assumptions for important variables and by using middle, low, and high values to appropriately express realistic, optimistic, and pessimistic scenarios, the policymaker may estimate the limits of errors in projected costs and establish minimum, maximum, and break-even costs for the program.

Better methods also are needed for measuring the health status of individuals and of groups and for valuing changes in health status. Any important ethical, legal, societal, and political implications of using the technology will need to be considered in the process of making policy decisions.

A problem of all comparative secondary analysis, including CEA/CBA, is the lack of standardization of primary component evaluations so that data from different sources cannot be appropriately combined. **The development of better organized and standardized data collection methods would greatly facilitate CEA/CBA, and the promulgation of standard preferred methods for analysis would encourage their wider use (Institute of Medicine, 1981).**

The usefulness of CBA/CEA can be increased by improved analytic methodology. **Better methods are needed for imputing or substituting for missing data.** Methodology used should be understandable by the policymakers who need the information to make their decisions, and conclusions or recommendations should be supported by the best data available.

The analytic methodology and the data used should be credible and presented in a form understandable to the decision makers. Data interpretation and recommendations should be separated from data analysis so decision makers can review the data and minimize possible biases introduced by the evaluator's conclusions. OTA (1980a) emphasizes that many methodological weaknesses of CEA/CBA may be hidden by the process of deriving a numerical cost-benefit or cost-effectiveness ratio and encourages the use of arranging all the elements that are included in the decisions. Thus, sometimes a tabular array of the data can enable useful comparisons and inferences.

Recommendations

Cost-effectiveness analysis and cost-benefit analysis are assessment methods for an economic analysis of the positive and the negative consequences from the use of alternative technologies. A formal series of steps usually followed in conducting a CEA/CBA: define the problem, determine the objectives for using the technology, identify the alternative technologies, analyze the intended effects and benefits and also all the important unintended consequences, analyze all costs, differentiate the prospective user of the analysis (i.e., policymaker, health care providers, patient), analyze uncertainties, and finally, interpret the results in a manner to decrease the uncertainty of decision making.

CEAs are more commonly done than CBAs. CEAs are more useful for making a choice as to the lowest cost technology to achieve a specified objective, benefit, or effect. CBAs are more difficult to do because all effects and benefits must be expressed in monetary terms. However, a CBA is most useful in making a choice between technologies producing different objectives, benefits, or effects. CEA/CBA are useful for aiding in policy-level decision making but have little relevance to clinical decision making in medical practice. CEA/CBA can be useful for planning and usually employ sensitivity analysis for uncertainties of the future, such as by testing the effects of a range of discount rates on results. Better methodology is still needed, for such tasks as valuing changes in health status.

The usefulness of CEA/CBA should be improved through studies to develop better methods for expressing the value of changes in health status and measuring the quality of life during years saved by the use of the technologies.

TECHNOLOGY ASSESSMENT: THE ROLE OF MATHEMATICAL MODELING*

A model is a representation of the real world. A mathematical model is characterized by the use of mathematics to represent the parts of the real world that are of interest in a particular problem and the reationships between those parts. With respect to technology assessment, mathematical models can help describe the relationship between a technology and the clinical conditions it is intended to affect and predict how the use of that technology will affect medically important outcomes.

Mathematical models have proved useful in a broad range of applications pertinent to the assessment of medical technologies. The analytical methods of statistics, economics, decision analysis, epidemiology, and cost-effectiveness analysis are all built on mathematical models. This section will focus on another category of applications: the use of mathematical models to describe the natural history of a medical condition and how the natural history is affected by the medical procedure. In this chapter, the term mathematical model will be restricted to this category of applications.

Mathematical models have been used successfully to assess a wide variety of med-

---

* This section was drafted by David M. Eddy.

ical technologies. Examples include an analysis of treatment and prevention of myocardial infarctions (Cretin, 1977), the value of continued stay certification (Averill and McMahon, 1977), a comparison of hysterectomy and tubal ligation for sterilization (Deane and Ulene, 1977), vaccination for swine influenza (Schoenbaum et al., 1976b), screening and treatment of hypertension (Weinstein and Stason, 1976; Stason and Weinstein, 1977), and screening for cancer (Eddy, 1980; Shwartz, 1978). Additional applications are described in several collections and reviews (Bunker et al., 1977; OTA, 1981d; Warner and Luce, 1982). Used properly, mathematical models can be powerful tools in the assessment of medical technologies.

Background

Because the use of mathematical models in medical technology assessment is comparatively new, it is important to understand how they relate to more traditional methods of technology assessment.

The task of technology assessment is to estimate the consequences of using a technology in a particular setting. Ideally, this would be accomplished by conducting an experiment, that is, applying the technology in the setting of interest and observing the results. For a number of reasons, however, this is not possible. Most important, there are too many possible settings. A medical technology is not a static item; it takes a variety of forms depending on who is using it, on whom, when, and how. A diagnostic test can be preceded or followed by other tests; can be used at different times in the course of a patient's condition; can be used on patients with different types of problems, different ages, and different risk factors; can be used with different techniques; can be interpreted against different criteria; and can be followed by different therapies. Therapeutic and other types of medical technologies can present in equally diverse ways. To study with traditional experimental methods only one manifestation of a technology in one particular setting is difficult, time-consuming, and expensive; to study all of its potential modes of use is impossible.

Even when a study is designed for one particular setting, other problems arise. One may have to wait years for results, leaving the question of what to do today. Furthermore, the disease or the technology could change while the study is in progress, raising new questions about the interpretation and applicability of the results.

Because of these problems, a technology assessment is usually conducted in two steps. In the first, the investigator gathers the available information about the performance of the technology, focusing in particular on its performance in circumstances that are related as closely as possible to the circumstances of interest. In the second, that information is processed to estimate how the technology would perform if it were applied in the actual circumstances of interest. Many methods are available for gathering information about the impact of a technology in a particular setting. These include randomized controlled trials (RCTs), community trials, case-control studies, and other experimental and epidemiological methods that are discussed elsewhere in this chapter. Each of these techniques makes observations and gathers primary data about how the technology behaved in a particular set of circumstances, but they do not tell how the technology will behave in new settings. To learn that requires the second step of a technology assessment. The main role of mathematical modeling in technology assessment is to assist in that step—to help investigators process the observations made in experimental and epidemiological studies to estimate what would be expected to happen in circumstances that either have not or cannot be observed.

An Example

As an example (see Appendix 3-B of this chapter for more detail), suppose one wanted to assess the value of Pap smears for asymptomatic women in San Diego in the mid-1980s. The list of possible circumstances in which the Pap smear could be used is long. Should it be done at all? If so, should it be done on women starting at age 18, 20, 25, 30, or any other age? Should it be done every 6 months, every year, every 5 years? Should the ages or frequencies be different depending on a woman's family history, sexual practices, smoking habits, age, or medical condition? Should the examination be performed by nurses, internists, or gynecologists? Should the examination be done in offices, special clinics, or mobile units? At what age might screening be stopped? Once all these questions are answered for San Diego, they can be reasked for Dallas. And so forth. These are all important questions; one way or another, implicitly or explicitly, correctly or poorly, each one must be and will be answered every time a recommendation to perform Pap smears is made.

It is clearly impossible to study all the possible applications of a Pap smear with experimental and epidemiological methods. For example, only to compare the effects of annual and triennial Pap smears on mortality in a randomized controlled trial (without trying to learn anything about the ages of screening, risk factors, or any other variables) would require a sample size of about one million women, followed for about two decades.

Because of these limitations, the assessment of the Pap smear today must be pieced together from information that exists, derived from many different sources. One source consists of more than a dozen studies of what happened when the Pap smear was introduced in large populations. For this source, there are usually no concurrent (much less randomized) controls, and issues like age, risk factors and the type of delivery system, even issues like which women are getting the test and how frequently, can rarely be studied with any precision. Other sources of information include scores of studies on age-specific incidence rates, risk factors, the natural history of the disease, the sensitivity and specificity of the Pap smear, the proportion of lesions detected in different stages in different programs, survival rates, mortality from other causes, the cost of the test, and the cost of treatment. By default, statements about the value of the Pap smear in San Diego and policies about the ages, risk categories, and frequency of screening must be based on an integration of all these pieces of information.

The Role of Models

Processing or integrating information from different sources requires a model, some method for representing how all the information fits together, and what it implies about the value of the technology.

Mental Models By far the most common model is the mental model, in which the person who is assessing the technology thinks about the pertinent information and mentally estimates the consequences of using the technology in the circumstances of interest. A common name for this is clinical judgment. The mental model may be a very simple one—for example, the assessor may be willing to assume that what happened in a Pap smear-screening program in Louisville, Kentucky, in the 1960s will apply to San Diego in the 1980s, and may be willing to ignore factors like age, risk, and technique—but it is still a model. Any physician or policymaker who recommends a particular program for a Pap smear must have considered some observations and must have made some estimates, however crude, of what would happen if that recommendation were followed.

Mathematical Models The drawbacks of mental models are obvious: the complexity of most medical technology assessment problems simply exceeds the capacity of the unaided human mind. It is impossible to keep all the factors and numbers straight and to perform all the calculations correctly in one's head. This raises the need for mathematical models. A mathematical model is a formalization of mental modeling. While not inherently different from mental models in intent or general approach, mathematical models have qualities that make them useful in the assessment of medical technologies. First, they can encompass a large number of variables, they permit the expression of complicated relationships between the variables, and they provide rules to ensure that calculations are correct. With the use of computers there is virtually no limit to the number of factors that can be included, the complexity of the formulas, or the number of computations. Second, because mathematical models are explicit, they force one to be precise in making definitions, stating assumptions, and stating numbers. Furthermore, they permit others to review the factors, assumptions, numbers, and reasoning. But the most important feature of mathematical models is that they transform the essential features of a problem into a symbolic language that, unlike English, can be manipulated to gain insights and see conclusions that are otherwise invisible. To appreciate the power of mathematical models compared with mental models, consider estimating your income tax without using addition or multiplication.

Uses of Mathematical Models in Technology Assessment

Estimating Outcomes The most important use of a mathematical model is to help integrate the results of more traditional methods of experimental and epidemiological studies to estimate the consequences or outcomes of applying a technology in a particular setting. Its potential for this use covers a broad spectrum, depending on the questions being asked and the number and quality of available studies. Toward one end of the spectrum, a mathematical model can extend the results of a particular research project, to examine its implications for a new setting that differs only slightly from the setting of the original project. For example, the Health Insurance Plan of Greater New York (HIP) conducted a randomized controlled trial of breast cancer screening, providing direct observations of the effect of an annual mammogram and an annual physical examination on a specific population of women in New York in the late 1960s. If one wanted to assess the value of breast cancer screening today in a 50-year-old woman in Oregon whose mother had breast cancer, or the value of doing a breast physical examination only, or the value of a biennial mammogram, it is possible to build a mathematical model that uses the observations of the HIP study to study these new issues. Indeed, mathematical modeling may be the best way to address these issues, being faster and less expensive than a new RCT and more accurate than simply assuming that what happened in New York 15 years ago will happen in Oregon today (ignoring factors such as age, risk factors, and mammography technique).

Toward the other end of the spectrum, mathematical models can be used to study assessment problems that have never been the subject of any comprehensive experimental studies. In these cases for which there are no results from closely related studies to examine (like the HIP study) the only available approach is to try to integrate the results of a variety of studies about particular parts of the problem. The assessment of the frequency of the Pap smear is a good example. A mathematical model can integrate information about dozens of factors to provide estimated outcomes that never have been observed in any study, such as the increase in probability of death from cervical cancer, long-term costs of screening and treatment, and so forth. A great number of medical technologies present assessment problems of this type and have been successfully addressed in studies such as those previously cited.

Additional Uses Although the main use of a mathematical model is to estimate the outcomes of applying a technology in various settings, there are other important uses. These include the analysis of disease dynamics, hypothesis testing, research planning, and communication.

First, mathematical models can use information from carefully designed experimental and epidemiological studies to improve our understanding of the etiology and natural history of diseases. For example, the duration and reversibility of carcinoma in situ of the cervix is an important determinant of screening, treatment, and prognosis for that disease. But neither the duration or reversibility can be observed directly. With a mathematical model it is possible to estimate the pertinent parameters for these variables from observable data (Shur, 1981).

A second, similar function of models is that they can be used to test or validate hypotheses about the natural history of a disease or the effects of a technology on the disease. In addressing such problems, an investigator typically faces a collection of observations and must formulate hypotheses about the underlying dynamics of the disease and the impact of the technology that explains the observations. Mathematical models can be created to describe the hypothesized dynamics, parameters can be fitted, and results can be predicted. The extent to which the values predicted by the model fit the observations provides evidence about the validity of the hypothesis.

Third, when models are used to estimate the outcomes of applying a technology in different settings, an investigator can explore the value of collecting additional information by noting the sensitivity of various outcome measures to variations in assumptions and input values and by identifying areas of a problem that deserve more research. By comparing the value of additional information about a parameter with the cost of obtaining that information, research priorities can be set.

Finally, irrespective of their value in calculating estimates of outcomes, mathematical models can be powerful communication tools. Mathematical models force investigators to be explicit and precise, to define their terms, and to express their ideas in unambiguous terms. Furthermore, the entire exercise is open to view and criticism. A related use of models is to provide a framework for consensus formation. It is often desirable to have many experts from a variety of backgrounds concentrate together on an assessment. Mathematical models can focus this energy, forcing participants to agree on such basic ingredients to an assessment as the objectives, options, definitions, structure of the problem, basic facts, and values—or to identify explicitly their differences of opinion (e.g., Barron and Richart, 1981; Eddy, 1981; Galliher, 1981; Richart, 1981).

Types of Mathematical Models

The principles of mathematical modeling are simple and follow closely the intuitive process that forms the basis of mental models. The first step is to identify the important factors or variables that determine the value of the technology. The next step is to define the relationships between those variables that determine how a change in one variable affects another. The distinguishing feature of a mathematical model is the use of mathematics to define the relationships between variables. Simple examples are the balance sheet of a bank account and formulas such as distance = rate × time, or total cost = unit cost × number of units.

Many different types of mathematical models can be used to assess a medical technology, depending on whether the problem can be modeled as discrete or continuous, deterministic or probabilistic, or static or dynamic, and depending on other modeling decisions such as the appropriate number of dimensions or distributional assumptions. The particular methods will not be cataloged here but range from techniques as simple as traditional "back of the envelope" arithmetic to far more complicated models that require a page, a pad, or a computer to store the variables and perform the calculations.

Like experimental and epidemiological methods, mathematical models can have varying degrees of detail and complexity, and their development can require different amounts of time and money. For example, to study the question of breast cancer screening in high-risk women, one might use a very simple mathematical model such as assuming that a positive family history of breast cancer implies a relative risk of two, and then multiplying the pertinent results of the HIP study by two. On the other hand, to address the same question, a much more complicated model could be developed, involving a detailed analysis of age-specific incidence rates in women with particular risk factors, incidence rates for other nonmalignant conditions in these women, participation rates of high-risk women in screening programs, compliance rates of such women to postscreening recommendations, response to treatment, and so forth.

As in the choice of an appropriate experimental or epidemiological study, the choice of an appropriate mathematical model depends on judgments about the likelihood that different methods will yield different conclusions and the expected importance of different conclusions in terms of the actions they imply and the consequences of those actions. These judgments about which factors should be included in a mathematical model, and how the relationships between the factors should be translated into the language of mathematics, form the art of mathematical modeling.

Validation of Mathematical Models

It is important to have some measure of how well a given model can predict a set of outcomes. The most obvious requirement is that the structure of the model makes sense to people who have good knowledge of the problem. Factors they consider to be important should be included in the model; the mathematical functions used should appeal to their intuitions. They should agree that the data sources are reasonable, and so forth. The concurrence of experts, therefore, might be considered a first-order validation.

The next approach is to compare estimates made by a model with actual observations. However, this is far more complicated than it appears because most good models are built from actual observations. Since the structure and parameters of the models are estimated to predict the observations, it should be no surprise when they do. Nonetheless, not all models pass this test, and it is reasonable to define a second-order validation: any model should be able to match the data used to estimate parameters. Failure to pass this test strongly suggests that the structure of the model is faulty.

A third-order validation could be made by comparing the predictions of a model with observations that were never used to construct the model. In theory, a model can be constructed using one set of existing data and tested against a different set of existing data (e.g., Shwartz, 1978). However, there may be a trade-off between using all the available data to construct the model, which yields a more accurate model (in the sense that it can replicate the observed data more closely) but prohibits this type of validation, or using only part of the data to construct the model (which may reduce its accuracy) and saving the remaining data for validation. Note that for validation, one might use only part of the data. Once that assessment is completed, and the investigator is satisfied with the method, the whole data set can be used to better estimate the required parameters for future work.

First- and second-order model validations are made even more complicated by two facts. First, some observations are far easier to match than others. It is possible to vary some model parameters drastically and still have the model generate some estimates that are always close to some observations. A close fit in such instances is almost meaningless, and the weight to be placed on a first- or second-order validation will depend not only the number of observations the model can predict and the accuracy of the predictions, but also on the sensitivity of predictions to the model parameters about which there is the greatest uncertainty. The second fact is that observations themselves could be wrong in the sense that they do not represent the population mean. A fourth-order validation could be defined by comparing the outcomes predicted by a model for a new and previously unobserved program with the actual outcomes of that program when it eventually is conducted. Unfortunately, this too may not be meaningful because the actual conditions under which a program is eventually conducted can be quite different from the operating conditions assumed when the model was constructed. Changes in the technology itself; the age, risk, and behavior of the patients; the institutional setting; and many other factors can make comparisons meaningless. Beyond this, the random component to the outcomes of any clinical trial can prevent the predicted and observed outcomes from matching, even if a model is perfect.

In brief, as important as this problem is, there is no simple and universally applicable procedure for validating a model. Each case must be considered by itself. In many cases only a first-order validation will be possible, and only in very rare cases will a fourth-order validation be possible. This should not, however, prohibit the use of models. The decision to use a model should be based on a comparison with the validity of the other techniques that might be used to assess the technology. For example, what is the validity of the mental models or clinical judgments that form the basis for the overwhelming majority of assessments?

Limitations

First, unlike the techniques for gathering primary information discussed in earlier chapters, a mathematical model does not provide any new observations. Because of this a mathematical model cannot assess or validate a technology in the sense of documenting its impact with calibrated observations.

Second, to the extent that a model is based on subjective clinical judgments about the pathophysiology and clinical dynamics of a problem, a mathematical model will perpetuate any errors in these judgments—a variation on the theme of "garbage in, garbage out." For example, a mathematical model based on the testimony of eighteenth century experts would have "confirmed" the value of leeching. Building models can expose gaps, inconsistencies, and errors in reasoning, but to the extent that current clinical knowledge is incorrect, the errors can appear in the models and an erroneous model will pass a first-order validation. Because of this, to the greatest extent possible, models should be based on observations from well-designed studies rather than subjective judgments, and the results of a mathematical model should never be preferred to the results of actual clinical experiments, when they are available. Needless to say, this problem is even more severe for mental models, which rely almost exclusively on subjective judgments.

Third, mathematical models can be poorly designed. Most medical technology assessment problems, especially those that require mathematical modeling, are complicated. Creating a mathematical model of such problems requires a good knowledge of medicine, technology, mathematics, and modeling. One must be able to sense the structure of the problem, identify the important factors, appreciate what simplifications are appropriate and what are not, and write reasonable equations. It is easy to make mistakes. The most common error is to make unreasonable simplifications. Any model must simplify reality; this by itself does not detract from a model's value, and indeed one of the main purposes of a model is to help separate the important from the unimportant. The problem arises not with simplification but with oversimplification, which can render a model not only useless, but harmful. The most common causes of oversimplification are to omit important variables and to attempt to squeeze a problem into a familiar or convenient mathematical form, rather than to create a form to fit the problem.

Fourth, the results even of a good model can be misinterpreted or misused. One of the most common errors is to take the results of a model too literally, failing to appreciate the degree of uncertainty that surrounds its results. It can be hard to resist the urge to construct a model, look around for data, insert some numbers when the data cannot be found, clearly state that these assumptions are made only to demonstrate the performance of the model, and then believe the output. Even if the author of the model remembers its weaknesses, others may not. Another error is to ignore the specifications and assumptions of a model and apply its results to situations it was not intended to address. Still another error is to assume that the outcomes addressed by the model are the only ones that need to be considered in making a decision about the technology. It should be recognized that misinterpretation and misuse are not problems inherent to models; they are problems with those who use the models. The solution is not to withdraw the model but to educate those who would use its results.

Finally, the accuracy of the results of a model is limited by the accuracy of the data it uses. It is important however not to overstate this limitation. First, this too is not a problem with models as such; it is a data problem. The structure of a model can accurately represent reality; it is the use of the model that will be limited by the poor data. Second, this limitation is not restricted to mathematical models. Whatever method is used to estimate the outcomes of applying a technology, the accuracy of its conclusions will be limited by the accuracy of the available data. A model does not by itself create the need for data that would not otherwise be important. But a model does make the data needs explicit and does focus attention on poor data (which might cause discomfort), but this is not a weakness of models; it is a strength. Ignoring important factors about which there are few good data does not make those factors unimportant; it merely ignores them. Third, models have several properties that make them the preferred method for studying problems for which the data are poor: (1) the explicitness of models focuses attention on gaps and biases in the information, raising cautions about conclusions that might otherwise pass unscathed. (2) Given that data problems cannot be willed away, models are still the best method to gain insights and make estimates based on the best information available. (3) Through sensitivity analyses, models can indicate the importance of uncertainty or poor data about a variable. (4) Models can be used to estimate the value of conducting research to get better data. While poor data spoil the quality of conclusions drawn by any method, the solution is not to discard models but to use models to squeeze the most information out of the data that do exist and to collect better data for the next application. In general, the worse the data, the greater the need for a model.

In judging the seriousness of these limitations, it is important to recall that all methods of technology assessment require judgments and simplifications, all methods can deliver wrong answers, all methods can be misused, and all methods depend on the quality of the available data. While a mathematical model can never be perfect, it can still increase our ability to understand a problem and make decisions.

Strengthening the Technique

The techniques of mathematical modeling (and the related techniques of computing) already have been developed in other fields to a high level of complexity. Mathematical models have been used for centuries in other fields with great success. Today mathematical models are used to help build bridges, design airplane wings, forecast weather, create video games, plan highways, analyze radiowaves, refract lenses, guide satellites, route shipments, search for oil, generate electrocardiographs, plan crops, control floods, compute tomograms, and carry out thousands of other activities. The results of this research already are available for application to the evaluation of medical technologies. In medicine the main needs are not to improve the techniques, but to apply them responsibly.

This suggests several priorities. First, efforts must be made to define and demonstrate the role of mathematical models in the technology assessment process. Clinicians, researchers, statisticians, health planners, and policymakers should be exposed to examples of technology assessments that demonstrate the strengths and weaknesses of mathematical models and that demonstrate how they fit with more traditional methods. In the end, the use of the method will depend on its helpfulness to decision makers; the first step is to provide decision makers with opportunities to make that assessment.

Second, there is a need for more education in the application of mathematical models to medical problems. Modelers must know more than a small number of methods; they must understand at a deep theoretical level the assumption behind and limitations of their methods, and they must be capable of modifying those methods to fit a particular problem. They must also learn how to communicate with people in medicine to develop a realistic model and to describe how it can be used. On the other side, people who want to use the results of models must learn their strengths and weaknesses.

Third, work is needed in the quality control of models and their applications. For example, mathematical models present special problems for the editors and readers of medical journals. The description of most models is too long to fit in the usual methods section of a paper, and few reviewers could understand them if they did. Yet the form of a model can drastically affect its validity and usefulness. **Related issues are the need to control misinterpretation and misuse, the need for a system for validating models, and the need to calibrate the probability that a model's results accurately represent reality.**

A start toward these goals can be made

by asking that each report of a technology assessment employing a mathematical model contain the following elements:

1. a statement of the problem;
2. a description of the relevant factors and outcomes;
3. a description of the model;
4. a description of data sources (including subjective estimates), with a description of the strengths and weaknesses of each source;
5. a list of assumptions pertaining to:
   a. the structure of the model (e.g., factors included, relationships, and distributions),
   b. the data;
6. a list of the parameter values that will be used for a base case analysis, and a list of the ranges in those values that represent appropriate confidence limits and that will be used in a sensitivity analysis;
7. the results derived from applying the model for the base case;
8. the results of the sensitivity analyses;
9. a discussion of how the modeling assumptions might affect the results, indicating both the direction of the bias and the approximate magnitude of the effect;
10. a description of the validation method and results;
11. a description of the settings to which the results of the analysis can be applied and a list of main factors that could limit the applicability of the results; and
12. a description of research in progress that could yield new data that could alter the results of the analysis.

If the analysis recommends a policy, the report should also contain:

13. a list of the outcomes that required value judgments;
14. a description of the values assessed for those outcomes;
15. a description of the sources of those values;
16. the policy recommendation;
17. a description of the sensitivity of the recommendation to variations in the values; and
18. a description of the settings to which the recommendations apply.

Finally, greater care should be taken in the collection of data. A tremendous amount of research is conducted by thousands of investigators on hundreds of clinically important questions every year. The fact that good data do not exist for building mathematical models, or even for constructing simpler structures like decision trees, is testimony that many of those conducting the research do not have a clear model in their minds of precisely how the data they are collecting should contribute to the analysis of the problem they are addressing. Because a model is the tool that converts data into insights, one can argue that every experimental and epidemiological study should be preceded by a model, every datum collected should have a place in that model, and attempts should be made to collect all the data needed for the model.

Conclusion

Mathematical models provide a method for synthesizing existing information to estimate the consequences of applying a technology in a particular set of circumstances. Mathematical models should not be viewed as an isolated technique that may or may not be used in a particular assessment, or as an alternative to, or worse, as a competitor of clinical judgment or experimental and epidemiological studies. Any assessment of any technology will require integrating information from experimental and epidemiological studies to estimate how a technology will perform in a particular setting. By their explicitness, power, and precision, mathematical models can provide a powerful aid to human judgment in the interpretation of data from clinical research.

SOCIAL AND ETHICAL ISSUES IN TECHNOLOGY ASSESSMENT*

A little-emphasized aspect of technology assessment is the examination of the social, ethical, and legal questions raised by the use of technology in clinical practice. Although these questions do not always lend themselves to quantitative measurement and analysis, they can be systematically identified and evaluated. The methods for accomplishing this will not be covered in detail here, but the following discussion will serve to illustrate possible approaches. Questions to be considered include the following: Who is affected or not affected by a technology? What ethical principles are involved in testing and use of a technology? What might be the unintended consequences or side effects of a technology? How does the technology fit into larger cultural political contexts? What values affect the application of the results?

An inquiry into the consequences of the use of a medical technology on social groups and relationships will require a study of the patient as a member of a family, of an organization, and of a community. Although the sociopolitical aspects of policy decision making have long been recognized, the increasing influence of the consumer/patient in policy decisions affecting the diffusion of medical technology only recently has been seen for its importance. Toffler describes a rising "third wave" in our society bringing a great increase in self-help and do-it-yourself activity that will powerfully affect our traditional health care delivery systems. Ferguson (1980) extrapolates from consumerism to a new "paradigm of health" in which the public increasingly embraces "holistic" or "alternative" medicine that employs less technology and uses the placebo effect, biofeedback, meditation, visualization, and forms of body manipulation as modes of self-therapy. Naisbitt (1982) explains that the more that machine-like technology is introduced into society, the more people value the human qualities, thus accounting for the trend to forms of home care rather than institutional care.

Another type of social consideration in the introduction of new technology has to do with its potential new manpower requirements. For instance, the change from manual to automated clinical laboratory methods required a major change in the training of laboratory technologists. The advent of coronary care units required the training and employment of highly specialized nurses. An Institute of Medicine study (Sanders, 1979) concluded that new technology often has important effects upon manpower in the community. It requires consideration of the need for new physicians, assistants, and technicians for the use of new equipment embodied technology. It may call for an increase in the training of new specialties, but also for a decrease in training and employment opportunities of outmoded specialties.

A consideration of social benefits and costs for a medical technology should include its opportunity costs—alternative uses for the money. Current examples of expensive programs that raise questions of opportunity costs include Medicare's end-stage renal disease patients of a kidney transplant or lifelong dialysis. Organ transplantation generally poses cost as a major social consequence, which also has large overlaps of ethical and legal ramifications.

Various of society's adjustments and accommodations in matters of health and safety affect assessments of technologies by altering their costs either in dollars or emotional stress or both. Structures of all kinds,

* This section was written by Morris Collen and Lincoln Moses.

and most any transportation system, can be modified for use by disabled persons; is the real question cost-effectiveness? There is nothing technologically difficult in removing nonsmokers from the effluvium of smokers, but there can arise serious questions of how far to carry the effort. Technology assessment in any of these matters of social, ethical, and legal import has great difficulties in determining net benefits and costs. Once the basic demands of humanitarianism have been met, much of the rationale for technology assessment is in the purview of economics. However, softening of that economic edge is a task for the components of assessment that are concerned with social and ethical issues.

OTA (1980a,b) observed that society has collective objectives that stem from its underlying values and traditions—objectives that are not strictly economic and not directly related to health status. These objectives may be concerned with the equitable distribution of medical care—ensuring that the poor have adequate access to health services—or with protecting the rights of the unborn, the mentally ill, or the comatose patient.

An economic approach to the problems of health and medical care is firmly rooted in three fundamental observations, according to Fuchs (1974): (1) resources are scarce in relation to human wants, (2) resources have alternative uses, and (3) people have different wants, with considerable variation in the relative importance they attach to them. The basic economic problem identified by Fuchs is "how to allocate scarce resources so as to best satisfy human wants."

Constraints on economic resources will necessitate decisions as to resource allocation and resource rationing, which, in turn, will raise ethical and related issues. Evans (1983) believes that in the future the major issues confronting not only medicine but this society as a whole will be the social, ethical, and legal implications of resource allocation and rationing. The resources available to meet the demand for health care already are limited; decisions already are being made; and priorities are being set as physicians allocate their time, hospitals ration beds, and fiscal intermediaries devise straitened reimbursement policies, he contends. It is only because those decisions are not publicized that they have not become a social issue, according to Evans, who suggests that within a society that has failed to come to grips with the meaning of death and the essence of life, rationing decisions will seem usually cruel. Yet, when these decisions are acknowledged as inescapable, he believes this society, this culture, will be more prepared to deal with the one event that is truly inevitable—death.

Once it is apparent that all who are in need cannot be treated, the rationing process attempts to determine which potential recipients are likely to derive the greatest benefits. This usually requires (1) the development of acceptable criteria for withholding treatment on a condition-by-condition basis and (2) identifying those who make the decisions about whom to treat.

End-stage renal disease (ESRD) provides an example of a medical condition for which there is a relatively long history of decisions about eligibility for treatment. The first successful treatment was hemodialysis. During the early years of dialysis, when very few machines were available, patient selection was made by physicians or community committees. At that time it was decided that although all patients with ESRD had a terminal condition, some had better prospects for treatment than others. The preferred candidates were selected on the basis of such criteria as age, medical suitability, mental acuity, family involvement, criminal record, economic status (income, net worth), employment record, availability of transportation, willingness to cooperate in the treatment regimen, likelihood of vocational rehabilitation, psychiatric status, marital status, educational background, occupation, and future potential. The eventual decision to extend Social Security disability benefits to patients with ESRD resolved the rationing problem by removing financial limits on treatment.

In general, how are criteria for the rationing of limited resources likely to be developed? As described elsewhere in this report, cost-effectiveness and cost-benefit analyses can be useful to compare various health care programs and determine which program could yield the greatest benefit at the least cost. For example, hemodialysis could be compared with heart transplantation to see which has the greatest benefits per dollar expended.

At some time, society will have to make some basic decisions about the allocation of economic resources between the aged and those younger. Even though they are based on explicit and even rational criteria, any plan that is eventually adopted is certainly debatable from the perspectives of others. To adopt a set of criteria including age of patients is to make a decision about limiting treatment. On the other hand, to treat all patients with a given disorder or within a given disease category, regardless of derived benefits, necessarily implies the withholding of treatment from patients with other disorders. The question is one of priorities. Data can be used to set priorities, but human judgment must be exercised to determine which priorities will hold. The conscious development of explicit allocation criteria, as a first step in the direction of wisely using limited resources, probably will strain our society as few issues have. Many of us will remember when such decisions did not have to be made and, short of cataclysm, will not understand a new imperative of calculated neglect.

Decisions must be made concerning which patients will best benefit from expensive health care technology. The problem, however, is that, in many respects, social and medical criteria are inextricably intertwined. People of low socioeconomic status are likely to be in poorer health and have multiple diseases. In part, this reflects poor nutritional habits, detrimental lifestyle, and the historical lack of resources to obtain proper health care. Consequently, if medical criteria were to be the basis on which rationing decisions are made, they might exclude the poor and disadvantaged because health and socioeconomic status are highly interdependent. For example, it is not unusual to find that of those persons with ESRD, those of lower socioeconomic status are likely to have multiple associated conditions such as diabetes, hepatitis, and hypertension. Not only are these patients less desirable candidates for dialysis and transplantation, but also they are among the more expensive patients to treat. Without careful planning and evaluation, the gulf between the haves and have-nots, as evidenced by formal selection criteria, is likely to widen.

In the above examples, interprogram analyses were applied only to health care programs. But such analysis also can be used to compare the expenditure of health care resources with other socially desirable uses of resources, such as a public assistance program. This requires conducting a cost-benefit analysis in which all expenditures and benefits are converted to monetary terms, after which direct comparisons can be made among diverse programs. The results of such an analysis may indicate that resources should be reallocated from social and other publicly financed programs to support health programs, or vice versa.

An analysis of benefits and costs of a medical technology to a community or a population group often involves political considerations. OTA (1980a) suggests that if benefits from a technology are controversial, nonscientific negotiations and compromise may be the best course for policymakers. The political process may respond better to community needs than the most careful cost-benefit analysis.

Decisions can be made on the basis of cost-effectiveness or cost-benefit analyses, or by political activities influenced by different lobbying groups. In any case, the first decision likely will be as to which patient groups will receive support (i.e., the resource allocation decision); then, as resources continue to dwindle, allocations will be made within programs and decisions will be made as to how clinicians might ration the limited resources made available to them. Increasingly, it is apparent that this scenario approximates the situation of the kidney disease program today.

The Institute of Medicine (1981) suggested that the public would accept controls on the diffusion of a technology until its effectiveness was proved if it were made clear that such controls ultimately would increase the overall quality of medical care, that lack of control could decrease the quality of care, and that these controls would be applied equitably.

Experience in Addressing Ethical Issues

Although no permanently established group currently addresses the ethical and social consequences of technology, several bodies have in the past been specially constituted to address those issues. For example, the National Commission for the Protection of Human Subjects was directed under section 203 of P.L. 93-348 to conduct a "special study" of the ethical, social, and legal implications of advances in biomedical and behavioral research and technology. This commission and its successor, the President's Commission for the Study of Ethical Problems in Medicine and Biomedical and Behavioral Research, attended explicitly to the ethical, social, and legal implications of advances in technology.

The National Commission for the Protection of Human Subjects (NCPHS) (1978) used several methods for assessing the social and ethical questions raised by technological innovation. In one approach investigators used the Delphi technique to examine such matters as systematic control of behavior, reproductive engineering, genetic screening, extension of life, and data bank-computer technology. In a second approach researchers used a case-study method for a colloquium to develop a historical and sociological perspective on recent advances in biomedical and behavioral research and services. Their colloquium explored the social impact of advances, of legal and institutional constraints, and of incentives governing the introduction of new technologies into medical practice. Finally the colloquium reviewed current knowledge about the public's understanding of and attitudes toward advances and their implications.

The President's Commission for the Study of Ethical Problems in Medicine and Biomedical and Behavioral Research (1983) approached its analysis of medical care by applying three basic principles:

- that the well-being of people be promoted;
- that people's value preferences and choices be respected; and
- that people be treated equitably.

However, they cautioned that medicine and research touch too many beliefs central to human existence to be summed up in a few principles. The commission's overall task was to help clarify the issues and highlight the facts that appear to be most relevant for informed decision making, to suggest improvements in public policy, and to offer guidance for the people who are making decisions. They issued 13 reports on issues in health care and biomedical and behavioral research, including the definition of death, life-sustaining treatments, genetic engineering, and compensation of subjects injured in research.

Although the NCPHS and the Presidential Commission were especially constituted to address ethical, social, and legal issues, there are other forums where these matters can be considered. The Office of Technology Assessment (OTA), for example, has taken up these issues in some of its reports (OTA 1978a; 1982b).

These examples are evidence that there is a desire and some effort to carry out technology assessment from ethical points of view. Nevertheless, in the committee's opinion the best methodologies for exploring such dimensions are still not well defined and more work is needed in this area.

Ethics of Investigation

The trial of new drugs, diagnostic procedures, and therapeutic maneuvers are keys to progress in health care. At the same time, these steps involve uncertainty and therefore risks. The risks are borne by patients in whom the new, uncertain methods are tried out, by the professionals who conduct these pioneer efforts, and by unknown future patients who may receive inferior care if the results of the investigative efforts are misleading. That can occur if an assessment lends support to a defective new idea or fails to reveal the worth of a genuinely good innovation. When an enterprise imposes risks on people who have differing interests, ethical issues are surely involved. Assessment of medical technology is such an enterprise.

Our consideration here of ethics of investigation is informed by our acceptance of two principles: First, it is unethical to exploit one person for the benefit of another. Second, to waste information that can benefit future patients is unethical, especially if that information has been obtained under conditions of risk.

We find it convenient to treat the ethical issues as those that attach to three temporal phases: initiation, conduct, and termination.

Initiation When is a new intervention promising enough to justify applying it to people in an experimental way? Who should judge that question and decide? What standards are applicable? Some would argue that a patient's own physician is the only one with ethical standing to decide. Others might prefer the advantages that can accompany collegial action and recourse to written protocol.

On whom shall the novel intervention be tried? Human subject committees, informed consent procedures, and written protocols all address this matter—but only where the novel intervention is owned to be part of an investigation. Some may find an ethical anomaly in the lack of any such parallel protections where the patient is simply undergoing treatment—with this same novel intervention.

Conduct Is the study so conducted that it must yield cogent information? Or is it so designed that on completion little trustworthy information can be salvaged? The ethical content of these questions sometimes leads to a policy of seating research-design experts on human subject committees.

Termination There are two ways to go wrong, and both are injurious to the interests of patients. If a trial is continued unnecessarily long, then unnecessarily many patients will receive an inferior treatment (the innovation, if it is inferior; the standard, if the innovation is an improvement). The same difficulty can arise if investigation of an innovation is carried forward in too long a sequence of separate studies, as Baum et al. (1981) have reported in a meta-analysis of studies of prophylactic antibiotic therapy for colon surgery.

The second way to go wrong in termination is to quit too soon—before an obtainable conclusive answer is on hand. Some of the controversy over the University Group Diabetes Program (UGDP) concerned the timing of its termination. The ethical issue in early termination is complicated by the need to weigh the relative responsibility of the investigators for the patients in the study and for all others with the disease in question. The decision was especially difficult for the UGDP investigators because they often had the dual role of physician to the patients in the study. To avoid that conflict most large-scale studies now have a data-monitoring committee of clinicians, biostatisticians, and laymen to decide when to inform the investigators that a decision to stop needs to be made.

This brief review is concluded with some ethical aspects of medical investigation with three general observations.

First, the problems cannot be avoided by some shortcut like setting a policy of only trying out good innovations and not trying out poor ones. Gilbert et al. (1977) reviewed 32 randomized trials of innovations in surgery and anesthesia. They found that these well-tested innovations were beneficial in 49 percent of the studies. There is no shirking the inconvenient fact that theory and opinion in medicine are not reliable guides to the value of new interventions; they must be tried, and in ways that can produce cogent answers.

Second, weak studies are not good enough. Many authors have found that the weaker the controls in a study, the better the innovation appears. Weak studies are not ethically sufficient to the task of helping beneficial new technologies enter the health care system. For example, Grace et al. (1966) found that in investigations of the portocaval shunt operation, the enthusiasm of the investigator at completion of the study was lower in those studies that were better controlled. In poorly controlled studies, 72 percent of the investigators reported "marked" improvement in patients. In well-controlled studies, the investigators were split 50-50 between "moderate" improvement and "none." Hugo Muench (Bearman et al., 1974) in a parody of statistical laws based on a lifetime of biostatistical consulting says, essentially, that nothing improves the performance of an innovation as much as lack of controls. Gilbert et al. (1977) found in poorly controlled trials that 64 percent of the innovations appeared to represent improvements as compared with 49 percent in well-controlled trials. Thus strong trials are needed lest the worth of an innovation be exaggerated.

Third, the scientific attitude of withholding judgment, of remaining skeptical, in the presence of inadequate evidence is commendable in medical investigations. We sometimes see controversies where adherents of one view insist that therapy A is better than therapy B for certain patients and will use only A, while adherents to the opposite view will only use B in such patients. This is an egregious failure of tempering opinion with science; it is ethically unsatisfactory and should constitute a warrant for the conduct of a controlled study. But the same theme—the ethical desirability of withholding judgment—arises in early termination and deferring widespread adoption of new methods until careful studies justify it.

CONCLUSIONS AND RECOMMENDATIONS

This chapter was begun with the point that technology assessment is important because it gives the bridge between basic research and development and prudent practical application of medical technology. Experience, not theory, must be the controlling factor in deciding whether to use a technology. Learning from experience requires formal plans, records, and analysis, not casual observation, and progress in health care depends on such learning.

To summarize, the foundation for assessing medical technology exists in the assembly of methodologies and the assessments that are available. But much work remains to be done before the enterprise is complete. Much of that work consists of research. In nearly every section of this chapter, research needs have been pointed out. Sometimes the needs are well formulated, as with the list of six questions concerning group judgment methods, and sometimes almost implicit, as with the need to more fully exploit sample surveys of the NCHS for technology assessment. But beyond the research problems of special methodologies, there is the special problem of assembling information from a variety of sources and integrating the results. We need to improve and widen the application of techniques like meta-analysis that can combine information from a number of studies intended to answer a common question about the safety and efficacy of a clinical practice. Also needed are improved methods for weighing information about clinical benefits along with economic and social consequences of medical practice, as in the techniques of cost effectiveness analysis, cost-benefit analysis, and technology assessment. These many needs justify three recommendations (in italics).

- *Increase research activity to improve and strengthen the varied methods that are applicable to the assessment of medical technology.*
- *Increase resources for training research workers in medical technology, both for advancing methodology and for applying those methods to the many unevaluated technologies.* (The reader is reminded that epidemiology and biostatistics have been and remain personnel shortage areas.)

It should be remarked at this point that need for another kind of training also flows from the underdeveloped state of medical technology assessment: biomedical personnel need training in the main ideas of technology assessment even if they are not carrying out the assessment themselves, because they must be able to appraise the strengths and merits of studies.

- *Invest greater effort and resources into obtaining evaluative primary data about medical technology in use.*

It can be seen that again and again not enough solid primary data are at hand to support cogent assessment. Recall that all respondents to OTA's (1980b) survey of CEA/CBA practitioners raised this complaint. Similarly, perusal of OHTA-OMAR reviews repeatedly point to the paucity of randomized clinical trials of other cogent primary data (NIH, 1983, 1984; Fink et al., 1984; K. E. Lasch, Synthesizing in HRST Reports, unpublished report, Harvard School of Public Health, 1985). Drawing up priorities for information building and then applying resources to the task are urgent needs of the U.S. health care system.

APPENDIX 3-A: EXAMPLE OF COST-BENEFIT ANALYSIS*

This example of cost-benefit analysis is adapted from one given by Swain (1981). It compares three alternatives for the reduction of lead poisoning in fictional "Kleen City." Lead poisoning of children under 5 due to ingestion of lead from painted surfaces is a major cause of death and severe brain damage for children in this age class.

The three candidate programs for reducing lead poisoning in Kleen City are

1. child screening and child treatment only;

* This appendix was prepared by Morris Collen and Clifford Goodman.

2. house testing and house deleading only;
3. both 1 and 2.

The CBA is based on the following assumptions:

- Planning period: 15 years
- Population aged 1 to 5: 17,000
- Annual births: 3,500
- Annual deaths of 1 to 5 population: 100
- Residences in the city: 10,000
- Proportion of residences with significant amounts of lead-painted surfaces accessible to children: 1/7
- Children with lead poisoning (levels of lead in the blood of greater than 50 micrograms per 100 milliliters): 6 percent
- Of those children with lead poisoning, those requiring chelation therapy to achieve adequate reductions in the level of lead: 35 percent
- Discount rate: 8 percent

The notation $(PV\ i\%, n)$ is a cash flow conversion factor used to determine the present value of n periodic \$1 payments at discount rate n. This is:

$$(PV\ i\%, n) = \frac{(1 + i)(\exp n) - 1}{(1 + i)(\exp n)i}$$

For example, the present value of 5 yearly \$1 payments at a discount rate of 10 percent is:

$$(PV\ 10\%, 5) = \frac{(1 + 0.1)(\exp 5) - 1}{(1 + 0.1)(\exp 5)\ 0.1} = \$3.79$$

For this CBA example, we will use the cash flow conversion factor $(PV\ 8\%, 15)$ to determine the present value of 15 yearly (our planning period) \$1 payments at our chosen discount rate, 8 percent. This is equal to:

$$(PV\ 8\%, 15) = \frac{(1 + 0.08)(\exp 15) - 1}{(1 + 0.08)(\exp 15)0.08} = \$8.559$$

For children aged 1 to 5 with a minimum of 50 micrograms per milliliter, the likely outcomes are

0.003	will die as a result of lead intoxication;
0.025	will exhibit permanent, severe brain damage as a result of lead intoxication;
0.072	will exhibit permanent, moderate brain damage as a result of lead intoxication; and
0.900	will return to acceptable lead levels with no signs of permanent damage under proper care.

The *costs* of child screening and child treatment of lead poisoning are estimated to be

\$8	for locating and testing an individual child,
\$9	for follow-up of children with excessive but not extreme lead levels, and
\$1,000	for chelation therapy of children found to have extreme levels of lead present in the blood.

The *costs* of house testing and house deleading are estimated to be

\$50	to test a house for lead paint
\$900	per dwelling deleaded by treatment of all surfaces found to have significant amounts of lead

The *benefits* associated with the results of lead-poisoning control programs fall into two categories.

1. Benefits due to the averted costs of treatment for children who would otherwise have been afflicted with the effects of lead poisoning. Given at a present value when discounted at 8 percent, these are

\$600	for children who would have died of lead poisoning;
\$130,000	for children who would have sustained severe, permanent brain damage;

\$17,430	for children who would have sustained moderate, permanent brain damage; and
\$1,800	for children with no permanent brain damage.

2. Benefits due to the increased income that can be gained by children who would otherwise have been afflicted by the effects of lead poisoning. Given at a present value when discounted at 8% these are

\$17,000	for children who would have died;
\$17,000	for children who would have sustained severe, permanent brain damage;
\$2,500	for children who have sustained moderate, permanent brain damage; and
\$1,600	for children who would have sustained no permanent damage.

Program 1: Child Screening and Child Treatment Only Screening must be repeated for the entire population for each of the 15 years. Assuming that there are approximately 100 deaths per year of children in the 1 to 5 age range, then the population of Kleen City will remain nearly constant during the 15-year period in the age range of concern. During each of the years, there will be approximately 17,000 children who must be screened for lead intoxication. Of that population, 6 percent will exhibit high lead levels and be subjected either to chelation therapy or follow-up testing during the year. Since under this program there is no significant removal of the original lead sources, each of the children will be subject to rescreening in the subsequent year, unless they are out of the population group being studied.

Costs (1): In each year of the program, 17,000 children will be screened (\$8 each), 6 percent of which will be treated (of treated: 65 percent with follow-up and 35 percent with chelation therapy). The present value of these screening and treatment costs are:

$$\begin{aligned} \text{Costs (1)} &= (PV\ 8\%,\ 15)17{,}000\{\$8 \\ &\quad + 0.06[(0.65 \times \$9) \\ &\quad + (0.35 \times \$1{,}000])} \\ &= (PV\ 8\%,\ 15)\ \$498{,}950 \\ &= \$4{,}270{,}513 \\ \text{Costs (1)} &= \$4{,}270{,}513 \qquad \text{(A)} \end{aligned}$$

Benefits (1): The average benefits per child screened in the first year due to the averted costs of treatment and the averted lost future income for the four outcomes can be combined into one expression:

$$\begin{aligned} &\text{Average benefits per child} \\ &\quad = 0.60\ [0.003(17{,}000 + 600) \\ &\qquad + 0.025(17{,}000 + 130{,}000) \\ &\qquad + 0.072(\ 2{,}500 + 17{,}430) \\ &\qquad + 0.900(\ 1{,}600 + 1{,}800)] \\ &\text{Average benefits per child} \\ &\quad = \$493.3656 \qquad \text{(B)} \end{aligned}$$

The benefits over the 15-year period can be calculated in two parts. For the 17,000 children screened in the first year, the benefits are:

$$\begin{aligned} &\text{Benefits in first year} \\ &= 17{,}000 \times \$493.3656 = \$8{,}386{,}440 \qquad \text{(C)} \end{aligned}$$

In each following year, a new group of 3,500 children will be screened. The benefits accruing to each of these groups are:

$$\begin{aligned} &\text{Benefits for each successive year} \\ &= 3{,}500 \times 493.3656 = \$1{,}726{,}780 \qquad \text{(D)} \end{aligned}$$

To determine the present value of these benefits accruing over the 15 years, we *do not* multiply this figure by 15, since the present value of the benefits of each successive year decreases. Thus, the present value of these benefits over the remainder of the planning period must be calculated:

$$\begin{aligned} &\text{Benefits for successive years} \\ &= (PV\ 8\%,\ 15)\$1{,}726{,}780 = \$14{,}780{,}370 \qquad \text{(D)} \end{aligned}$$

Benefits (1) = \$8,386,440 (C) + \$14,780,370 (D) = \$23,166,810

Net Gain (1) = Benefits (1) − Costs (1)
= \$23,166,810 − \$4,270,513

Net Gain (1) = *\$18,896,297*

Benefit (1)/Cost (1) ratio

$$= \frac{\$23{,}166{,}810}{\$\ 4{,}270{,}513} = 5.42$$

Program 2: House Testing and House Deleading Only For this program, it is assumed that house testing and deleading will be completed in the first year of the planning period. Given that assumption, then all the benefits of the house-screening process will be received after 1 year. A conservative estimate of the benefits would allow for the fact that without any child screening and treatment, all of the initial child population (17,000) might be susceptible to lead poisoning during the first year. Thus, the population receiving the benefits of house testing and deleading would be the children entering the 1 to 5 year age category after 1 year, i.e., 3,500 each year.

Costs (2): The costs associated with lead removal from residences are the cost of testing (\$50 each) the 10,000 residences for lead, plus the cost of removal of lead from those (\$900 for one out of every seven) houses found to have leaded surfaces.

Costs (2) = 10,000 × [\$50 + (1/7) × \$900] = \$1,785,714 (E)

Benefits (2): The benefits of averted cost of treatment and averted lost future income of the yearly group of 3,500 children are

Benefits (2) = (*PV* 8%, 15) 3,500 × \$493.3656 [from (B) above]
= (*PV* 8%, 15) \$1,726,780

Benefits (2) = \$14,780,370 (F)

Note that Benefits (2), the benefits of the home testing/deleading program (F), are the same as the benefits of the child screening/treatment program for successive years (D). As a result of Program 2 house testing/deleading in the first year, 3,500 children per year benefit by averting the costs of treatment and lost future income. The same 3,500 children per year achieve the same benefits from Program 1 annual screening/treatment.

Net Gain (2) = Benefits (2) − Costs (2)
= \$14,780,370 − \$1,785,714

Net Gain (2) = *\$12,994,656*

Benefit (2)/Cost (2) ratio

$$= \frac{\$14{,}780{,}370}{\$\ 1{,}785{,}714} = 8.23$$

Program 3: Combined Program The program combines child screening and treatment with house testing and deleading. Under this program, child screening/treatment needs to be carried out only until the removal of lead from houses is completed. If this task is completed by the end of the first year, then the only cost for child screening is that of screening the current population in the first year. This costs has been determined to be \$498,950 [see (A)]. The benefits accruing to the current population from the child screening and treatment are estimated to be \$8,386,440 [see (C)] Since the house testing and deleading has been assumed to impact on the new population, its benefits can be added to those for the single year of child screening to give a total set of benefits over the 15-year period of \$23,166,810. The combined cost of the two programs will be \$2,284,664.

Costs (3):

Costs (3) = (cost of child screening/treatment in first year) + (cost of house testing/deleading)
= \$498,950 (A) + \$1,785,714

Costs (3) = \$2,284,664 (E)

Benefits (3):

Benefits (3) = (benefits of child treatment/screening for first year population [17,000]) + (benefits of house testing/deleading)

Benefits (3) = \$8,386,440 (C) + \$14,780,370 (F)

Benefits (3) = \$23,166,810

Net Gain (3) = Benefits (3) − Costs (3)
= \$23,166,810 − \$2,284,664

Net Gain (3) = \$20,882,146

Benefit (3) ratio

$$= \frac{\$23,166,810}{\$\ 2,284,664} = 10.14$$

Comparison of Programs The following comparison shows that the combination program of child screening/treatment and house testing/deleading has a greater net gain as well as a higher benefit/cost ratio than either individual program. A choice between 1 and 2 would depend upon preference for the one with the greater benefit/cost ratio.

	Net Gain	Benefit/Cost Ratio
1. Child screening/treatment	\$18,896,297	5.42
2. House testing/deleading	12,994,656	8.23
3. Combination of 1 and 2	20,882,146	10.14

APPENDIX 3-B: AN EXAMPLE OF A MATHEMATICAL MODEL OF MEDICAL TECHNOLOGY*

This appendix illustrates some of the points raised in this chapter by describing briefly a mathematical model developed to assess the value of cancer screening tests.

As an example, imagine an asymptomatic, average-risk, 40-year-old woman who had a Pap smear a year ago, and suppose we wanted to estimate the effect of repeating the Pap smear today on the chance she will die of cervical cancer, or on her life expectancy. How much difference would it make to wait 2 more years?

To estimate the effect of a Pap smear on those and similar outcomes requires estimating a chain of probabilities: (1) the probability such a woman has a cervical cancer or precancerous lesion (dysplasia or carcinoma in situ) that could potentially be detected; (2) the probability that a Pap smear would detect such a lesion if it were present; (3) the probability that such a lesion would be detected in various stages; (4) the probability that if a cancer is not detected at this screening examination, a cancer will cause signs and symptoms in the interval before the next scheduled examination (and the probability that event will occur at various times in the interval); (5) the probability of any interval-detected cancer occurring in various stages; (6) case-survival rates that describe the woman's prognosis, given the stage in which the lesion is detected; and (7) the probabilities that the woman will die of other causes each year in the future. All these probabilities must be calculated conditional on the fact that this woman is a 40-year-old, average-risk, asymptomatic individual who had a negative Pap smear a year ago; the probabilities would change if she were a different age, had high-risk factors, had symptoms, or had had a negative Pap smear at another time in the past.

The power of mathematical models lies in the fact that formulas can be written for each of these probabilities. For example, the first probability is given approximately by

$$\int_{\infty}^{\infty} [1 - P(-t)]\{[F(t + I) - F(t)] + [1 - F(t + I)]FN\} r(t)\exp[-\textstyle\int_{\infty}^{t} r(x)dx]dt, \qquad (1)$$

* This appendix was prepared by David M. Eddy.

where I is the interval of time since the last Pap smear (in this example 1 year), $F(t)$ is the cumulative distribution for the length of time from the moment a lesion is first detectable by a Pap smear until it becomes an invasive cancer, $P(t)$ is the cumulative distribution for the length of time from the first moment of invasion to the appearance of signs and symptoms that would cause the patient to seek care in the absence of screening, $r(t)$ is the instantaneous incidence rate of invasive cancers [$r(0)$ is the rate in 40-year-old average-risk women], and FN is the random false-negative rate of the Pap smear.

Each of the elements in Equation 1 has an intuitive interpretation. The variable of integration, t, denotes the possible times that the woman might develop an invasive cancer of the cervix ($t = 0$ is now). By integrating from negative infinity to positive infinity, this formula considers all the possible times that an invasive cancer might occur. For any particular time that an invasive cancer might occur (call this time t'), the expression $1 - P(-t')$ gives the probability that the woman is currently asymptomatic and has not yet detected or sought care for signs or symptoms of the cancer. $F(t' + I) - F(t')$ gives the probability that the cancer was not potentially detectable until after the last Pap smear was done a year ago. The expression $1 - F(t' + I)$ gives the probability that the lesion was detectable before last year's Pap smear. This last expression must be multiplied by FN, the chance that that Pap smear was falsely negative and missed it. The expression $r(t') \exp[-\int_{\infty}^{t'} r(x)dx]$ is the probability that this woman will in fact develop an invasive cancer at the time t'.

A formula for the second probability is the same as Equation 1 except that Equa-

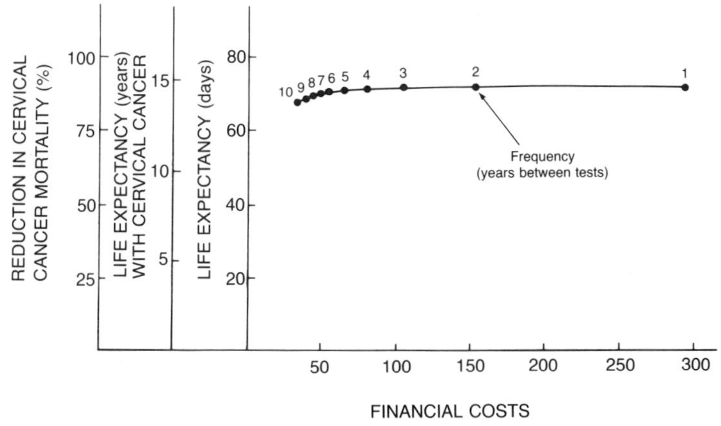

FIGURE 3-6 Effect of Pap test frequency on financial cost and three measures of benefit for a 20-year-old average-risk woman. Main assumptions are as follows: (1) testing is begun at age 20; (2) a woman will have a checkup every 3 years for other malignant diseases from ages 20 to 40, and then annually thereafter; (3) the marginal cost of a Pap test is $10; (4) Pap test-detectable dysplasia and carcinoma in situ precede invasive cervical carcinoma by an average of 17 years (range, 0 to 34 years); (5) 2.5 percent of invasive cervical cancers develop very rapidly, requiring less than 2 years to pass through dysplasia and CIS; (6) no cases of dysplasia or CIS regress spontaneously; (7) no Pap tests are falsely read as positive or suspicious; and (8) 5-year relative survival rates from time or detection (lead time adjusted) are dysplasia and CIS, 98 percent; local invasive, 78 percent; and regional invasive, 43 percent. If a woman must also pay a $25 office visit fee for the separate visits for the Pap test, the costs increase to about $700 for an annual Pap test and $1,700 for a biannual Pap test (Eddy, 1981).

tion 1 must be multiplied by $1 - FN$, the probability that the Pap smear will not be falsely negative. In similar fashion formulas can be written for the other important probabilities. These formulas are more complicated if one wants to consider the use of more than one type of test, a series of previous examinations done at various frequencies, and other factors, but the concepts are similar.

To estimate the value of a Pap smear done at various frequencies one can apply formulas to calculate the probabilities of important clinical and economic outcomes relating to cervical cancer for each year in a woman's life, constantly updating the parameters of the formulas to keep track of the woman's changing age and screening history. The calculations can be performed for each screening strategy being evaluated: for example, no screening at all, screening every year, screening every 3 years, screening every year for three negative examinations and then every 3 years, and so forth. Parameters for the equations, such as age-specific incidence rates $[r(t)]$ and parameters for the functions $P(t)$ and $F(t)$, are estimated from the data collected in clinical and epidemiological studies.

The results of an analysis using parameter values estimated from such studies are illustrated in Figure 3-6 (Eddy, 1981). This figure shows the estimated effect of screening a woman with a Pap smear at various frequencies from age 20 to 75. The figure indicates three measures of benefit: the decrease in the probability that the woman will die of cervical cancer; the increase in her life expectancy, given that the woman is destined to get invasive cancer; and the increase in life expectancy for the average-risk woman who may (with about a 1 percent probability) or may not get invasive cervical cancer. The horizontal axis gives the present value (at age 20) of a lifetime series of screening examinations minus the present value of expected savings in treatment costs.

The calculations indicate that the 3-year Pap smear is about 99 percent as effective as an annual Pap smear. If the 40-year-old, average-risk woman in the original example postponed her Pap smear another 2 years, the increased annual risk she would run of dying of cervical cancer would be on the order of 1 per 100,000, about the same as the risk of death from one round-trip transcontinental airplane flight.

REFERENCES

American College of Surgeons, Commission on Cancer. 1974. Cancer Program Manual. Chicago: American College of Surgeons.

American Public Health Association. 1981. Control of Communicable Diseases in Man, A. Beneson, ed. Washington, D.C.

Arnstein, S. R. 1977. Technology assessment: Opportunities and obstacles. IEEE Trans. Syst. Man and Cybern. SM-7:571–582.

Averill, R. F., and L. F. McMahon. 1977. A cost-benefit analysis of continued stay certification. Med. Care 15:158.

Bailar J. C. 1970a. Periodical incidence surveys: I. Organization. Seminar on Cancer Registries in Latin America, Pan American Health Organization-World Health Organization, 41–100.

Bailar J. C. 1970b. Periodical incidence surveys: II. Basis for the selection of survey areas. Seminar on Cancer Registries in Latin America, Pan American Health Organization-World Health Organization, 101–110.

Bailar, J. C., III, T. A. Louis, P. W. Lavori, and M. Polansky. 1984. A classification for biomedical research reports. N. Engl. J. Med. 311:1482–1487.

Banta, D. H., C. J. Behney, and J. S. Willems. 1981. Costs and their evaluation. In Toward Rational Technology in Medicine. New York: Springer Publishing.

Barron, B. A., and R. M. Richart. 1981. Screening protocols for cervical neoplastic disease. Gynecol. Oncol. 12:S156.

Baum, M. L., D. S. Anish, T. C. Chalmers, et al. 1981. A survey of clinical trials of antibiotic prophylaxis in colon surgery: Evidence against further use of no-treatment controls. N. Engl. J. Med. 305:795–798.

Bearman, J. E., R. B. Lowenson, and W. H. Gullen. 1974. Muench's Postulates, Laws and Corollaries, Biometrics Note #4, National Eye Institute, DHEW, Bethesda.

Bell, R. L., and E. O. Smith. 1982. Clinical trials in post-marketing surveillance of drugs. Controlled Clinical Trials 3:61–68.

Berk, A. A., and T. C. Chalmers. 1981. Cost and efficacy of the substitution of ambulatory for inpatient care. N. Engl. J. Med. 304:393–397.

Bernstein, L. M., E. R. Siegel, and C. M. Goldstein. 1980. The hepatitis knowledge base: A prototype information transfer system. Ann. Intern. Med. 93:169–181.

Berwick, D. M., and A. L. Komaroff. 1982. Cost effectiveness of lead screening. N. Engl. J. Med. 306:1392–1398.

Blum, R. L. 1982. Discovery, confirmation, and incorporation of causal relationships from a large time-oriented clinical data base: The RX project. Comp. Biomed. Res. 15:164–187.

Boruch, R. F. 1985. Enhancing the usefulness of longitudinal data by coupling longitudinal surveys and randomized experiments. Draft Report for DOL, Center for Statistics and Probability, Northwestern University.

Boruch, R. F., and J. S. Cecil. 1979. Assuring confidentiality of social research data. Philadelphia: University of Pennsylvania Press.

Boston Collaborative Drug Surveillance Program. 1973. Oral contraceptives and venous thromboembolic disease, surgically confirmed gallbladder disease and breast tumors. Lancet 1:1399–1404.

Braakman, R. 1978. Data bank of head injuries in three countries. Scott. Med. J. 23:107–108.

Bruce, R. A., et al. 1974. Seattle Heart Watch: Initial clinical circulation and electrocardiographic responses to maximal exercise. Am. J. Cardiol. 33:459–469.

Bruce, R. A., et al. 1981. A computer terminal program to evaluate cardiovascular functional limits and estimate coronary event rates. West. J. Med. 135:342–350.

Bunker, J. P., B. J. Barnes, and F. Mosteller. 1977. Costs, Risks and Benefits of Surgery. New York: Oxford University Press.

Burke, J. F., H. S. Jordan, C. B. Boyle, and E. Vanner. 1981. An Impact Study of the 1978 Consensus Conference on Supportive Therapy in Burn Care. Massachusetts Health Research Institute.

Byar, D. P., R. M. Simon, W. T. Friedewald, et al. 1976. Randomized clinical trials: Perspectives on some recent ideas. N. Engl. J. Med. 295:74–80.

Campbell, D. T., and J. C. Stanley. 1963. Experimental and Quasi-Experimental Designs for Research. Chicago: Rand McNally College Publishing.

Centers for Disease Control. 1979. Abortion Surveillance 1977. Atlanta, Ga.: Department of Health, Education, and Welfare.

Centers for Disease Control. 1982a. Annual Summary, 1981. Reported morbidity and mortality in the United States. Morbid. Mortal. Weekly Rep. 30(54).

Centers for Disease Control. 1982b. Annual Summary, 1981. Morbid. Mortal. Weekly Rep. 30:126–127.

Centor, R. A., and J. S. Schwartz. In press. Calculation of the area under a ROC curve using microcomputers. Med Decision Making.

Chaitman, B. R., et al. 1981. Angiographic prevalence of high-risk coronary artery disease in patient subsets (CASS). Circulation 64:360–367.

Chalmers, T. C. 1975. Randomizing the first patient. Med. Clin. North Am. 59:1035–1038.

Chalmers, T. C. 1981. The Clinical Trial. Milbank Mem. Fund Q. 59:324–339.

Cochran, W. G. 1954. The combination of estimates from different experiments. Biometrics 10:101–129.

Cohen, S. N., M. F. Armstrong, R. L. Briggs, et al. 1974. Computer-based monitoring and reporting of drug interactions. Medinfo 1974:889–894.

Collen, J. F., R. Feldman, A. Siegelaub, and D. Crawford. 1970. Dollar cost per positive test for automated multiphasic screening. N. Engl. J. Med. 283:459–463.

Collen, M. F. 1979a. A case study of mammography. In Medical Technology and the Health Care System: A Study of the Diffusion of Equipment-Embodied Technology. Prepared by the Committee on Technology and Health Care, National Academy of Sciences, Washington, D.C.

Collen, M. F. 1979b. A study of multiphasic health testing. In Medical Technology and the Health Care System: A Study of the Diffusion of Equipment-Embodied Technology. Prepared by the Committee on Technology and Health Care, National Academy of Sciences, Washington, D.C.

Collen, M. F. 1979c. A guideline matrix for technological system evaluation. J. Med. Systems 2:249–254.

Collen, M. F. 1979d. Cost effectiveness of automated laboratory testing. In Clinician and Chemist, D. S. Young, et al., ed., Proceedings of the First A.O. Beckman Conference in Clinical Chemistry, American Association of Clinical Chemists, Washington, D.C.

Collen, M. F. 1983. Utilization of Diagnostic X-ray Examinations. HHS Pub. FDA 83-8208. Washington, D.C.: U.S. Government Printing Office.

Collen, M. F., L. G. Dales, G. D. Friedman, et al. 1973. Multiphasic health checkup evaluation study. 4. Preliminary cost benefit analysis for middle-aged men. Prev. Med. 2:236–246.

Collen, M. F., S. R. Garfield, R. H. Richart, et al. 1977. Cost analyses of alternative health examination modes. Arch. Int. Med. 137:73–79.

Commission on Cancer. 1974. Cancer Program Manual. Chicago: American College of Surgeons.

Cook, T. D., and L. C. Leviton. 1980. Reviewing the literature: A comparison of traditional methods with meta-analysis. J. Pers. 48:449–472.

Cooper, B. S., and D. P. Rice. 1976. The economic cost of illness revisited. Soc. Secur. Bull. 39:21–36.

Cowley, R. A., W. J. Sacco, W. Gill, et al. 1974. A prognostic index for severe trauma. J. Trauma 14:1029–1035.

Cox, E. B., and W. Stanley. 1979a. Schema driven time-oriented record on minicomputer. Comp. Biomed. Res. 12:503–516.

Cox, E. B., J. Laszlo, and A. Freiman. 1979b. Classification of cancer patients: Beyond TNM. J. Am. Med. Assoc. 242:2691–2695.

Cretin, S. 1977. Cost-benefit analysis of treatment and prevention of myocardial infarction. Health Serv. Res. 12:174.

Cutler, S. J., J. Scotto, S. S. Devesa, and R. R. Connelly. 1974. Third National Cancer Survey—An overview of available information. J. Natl. Cancer Inst. 53:1565–1575.

Dalkey, N. C. 1969. The Delphi Method: An Experimental Study of Group Opinion. Santa Monica, Calif.: Rand Corporation.

Dannenberg, A. L., R. Shapiro, and J. F. Fries. 1979. Enhancement of clinical predictive ability by computer consultation. Meth. Inform. Med. 18:10–14.

Deane, R., and A. Ulene. 1977. Hysterectomy or tubal ligation for sterilization: A cost-effectiveness analysis. Inquiry 14:73.

Delbecq, A., A. H. Van de Ven, and D. H. Gustafson. 1975. Group Techniques for Program Planning. Glenview, Ill.: Scott, Foresman.

Demographic Analysis Section, Biometry Branch, National Cancer Institute. 1976. Code Manual—The SEER Program. DHEW Pub. No. (NIH)-79-1999. Bethesda, Md.: National Cancer Institute.

DerSimonian, R., L. J. Charrette, B. McPeek, and F. Mosteller. 1982. Reporting on methods in clinical trials. N. Engl. J. Med. 306:1332–1337.

DerSimonian, R., and N. Laird. 1982. Evaluating the effectiveness of coaching for SAT exams, a meta-analysis. Pp. 1–15 in Harvard Educational Review.

Devine, E. C., and T. D. Cook. 1983. Effects of psychoeducational intervention on length of hospital stay: A meta-analytic review of 34 studies, American Journal of Nursing. Reproduced in R. J. Light, ed. 1983. Evaluation Studies, Review Annual, Vol. 8, pp. 417–432. Beverly Hills, Calif.: Sage Publications.

Dixon, R. E. 1978. Effects of infections on hospital care. Ann. Intern. Med. 89 (part 2):749–753.

Drazen, E., and J. Metzger. 1981. Methods for evaluating costs of automated hospital information systems. DHHS Publ. No. (PHS) 81-3283. Washington, D.C.: U.S. Government Printing Office.

Dyke, F. J., F. A. Murphy, J. K. Murphy, et al. 1974. Effect of surveillance on the number of hysterectomies in the province of Saskatchewan. N. Engl. J. Med. 296:1326–1328.

Eddy, D. M. 1980. Screening for Cancer: Theory, Analysis and Design. Englewood Cliffs, N.J.: Prentice-Hall.

Eddy, D. M. 1981. Appropriateness of cervical cancer screening. Gynecol. Oncol. 12:S168.

Eddy, D. M. 1982. Clinical policies and the quality of clinical practice. N. Engl. J. Med. 307:343–347.

Emerson, J. D., B. McPeek, and F. Mosteller. 1984. Reporting clinical trials in general surgical journals. Surgery 95:572–579.

Evans, R. W. 1983. Health care technology and the inevitability of resource allocation and rationing decisions. J. Am. Med. Assoc. 149:2208–2219.

Evenson, R. C., H. Altman, I. W. Sletten, and D. W. Cho. 1975. Accuracy of actuarial and clinical predictions for length of stay and unauthorized absence. Dis. New. Syst. 36:250–252.

Eysenck, H. J. 1978. An exercise in mega-silliness. Am. Psychol. 33:517.

Farber, M. E., and S. N. Finkelstein. 1979. A cost-benefit analysis of a mandatory premarital rubella-antibody screening program. N. Engl. J. Med. 300:856–859.

Feigl, P., N. E. Breslow, J. Laszlo, et al. 1981. The U.S. centralized cancer patient data system for uniform communication among cancer centers. J. Natl. Cancer Inst. 67:1017–1024.

Feinstein, A. R. 1977. Clinical Biostatistics, pp. 214–226. St. Louis: C. V. Mosby.

Feinstein, A. R. 1978. Clinical biostatistics XLIV. Clin. Pharmacol. Ther. 24:117–25.

Ferguson, M. 1980. The Aquarian Conspiracy. Los Angeles: J. P. Tarcher, Inc.

Fineberg, H. V. 1979. Gastric freezing: A study of diffusion of a medical innovation. Pp. 173–200 in Medical Technology and the Health Care System: A Study of the Diffusion of Equipment-Embodied Technology. Washington, D.C.: National Academy Press.

Fineberg, H. V., R. Bauman, and M. Sosman. 1977. Computerized cranial tomography: Effect on diagnostic and therapeutic plans. J. Am. Med. Assoc. 238:224–230.

Fink, A., J. Kosecoff, M. Chassin, and R. H. Brook. 1984 Consensus methods: Characteristics and guidelines for use. Am. J. Public Health 74:979–983.

Finkler, S. A. 1982. The distinction between cost and charges. Ann. Intern. Med. 96:102–1099.

Finney, D. J. 1965. The design and logic of a monitor of drug use. J. Chronic Dis. 18:77–98.

Finney, D. J. 1966. Monitoring adverse reactions to drugs—its logic and its weakness. Pp. 198–207 in Medical Foundation, International Congress Series No. 115. Proceedings of the European Society for the Study of Drug Toxicity, Vol. VII.

Fisher, R. A. 1938. Statistical Methods for Research Workers. London: Oliver & Boyd.

Fisher, R. A. 1948. Combining independent tests of significance. Am. Stat. 2:30.

Fletcher, R. H., and S. W. Fletcher. 1979. Clinical

research in general medical journals: A 30 year perspective. N. Engl. J. Med. 301:108–183.

Foege, W. H., J. D. Millar, and J. M. Lane. 1971. Selective epidemiologic control in smallpox eradication. Am. J. Epidemiol. 94:311–315.

Freiman, J. A., T. C. Chalmers, H. Smith, Jr., and R. R. Kuebler. 1978. The importance of the type II error and the sample size in the design and interpretation of the randomized control trial. N. Engl. J. Med. 299:690–694.

Friedman, G. D. 1972. Screening criteria for drug monitoring: The Kaiser-Permanente drug reaction monitoring system. J. Chronic Dis. 25:11–20.

Friedman, G. D. 1983a. Rauwolfia and breast cancer: No relation found in long term users age fifty and over. J. Chronic Dis. 36:367–370.

Friedman, G. D., and H. K. Ury. 1983b. Screening for possible drug carcinogenicity: Second report of findings. J. Natl. Cancer Inst. 71:1165–1175.

Friedman, L. F., C. D. Furberg, and D. L. DeMets. 1981. Fundamentals of Clinical Trials, ix, 225. Boston: John Wright, PSG.

Fries, J. F., S. Weyl, and H. R. Holman. 1974. Estimating prognosis in systemic lupus erythematosus. Am. J. Med. 57:561–565.

Fuchs, V. R. 1974. Who Shall Live? Health, Economics and Social Choice. New York: Basic Books.

Galbraith, S. L. 1978. Prognostic factors already known. Scott Med. J. 23:108–109.

Galliher, H. P. 1981. Optimizing ages for cervical smear examinations in followed healthy individuals. Gynecol. Oncol. 12:S188.

Garber, A. M., V. R. Fuchs, and J. F. Silverman. 1984. Case mix, costs, and outcomes: differences between faculty and community services in a university hospital. N. Engl. J. Med. 310:1231–1237.

Gershman, S. T., H. Barrett, J. T. Flannery, et al. 1976. Development of the Connecticut tumor registry. Conn. Med. 40:697–701.

Gilbert, J. P., B. McPeek, and F. Mosteller. 1977. Progress in surgery and anesthesia: Benefits and risks of innovative therapy. In Costs, Risks, and Benefits of Surgery, J. Bunker, B. Barnes, and F. Mosteller, eds. New York: Oxford University Press.

Gittelsohn, A. M., and J. Wennberg. 1977. On the incidence of tonsillectomy and other common surgical procedures. Pp. 91–106 in Costs, Risks and Benefits of Surgery, J. P. Bunker, B. A. Barnes, and F. Mosteller, eds. New York: Oxford University Press.

Glaser, E. M. 1980. Using behavioral science strategies for defining the state-of-the-art. J. Appl. Behav. Sci. 16:79–82.

Glass, G. V. 1976. Primary, secondary and meta-analysis of research. Educ. Res. 5:351–379.

Glass, G. V., B. McGaw, and M. L. Smith. 1981. Meta-Analysis in Social Research. Beverly Hills, Calif.: Sage Publications.

Globe, S., G. N. Levy, and C. M. Schwartz. 1967. Science, Technology, and Innovation. Contract NSF-C667 (Battelle-Columbus Laboratories). Washington, D.C.: National Science Foundation.

Grace, N. D., H. Muench, and T. C. Chalmers. 1966. The present status of shunts for portal hypertension in cirrhosis. Gastroenterology 50:684.

Graham, G. F., and F. J. Wyllie. 1979. Prediction of gall-stone pancreatitis by computer. Br. Med. J. 1:515–517.

Groot, L. M. J. 1982. Advanced and Expensive Medical Technology in the Member States of the European Community: Legislation, Policy and Costs. Commissioned by the European Community. Mimeograph; Roermond, The Netherlands.

Grossman, L. B. 1981. Beads and balloons. Pp. 2–6 in Pacemaker, Vol. 6, No. 3. Detroit: Harper Grace Hospitals.

Gustafson, D. H., A. L. Delbecq, M. Hansen, and R. F. Myers. 1975. Design of a health policy research and development system. Inquiry 12:251–262.

Haley, R. W., D. Quade, H. E. Freeman, et al. 1980. The Senic Project: Study on the efficacy of nonsocomial infection control. Am. J. Epidemiol. 111:472–485.

Hanley, J. A., and B. J. McNeil. 1982. The meaning and use of the area under a receiver operating characteristic (ROC) curve. Diag. Radiol. 143:29–36.

Health and Social Service Journal, May 30, 1980, pp. 702–704.

Hedges, L. V., and I. Olkin. 1980. Vote-counting methods in research synthesis. Psychol. Bull. 88:359–369.

Herbert, T. T., and E. B. Yost. 1979. A comparison of decision quality under nominal and interacting consensus group formats: The case of the structured problem. Decision Sci. 10:358–370.

Herbst, A. L., M. Ulfelder, and D. C. Poskaner. 1971. Association of maternal stilbestrol therapy with tumor appearance in young women. N. Engl. J. Med. 284:878–881.

Heyman, A., J. G. Burch, R. Rosati, et al. 1979. Use of a computerized information system in the management of patients with transient cerebral ischemia. Neurology 29:214–221.

Hiltz, S. R., and M. Turoff. 1978. The Network Nation. Reading, Mass: Addison-Wesley.

Hoaglin, D. C., R. J. Light, B. McPeek, et al. 1982. Data for Decisions. Cambridge, Mass: Abt Books.

Hodgkin, J. E., ed. 1979. Chronic Obstructive Pulmonary Diseases: Current Concepts in Diagnosis and Comprehensive Care. Park Ridge, Ill.: American College of Chest Physicians.

Hodgkin, J. E., O. J. Balchum, I. Kass, et al. 1975. Chronic obstructive airway diseases: Current concepts in diagnosis and comprehensive care. J. Am. Med. Assoc. 232:1243–1260.

Hook, E. B., D. M. Schreinemachers, and P. K. Cross. 1981. Use of prenatal cytogenic diagnosis in New York State. N. Engl. J. Med. 305:1410–1413.

Horn, S. D., and J. W. Williamson. 1977. Statistical methods for reliability and validity testing: An application to nominal group judgments in health care. Med. Care 15:922–928.

Hovrocks, J. C., D. E. Lambert, W. A. McAdams, et al. 1976. Transfer of computer aided diagnosis of dyspepsia from one geographical area to another. Gut 17:640–644.

Hunter, J. E. 1982. Meta-Analysis: Cumulating Research Findings Across Studies. Beverly Hill, Calif.: Sage Publications.

IMS America Ltd. 1978. Report of the Joint Commission on Prescription Drug Use, Contract 223-78-3007. Department of Health, Education, and Welfare, Food and Drug Administration.

Inglefinger, J. A., F. Mosteller, L. A. Thibodeau, and J. H. Ware. 1983. Biostatistics in Clinical Medicine, Section 11-6, pp. xiii, 316. New York: Macmillan.

Institute of Medicine 1981. Evaluating Medical Technologies in Clinical Use. Washington, D.C.: National Academy Press.

Jackson, G. B. 1980. Methods for integrative reviews. Rev. Educ. Res. 50:438–460.

Jacoby, I. 1983. Biomedical technology: Information dissemination and the NIH consensus development process. Knowledge: Creation, Diffusion. Utilization 5:245–261.

Jeans, W. D., and A. F. Morris. 1976. The accuracy of radiological and computer diagnoses in small bowel examinations in children. Br. J. Radiol. 49:665–669, 1976.

Jennett, B., G. Teasdale, R. Brackman, et al. 1976. Predicting outcome in individual patients after severe head trauma. Lancet 1:1031–1034.

Jick, H., A. M. Walker, and C. Spriet-Pourra. 1979. Postmarketing follow-up. J. Am. Med. Assoc. 242:2310–2314.

Jillson, I. A. 1975. The national drug-abuse policy delphi: Progress report and findings to date. In The Delphi Method: Techniques and Applications, H. Linstone and M. Turoff, eds. Reading, Mass.: Addison-Wesley.

Kennedy, M. M. 1979. Generalizing from single case studies. Eval. Q. 3:661–678.

Kimball, A. M., S. B. Thacker, and M. E. Levy. 1980. Shigella surveillance in a large metropolitan area: Assessment of a passive reporting system. Am. J. Public Health 70:164–166.

Klarman, H. E. 1973. Application of cost-benefit analysis of health systems technology. In Technology and Health Care Systems in the 1980's, M. F. Collen, ed. DHEW Publ. (HMS) 73-3016. Washington, D.C.: U.S. Government Printing Office.

Knill-Jones, R. 1978. New statistical approach to prediction. Scott. Med. J. 23:102–110.

Kolata, G. 1985. Heart panel's conclusions questioned. Science 227:40–41.

Koplan, J. P., and L. S. Farer. 1980. Choice of preventive treatment for Isoniazid-resistant tuberculous infection. J. Am. Med. Assoc. 244:2736–2740.

Koplan, J. P., and S. R. Preblud. 1982. A benefit-cost analysis of mumps vaccine. Am. J. Dis. Child. 136:362–364.

Koplan, J. P., S. C. Schoenbaum, M. C. Weinstein, et al. 1979. Pertussis vaccine: An analysis of benefits, risks and costs. N. Engl. J. Med. 301:906–911.

Kruskal, W., and F. Mosteller. 1980. Representative sampling IV: The history of the concept in statistics, 1895–1939. Int. Stat. Rev. 48:169–195.

Kurland, L. T., and C. A. Molgaard. 1981. The patient record in epidemiology. Sci. Am. 245:54–63.

Lane, J. M., F. L. Ruben, J. M. Neff, et al. 1969. Complications of smallpox vaccination, 1968. National surveillance in the United States. N. Engl. J. Med. 281:1201–1208.

Laszlo, J. 1984. In press. Two long-range clinical data bases are terminated—bang, whimper, or ripple? J. Clin. Oncol.

Laszlo, J. Healthy registry and clinical data base terminology, with special reference to cancer registries. Submitted for publication.

Laszlo, J., C. Angle, and E. Cox. 1976. The hospital tumor registry: Present status and future prospects. Cancer 38:395.

Lave, J., A. Dobson, and C. Walton. 1983. The potential use of Health Care Financing Administration data tapes for health care services research. Health Care Financing Rev. 5:93–98.

Layde, P. M., S. D. Von Allman, and G. P. Oakley. 1979. Maternal serum alpha-fetoprotein screening: A cost-benefit analysis. Am. J. Publ. Health 69:566–573.

Lembcke, P. A. 1956. Medical auditing by scientific methods, illustrated by major female pelvic surgery. J. Am. Med. Assoc. 162:646–655.

Lenfant, C., B. Rifkind, and I. Jacoby. 1985. Heart panel's conclusions (letter). Science 227:582–583.

Light, R. J., ed. 1983. Evaluation Studies Review Annual, Vol. 8. Beverly Hills: Sage Publications.

Light, R. J., and P. V. Smith. 1971. Accumulating evidence: Procedures for resolving contradictions among different research studies. Harv. Ed. Rev. 41:429–471.

Linstone, H., and M. Turoff, eds. 1975. The Delphi Method: Techniques and Applications. Reading, Mass.: Addison-Wesley.

Lips, K. J. M., V. D. S. Veer, A. Struyvenberg, and R. A. Geerdink. 1982. Genetic predisposition to cancer in man. Am. J. Med. 73:305–307.

Louis, P. 1836. Researches on the Effects of Blood Letting on Some Inflammatory Disease and on the Influence of Tartarized Antimony and Vesication in Pneumonia (translated by C. G. Putman). Boston: Hilliard Gray and Company.

Louis, T. A., H. Fineberg, and F. Mosteller. 1985. Findings for public health from meta-analysis, pp. 1–20. Annual Review of Public Health. Palo Alto, California: Annual Reviews, Inc.

Lusted, L. B. 1969. Perception of roentgen image: Applications of signal detection theory. Rad. Clinics N. Am. 7:435–445.

Maclennan, R., C. Muir, and A. Winkler. 1978. Cancer Registration and Its Techniques. Lyon: International Association for Cancer Research.

Mantel, N., and W. Haenszel. 1959. Statistical aspects of the analysis of data from retrospective studies of disease. J. Natl. Cancer Inst. 22:719–748.

McNeil, B. J. 1979. Pitfalls in and Requirements for Evaluations of Diagnostic Technologies in Medical Technology. DHEW Publ. No. (PHS) 79-3254. Urban Institute Conference.

McNeil, B. J., P. D. Varady, B. A. Burrows, and S. J. Adelstein. 1975. Cost-effectiveness calculations in the diagnosis and treatment of hypertensive renovascular disease. N. Engl. J. Med. 293:216–221.

McShane, D. J., J. Porta, and J. F. Fries. 1978. Comparison of therapy in severe systemic lupus erythematosus employing stratification techniques. J. Rheumatol. 5:51–58.

Meier, P. 1975. Statistics and medical experimentation. Biometrics 31:511–530.

Metz, C. E. 1978. Basic principles of ROC analysis. Semin. Nucl. Med. 7:283–298.

Metz, C. E., D. J. Goodenaugh, and K. Rossman. 1973. Evaluation of receiver operating characteristic curve data in terms of information theory, with applications in radiology. Radiology 109:297–303.

Moscovice, I., P. Armstrong, S. Shortell, and R. Bennet. 1977. Health services research for decision-makers: The use of the Delphi technique to determine health priorities. J. Health Politics, Policy and Law 2:388–410.

Mosteller, F. M., and R. R. Bush. 1954. Selected quantitative techniques. In Handbook of Social Psychology, Vol. I, Theory and Method, G. Lindzey, ed. Cambridge, Mass.: Addison-Wesley.

Mulley, A. G., M. D. Silverstein, and J. L. Dienstag. 1982. Indications for use of hepatitis B vaccine, based on cost-effectiveness analysis. N. Engl. J. Med. 307:644–652.

Mullner, R. M., C. S. Byre, and C. L. Killingsworth. 1983. An inventory of the U.S. health care data bases. Review of Public Data Use 11:79–192.

Naisbitt, J. 1982. Megatrends. New York: Warner Books.

Nance, F. C., and I. Cohn, Jr. 1969. Surgical judgment in the management of stab wounds of the abdomen. A retrospective and prospective analysis based on a study of 600 stabbed patients. Annals of Surgery 170:569.

National Academy of Sciences. 1978. Personnel Needs and Training for Biomedical and Behavioral Research Personnel. Washington, D.C.: National Academy Press.

National Academy of Sciences. 1981. Personnel Needs and Training for Biomedical and Behavioral Research. Washington, D.C.: National Academy Press.

National Academy of Sciences/Institute of Medicine. 1983. Personnel Needs and Training for Biomedical and Behavioral Research. Washington, D.C.: National Academy Press.

National Academy of Sciences. 1985. Sharing Research Data, S. E. Fineberg, M. E. Martin, and M. L. Straf, eds. Washington, D.C.: National Academy Press.

National Center for Health Care Technology. 1981. Coronary artery bypass surgery. J. Am. Med. Assoc. 2246:1643.

National Center for Health Statistics. 1980a. Catalog of Public Use Data Tapes from the National Center for Health Statistics. Public Health Service, DHHS Publ. No. (PHS) 81-1213. Washington, D.C.: U.S. Government Printing Office.

National Center for Health Statistics. 1980b. Data Systems of the National Center for Health Statistics. Pp. 28–30 in Public Health Service, DHHS Publ. No. (PHS) 80-1247. Washington, D.C.: U.S. Government Printing Office.

National Center for Health Statistics. 1980c. Long-Term Health Care: Minimum Data Set. Report of the National Committee on Vital and Health Statistics. Public Health Service, DHHS Publ. No. (PHS) 80-1158. Washington, D.C.: U.S. Government Printing Office.

National Center for Health Statistics. 1980d. The collection and processing of drug information, National Ambulatory Medical Care Survey, United States. Prepared by H. Koch. In Vital and Health Statistics, Series 2, No. 90. Public Health Service. Washington, D.C.: U.S. Government Printing Office.

National Center for Health Statistics. 1980e. Trends and variations in cesarean section delivery. Prepared by P. J. Placek, S. M. Taffel, and J. C. Kleinman. Pp. 73–36 in Health, United States, 1980. Public Health Service, DHHS Publ. No. (PHS) 81-1232. Washington: U.S. Government Printing Office.

National Center for Health Statistics. 1980f. Uniform Hospital Discharge Data: Minimum Data Set. Report of the National Committee on Vital and Health Statistics. Public Health Service, DHEW

Publ. No. (PHS) 80-1157. Hyattsville, Md.: U.S. Government Printing Office.

National Center for Health Statistics. 1981a. Inpatient utilization of short-stay hospitals by diagnosis, United States, 1978. Prepared by E. McCarthy. P. 24 in Vital and Health Statistics, Series 13, No. 55. Public Health Service, DHHS Publ. No. (PHS) 81-1716. Washington, D.C.: U.S. Government Printing Office.

National Center for Health Statistics. 1981b. NMCES Household Interview Instruments: Instruments and Procedures 1. Prepared by G. S. Bonham and L. T. Corder. Public Health Service, DHHS Publ. No. (PHS) 81-3280. Washington, D.C.: U.S. Government Printing Office.

National Center for Health Statistics. 1981c. Uniform Ambulatory Medical Care: Minimum Data Set. Report of the National Committee on Vital and Health Statistics. Public Health Service, DHHS Publ. No. (PHS) 81-1161. Hyattsville, Md.: U.S. Government Printing Office.

National Center for Health Statistics. 1983a. Data Systems of the National Center for Health Statistics, pp. 63–75. Public Health Service, DHHS Publ. No. (PHS) 80-1247. Washington, D.C.: U.S. Government Printing Office.

National Center for Health Statistics. 1983b. Drug utilization in office-based practices: Summary of findings. National Ambulatory Medical Care Survey. United States, 1980. Prepared by H. Koch. In Vital and Health Statistics, Series 13, No. 65. Public Health Service, DHHS Publ. No. (PHS) 83-1726. Washington, D.C.: U.S. Government Printing Office.

National Center for Health Statistics. 1983c. Health, United States, 1983, p. 13. Public Health Service, DHHS Publ. No. (PHS) 84-1232. Washington, D.C.: U.S. Government Printing Office.

National Center for Health Statistics. 1983d. Procedures and questionnaires of the National Medical Care Utilization and Expenditure Survey. Prepared by G. S. Bonham. In Series A, Methodological Report No. 1. Public Health Service, DHHS Publ. No. 83-20001. Washington, D.C.: U.S. Government Printing Office.

National Center for Health Statistics. 1983e. Utilization of shortstay hospitals: United States, 1981 annual summary. In Vital and Health Statistics, Series 13, No. 72. Public Health Service, DHHS Publ. No. (PHS) 83-1733. Washington D.C.: U.S. Government Printing Office.

National Center for Health Statistics. 1983f. Variation in use of obstetric technology. Prepared by J. C. Kleinman, M. Cooke, S. Machlin, and S. S. Kessel. Pp. 63–75 in Health, United States, 1983. Public Health Service, DHHS Publ. No. (PHS) 84-1232. Washington, D.C.: U.S. Government Printing Office.

National Commission for the Protection of Human Subjects. 1978. Report and Recommendations. Washington, D.C.: U.S. Government Printing Office.

National Institutes of Health. 1983. Liver transplantation consensus development. Conference Summary. Volume 4, Number 7.

National Institutes of Health. 1984. Diagnostic ultrasound imaging in pregnancy. Consensus Development Conference. Volume 5, Number 1.

NHLBI Angioplasty, Kent et al. 1982. Percutaneous transluminal coronary angioplasty: Report from the registry of the National Heart, Lung, and Blood Institute. Am. J. Cardiol. 49:2011–2018.

Needleman, H. L, S. K. Geiger, and R. Frank. 1985. Lead and IQ scores: a reanalysis. Science 227:701–702.

Needleman, H. L., C. Gunnoe, A. Leviton, et al. 1979. Deficits in psychologic and classroom performance of children with elevated dentine lead levels. N. Engl. J. Med. 300:689–695.

Neustadt, R., and H. V. Fineberg. 1983. The Epidemic That Never Was: Decision Making in the Swine Flu Scare. 1983. New York: Vintage Books.

Neutra, R. R., S. E. Fienberg, S. Greenland, and E. A. Friedman. 1978. Effect of fetal monitoring on neonatal death rates. N. Engl. J. Med. 299:324–326.

Office of Health Research Statistics and Technology. 1981. U.S. Department of Health and Human Services. Transsexual surgery. Assessment Report Series 1(4). Washington, D.C.: U.S. Department of Health and Human Services.

Office of Technology Assessment, U.S. Congress. 1978a. Assessing the efficacy and safety of medical technologies. Washington, D.C.: U.S. Government Printing Office.

Office of Technology Assessment, U.S. Congress. 1978b. Policy implications of the computed tomography (CT) scanner. GPO Stock No. 052-003-00565-4. Washington, D.C.: U.S. Government Printing Office.

Office of Technology Assessment, U.S. Congress. 1980a. The implications of cost-effectiveness analysis of medical technology. Stock No. 051-003-00765-7. Washington, D.C.: U.S. Government Printing Office.

Office of Technology Assessment, U.S. Congress. 1980b. The implications of cost-effectiveness analysis of medical technology/background paper #1: Methodological issues and literature review. Washington, D.C.: U.S. Government Printing Office.

Office of Technology Assessment, U.S. Congress. 1980c. The implications of cost-effectiveness analysis of medical technology/background paper #3: The efficacy and cost effectiveness of psychotherapy. Washington, D.C.: U.S. Government Printing Office.

Office of Technology Assessment, U.S. Congress. 1981a. Cost effectiveness of influenza vaccination.

Washington, D.C.: U.S. Government Printing Office.

Office of Technology Assessment, U.S. Congress. 1981b. The implications of cost-effectiveness analysis of medical technology/background paper #2: Case studies of medical technologies/care study #2: The feasibility of economic evaluation of diagnostic procedures: The case of CT scanning. Washington, D.C.: U.S. Government Printing Office.

Office of Technology Assessment, U.S. Congress. 1981c. The implications of cost-effectiveness analysis of medical technology/background paper #2. Case studies of medical technologies/case study #1: Formal analysis, policy formulation, and end-stage renal disease. Washington, D.C.: U.S. Government Printing Office.

Office of Technology Assessment, U.S. Congress. 1981d. The implications of cost-effectiveness analysis of medical technology/background paper #2: Case studies of medical technologies/case study #3: Screening for colon cancer: A technology assessment. Washington, D.C.: U.S. Governmment Printing Office.

Office of Technology Assessment, U.S. Congress. 1982a. Postmarketing Surveillance of Prescription Drugs. Washington, D.C.: U.S. Government Printing Office.

Office of Technology Assessment, U.S. Congress. 1982b. Strategies for Medical Technology Assessment. Washington, D.C.: U.S. Government Printing Office.

Office of Technology Assessment, U.S. Congress. 1982c. Technology and Handicapped People, p. 22. OTA-H-179. Washington, D.C.: U.S. Government Printing Office.

Office of Technology Assessment, U.S. Congress. 1983a. Abstracts of Case Studies in the Health Technology Case Study Series. OTA-P-225. Washington, D.C.: U.S. Government Printing Office.

Office of Technology Assessment, U.S. Congress. 1983b. Variations in Hospital Length of Stay: Their Relationship to Health Outcomes. Health Technology Case Study 24. OTA-HCS-24. Washington, D.C.: U.S. Government Printing Office.

Olsen, S. A. 1982. Group Planning and Problem Solving Methods in Engineering Management. New York: John Wiley & Sons.

Patrick, K. M., and R. Woolley. 1981. A cost-benefit analysis of immunization for pneumococcal pneumonia. J. Am. Med. Assoc. 245:473–477.

Pauker, S., and J. Kassirer. 1975. Therapeutic decision making: A cost-benefit analysis. N. Engl. J. Med. 293:229–234.

Pearson, E. S. 1938. The probability integral transformation for testing goodness of fit and combining independent tests of significance. Biometrika 30:134–148.

Pearson, E. S. 1950. On questions raised by the combination of tests based on discontinuous distributions. Biometrika 37:383–398.

Perry, S., and J. T. Kalberer. 1980. The NIH Consensus-Development Program and the assessment of health-care technologies: The first two years. N. Engl. J. Med. 303:169–172.

Pillemer, D. B., and R. J. Light. 1980. Synthesizing outcomes: How to use research evidence from many studies. Harvard Educ. Rev. 50:176–195.

Pocock, S. J. 1976. The combination of randomized and historical controls in clinical trials. J. Chronic Dis. 29:175–188.

Policy Research Incorporated. 1975a. National Drug Abuse Policy Delphi Study: Questionnaires and Summaries of Results. Baltimore.

Policy Research Incorporated. 1975b. National Drug Abuse Policy Report: Final Report. Baltimore.

Policy Research Incorporated. 1977. A Comprehensive Study of the Ethical, Legal, and Social Implications of Advances in Biomedical and Behavioral Research and Technology: Summary of the Final Report. Baltimore.

Policy Research Incorporated. 1979a. Medical Practice Information Demonstration Project: Depression Project: First Series of Instruments. Baltimore.

Policy Research Incorporated. 1979b. Medical Practice Information Demonstration Project: Bipolar Disorder: A State-of-the-Science Report. Baltimore.

Pollack, E. S. 1982a. Monitoring cancer incidence and patient survival in the United States. Proceedings, Social Statistics Section. Washington, D.C.: American Statistical Association.

Pollack, E. S. 1982b. SEER cost study. Printed for private distribution, Natonal Cancer Institute.

President's Commission for the Study of Ethical Problems in Medicine and Biomedical and Behavioral Research. 1983. Summing up: Final Report on Studies of the Ethical and Legal Problems in Medicine and Biomedical and Behavioral Research. Washington, D.C.: U.S. Government Printing Office.

Principal investigators of CASS and their associates. 1981. National Heart, Lung, and Blood Institute Coronary Artery Surgery Study. Circulation 63(suppl. I):1–81.

Queram, C. J. 1977. Cancer Registries and Reporting Systems in the United States. Madison, Wis.: Department of Health and Social Services, Bureau of Health Statistics, Division of Health.

Rand Corporation. 1983. Submission to the Office of Management and Budget of Supporting Statement and Data Collection Instruments for Assessing the Effectiveness of the NIH Consensus Development Program.

Ransahoff, D. F., and A. R. Feinstein. 1978. Problems of spectrum and bias in evaluating the efficacy of diagnostic tests. N. Engl. J. Med. 299:926–930.

Re, R., R. Novelline, M. T. Escourrou, et al. 1978.

Inhibition of angiotensin-converting enzyme for diagnosis of renal artery stenosis. N. Engl. J. Med. 298:582–586.

Remington, R. D. 1976. Recommendations. Pp. 141–150 in Assessing Drug Reactions—Adverse and Beneficial, Vol. 7, Philosophy and Technology of Drug Assessment, F. N. Allen, ed. Washington, D.C.: The Interdisciplinary Communications Associates.

Rennie, D. 1981. Consensus Statements. N. Engl. J. Med. 304:665–666.

Richart, R. H. 1974. Evaluation of a hospital computer system, in Hospital Computer Systems, M. Collen, ed. New York: John Wiley & Sons, Inc.

Richart, R. M. 1981. Discussion of session III: Screening of cervical neoplasia. Gynecol. Oncol. 12:S212.

Robertson, A., and M. H. Zweig. 1981. Use of receiver operating characteristic curves to evaluate the clinical performance of analytical systems. Clin. Chem. 77:1568–1574.

Romm, F. J., and B. S. Hulka. 1979. Developing criteria for quality of care assessment: Effect of the Delphi technique. Health Services Res. 14:309–312.

Roos, L. L., Jr. 1979. Alternative designs to study outcomes. Med. Care 17:1069–1087.

Rosati, R. A., A. G. Wallace, and E. A. Stead. 1973. The way of the future. Arch. Intern. Med. 131:285.

Rosenthal, R. 1978a. Combining results of independent studies. Psychol. Bull. 85:185–193.

Rosenthal, R., and D. B. Rubin. 1978b. Interpersonal expectancy effects: The first 345 studies. Behavioral and Brain Sciences 3:377–415.

Russell, L. B. 1979. Technology in Hospitals: Medical Advances in Their Diffusion. Washington, D.C.: The Brookings Institution.

Sackman, H. 1975. Delphi Critique. Lexington, Mass.: Lexington Books.

Sanders, C. A. 1979. Medical technology and the health care system: A study of the diffusion of equipment-embodied technology, by the Committee on Technology and Health Care. Washington, D.C.: National Academy of Sciences.

Schaffarzick, R., cited by Wennberg and Gittelsohn, 1973.

Schneiderman, M. A. 1966. Looking backward: Is it worth the crick in the neck? Or: pitfalls in using retrospective data. Am. J. Roentgenol. Radium Ther. Nucl. Med. 96:230–235.

Schoenbaum, S., J. N. Hyde, L. Bartoshesky, and K. Crampton. 1976a. Benefit-cost analysis of rubella vaccination policy. N. Engl. J. Med. 294:306–310.

Schoenbaum, S. C., B. J. McNeil, and J. Kavet. 1976b. The swine-influenza decision. N. Engl. J. Med. 295:759–765.

Schwartz, J. S., P. J. Weinbaum, C. Nesler, et al. 1983. Assessment of tests to identify infants at high risk of respiratory distress syndrome (RDS) using receiver operating characteristic (ROC) curve analysis. Med. Decision Making 3:365.

Scitovsky, A. A. 1979. Changes in the use of ancillary services for 'common' illness. Pp. 39–56 in Medical Technology: The Culprit Behind Health Costs? Proceedings of the 1977 Sun Valley Forum on National Health Insurance, Stuart H. Altman and Robert Blendon, eds. DHEW Publ. No. (PHS) 79-3216. New York: John Wiley.

Shapiro, M., et al. 1983a. Benefit-cost analysis of antimicrobial prophylaxis in abdominal and vaginal hysterectomy. J. Am. Med. Assoc. 249:1290–1294.

Shapiro, S. H., and T. A. Louis. 1983. Clinical Trials: Issues and Approaches, pp. ix, 209. New York: Marcel Dekker.

Sherins, R. J., C. L. Olivery, and J. L. Ziegler. 1978. Gynecomastia and gonadal dysfunction in adolescent boys treated with combination chemotherapy for Hodgkin's disease. N. Engl. J. Med. 299:12–16.

Showstack, J., et al. 1981. Evaluating the costs and benefits of a diagnostic technology: The case of upper gastrointestinal endoscopy. Med. Care 19:498–509.

Shur, R. D. 1981. Estimating the natural history of cancer from cross-sectional data. Ph.D. Dissertation, Engineering-Economic Systems, Stanford University.

Shwartz, M. 1978. An analysis of the benefits of serial screening for breast cancer based upon a mathematical model of the disease. Cancer 51:1550.

Siegel, E. R., 1980. Use of computer conferencing to validate and update NLM's hepatitis knowledge base, in The Future of Electronic Communications, M. M. Henderson, and M. J. MacNaughton, eds. Washington, D.C.: American Association for the Advancement of Science.

Snow, J. 1847. On the Inhalation of the Vapor of Ether in Surgical Operations. (Reproduced by Lea & Febiger, Philadelphia, 1959.)

Stange, P., and A. T. Summer. 1978. Predicting treatment costs and life expectancy for end-stage renal disease. N. Engl. J. Med. 298:372–378.

Stason, W,. and M. Weinstein. 1977. Allocation of resources to manage hypertension. N. Engl. J. Med. 296:732.

Steinberg, D. 1985. Heart panel's conclusions (letter). Science 227:582.

Swain, R. W. 1981. Health Systems Analysis. Columbus, Ohio: Grid Publishing.

Swets, J. A. 1979. ROC analysis applied to the evaluation of medical imaging techniques. Invest. Radiology 14:109–121.

Swets, J. D., and R. M. Pickett. 1982. Evaluation of Diagnostic Systems. New York: Academic Press.

Tatro, D. S., T. N. Moore, and S. N. Cohen. 1979. Computer-based system for adverse drug detection and prevention. Am. J. Hosp. Pharm. 36:198–201.

Teasdale, G. 1978. Prediction in action. Scott. Med. J. 23:111.

The Lancet Commission on Anesthesia. 1893. Lancet 1:629–638, 693–708, 761–776, 899–914, 971–978, 1236–1240, 1479–1498.

Thornell, C. A. 1981. Comparison of Strategies for the Development of Process Measures in Emergency Medical Services, NCHSR Research Summary Series. Hyattsville, Md.: National Center for Health Services Research.

Turoff, M., and S. R. Hiltz. 1982. Computer support for group versus individual decisions. IEEE Trans. Comm. COM-30(1):82–91.

U.S. Consumer Product Safety Commission. 1982. National Electronic Injury Surveillance System. NEISS Data Highlights 6:1–4.

U.S. Public Health Service. 1964. Smoking and Health. Report of the Advisory Committee to the Surgeon General of the Public Health Service. Washington, D.C.: U.S. Department of Health, Education, and Welfare.

Warner, K. E., and R. C. Hutton. 1981. Cost-benefit and cost-effectiveness analysis in health care. Med. Care 19:498–509.

Warner, K. E., and B. R. Luce. 1982. Cost-Benefit and Cost-Effectiveness Analysis in Health Care. Ann Arbor, Mich.: Health Administration Press.

Weinstein M., and W. Stason. 1976. Hypertension: A Policy Perspective. Cambridge, Mass.: Harvard University Press.

Weinstein, M. C., and H. V. Fineberg. 1980. Clinical Decision Analysis. Philadelphia: W. B. Saunders.

Weinstein, M. C., and B. Stason. 1977. Foundations of cost-effectiveness analysis for health and medical practices. N. Engl. J. Med. 296:716–721.

Wennberg, J. 1984. Dealing with medical practice variations: A proposal for action. Health Affairs 3:6–32.

Wennberg, J., and A. Gittlesohn. 1973. Small area variations in health care delivery. Science 182:1102–1108.

Wennberg, J. E. 1981. A strategy for the post-marketing surveillance and evaluation of health care technology. Department of Community and Family Medicine, Dartmouth Medical School.

Wennberg, J. E., J. P. Bunker, and B. Barnes. 1980. The need for assessing the outcome of common medical practices. Ann. Rev. Public Health 1:277–295.

White, C., and J. C. Bailar. 1956. Retrospective and prospective methods of studing association in medicine. Am. J. Public Health 46:35–44.

White, J. J., and N. W. Axnick. 1975. The benefits from 10 years of measles immunization in the United States. Public Health Rep. 90:205–207.

Willems, J. S., R. Sanders, A. Riddiough, and C. Bell. 1980. Cost-effectiveness of vaccination against pneumococcal pneumonia. N. Engl. J. Med. 303:553–559.

Williamson, J. W. 1978. Formulating priorities for quality assurance activity. J. Am. Med. Assoc. 239:631–637.

Wilson, D. H. 1979a. The acute abdomen in the accident and emergency department. Practitioner 222:480–485.

Wilson, S. 1979b. Explorations of the usefulness of case study evaluations. Evaluation Q. 3:446–59.

World Health Organization. 1976a. WHO Handbook for Standardized Cancer Registrations. Geneva.

World Health Organization. 1976b. ICD-O, International Classification of Diseases for Oncology, lst ed. Geneva.

Wortman, P. M. 1983. Evaluation research: A methodological perspective. Ann. Rev. Psychol. 34:223–260.

Wortman, P. M., and L. Saxe. 1982a. Assessment of medical technology: Methodological considerations (Appendix C). In Strategies for Medical Technology Assessment, prepared by the Office of Technology Assessment, U.S. Congress. Washington, D.C.: U.S. Government Printing Office.

Wortman, P. M., and A. Vinokur. 1982b. Evaluation of NIH Consensus Development Process. Phase I: Final Report. Ann Arbor, Mich.: Center for Research on Utilization of Scientific Knowledge, University of Michigan.

Yin, R. K. 1984. Cast Study Research, Deisgn and Methods. Beverly Hills: Sage Publications.

Young, J. L., Jr., A. Asire, and E. Pollock. 1976. SEER Program: Cancer Incidence and Mortality in the United Stats 1973–1976. DHEW Pub. No. (NIH) 78-1837. Bethesda, Md: National Cancer Institute.

Young, J. L., C. L. Percy, A. J. Asire, eds. 1981. SEER Program: Incidence and Mortality Data, 1973–77. National Cancer Institute Monograph 57, USG 80, NIH Pub. No. 81-2330. Washington, D.C.: National Cancer Institute.

4 Effects of Clinical Evaluation on the Diffusion of Medical Technology

Patterns of medical practice often diverge from recommendations based on controlled clinical evaluations. This chapter views such discrepancies in light of the many forces in addition to clinical evaluation that influence the adoption and abandonment of medical technology.

The central question for the chapter can be stated simply: What effect does the evaluation of medical technologies have on their diffusion? The next two sections of the chapter introduce some of the complexities of this question and present an approach to assessing the literature that tries to answer it. Following a review of literature about the effect of evaluation on the diffusion of medical technology, the chapter summarizes its principal conclusions and offers a few recommendations.

The relation between evaluation and diffusion is part of a larger issue of the contribution of technology assessment to improved health. This review emphasizes the connection between evaluations and physician behavior, although recognizing that health benefits in many medical situations ultimately depend on the behavior of patients as much as or more than that of physicians.

Harvey V. Fineberg prepared this chapter.

EVALUATION

In this review, the impact of two general types of evaluation are considered: (1) primary assessments of the consequences of a medical technology and (2) synthetic assessments of the implications for clinical practice of the available primary evidence. Both primary and synthetic assessments take a variety of forms. Primary assessments range from judgments based on personal experience to multicenter randomized clinical trials. Synthetic activities range from review articles to meetings of experts for the purpose of reaching consensus on a controversial issue.

This section deals with the effect of evaluation on medical care decisions, usually the decisions of physicians. Relatively few studies quantitatively assess the influence of community-based epidemiological studies, data banks, or case studies on changes in physician practice. Many primary and synthetic evaluations are used by regulatory bodies like the Food and Drug Administration or by third-party payers in reaching their policy decisions; these evaluations indirectly and powerfully impinge on clinical practice and should be considered by someone. In this chapter no attempt was made to cover the effect of evaluations on decisions about the organization, administration, and support systems of health institutions, although these too have an indirect bearing on medical practices. Nor has an attempt been made to catalog the impact of epidemiologic assessments on social policy (as in the areas of toxicology and environmental health) or on public behavior (as in the decline in cigarette smoking) related to health. The emphasis is on physician practices and on the influence of various forms of clinical evaluation in changing those practices.

Primary clinical evaluations could be arranged in a hierarchy according to their freedom from bias, for instance, with the randomized clinical trial (RCT) at the top and then, moving downward, controlled (nonrandomized) studies, series of patients without controls, and personal recollection unaided by systematic record keeping. If even the weakest forms of evaluation count in our lexicon of evaluation, then most clinical practice is based on an evaluation. To refine the question posed at the outset of the chapter, we would like to know whether (and, possibly, to what extent) the more rigorous and powerful forms of primary clinical assessment are more influential than less rigorous forms in shaping medical practice and the policy decisions that affect the use of medical technology. In some instances, of course, a particular technology cannot be studied using the stronger methods, for example, when an RCT is not feasible because of sample size.

DIFFUSION

Diffusion refers to the spread of an innovation over time in a social system (Rogers and Shoemaker, 1971). The concept includes new practices being adopted and old practices being abandoned. Built into the notion of diffusion is the expectation that social change is not instantaneous and that some difference in practice among physicians at a moment in time is therefore reasonable and likely. Many studies of diffusion in the social sciences examine situations in which measurable expansion or contraction in a practice occurs over the duration of the study rather than where patterns of practice (possibly including marked variation across individuals, institutions, or geography) are relatively stable.

In many studies of diffusion, the correctness of knowledge available to the potential adopter is taken for granted. An innovation or practice is regarded as objectively and knowably good or bad. The majority of these studies do not relate the nature and quality of evaluative evidence to the spread of a practice over time. Instead, diffusion studies tend to focus on characteristics of the innovation, characteristics of the potential adopters, communication channels (bringing information to the adopter), the decision-making process, institutional features, and environmental forces that bear on the spread of a practice. Notions of evaluation, if introduced at all, tend to enter as attributes of the innovation (for example, the ease with which it can be tried on an interim basis) rather than as an independent determinant of the rate or extent of diffusion.

Investigators concerned with the impact of scientific evidence on physician beliefs and practices frequently examine the state of practice at a single point in time rather than as a diffusion process over time. The prime interest in many of these studies has been to assess the knowledge and judgment of physicians rather than to judge critically the effectiveness of a clinical trial in reaching or convincing physicians. This discussion is especially concerned with studies that relate evaluation and specific evaluation methods to changes in practice over time.

Determinants of Diffusion

Many factors bear on the adoption and abandonment of medical technology. The following discussion identifies 10 sources of influence. The first 4 (prevailing theory, attributes of the innovation, features of the clinical situation, and the presence of an advocate) are relatively insensitive to change by policymakers. The next 3 (practice setting, decision-making process, and characteristics of the potential adopters) may be subject over time to some policy influence. The remaining 3 (environmental constraints and incentives, conduct and methods of evaluation, and channels of communication) are relatively susceptible to influence by policymakers. Each factor is discussed briefly, with the greatest attention given to the last group.

Prevailing Theory Prevailing theory and accepted explanations for empirical phenomena appear to have a strong influence on the acceptance of new ideas. Prevailing theories may delay the acceptance of ultimately proved innovations. Stern (1927) cites a number of classic examples, such as the resistance to smallpox vaccination by those who held that improved sanitation was the main cause of a decline in the smallpox rate, disbelief in the manifold consequences of syphilis by those who held to the theory of duality of tuberculosis; and refusal to recognize puerperal fever as a contagious disease by those who subscribed to atmospheric, cosmic, and telluric influences on health. Twentieth century examples include long-delayed acceptance of salicylates in the treatment of rheumatoid arthritis (Goodwin and Goodwin, 1982) and a number of advances in cardiopulmonary medicine and surgery (Comroe, 1976). In other cases, appeals to prevailing theory as a rational basis for belief about etiology and treatment of disease appeared to have hastened the acceptance of unsubstantiated practices that were ultimately discarded. This occurred, for example, in the case of gastric freezing for the treatment of duodenal ulcers (Fineberg, 1979) and the conduct of subsequently discarded operations such as surgery for the endocrine glands and surgery for constipation (Barnes, 1977). Marks (Ideas as Social Reforms: The Legacies of Randomized Clinical Trials, unpublished report, 1983) argues that relatively new methods of evaluation (like RCTs) are themselves an innovation whose acceptance is influenced by prevailing theory about the nature of clinical evaluation and its role in medical decision making.

The Innovation Innovations vary in the benefits and costs they offer the physician and in their compatibility with the physician's experience and style of practice. Diffusion of new practices is presumably enhanced by the extent to which they are easy to use, require little effort to learn, impose little change in practice style, are highly remunerative and satisfying, and have no clinically worthy competitors.

The Clinical Situation An innovation that solves an important clinical problem and is seen as highly pertinent to practice is likely to be adopted more readily than an otherwise equally attractive innovation that addresses a less pressing or pertinent situation.

Advocacy Successful diffusion of new practices often has been attributed to an authoritative advocate who promotes the innovation (Globe et al., 1967; Barnes, 1977; Fineberg, 1979). Forceful advocates have wrongly encouraged practices that were subsequently abandoned as ineffective as well as practices that were eventually proved effective. An authority figure who is correct in strongly promoting or opposing one innovation may turn out to be wrong about a later innovation (Stern, 1927; Comroe, 1976; Fineberg, 1979).

The Potential Adopter Many studies of diffusion and of variation in medical practices seek to explain patterns of practice in terms of physician attributes such as their technical skills, demographic characteristics, professional characteristics, sociometric status, and attitudes toward innovation. In principle, changes in medical school admissions policies and in access to various types of specialty training could in time alter attributes of the physician population.

The Practice Setting Several features of the setting and environment in which physicians practice can influence their use of medical technology. Physicians in group practices appear to adopt innovations more rapidly than physicians in solo practice (Williamson, 1975). The size and teaching status of hospitals appear to influence hospital acquisition of equipment, making possible new physician practices (Russell, 1979). The pattern of practice among colleagues influences the way physicians use available medical technology (Freeborn et al., 1972).

The Decision-Making Process Some medical practice decisions are wholly within the domain of the individual practitioner. Others are group decisions, and yet others require a concomitant or prior institutional decision. A decision-making process that involves more people is likely to require a longer time to reach a conclusion. In a study of three anesthetic practices, the one that required a collective and institutional decision (scavenging for waste anesthetic gases) entailed several years longer delay between awareness and change in practice than was the case for the other two practices in which the physician could take action as an individual (Fineberg et al., 1978, 1980).

Environmental Constraints and Incentives Regulatory agencies and medical care insurers exercise direct and indirect control over the diffusion of many medical practices. Examples may be cited at the federal, state, and local levels. At the federal level, the Food and Drug Administration sets standards for the approval of new drugs and medical devices; the Health Care Financing Administration makes insurance coverage decisions for Medicare patients that may prompt similar action by other third-party payers; and the Centers for Disease Control set the antigenic content and recommended usage of vaccines, among other recommendations for practice. At the state level, certificate-of-need programs, at least in principle, directly influence hospital equipment and services, many of which impinge on clinicians' practices. Locally, institutional review bodies and quality assurance efforts affect decisions about medical practices. The climate of malpractice litigation also may alter a clinicians' reliance on certain medical procedures. All such environmental forces shape the opportunities and incentives for change in medical practice.

Evaluation and Methods of Evaluation The factor that is of central concern in this chapter is the role of formal evaluation in shaping the behavior of physicians. Evaluation may act directly on the perceptions of physicians; it may influence experts who in turn influence physicians (through a channel of communication); or it may influence the policy decisions of regulatory bodies (such as the Food and Drug Administration), or of third-party payers (such as the Health Care Financing Administration), and hence alter the environment in which medical practice decisions are made. In this chapter, all three possible chains of influence on physician practices are examined.

Many clinicians are not well prepared to deal with quantitative methods in formal evaluations (Berwick et al., 1981). Debates about the merits of particular evaluations may be the expression of fundamental disagreement about the nature and role of controlled clinical trials in medicine (Feinstein, 1983; Bonchek, 1979; Marks, unpublished report, 1983).

Channels of Communication A substantial number of diffusion studies in medicine have examined the ways in which physicians learn about new practices. Investigators are interested in which sources of information and which channels of communication are most influential. Because different channels of communication can to a degree be selected by clinical investigators and potentially enhanced by policymakers, research in this area warrants elaboration.

A large body of early work on channels of communication concerned the dissemination of drugs among medical practitioners, especially the influence of face-to-face sales representatives and of social networks among physicians (Sherrington, 1965). These early studies found that direct person-to-person contacts by drug company representatives were more influential than other forms of advertising (Caplow, 1954). This finding has been reaffirmed in recent studies showing that personal representation by pharmacists or, even more effectively, by other physicians can influence doctors to be more prudent drug prescribers (Avorn and Soumerai, 1983; Schaffner, 1983).

Studies of how doctors learn about new medical practices, based on physician surveys, have found medical journals, discussion with colleagues, and continuing education each to be regarded as important sources, with journals most consistently cited as high (Fineberg et al., 1978; Manning and Denson, 1979, 1980; Stross and Harlan, 1981; Market Facts, 1982; Jordan et al., 1983). One study of physician awareness of pertinent findings published in a journal of a specialty different from their own found that most of those who were aware of the findings learned about them from consultants or colleagues (Stross, 1979). In a study of three practices in anesthesiology, the channels of communication (papers published in journals, colleagues, and continuing education) differed more in how many physicians they reached than in their persuasiveness to change practice (Fineberg et al., 1978). Persuasiveness depended more on the nature of the clinical finding being communicated than on the channel of communication. Whether formal medical training appears relatively important in conveying new knowledge (Jordan et al., 1983) or relatively unimportant (Manning and Denson, 1979) may depend mainly on the recency of the innovation and on the age of the potential adopter. Other studies are beginning to assess the influence of National Institutes of Health (NIH) consensus conferences on specific physician practices (The Rand Corporation, 1983; Jacoby, Biomedical Technology Information Dissemination and the NIH Consensus Development Process, unpublished report, 1983).

In thinking about the implications of these studies, several additional points should be borne in mind. First, channels of communication that are perceived to be most effective may be specific to particular types of innovation (e.g., different for drugs than for surgical procedures) and the particular physician audiences (specialists or younger practitioners may be attuned to different channels than generalists or older physicians).

Second, what physicians say or believe

influences them may differ from what actually influences them (Avorn et al., 1982).

Third, investigators are unlikely to draw favorable conclusions about the importance of channels of communication that they omit from their survey instruments. If, for example, a survey questionnaire lists "journals, books, conferences, and continuing education" as possible responses, then "talking with colleagues" is unlikely to be found important. If a study restricts itself to the social network of physicians in the transmission of information, then the role of journals is not likely to appear very prominent.

Fourth, if a channel of communication has been less effective, it may be because few physicians have been exposed to that channel or because that channel is intrinsically unconvincing compared with other sources of information. Continuing medical education, for example, appears to have lesser perceived impact than medical journals. The policy implications are quite different if one believes that the weak showing is because of low exposure to continuing education than if one believes that physicians are not convinced by what they see and hear at such educational programs.

Fifth, as time passes after the initial release of new information, different channels of communication may become relatively more important as conveyors of information to physicians. The initial release of new findings usually come in the form of a publication or presentation at a professional meeting. Soon after the release of new findings, then, journals (or public news media) may be especially prominent sources (Stross and Harlan, 1981; Market Facts, 1982). Later, colleagues and medical teaching conferences may become more prominent than they were earlier (Fineberg et al., 1978; Stross and Harlan, 1979; Jordan et al., 1983). Thus, in a study of the importance of different channels of communication, findings may depend in part on the timing of the study relative to the time the innovation was introduced.

All physicians are challenged to discern what they need to know from the sea of new medical information that surges around them. Physicians do appear open to the idea of receiving direct mail summaries of new medical findings (Market Facts, 1982). The success of the brief monthly, *The Medical Letter*, has spawned a flock of imitators, and at least one medical textbook (*Scientific American Medicine*) provides monthly updates with short summaries of key findings relevant to practice. Channels of communication that convey pertinent, concise information would seem to have a comparative advantage. The expanding availability of personal computers in physician homes and offices offers a new medium that can potentially convey evaluative information on new and current medical practices. Of course, the physicians most resistant to changing their medical practices may also be the last ones to install a home computer.

Measures of Diffusion and Sources of Data

Studies of diffusion and evaluation involve a variety of dependent variables, partly determined by the specific objectives of the study, partly by the nature of the medical practice being studied, and partly by the data available to the investigator.

Interest here is in evidence about the direct and indirect effects of evaluation on (1) physician beliefs, (2) expert opinion, and (3) clinical practices. Measures of the first typically rely on surveys or interviews with practitioners and express results as a proportion who adhere to certain beliefs at a particular time or at different points in time. Studies of expert opinion may also use survey methods or rely on literature reviews or on recommendations in textbooks, review articles, or other guidelines written by experts. Studies of medical practices may draw upon many data sources: (1) surveys of physicians or of institutions; (2) information gathered from patients or from the general public, as in the Health Interview Survey of the National Center for Health Statistics (NCHS); (3) patient medical records; (4) pharmaceutical records; (5) information from manufacturers of equipment or of medical devices; (6) national practice registries, such as the National Disease and Therapeutic Index; (7) insurance payment records; and (8) information from state and national data files on hospitalization and medical procedures, such as the NCHS Hospital Discharge Survey, reports of the Commission on Professional Hospital Activities, and several statewide data consortia.

While admiring the ingenuity of many investigators in finding pertinent data, we should bear in mind limitations and biases lurking in these various measures. Surveys are subject to selection and recall biases. Manufacturer sales data may trace the dissemination of new equipment, although that is not necessarily coincident with the extent of its use. Records from selected insurers may be incomplete, and national registries may fail to reflect changing patterns of disease classification and new, important though less than major, changes in patient management.

The dependent variable in a diffusion study may be expressed as a count or as a proportion. For example, a certain *number* of pills, *number* of prescriptions, or *number* of devices is supplied each year; or a certain *fraction* of physicians used a drug or a *fraction* of hospitals have purchased a new piece of equipment. Embedded in each of these dependent variables is a population of potential adopters of the practice being studied. The potential target population is explicitly the denominator in a fraction and is left unspecified in the case of counts. In either case, the interpretation of a study depends on an appropriately defined target population that is either stable over time or is correctly adjusted over time, as, for example, the target pool of patients varies or the number of trained clinicians changes.

Diffusion as Affected by Evaluation

Diffusion may be considered a process of growth and decay over time. In an idealized case, unambiguous new findings of an unequivocally superior innovation, or clear-cut determination of a definitively inferior current practice, would be instantaneously communicated to all pertinent adopters who would promptly make the appropriate change in practice without any constraints or disincentives. The diffusion pattern would be an extremely sharp rise in the case of adoption and an extremely sharp fall in the case of abandonment (Figure 4-1A and 4-1B).

Evaluations often are not clear-cut, and any of the 10 factors that influence diffusion can introduce friction into the system. Empirically, a number of innovations have been found to follow an S-shaped pattern of diffusion (Figure 4-2A). A traditional sociometric model accounting for such a pattern postulates early adopters and opinion leaders who influence increasing numbers of other physicians to adopt a new practice, leaving some resisters in the end who fail to adopt the innovation (Rogers and Shoemaker, 1971). Other models invoking different determinants of diffusion (features of the innovation itself, of the setting for use, of the decision making process, etc.) could also be constructed to account for an observed S-shaped pattern of diffusion. Thus, an observed pattern of diffusion does not typically indicate the relative contributions of the various possible determinants of diffusion.

Several studies of the spread of medical equipment and institutional innovations have shown approximately S-shaped patterns of spread with slower initial rise fol-

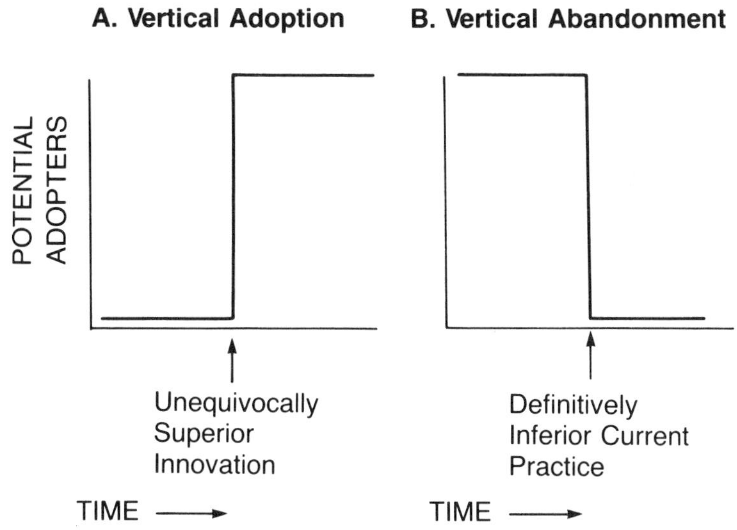

FIGURE 4-1A and 4-1B Idealized diffusion pattern.

lowed by an accelerated phase (Fineberg et al., 1977; Fineberg, 1979; Russell, 1979; Office of Technology Assessment [OTA], 1981). Some studies of the diffusion of new drugs have found a pattern of spread that is initially very rapid (Figure 4-2B) (Warner, 1975; Fineberg and Pearlman, 1981). Fewer empirical studies have examined the phase of abandonment. Some cases show gradual abandonment (Figure 4-2C) (Fineberg et al., 1980); others, involving drugs found to be unsafe, show rapid decline in usage shortly after release of the findings (Figure 4-2D) (Finkelstein and Gilbert, 1983).

An assessment of the impact of evaluation on practice requires a standard for judging impact. Two standards seem plausible, one that might be called *rational behavior*, and a second that might be called *expected behavior*. With rational behavior as the standard, emphasis is on the extent to which practice conforms to the findings of evaluation, meaning *all adopt* for positive evaluations and *all abandon* for negative evaluations. With expected behavior as the standard, emphasis is on changes in the pattern of diffusion that can be related to evaluation.

A clinical evaluation might affect both the rate of adoption or abandonment of a practice and the extent of its ultimate use. Since these changes may be in a direction consistent with the findings of evaluation, though falling short of full conformance, the expected behavior standard is less demanding than the rational behavior standard. Investigators who base their conclusions on a rational standard often intend to judge the behavior of physicians, not the credibility of an evaluation method. An expected behavior standard implicitly recognizes that evaluation is only one of many determinants of diffusion.

Seeking to establish a relation between an evaluation and a change in diffusion can take the form of answering five kinds of questions:

1. What is the baseline pattern of diffusion? In other words, what pattern of adoption or abandonment of pertinent

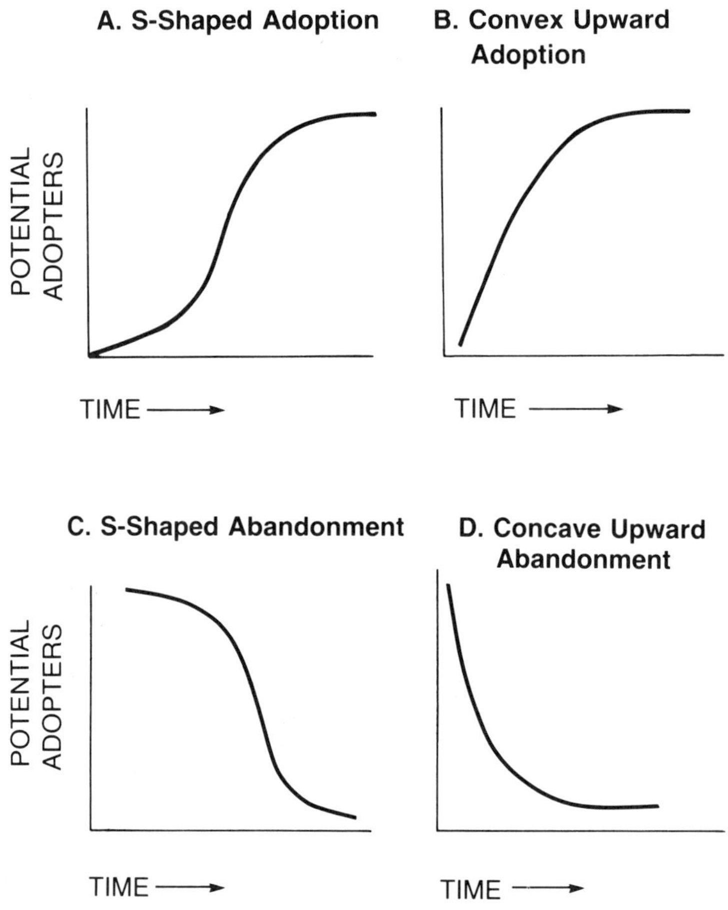

FIGURE 4-2A through 4-2D Empirical diffusion patterns.

clinical practices would be expected to occur over time if the evaluation in question had not been carried out?

2. What do results of the evaluation, when correctly interpreted, imply about what constitutes appropriate medical care? Do the implications require a change in the use of a medical technology? In efforts to discriminate among the effects of different types of evaluation, are the implications from one type of evaluation different from the implications of others?

3. Are there changes in physician awareness and in the pattern of practice that are consistent with the findings of evaluation (or of one type of evaluation)?

4. What is the temporal relation between evaluation and changes, if any, in the pattern of practice?

5. Is there additional evidence (such as interviews, bibliographic citations, opinion surveys, etc.) supporting a connection between an evaluation and change in practice?

Answers to these questions can provide circumstantial evidence about the relation between evaluation and practice, making a connection seem plausible or implausible, though not established in a rigorous way. A controlled trial of the effectiveness of controlled trials has not been done and is hard to imagine.

EVIDENCE ABOUT THE EFFECTS OF EVALUATION ON DIFFUSION

The principle body of work used in this analysis consists of 48 papers, reports, books, and other documents that assess the relation between evaluation and medical practice. This highly diverse literature cuts across many medical specialty areas. (A summary of the literature is appended.) Though doubtless incomplete, this collection is sufficiently rich to provide a basis for discussion. Several recent reviews concerned with the effects of clinical trials on medical practice aided the bibliographic search (Controlled Clinical Trials, September 1982; OTA, 1983; Hawkins, Evaluating the Benefit of Clinical Trials to Patients, unpublished report, 1983).

The terminology in referring to this literature can be confusing because it consists of studies of the effects of other studies. In the remainder of this chapter, the term *study* will be reserved for an analysis of the effects of one or more clinical trials, consensus exercises, or other forms of clinical evaluation on physician behavior in a particular clinical situation. We use the words practice or clinical practice to mean physician behavior. When referring to a clinical evaluation that is the subject of a study, we will refer to it as a clinical trial or, when appropriate, as a randomized clinical trial (RCT).

The discussion is organized in two major categories depending on the directly measured effect of evaluation: (1) effects directly on physician behavior and (2) effects directly on regulators or third-party payers.

Evaluation and Physician Behavior

All but two of the reviewed studies deal at least in part with the relation between clinical evaluation and the knowledge, beliefs, and decisions of physicians. The kinds of evaluation whose effects are examined in these studies fall into two broad groups: primary evaluations, such as randomized clinical trials, which acquire and present new clinical findings; and synthetic evaluations, such as consensus conferences, which integrate and interpret available primary evidence. Thirty-eight studies deal at least in part with primary evaluations.

The Impact of Primary Evaluations on Physicians In attempting to organize evidence about the relation between clinical trials and physician decision making, it is useful to distinguish two analytic strategies that may be adopted in a study (Garnier et al., 1982; OTA, 1983; Hawkins, unpublished report, 1983). The first strategy begins with a clinical trial or trials and attempts to trace its effects on physician awareness or behavior. The second begins with a set of practices or innovations and traces back to the various kinds of evaluation that contributed to its development, dissemination, or abandonment. The next two subsections discuss studies that follow the first strategy and examine the effects of clinical trials on physician awareness and clinical decisions. The third subsection reviews studies that follow the second strategy and attempt to trace the origin of medical opinion or practices.

Effects of Clinical Trials on Physician Awareness Two studies are devoted mainly to assessing physician awareness of findings from RCTs (Stross and Harlan, 1979, 1981). In the first, family physicians and internists attending a continuing medical education (CME) course (on an unspecified subject) were asked whether they were aware of findings about the treatment of diabetic retinopathy that had been published 18 months earlier in the *American Journal of Ophthalmology*. Two-thirds were not (72 percent of family practitioners and 54 percent of internists). Of the minority who did know about the study, two-thirds said they learned about it from an ophthalmologist or colleague. Although 70 citations to the controlled trial of treatment for diabetic retinopathy appeared in the medical literature between 1976 and 1979, none before 1978 was published in a general American medical journal unrestricted in geographical or subject scope (Dunn, 1981). In this case, numerous citations did not ensure the effective communication of a scientific finding. Moreover, physician awareness would turn out to be no guarantee of improved medical practice. A later evaluation found that 60 percent of internists could not properly diagnose proliferative diabetic retinopathy and so would be unable to recognize patients to whom the initial RCT applies (Sussman et al., 1982).

In a second study of physician awareness, Stross and Harlan (1981) surveyed physicians attending CME courses about their knowledge of results from the Hypertension Detection and Follow-up Program (HDFP). This time, 40 percent of family physicians and 60 percent of internists, respectively 2 months and 6 months following publication of the RCT in the *Journal of the American Medical Association* in 1979, said they were aware of the findings, and most of those had learned about it from the literature. These figures represent awareness among physicians at single points in time for each physician group. Hence, the figures are not revealing about the diffusion over time of knowledge about this RCT, much less about its impact on clinical practices. As in the case of diabetic retinopathy, a later study would raise questions about the translation of this RCT into effective clinical practice, in part because of inappropriate medication prescribed by physicians and in part because of patient nonadherence to prescribed medication regimens (Wagner, 1981).

The management of hypertension illustrates some of the pitfalls in attempting to draw conclusions about the effects of clinical evaluations on physician awareness and medical practice. In 1977, the Joint National Committee on Detection, Evaluation, and Treatment of High Blood Pressure recommended an individualized approach to treating patients with mild hypertension. A 1978 survey of physicians in New York City found that 92 percent were routinely starting antihypertensive medication for patients with mild hypertension, a far more aggressive treatment strategy than recommended by the National Committee (Thomson, 1981). Results from the Hypertension Detection and Follow-up Program subsequently lent support to the more aggressive treatment strategy previously followed by more than nine out of ten physicians in New York City. In this case, a widespread practice that appeared unjustified at one time was borne out by a subsequent randomized trial; thus, demonstration of efficacy by an RCT may follow as well as precede prevailing patterns of practice. The optimal strategy for treatment of mild hypertension continues to be controversial, and value judgments about the conformance of physician practices to a particular management strategy would seem more hazardous today than perhaps they once appeared.

A set of surveys recently commissioned by the National Heart, Lung, and Blood Institute (NHLBI) investigated physician awareness of findings from two specific RCTs and their effects on practice (Market Facts, 1982). This study design is noteworthy in that it represents an exceptional effort to obtain data on physician knowledge and attitudes both before and after release of findings in 1980 from an RCT (the Aspirin Myocardial Infarction Study [AMIS] trial) that examined whether aspirin prevents recurrence of myocardial infarction. This RCT found no benefits to aspirin, in contrast to some earlier clinical trials of antiplatelet therapy (Friedewald and Schoenberger, 1982). The majority of physicians in the survey remained unaffected by findings from the AMIS trial and continued to recommend aspirin for patients following a myocardial infarction. The second subject of the survey was an RCT, the Coronary Drug Project (CDP), that had been published more than 4 years before the initial survey. This RCT had raised doubts about the efficacy and safety of lipid-lowering drugs in preventing recurrence of myocardial infarction. The majority of physicians in the survey either never prescribed lipid-lowering drugs (14 percent) or used them only as secondary therapy (72 percent), and physicians who were aware of the CDP results were less likely than other physicians to use these drugs.

A recent paper about the impact of the CDP draws in part on pertinent findings from the surveys sponsored by the NHLBI (Friedman et al., 1983). Of the more than 1,700 physicians interviewed, 45 percent said they had no familiarity with the CDP, 39 percent said they were familiar with the CDP in general, and 17 percent said they were familiar with its specific findings. When sorted by specialty group, 16 percent of cardiologists, 46 percent of internists, and 70 percent of general practitioners had no familiarity with the CDP. Physicians claiming some or full familiarity with CDP were approximately twice as likely as physicians with no familiarity with CDP to believe that specific lipid lowering drugs are not effective or safe.

Another survey of physician awareness of new clinical knowledge focused on three well-established findings in anesthesiology (Fineberg et al., 1978). In this study there appeared to be a marked acceleration in the spread of knowledge among anesthesiologists, following initial publication of one finding, though not for the other two. Change in practice lagged to varying degrees after awareness and was longest for the one practice (scavenging waste gases) requiring institutional action.

Effects of RCTs on Physician Practices Twenty papers attempt to assess the effect of specific randomized clinical trials on medical practice (see Appendix A). This group of papers is of particular interest because RCTs are technically the strongest form of evaluation. Several papers cover more than one clinical practice, and a number of practices are covered in more than one paper. On balance, the 20 papers deal with the effects of RCTs on 19 clinical practices.

If we count as one study each instance in which a paper assesses the effects of one or more RCTs on a particular clinical practice, the 20 papers represent 28 studies (Table 4-1). One paper (Chalmers, 1974) assesses the effects of randomized clinical trials on four medical practices. Three other papers (Friedewald and Schoenberger, 1982; Fisher and Kennedy, 1982; Market Facts, 1982), respectively, cover four, two, and two practices in the area of cardiovascular disease, accounting for a total of 8 studies. The remaining 16 papers each deal with a single clinical practice. Five clinical practices (internal mammary artery ligation, gastric freezing, treatment of breast cancer, antiplatelet agents for the prevention of recurrent myocardial infarction, and management of mild hypertension) are each examined in 2 papers. The effect of the Coronary Drug Project on the use of lipid-lowering drugs and of the University Group Diabetes Project (UGDP) on the use of oral hypoglycemics are each covered in 3 studies.

Examination of these 28 studies proceeds along a line of questioning like that outlined at the end of the section on diffusion

TABLE 4-1 Studies of the Effects of Randomized Controlled Trials on Medical Practice

Study No.	References	Date	Practices: Action	Medical Condition
1	Barsamian	1977	Internal mammary artery ligation	Angina pectoris
2	Chalmers	1974	Stilbestrol	Pregnancy
3	Chalmers	1974	Bed rest	Viral hepatitis
4	Chalmers	1974	Bland diet	Duodenal ulcer
5	Chalmers	1974	Oral hypoglycemics	Diabetes mellitus
6	Chassin	1983	Length of hospital stay	Myocardial infarction
7	Combs et al.	1983	Referral for treatment	Senile macular degeneration
8	Fineberg	1979	Artificial lung	Respiratory failure
9	Fineberg and Hiatt	1979	Gastric freezing	Ulcer disease
10	Finkelstein and Gilbert	1983	Tolbutamide	Diabetes mellitus
11	Fisher and Kennedy	1982	Coronary artery bypass graft surgery	Cardiovascular disease
12	Fisher and Kennedy	1982	Internal mammary artery ligation	Angina pectoris
13	Friedewald and Schoenberger	1982	Drug prescription	Mild hypertension
14	Friedewald and Schoenberger	1982	Antiplatelets	Cardiovascular disease
15	Friedewald and Schoenberger	1982	Beta-blockers	Cardiovascular disease
16	Friedewald and Schoenberger	1982	Lipid-lowering drugs	Cardiovascular disease
17	Friedman et al.	1983	Lipid-lowering drugs	Cardiovascular disease
18	Haines	1983	Neurosurgery	Neurosurgical conditions
19	Market Facts	1982	Lipid-lowering drugs	Cardiovascular disease
20	Market Facts	1982	Antiplatelets	Cardiovascular disease
21	McPherson and Fox	1977	Treatments	Breast cancer
22	Miao	1977	Gastric freezing	Ulcer disease
23	Moskowitz et al.	1981	Treatment	Alcohol withdrawal
24	OTA	1978	Hyperbaric oxygen	Cognitive deficits
25	OTA	1983	Treatments	Breast cancer
26	Thomson et al.	1981	Drug prescription	Mild hypertension
27	Warner et al.	1978	Oral hypoglycemics	Diabetes mellitus
28	Wilson et al.	1982	Antimicrobial prophylaxis	Gastrointestinal surgery

as affected by evaluation. Based on the view of the authors of 25 studies, 17 practices have had RCTs with clear implications for medical practice. Of these 25 studies, 5 deal with two RCTs (UGDP study of treatments of diabetics and the HDFP study of hypertension) where the clinical implications of the RCT are controversial, though not in the view of the authors of the papers cited. The RCTs in two areas (use of antiplatelet agents to prevent recurrent myocardial infarction and a collection of randomized trials on neurosurgical procedures) do not have clear implications for practice in the views of the authors of the 3 studies that deal with RCTs in these two areas (see Table 4-2).

Among the 25 studies in which RCTs are judged to have had clear implications for practice, 17 (dealing with 13 practices) provide some quantitative information about the frequency of use of the medical practice in question. Of these 17 studies, 7 describe the use of a practice at one point in time. The remaining 10 studies report quantitative information about patterns of

TABLE 4-2 Effects of Specific RCTs on Medical Practice

A. Does RCT have clear implications for practice:					
No—(3) [2]					
Yes—(27) [17]					
B. Is practice pattern quantitatively reported?					
No—(8) [7]					
Yes—(17) [13]					
C. Is practice measured over time or only at one point in time?					
Over Time		One Point			
(10) [7]		(7) [7]			
D. Does practice level or pattern conform to RCT findings?					
		(1)[1]	No	(4)[4]	
		(5)[4]	Somewhat	(1)[1]	
	(9)[7]	(4)[4]	Yes	(2)[2]	(3)[3]
E. Did RCT precede measured change in pattern of practice?					
		(1)[1]	No	(1)[1]	
		(1)[1]	Probably not		
		(1)[1]	Probably yes		
	(7)[5]	(6)[4]	Yes	(2)[2]	(2)[2]
F. Do RCT results differ from results of other (less strong) forms of evaluation or from traditional practice?					
			Uncertain	(2)[2]	
		(4)[3]	Somewhat		
	(7)[5]	(3)[4]	Yes		

NOTE: A total of 28 studies (in parentheses) and 9 practices (in brackets) are considered here.

practice over time and thus provide evidence about the relation between RCTs and diffusion of medical technology.

This latter group of 10 studies covers seven medical practices: oral hypoglycemics for diabetics (Chalmers, 1974; Warner et al., 1978; Finkelstein and Gilbert, 1983); referrals for treatment of senile macular degeneration (Combs et al., 1983); gastric freezing (Fineberg, 1979); lipid-lowering drugs (Market Facts, 1982; Friedman et al., 1983); length of hospital stay for myocardial infarction (Chassin, 1983); coronary artery bypass graft surgery (Fisher and Kennedy, 1982); and treatment of breast cancer (OTA, 1983). One study found no change in practice consistent with the findings of an RCT; this study examined application of the UGDP study in 1970 (Chalmers, 1974). Five studies found a moderate shift in practice consistent with the findings of previous RCTs. These dealt with the treatment of breast cancer between 1972 and 1981 (OTA, 1983); with coronary artery bypass graft surgery between 1974 and 1979 (Fisher and Kennedy, 1982); with the use of lipid-lowering agents between 4 and 6 years after publication in 1975 or the CDP results (Market Facts, 1982; Friedman et al., 1983); and with prescriptions for oral hypoglycemic agents between 3 and 7 years after publication of the UGDP study (Warner et al., 1978). In the first two of these four cases (treatment of breast cancer and coronary artery bypass graft surgery), some evidence from non-RCTs favored the same directions of practice as did the RCTs. Four studies (Fineberg, 1979; Finkelstein and Gilbert, 1983; Combs et al., 1983; Chassin, 1983) found a marked shift in practice consistent with the findings of RCTs, though in the two cases of gastric freezing (Fineberg, 1979) and length of stay for myocardial infarction (Chassin, 1983) evaluation by RCT did not precede the change in the pattern of practice.

After applying all of these analytic filters, there remain 2 of the original 28 studies of the effects of specific RCTs on medical practices in which the RCT has clear implications for practice, the pattern of practice reported quantitatively over time conforms fully to the RCT findings, the RCT preceded the change in the pattern of practice, and findings from the RCT differ from the results of other forms of evaluation. One of these is an unpublished study of referrals of patients with senile macular degeneration at one opthalmological treatment center (Combs et al., 1983). Twice as many patients with treatable disease were referred in the 6 months following release of the results of the senile macular degeneration trial as had been seen in the 6 months before the trial. The second study found that the use of tolbutamide began to decline promptly and sharply after release of the UGDP results in 1970 (Finkelstein and Gilbert, 1983).

Studies of oral hypoglycemics, of treatment for breast cancer, and of lipid-lowering drugs highlight the importance of the passage of time in drawing conclusions about the effects of RCTs on clinical practices. In the first few years after release of the UGDP study, doctors apparently substituted other hypoglycemic agents for tolbutamide, because the use of all hypoglycemics remained steady through 1973 (Chalmers, 1974) despite the fall in use of tolbutamide beginning in 1971 (Finkelstein and Gilbert, 1983). By 1977, use of all hypoglycemics had declined by half (Warner et al., 1978; Chalmers, 1982). Similarly, conclusions about the effect of RCTs on the treatment of breast cancer that are based on the pattern of treatment in 1970 (McPherson and Fox, 1977) differ from conclusions based on trends during the subsequent decade (OTA, 1983). In the period between 4 and 6 years after publication of results of the CDP in 1975, the proportion of physicians who said they never prescribe lipid-lowering drugs rose from 10 to 18 percent (Market Facts, 1982). This occurred despite the fact that the proportion of physicians demonstrating full knowledge of CDP findings remained low (6 percent of all cardiologists and 3 percent of all physicians). Such results support the importance of secondary spread of new findings from one or multiple primary publications through such channels as medical conferences and interaction with colleagues.

The relation between the level or pattern of a clinical practice and the results of a clinical trial can reasonably be described only *as of a given time* after the release of findings from the trial. The full effects of an RCT on practice may take some years to manifest. The occurrence of other events (new technical developments, evaluations, environmental changes, etc.) in the interim may make it more difficult to connect changes in practice with an RCT that has in fact been influential.

Some difficulties in discerning temporal and causal connections between clinical evaluations and changes in medical practice are illustrated by the case of length of hospital stay for myocardial infarction. In this instance of medical decision making, changing patterns of practice, randomized trials, and evidence from nonrandomized studies all overlap in time in a way that defies inferences of causal relations. The average length of hospital stay for myocardial infarction has declined steadily in the United States, falling from almost 19 days in 1968 to less than 13 days in 1980 (Figure 4-3). During this time, marked variation in length of stay from one region of the country to another persisted.

Superimposed on the trend line for hospital length of stay in Figure 4-4 are the durations of hospitalization examined in randomized and nonrandomized controlled trials of hospital stay for myocardial infarction (Chassin, 1983; Pryor et al., 1983). Virtually all studies have found no statistically significant differences in outcome between shorter and longer hospital stays (Chassin, 1983; Pryor et al., 1983). Because the evidence from all trials points in the same direction, it is impossible to distinguish the impact of one or another trial on clinical practice. Moreover, because of the limited size of available trials, it is possible that earlier hospital discharge may pose some health hazard despite the array of evidence showing no statistically significant differences between shorter and longer hospital stays (Chassin, 1983). On the other hand, it is also possible that earlier discharge confers as yet unestablished benefits. The trend in practice may be the result of multiple factors, including changing theories about cardiovascular healing and external pressures to shorten hospital

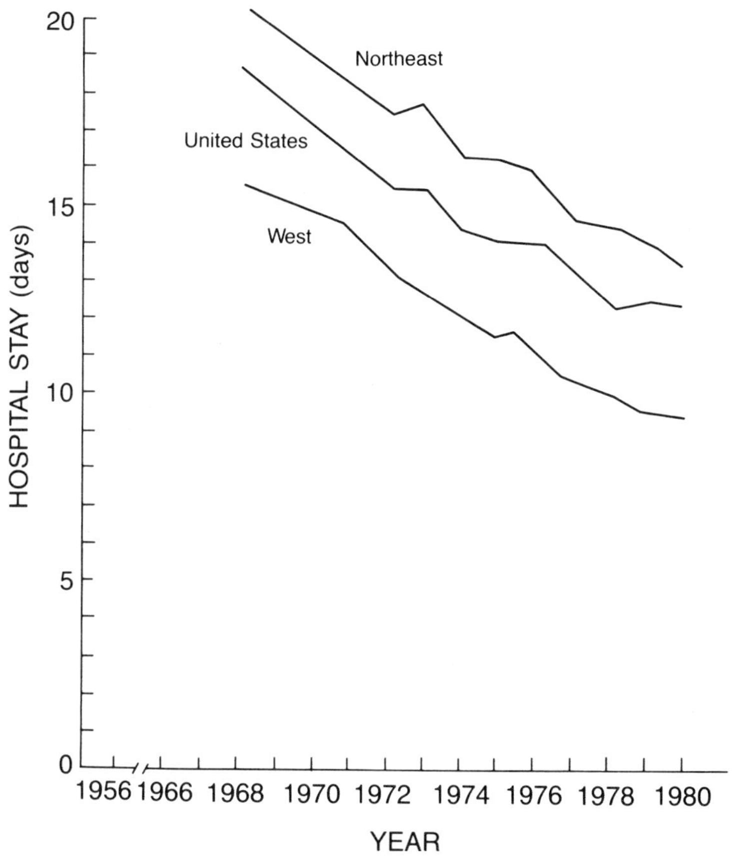

FIGURE 4-3 Average length of hospital stay for myocardial infarction.

stays, quite apart from evidence produced by controlled clinical trials. It is evident from inspection of Figure 4-4 that many physicians have been discharging patients with myocardial infarction earlier than had yet been demonstrated as safe by randomized trials.

Simply because a study fails to demonstrate beyond a reasonable doubt that a clinical trial has influenced the diffusion of a practice does not mean that the clinical trial was not actually influential. For example, it is possible that early randomized trials helped to prevent the unwarranted diffusion of the artificial lung (Fineberg and Hiatt, 1979) and of hyperbaric oxygen to treat cognitive deficits in the elderly (OTA, 1978). When an RCT reinforces the value of an existing practice, this may be beneficial in preventing unwarranted departures from the standard practice and in influencing nonconfirming physicians to adopt the demonstrably superior practice.

In some cases the patterns of practice over time conform partially to the findings of randomized trials. In some of these cases, such as coronary artery surgery, treatment of breast cancer, and use of lipid-lowering drugs, it seems highly likely that RCTs have influenced clinical practices. When multiple RCTs and possibly other studies as well all suggest changes in practice in a similar direction, it may be difficult to discern the particular effect of a

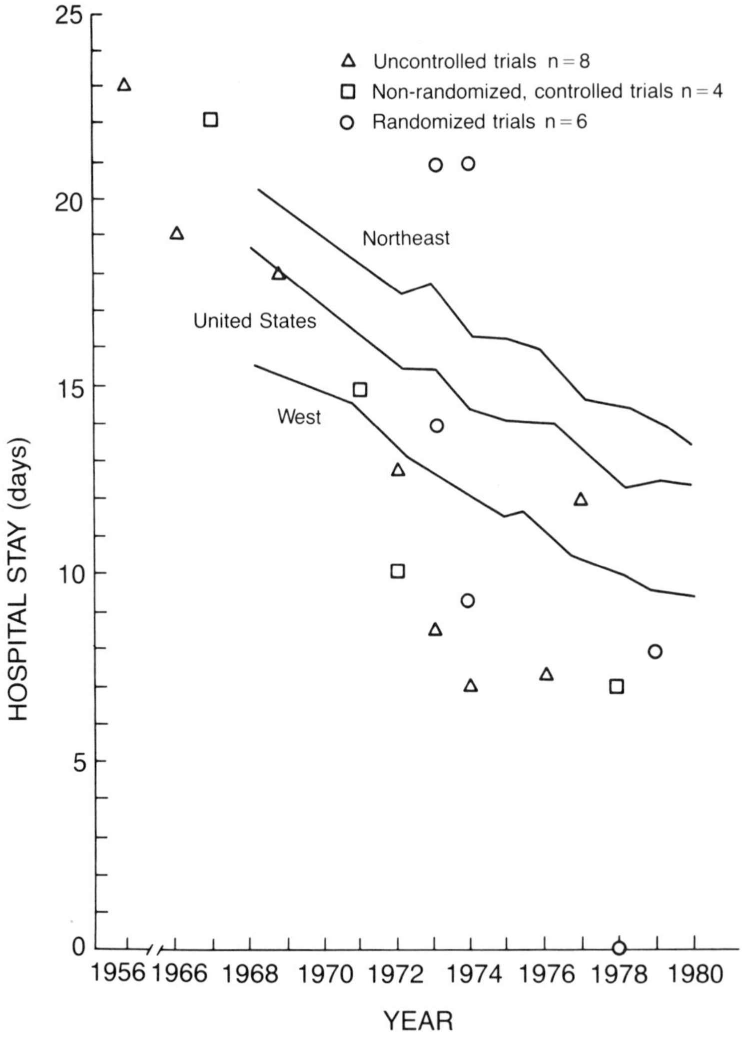

FIGURE 4-4 Average length of hospital stay for myocardial infarction.

single study; yet, circumstantial evidence supporting the eventual influence of the collection of studies can be strong.

The Coronary Artery Surgery Study enrolled nearly 25,000 patients undergoing angiography at 15 institutions (Fisher and Kennedy, 1982). The proportion of patients with one-vessel disease who underwent surgery declined from 38 percent in 1974–1975 to 30 percent in 1978–1979, a result consistent with the findings of randomized trials that had appeared in the interim. Perhaps more striking than the overall effects of these randomized trials is the marked variation in reliance on surgery at participating hospitals. The proportion of angiographically examined patients undergoing surgery ranged from 31 to 70 percent at the different hospitals, an observation consistent with highly variable responsiveness to randomized trials in different settings.

In the case of breast cancer, *radical* mastectomy declined from 70 percent of operative procedures in 1970 (McPherson and Fox, 1977) to about 3 percent in 1981 (OTA, 1983). The dominant practice in 1981, accounting for 70 percent of operative procedures, was the *modified* radical mastectomy, though randomized trials suggested that simple mastectomy with local irradiation would be equally effective (OTA, 1983).

The number of prescriptions for lipid-lowering agents rose between 1970 and 1975, then declined by more than 50 percent between 1975 and 1980 (Friedman et al., 1983). A number of RCTs reported between 1970 and 1980 support the overall conclusions that lipid-lowering drugs do not demonstrably improve the course of cardiovascular disease (Buchwald et al., 1982). Prominent among these trials are the CDP discussed earlier and the World Health Organization (WHO) (European) trials published in 1978 and 1980 showing that clofibrate, the most widely used lipid-lowering agent, is ineffective in the primary prevention of myocardial infarction and possibly adds to the risk of mortality (Buchwald et al., 1982; Friedman et al., 1983). Among these RCTs, only the CDP has been the subject of a specific inquiry about awareness among U.S. physicians, and it is uncertain which trials have had the greatest impact on physician practices. While physician familiarity with CDP findings is limited, and many continue to prescribe lipid-lowering agents, there has been a gradual shift in practice along the lines suggested by these RCTs.

Types of Evaluation That Precede Accepted Medical Practices A number of studies attempt to assess the roles played by different types of evaluation prior to the general acceptance of a medical practice. Of special interest are studies that compare the influence of randomized and of nonrandomized clinical trials. According to an opinion expressed by the Office of Technology Assessment, randomized clinical trials have been applied to 10 or 20 percent of medical practices (OTA, 1983). In some areas of medical practice, such as the development of cancer chemotherapy, thousands of randomized trials have been conducted (Armitage et al., 1978). The frequency of randomized trials in other areas of medicine has been increasing (Chalmers et al., 1979).

In the opinion of many oncologists and researchers involved in evaluations of cancer treatment, randomized trials have generally been more useful than nonrandomized trials in the development of cancer therapies (Armitage et al., 1978; Rockette et al., 1982). However, several studies that have looked quantitatively at the origins of current therapeutic practices in several types of cancer found nonrandomized studies to have played a dominant role in the development of therapy. For example, Gehan (1982) found that nonrandomized trials, more frequently than RCTs, were the source of currently accepted treatments for acute leukemia. In their oncology center, Garnier et al. (1982) found the greatest consensus around treatments for head and neck cancer that had not been evaluated by randomized trials. Part of the reason may be that randomized studies are especially likely to be applied to areas of controversy.

Other studies also suggest a nondominant role for randomized studies in shaping medical practices. Ingelfinger et al. (1974) reviewed 23 controversies in internal medicine that had been debated in print 8 years earlier. Though interest in some had waned, few if any had been resolved by a clear-cut clinical trial. Gilbert et al. (1977) traced the introduction of 107 innovations in surgery and anesthesia and found that one-third were randomized trials. In reviewing the literature about four discarded surgical practices, Barnes (1977) noted a lack of randomized trials at both the beginning and end of the life cycles of the discarded procedures. Christensen et al. (1977) compared the treatments for duodenal ulcer recommended in textbooks with evidence from randomized trials. They found a number of treatments, including the use of antacids, continued to be recommended without having been demonstrated effective in randomized studies. Antacids in sufficient amounts subsequently were shown to be more effective than placebo in promoting ulcer healing (Peterson et al., 1977). Like the earlier example of treatment for mild hypertension, this sequence of studies shows that acceptance of a medical practice sometimes precedes a demonstration of efficacy in randomized trials.

The Impact of Synthetic Evaluations Synthetic evaluations encompass a variety of efforts to interpret and integrate information obtained from primary evaluations. Synthetic evaluations include review articles, decision analyses, cost-effectiveness assessments, informal and formal group processes to reach consensus, and many more. It is, of course, difficult to discern the effects on practice of review papers apart from the primary evaluations on which they are based. Although decision analysis and cost-effectiveness analysis are being applied to medical problems with increasing frequency, much more has been written about the methods and limitations of such analyses than has been written about the adoption of their results by physicians. Because this chapter concerns the effects of evaluation on clinical practices, evidence will not be reviewed about the effects of programs that entail regulatory sanctions, like hospital utilization review. Our primary focus in this section is on studies of the impact on physician knowledge and practice of expert consensus and guidelines.

A major study of the effectiveness of the National Institutes of Health Consensus Development Program is currently under way (The Rand Corporation, 1983). This study is intended to trace the dissemination of conclusions from NIH consensus conferences into the medical community and to measure changes over time in reliance on practices that have been the subject of a consensus conference. Its results are expected to be available in 1985.

At least one survey has measured physician awareness of the occurrence and conclusions from two NIH consensus conferences by means of telephone surveys 2 weeks before each conference and 6 weeks after publication of conclusions in the *Journal of the American Medical Association* (Jacoby, unpublished report, 1983). Approximately 9 percent of physicians in the survey were aware of the consensus development program at NIH. Two weeks before the consensus conference on computed tomography, 16 percent of physicians in pertinent specialties said they knew about the upcoming conference. At a similar time before the consensus conference on hip joint replacement, 7 percent of pertinent specialists reported being aware of the upcoming conference. Six weeks after publication of results, 4 percent of surveyed physicians reported being aware of conclusions from the conference on computed tomography, and 1 percent said they were aware of the conclusions from the conference on hip replacement. Most of those who knew about conference conclusions said they had read about them in a professional journal.

An earlier section described a study of physician attitudes and practices following a consensus conference on hypertension (Thomson et al., 1981). Physicians were more aggressive in treating mild hypertensives than was recommended by the consensus conference, though such practice was consistent with the findings of the subsequently published HDFP trial.

Since the mid-1970s, the Blue Cross and Blue Shield Association has sponsored a program designed to produce medical consensus on appropriate practices and to improve physician use of medical resources. In 1977, this Medical Necessity Program announced consensus on 42 outmoded diagnostic tests and surgical procedures that should no longer be performed. Member Blue Cross and Blue Shield Plans were advised to discontinue routine payment for these procedures and to require physicians requesting reimbursement to provide a medical justification. A review of insurance claims for the federal employee health benefits program in 1975 and 1978 revealed a decline in claims for listed surgical procedures of 26 percent and a decline in diagnostic test claims of 85 percent (Blue Cross and Blue Shield Association, 1982). These results are suggestive of an effect, though without any earlier points of reference, it is difficult to know how much of the decline in tests and surgery might be attributable to the pronouncement by the Medical Necessity Program in 1977. In early 1979, the Medical Necessity Program discouraged routine use of admission test batteries, and most Blue Cross and Blue Shield Plans are reportedly working with hospitals to implement this policy (Blue Cross and Blue Shield Association, 1982). In October 1982, the Medical Necessity Program announced and widely disseminated new guidelines for respiratory care that were developed in association with the American College of Physicians, the American College of Surgeons, and the American Academy of Pediatrics. The aim of this new phase of the program is to reduce unnecessary reliance on respiratory care services, estimated to account for two to four billion dollars of annual hospital costs (Blue Cross and Blue Shield Association, 1982). More recently (1984), Diagnostic Imaging Guidelines were released in association with a number of medical specialty societies, primarily the American College of Radiology.

A number of professional associations have undertaken programs to improve the use of medical resources, relying heavily on guidelines generated by expert panels. One of these, the Clinical Efficacy Assessment Project of the American College of Physicians (ACP), uses expert committees, consultants, review by relevant medical professional societies, and approval by the Board of Governors and Regents of ACP to synthesize the literature and prepare position papers on the safety and efficacy of a variety of clinical practices. These papers have begun to appear periodically in the *Annals of Internal Medicine*.

The Public Health Service publishes a variety of clinical guidelines for prevention, diagnosis, and treatment of diseases of public health importance. Such recommendations appear, for example, in *Morbidity and Mortality Weekly Reports*. Widely distributed to subscribers, these recommendations are surely influential, though their overall effects on the diffusion of new practices has not been systematically assessed. One survey of public health physicians responsible for tuberculosis control found greater conformity to public health service guidelines on chemoprophylaxis than on diagnosis and treatment (Leff et al., 1979, 1981).

EVALUATION AND POLICY ON REGULATION AND REIMBURSEMENT

Requirements of the Food and Drug Administration (FDA) to establish the safety and efficacy of new drugs are doubtless among the strongest promoters of controlled clinical trials in the United States. Until the FDA approves a new pharmaceutical, it is not generally available for use by physicians. FDA's insistence and reliance on randomized controlled trials in the licensing of new drugs probably constitute the most potent source of influence of RCTs on the diffusion of new medical technology in the United States.

Although the FDA approves particular uses of a new drug, physicians are generally free to prescribe a licensed drug as they see fit. Studies of specific new drugs, such as cimetidine, have found them to be used frequently in ways that are not explicitly approved by the FDA (Cocco and Cocco, 1981; Schade and Donaldson, 1981; Fineberg and Pearlman, 1981).

Friedman et al. (1983) reviewed changes in FDA labeling for the lipid-lowering drug, clofibrate, between 1969 and 1982. During this period, indications for the drug were progressively restricted and warnings of adverse reactions expanded. The authors ascribe major changes in 1979 both to the Coronary Drug Project published in 1975 and to the WHO (European) clofibrate trial published in 1978. Further labeling changes in 1982 were due primarily to new findings in the WHO trial published in 1980.

When the Health Care Financing Administration receives a request for reimbursement of a new medical procedure about which it is undecided, it may seek the advice of the Office of Health Technology Assessment of the Public Health Service about the medical acceptability of the practice. During 1979 and 1980, the Public Health Service made recommendations of nonreimbursement for 21 of 50 procedures it reviewed. The Health Care Financing Administration accepted all these recommendations. One study commissioned in 1980 by the now defunct National Center for Health Care Technology estimated that decisions not to reimburse four procedures (dialysis for schizophrenia, hyperthermia for cancer, radial keratotomy for myopia, and endothelial cell photography) produced savings to the Medicare program of $312 million over a 10-year period (Center for the Analysis of Health Practices, 1981). We are aware of no systematic review of the contribution of various types of clinical evaluation to the recommendations produced by the Public Health Service. According to the OTA, an RCT showing no benefit from hyperbaric oxygen treatment for cognitive deficits in the elderly contributed to decisions by Medicare and other insurers not to reimburse for the procedure (OTA, 1978).

CONCLUSIONS AND RECOMMENDATIONS

Clinical evaluation is one among many factors bearing on the diffusion of medical technology. Evaluations often seem to be overwhelmed by the other nine determinants of physician behavior discussed in this chapter. Improving the care of patients requires both improved methods of evaluation and more effective translation of the results of evaluation into practice. Evaluations are likely to exert a greater impact on diffusion if they are buttressed by attention to other controllable factors, such as channels of communication and environmental constraints and incentives, that affect the adoption and abandonment of medical technology.

The discussion in this chapter leads to the following recommendations (in italics).

- *Strengthen the weaker methods of evaluating medical practice and increase use of stronger methods.* Those who are working to improve methods for evaluating medical practices should attend to strengthening the weaker methods, such as case studies and nonrandomized trials, in order to enhance their reliability as guides to clinical action. At present, stronger forms of evaluation, such as controlled trials, are not notably more successful than weaker forms in shaping medical practices. Recognizing the widespread use and apparent influence of these weaker methods of evaluation, efforts to improve both the methods and their execution might have a substantial impact on clinical care. The advantage of scientifically stronger forms of evaluation is not that they ensure greater impact on clinical practice; the advantage is that whatever impact the evaluation carries will be more likely to benefit the patient.

• *Study the diffusion of medical practice concepts and procedures so as to understand how to speed adoption of good practices and discourage use of those that are less effective or harmful.* Government agencies, private foundations, and other interested organizations should support research to enhance understanding of the process of diffusion of medical practices. Instances of successful and of unsuccessful dissemination and instances in which evaluation does and does not prominently appear to influence diffusion should offer guidance. The research program should place special emphasis on those factors affecting diffusion, such as the channels of communication and the environmental constraints, that are at least partially controllable by public policy and organizational decisions.

Researchers and funding agencies should support research to develop and test more acceptable and effective ways to hasten dissemination of demonstrably beneficial practices and to promote abandonment of inappropriate practices. This research is aimed also at finding how current policies and programs influence medical practices. The range of possible interventions that might be assessed includes (1) education of physicians and medical students about evaluation methods, principles of decision making, and the effects of specific clinical practices; (2) innovative methods of communicating the results of clinical evaluations to physicians and other decision makers, including the possible use of electronic media such as home computers and medically oriented cable television stations; (3) feedback to physicians about their performance compared with established standards of practice or peer performance; (4) changes in administrative procedures, affecting such practices as standing orders, test requests, and use of prophylactic antimicrobials, that can lead to more thoughtful clinical decisions; (5) changes in reimbursement policy, including the possibility of material rewards to medical institutions and to physicians as incentives to improve the use of medical resources; (6) requirements or quotas limiting access to medical practices that are used excessively, that are unproved, or that require special facilities or training to use optimally; and (7) changes in the regulatory authority or procedures of such agencies as the federal Food and Drug Administration and state Determination of Need programs.

• *Establish lines of responsibility for making better medical practice a consequence of evaluation of medical technology.* Responsibility for promoting a closer connection between the results of evaluation and medical practice is widely shared among clinicians, medical educators, researchers, professional bodies, research organizations, journal editors and publishers, medical care institutions, equipment and pharmaceutical manufacturers, third-party payers, and regulatory agencies. These individuals and organizations have mixed interests and differing perspectives, though all are in principle dedicated to improved health care for the public. The diffuseness of responsibility for translating the results of evaluation into improved health care is one motivation behind proposals for a public-private entity sponsored by the Institute of Medicine and for additional forms of organization discussed in this report.

Each responsible party can and should take action that would strengthen the link between the results of evaluation and practice. For example, medical educators can place greater emphasis on training medical students and physicians to be discerning consumers of clinical evaluations and to be knowledgeable about medical decision making. Editors of professional journals can enhance the technical review of submitted papers by involving more statisticians, epidemiologists, and other methodologists in their review processes. Medical specialty societies can develop and disseminate authoritative guidelines for the use of medical technology within the purview of their clinical expertise. Third-party payers can support demonstration projects to reduce the inappropriate use of clinical practices.

Many of these recommended actions are already under way in some degree, though they need to be extended, reinforced, and coordinated. A public or public-private body charged with responsibility can identify priorities, enhance communication among the interested organizations, and promote systematic efforts to strengthen the connection between sound evaluation and the diffusion of medical technology.

APPENDIX 4-A: SUMMARIES OF STUDIES

Topic	Reference (Year)	Type of Evaluation Studied	Source of Data on Effects	Findings
Studies of Patterns of Clinical Evaluation and of the Effect of Clinical Evaluations on the Opinions of Experts				
Drugs to lower blood lipoproteins	Market Facts (1982)	Specific RCT: Coronary Drug Project (CDP) of NHLBI	Survey of 1,700 physicians before and after release of AMIS results; all interviews followed publication of CDP results.	Physicians aware of CDP results were less likely to prescribe lipid-lowering drugs (consistent with study results).
Aspirin to reduce recurrence of myocardial infarction	Market Facts (1982)	Specific RCT: Aspirin Myocardial Infarction Study (AMIS) of NHLBI	Survey of 1,700 physicians before and after release of AMIS results; all interviews followed publication of CDP.	Knowledge of AMIS not clearly related to attitudes toward aspirin use (AMIS results showed no benefit to aspirin; other studies had shown positive trends favoring aspirin).
Three practices in anesthesiology	Fineberg et al. (1978)	Epidemiologic surveys; physiologic findings nonrandomized controlled trial	Mailed questionnaires to anesthesiologists, at least 5 years after publication of evaluations.	Marked acceleration in spread of knowledge following initial publication of one finding, not for the other two findings. Journals dominated as source of information for this one finding. Colleagues were equally important for the other two findings.
Treatment of diabetic retinopathy	Stross and Harlan (1979)	Specific RCT: Diabetic Retinopathy Study	Survey of physicians attending CME course 18 months after publication of study.	28% of family practitioners and 46% of internists were aware of study finding. Two-thirds of those aware learned from an opthalmologist or colleague.

Hypertension	Stross and Harlan (1981)	Specific RCT: Hypertension Detection and Follow-up Program	Survey of physicians attending CME course.	40% of family physicians and 60% of internists were aware of study findings, respectively, 2 months and 6 months following release of study findings.
Drugs to lower blood lipoproteins	Friedman et al. (1983)	Coronary Drug Project (main results published in 1975)	Personal interviews with 1,785 physicians (587 cardiologists, 584 internists, 614 general practitioners [GPs]) (See Market Facts, 1982).	55% of all physicians (84% of cardiologists; 54% of internists; 30% of GPs) were aware of CDP in general or familiar with its specific findings. Physicians with some or full knowledge of CDP are approximately twice as likely as those with no familiarity of CDP to believe lipid-lowering drugs are non-effective or safe.
Discharge of low-weight infants	Berg and Salisbury (1971)	Nonrandomized trial with comparison group (supplemented by absence of contradictory evidence in literature)	Telephone survey of 102 board-certified pediatricians.	73% have inappropriate criteria for hospitalization, 2 years after initial study published.
Stilbestrol in pregnancy to prevent abortion	Chalmers (1974)	Controlled versus uncontrolled studies	7 textbooks of obstetrics, 10 years after controlled trials	6 of 7 textbooks have recommendations in agreement with controlled studies showing no benefit of stilbestrol.
Treatment of duodenal ulcer	Christensen et al. (1974)	Randomized controlled trials conducted between 1964 and 1974	Recommendations of textbooks in 1964 compared to 1974	Treatments not demonstrated to be effective in clinical trials (antacids and anticholinergics continue to be recommended, and other drugs (demonstrated to be effective in RCTs) are ignored.
23 controversies in internal medicine	Ingelfinger et al. (1974)	Variety, 10 years after initially published	Literature review	Few if any controversies were resolved by a clear-cut clinical trial.
Oral hypoglycemic agents in diabetics	Marks, unpublished report (1983)	UGDP	Published articles, reviews, editorials, letters.	Views persistent controversies as disputes over criteria for judging evidence, weights accorded different types of evidence (RCTs and other), and convictions about RCTs as the single proper standard for judging merit of practices.

APPENDIX 4-A ***Continued***

Topic	Reference (Year)	Type of Evaluation Studied	Source of Data on Effects	Findings
Studies of Patterns of Clinical Evaluation and of the Effect of Clinical Evaluations on the Opinions of Experts				
Secondary prevention of myocardial infarction	Marks, unpublished report (1983)	7 RCTs	Published articles, reviews, editorials, letters.	Views persistent controversies as disputes over criteria for judging evidence, weights accorded different types of evidence (RCTs and other), and convictions about RCTs as the single, proper standard for judging merit of practices.
Antiplatelet agents to prevent recurrent myocardial infarction	Friedwald and Schoenberger (1982)	2 RCTs (aspirin myocardial infarction study and anturane reinfarction trial)	Views of authors.	Aspirin not demonstrably effective; methodologic controversies dominate anturane trial.
Cancer therapy	UICC reports; Armitage et al. (1978)	RCTs and other controlled trials	Views of authors.	RCTs have been more useful than non-RCTs in developing cancer treatments.
Treatment of breast cancer	Rockette et al. (1982)	RCTs	Views of authors.	RCTs have strong effect on shaping breast cancer treatment.
Neurosurgical procedures	Haines (1983)	51 RCTs in the literature published since 1944	Views of authors.	Many trials have serious methodologic shortcomings and few if any have resolved important clinical questions.
Therapy for acute leukemia	Gehan (1982)	Published trials	Review of literature.	Nonrandomized (rather than randomized) studies have been the primary means of establishing effectiveness of new therapies between 1948 and 1971.
Therapy for head and neck cancer	Garnier et al. (1982)	Available literature	Opinion of hospital experts plus review of literature.	In most cases where there is a consensus about treatment at the investigators' hospital, it is the result of nonrandomized studies.
Innovations in surgery and anesthesia	Gilbert et al. (1977)	Published evaluations of innovations in surgery and anesthesia	Literature review.	Of 107 papers assessing innovation, approximately one-third are RCTs. Less well-controlled studies are more positive about innovation.

Discharge of low birth weight	Berg and Salisbury (1971)	Comparison group (concomitant) nonrandomized trial (plus absence of contradictory evidence in literature)	(Blue Cross) Insurance records.	90% of low-birth-weight infants are kept in hospital longer than necessary; 2 years after publication of initial study.
Oral hypoglycemic agents in diabetics	Chalmers (1974)	RCT (University Group Diabetes Project)	National Disease and Therapeutic Index (NDTI).	No decline in use of all oral hypoglycemics 3 years after UGDP results published in 1970.
	Warner et al. (1978); Finkelstein and Gilbert (1983)			Use of all hypoglycemics drops by 50% between third and seventh years after UGDP results published. Use of tolbutamide shows prompt and sharp decline soon after publication of UGDP results.
Stilbestrol in pregnancy to prevent abortion	Chalmers (1974)	6 controlled trials, one randomized between 1946 and 1955, show no effect; uncontrolled studies report positive results	Reported marketing studies.	50,000 women per year received stilbestrol in late 1960s.
Bedrest in viral hepatitis	Chalmers (1974)	2 controlled trials (randomization unspecified) show no benefit to bed rest	Medical records of hospitalized patients.	10–15 years after the first definitive study 49% of university hospital patients and 67% of community hospital patients still being kept at bed rest.
Bland diet for duodenal ulcer	Chalmers (1974)	8 studies (type unspecified) show no benefit for ulcer healing from bland diet	Medical records of hospitalized patients.	35 of 38 physicians admitting patients with diagnosis of ulcer order bland diets (a practice not substantiated by studies).
Tetracyclines in children	Ray et al. (1977)	Reports of drug toxicity in children	Insurance (Medicaid) records in Tennessee.	5% of all prescriptions (7,000 prescriptions) for children under 8 years of age were for tetracyclines.

APPENDIX 4-A *Continued*

Topic	Reference (Year)	Type of Evaluation Studied	Source of Data on Effects	Findings
Studies of Patterns of Clinical Evaluation and of the Effect of Clinical Evaluations on the Opinions of Experts				
Coronary artery bypass graft surgery	Fisher and Kennedy (1982)	7 RCTs	Referrals to surgery for CASS Registry within 4 years of Veteran's Administration (VA) RCT.	Following publication of VA RCT results in 1975, there was a slight decline in the proportion of patients with 1-vessel and 2-vessel disease referred for surgery (an effect consistent with findings of the study): — 1974–1975 / 1978–1979 1-vessel: 38% / 29.6% 2-vessel: 53% / 46.7% 3-vessel: 63.9% / 64.3%
Prophylactic antimicrobials in gastrointestinal surgery	Wilson et al. (1982)	RCTs	Survey of surgeons in Scotland.	Most use prophylactic antimicrobiotics in accordance with RCTs; 25% believe definitive proof lacking.
Three practices on anesthesiology	Fineberg et al. (1978)	Epidemiologic surveys; physiologic findings; nonrandomized controlled trials	Mailed questionnaire to anesthesiologists, at least 5 years after publication of evaluations.	Proportion who had adopted new practices at time of survey ranged from 65 to 85%. Delay between awareness and change was longest for the one practice requiring institutional action (scavenging waste gases).
Referrals for treatment of senile macular degeneration	Combs (1982)	RCT showing benefit of treatment	Records of Witmer Ophthalmological Institute.	In 6 months following announcement of study results compared to 6 months previous, the number of patient referrals tripled and the number of treatable cases doubled.
Internal mammary artery ligation	Barsamian (1977); Fisher and Kennedy (1982)	RCT	Views of authors.	RCT definitively showed procedure to be ineffective. (No quantitative data on utilization of the procedure before definitive studies.)
Gastric freezing	Miao (1977)	RCTs and other studies		RCT definitively showed procedure to be ineffective.
	Fineberg (1979)		Manufacturer records.	Sale of devices stopped several years prior to appearance of definitive study.

CT scanning	Creditor and Garrett (1979)	Available literature	Hospital records.	Acceptance of computed tomographic (CT) scanning preceded controlled evaluation.
Extracorporeal support for respiratory insufficiency	Fineberg and Hiatt (1979)	RCT	Views of authors.	Early randomized trial said to prevent spread of technology.
Amniocentesis	Omenn (1978)	Multi-center controlled trial	Views of authors.	Early multicenter trials said to promote wider dissemination.
Hyperbaric O_2 for cognitive deficits in the elderly	OTA (1978, 1983)	RCT	Views of authors.	RCT finds procedure ineffective and dampens physician use.
Treatment of breast cancer	McPherson and Fox (1977)	RCTs	National rates of surgery cited in other works.	Physicians persist in using radical mastectomy despite evidence from RCTs that simple mastectomy plus irradiation is at least as successful.
Treatment of breast cancer	OTA (1983)	RCTs	Survey of surgical patterns by American College of Surgeons.	Practice has changed in the direction, though not the degree, indicated by RCTs, Percent of breast cancer patients: 1972 / 1981 Radical mastectomy: 50% / 3% Modified radical: 30% / 70% Lumpectomy: 3% / 8% (Remainder) presumably represents simple mastectomy and possibly other treatments.
Beta-blockers after myocardial infarction	OTA (1983); Friedwald and Schoenberger (1982)	41 RCTs	Views of authors.	Small RCTs all show trend favoring use of beta-blockers. Widespread use probably preceded evidence from RCTs.
Length of stay (LOS) for myocardial infarction	Chassin (1983)	RCTs other controlled studies and non-RCTs	NCHS Hospital Discharge Survey.	LOS for myocardial infarction (MI) in the United States declined by one-third between 1968 and 1980. Many studies find shorter stays as safe as longer, though results are not conclusive.

APPENDIX 4-A ***Continued***

Topic	Reference (Year)	Type of Evaluation Studied	Source of Data on Effects	Findings
Studies of Patterns of Clinical Evaluation and of the Effect of Clinical Evaluations on the Opinions of Experts				
Treatment of alcohol withdrawal	Moskowitz et al. (1981)	RCTs	Survey of physicians.	Physicians practice was consistent with findings in RCTs prior to appearance of review articles making same recommendations.
Drugs to lower blood lipids (CDP)	Friedewald and Schoenberger (1982)	RCT (CDP)	Views of authors.	Gradual reduction in use of clofibrate consistent with findings in study.
Hypertension detection and follow-up	Friedewald and Schoenberger (1982)	RCT (HDFP)	Views of authors.	Study should have broad impact, leading to more aggressive treatment of hypertension.
Drug to lower blood lipids (Coronary Drug Project)	Market Facts (1982)	RCT	Survey of physicians 4–5 years after trial showing risks and lack of benefit from lipid-lowering agents.	Majority of physicians either never prescribe lipid-lowering drugs (14%) or use them only as secondary therapy (72%). 47% said they were using lipid-lowering drugs less often than in the past; 67% use these drugs more often.
Aspirin to reduce recurrence of myocardial infarction (AMIS)	Market Facts (1982)	RCT	Survey of physicians before and after study showing no benefit from aspirin following myocardial infarction.	Majority of physicians remained unaffected by AMIS findings, continuing to prescribe aspirin for patients following myocardial infarction.
Modern medical mistakes	Lambert (1978)	Varied	Review of literature.	Many medical mistakes occur because of the absence of proper early evaluation.
Discarded surgical procedures	Barnes (1977)	Evaluations in literature	Literature between 1880 and 1942.	Eventually discarded operations were characterized by lack of control experience and in several cases were sustained in the literature over decades.
Drugs to lower blood lipids (Coronary Drug Project)	Friedman et al. (1983)	RCT (CDP)	National Disease and Therapeutic Index.	Prescriptions for all lipid-lowering drugs in the United States rose from 1.5 million in 1970 to 2.3 million in 1975 then fell to 1 million in 1980.

			Personal interviews with 1,785 physicians from 1979 through 1981 (see Market Facts, 1982).	Percentage of physicians prescribing lipid-lowering drugs for post-MI patients: (1979 / 1980 / 1981) Never prescribe: 10.2 / 17.2 / 18.0 Rx only as 2° therapy: 73.8 / 74.0 / 69.2 Sometimes Rx as 1° therapy: 15.9 / 8.8 / 12.7 Number of physicians: 859 / 296 / 621
Studies of the Effect of Synthetic Assessment on Knowledge of Physicians				
NIH consensus conferences on CT scanning and total hip replacement	Jacoby, unpublished report (1983)	Consensus conference	Telephone surveys of 700 physicians in pertinent specialty areas 2 weeks prior to conference and 6 weeks after publication of conference results in the *Journal of the American Medical Association*.	8–9% of physicians were aware of the Consensus Development Program at NIH. Two weeks before each conference, 16% of physicians knew about the upcoming conference on CT; 7% knew about the conference on hip joint replacement. Six weeks after publication of results, 14% were aware of the conference on CT and 4% aware of the conclusions; 7% were aware of the conference on hip joint replacement and 1% aware of its conclusions. Most of those aware of study findings had read about them in professional journals.
Studies of Effect of Synthetic Assessments on Clinical Practices				
Guidelines for tuberculosis control	Leff et al. (1979); Leff and Brewin (1981)	Recommendation from Public Health Service, American Thoracic Society, American Lung Association	Mail survey of 28 municipal tuberculosis control officers.	Greater conformity to guidelines on chemoprophylaxis than on diagnosis and treatment.
Medical necessity, Blue Cross and Blue Shield	Blue Cross and Blue Shield Association (1982)	Consensus on 42 outmoded practices, announced and disseminated in 1977	Insurance claims in 1975 and 1978 for Federal Employee Health Benefits Program offered by Blue Cross and Blue Shield.	Number of claims paid for tested surgical procedures declined 26%; claims paid for listed diagnostic procedures declined 85%.

APPENDIX 4-A *Continued*

Topic	Reference (Year)	Type of Evaluation Studied	Source of Data on Effects	Findings
		Studies of Effect of Synthetic Assessments on Clinical Practices		
Approved uses for cimetidine	Fineberg and Pearlman (1981)	FDA-approved uses	NDTI data on drug use.	Many uses of cimetidine in practice are not approved by FDA.
	Schade and Donaldson (1981)		Medical records.	Many uses of cimetidine in practice are not approved by FDA.
	Cocco and Cocco (1981)			Many uses of cimetidine in practice are not approved by FDA.
NIH consensus conference on high blood pressure, held in 1977	Thomson et al. (1981)	Consensus conference	Survey of physicians in ambulatory settings in New York City.	90% of respondents were routinely treating patients with mild hypertension in contrast to individualized approach advocated by consensus statement.
Treatment of alcohol withdrawal	Moskowitz et al. (1981)	Review articles	Survey of physicians.	Physician use practices that were found effective in RCTs and use them before they are recommended in review articles.
		Studies of the Effects of Clinical Evaluations and Synthetic Assessments on Regulation and Reimbursement		
PHS advisories to HCFA	Center for Analysis of Health Practices (1981)	Review by PHS	Estimates of authors.	The PHS through National Center for Health Care Technology made recommendations of nonreimbursement for 21 of 50 procedures reviewed during 1979–1980. All recommendations were accepted by HCFA, though procedures at HCFA did not necessarily assure uniform application throughout the country. Decisions not to reimburse four procedures (dialysis for schizophrenia, hyperthermia for cancer, radial keratotomy for myopia, and endothelial cell photography) are estimated to produce savings of $312 million to the Medicare program over a 10-year period.

Hyperbaric oxygen for cognitive deficits in the elderly	OTA (1978, 1983)	RCT	Views of authors.	RCT shows procedure ineffective; facilitates decision by Medicare and other insurers not to reimburse.
Drugs to lower blood lipids	Friedman et al. (1983)	RCTs (CDP and WHO clofibrate trial)	Review of FDA labeling changes for clofibrate (Atromid-S) between 1969 and 1982.	Changes in labeling, identifying more side effects and progressively restricting indications for use, are believed due in part to CDP (which assessed use in patients with previous MI; results with clofibrate published 1975) and to WHO clofibrate trial (which assessed primary prevention of MI; results published 1978 and 1980). Major labeling changes in 1979 are attributed to both CDP and WHO trial; further restrictions in 1982 reflect most recent findings from WHO trial, with CDP results serving as background.

REFERENCES

Armitage, P., D. Bardelli, and D. A. G. Galton, et al. 1978. Methods and Impact of Controlled Therapeutic Trials in Cancer, Part I. UICC Technical Report Series, 36, Geneva.

Avorn, J., M. Chen, and R. Hartley. 1982. Scientific versus commercial sources of influence on the prescribing behavior of physicians. Am. J. Med. 73:4–8.

Avorn, J., and S. B. Soumerai. 1983. Improving drug-therapy decisions through educational outreach: A randomized controlled trial of academically based "detailing." N. Engl. J. Med. 308:1457–1463.

Barnes, B. 1977. Discarded operations: surgical innovation by trial and error. Pp. 109–123 in Costs, Risks and Benefits of Surgery, J. P. Bunker, B. A. Barnes, and F. Mosteller, eds. New York: Oxford University Press.

Barsamian, E. M. 1977. The rise and fall of internal mammary artery ligation in the treatment of angina pectoris and the lessons learned. Pp. 212–220 in Costs, Risks and Benefits of Surgery, J. P. Bunker, B. A. Barnes, and F. Mosteller, eds. New York: Oxford University Press.

Berg, R. B., and A. J. Salisbury. 1971. Discharging infants of low birth weight: Reconsideration of current practice. Am. J. Dis. Child. 122:414–417.

Berwick, D. M., H. V. Fineberg, and M. C. Weinstein. 1981. When doctors meet numbers. Am. J. Med. 71:991–998.

Blue Cross and Blue Shield Association. 1982. Announcement of new phase of medical necessity program. October 12. Memorandum. Chicago, Ill.

Bonchek, L. 1979. Are randomized trials appropriate for evaluating new operations? N. Engl. J. Med. 301:44–45.

Buchwald, H., L. Fitch, and R. B. Moore. 1982. Overview of randomized clinical trials of lipid intervention for atherosclerotic cardiovascular disease. Controlled Clinical Trials 3:271–83.

Caplow, T. 1954. Market attitudes: A research report from the medical field. Harvard Bus. Rev. 30:105–12.

Center for the Analysis of Health Practices, Harvard School of Public Health. 1981. Impact on health costs of NCHCT recommendations for nonreimbursement for medical procedures. Monograph Series. Washington, D.C.: National Center for Health Care Technology.

Chalmers, T. C. 1974. The impact of controlled trials on the practice of medicine. Mt. Sinai J. Med. (NY) 41:753–759.

Chalmers, T. C., B. Silverman, E. P. Shareck, A. Ambroz, B. Schroeder, and H. Smith, Jr. 1979. Randomized controlled trials in gastroenterology with particular attention to duodenal ulcer. Pp. 223–255 in Report to the Congress of the United States of the National Commission on Digestive Diseases, Vol. 4, part 2B, DHEW Pub. No. (NIH) 79-2885. Washington, D.C.: Department of Health, Education, and Welfare.

Chalmers, T. C. 1982. A potpourri of RCT topics. Controlled Clinical Trials 3:285–98.

Chassin, M. P. 1983. Health Technology Case Study, 24: Variations in Hospital Length of Stay: Their Relationship to Health Outcomes. OTA-HCS 23. Washington, D.C.: U.S. Congress, Office of Technology Assessment.

Christensen, E., E. Juhl, and N. Tygstrup. 1977. Treatment of duodenal ulcer: Randomized clinical trials of a decade (1964–1974). Gastroenterology 73:1170–1178.

Cocco, A. E., and D. V. Cocco. 1981. A survey of cimetidine prescribing. N. Engl. J. Med. 304:1281.

Combs, J. L., S. M. Cohen, S. L. Fine, R. P. Murphy, and A. Patz. 1983. The spectrum of senile macular degeneration (SMD) at the retinal vascular center. Presented at the Forty-second Scientific Meeting of the Residents Association of the Wilmer Ophthalmological Institute, Baltimore, April 20–22, 1983. Cited by Hawkins (1983).

Comroe, J. H., Jr. 1976. Lags between initial discovery and clinical application to cardiovascular pulmonary medicine and surgery. Report of the President's Biomedical Research Panel, Appendix B, Part I. DHEW Pub. No. (OS) 76-502. Washington, D.C.: U.S. Government Printing Office.

Creditor, M. C., and J. B. Garrett. 1977. The information base for diffusion of technology: Computed tomography scanning. N. Engl. J. Med. 297:49–52.

Dunn, D. R. F. 1981. Dissemination of the published results of an important clinical trial: An analysis of the citing literature. Bull. Med. Libr. Assoc. 69:301–306.

Feinstein, A. R. 1983. An additional basic science for clinical medicine: II. The limitations of randomized trials. Ann. Intern. Med. 99:544–550.

Fineberg, H. V., G. S. Parker, and L. A. Pearlman. 1977. CT scanners: Distribution and planning status in the United States. N. Engl. J. Med. 297:216–218.

Fineberg, H. V., R. Gabel, and M. Sosman. 1978. The acquisition and application of new medical knowledge by anesthesiologists: Three recent examples. Anesthesiology 48:430–436.

Fineberg, H. V. 1979. Gastric freezing: A study of diffusion of a medical innovation. Pp. 173–200 in Medical Technology and the Health Care System: A Study of the Diffusion of Equipment-embodied Technology. Washington, D.C.: National Academy of Sciences.

Fineberg, H. V., and H. H. Hiatt. 1979. Evaluation of medical practices: The case for technology assessment. N. Engl. J. Med. 301:1086–1091.

Fineberg, H. V., L. A. Pearlman, and R. A. Gabel. 1980. The case for abandonment of explosive anesthetic agents. N. Engl. J. Med. 303:613–617.

Fineberg, H. V., and L. A. Pearlman. 1981. Surgery for peptic ulcer disease in the United States: Trends before and after the introduction of cimetidine. Lancet 1:1305–1307.

Finkelstein, S. N., and D. L. Gilbert. 1983. Scientific evidence and the abandonment of medical technology: Study of eight drugs. Working Paper #1419-83. Alfred P. Sloan School of Management, Massachusetts Institute of Technology, Cambridge, Massachusetts.

Fisher, L. D., and J. W. Kennedy. 1982. Randomized surgical clinical trials for treatment of coronary artery disease. Controlled Clinical Trials 3:235–58.

Freeborn, D. K., D. Baer, M. R. Greenlick, and J. W. Bailey. 1972. Determinants of medical care utilization: Physicians' use of laboratory services. Am. J. Public Health 62:846–53.

Friedewald, W. T., and J. A. Schoenberger. 1982. Overview of recent clinical and methodological advances from clinical trials of cardiovascular disease. Controlled Clinical Trials 3:259–270.

Friedman, L., N. K. Wenger, and G. L. Knatterud. 1983. Impact of the coronary drug project findings on clinical practice. Controlled Clinical Trials 4:513–22.

Garnier, H. S., R. Flamant, and C. Fohanno. 1982. Assessment of the role of randomized clinical trials in establishing treatment policies. Controlled Clinical Trials 3:227–34.

Gehan, E. A. 1982. Progress in therapy in acute leukemia 1948–1981: Randomized versus nonrandomized clinical trials. Controlled Clinical Trials 3:199–208.

Gilbert, J., B. McPeek, and F. Mosteller. 1977. Progress in surgery and anesthesia: Benefits and risks of innovative therapy. Pp. 124–169 in Costs, Risks, and Benefits of Surgery, J. P. Bunker, B. A. Barnes, and F. Mosteller, eds. New York: Oxford University Press.

Globe, S., G. W. Levy, and C. M. Schwartz. 1967. Science, Technology, and Innovation. Contract NSF 8667 (Battelle-Columbus Laboratories). Washington, D.C.: National Science Foundation.

Goodwin, J., and J. M. Goodwin. 1982. Failure to recognize efficacious treatments: A history of salicylate therapy in rheumatoid arthritis. Perspect Biol. Med. 25:78–92.

Haines, S. J. 1983. Randomized clinical trials in neurosurgery. J. Neurosur 12:259–264.

Ingelfinger, F. J., R. V. Ebert, M. Finland, and A. S. Relman, eds. 1974. Controversy in Internal Medicine II. Philadelphia: W. B. Saunders.

Jordan, H. S., J. F. Burke, H. V. Fineberg, and J. S. Hanley. 1983. Diffusion of innovations in burn care: Selected findings. Burns 9:271–279.

Lambert, E. C. 1978. Modern Medical Mistakes. Bloomington: Indiana University Press.

Leff, A. R., D. Herskowitz, J. Gilbert, and A. Brewin. 1979. Tuberculosis chemoprophylaxis practices in metropolitan clinics. Am. Rev. Respir. Dis. 119:161–164.

Leff, A. R., and A. Brewin. 1981. Tuberculosis chemotherapy practices in major metropolitan health departments in the United States. Am. Rev. Respir. Dis. 123:176–180.

Manning P. R., and T. A. Denson. 1979. How cardiologists learn about echocardiography: A reminder for medical educators and legislators. Ann. Intern. Med. 91:496–471.

Manning, P. R., and T. A. Denson. 1980. How internists learned about cimetidine. Ann. Intern. Med. 92:690–692.

Market Facts. 1982. The Impact of Two Clinical Trials on Physician Knowledge and Practice. Contract No1-HV-82940. Washington, D.C.: National Heart, Lung, and Blood Institute.

McPherson, K., and M. S. Fox. 1977. Treatment of breast cancer. Pp. 308–322 in Costs, Risks, and Benefits of Surgery, J. P. Bunker, B. A. Barnes, and F. Mosteller, eds. New York: Oxford University Press.

Miao, L. L. 1977. Gastric freezing: An example of the evaluation of medical therapy by randomized clinical trials. Pp. 198–211 in Costs, Risks, and Benefits of Surgery, J. P. Bunker, B. A. Barnes, and F. Mosteller, eds. New York: Oxford University Press.

Moskowitz, G., T. C. Chalmers, H. S. Sacks, R. M. Fagerstrom, and H. Smith, Jr. 1981. Deficiencies of clinical trials of alcohol withdrawal. Alcoholism Clin. Exp. Res. 5:162–166.

Office of Technology Assessment, U.S. Congress. 1978. Assessing the Efficacy and Safety of Medical Technologies. Stock No. 052-003-00593-0. Washington, D.C.: U.S. Government Printing Office.

Office of Technology Assessment, U.S. Congress. 1981. Policy Implications of the Computed Tomography (CT) Scanner: An update. OTA-BP-H-8. Washington, D.C.: U.S. Government Printing Office.

Office of Technology Assessment, U.S. Congress. 1983. The Impact of Randomized Clinical Trials on Health Policy and Medical Practice. OTA-BP-H-22. Washington, D.C.: U.S. Government Printing Office.

Omenn, G. S. 1978. Prenatal diagnosis of genetic disorders. Science 200:952–958.

Peterson, W. L., R. A. L. Sturdevant, H. D. Frankl, C. T. Richardson, J. I. Isenberg, J. D. Elashoff, J. Q. Sones, R. A. Gross, R. W. McCallum, and J. S. Fordtran. 1977. Healing of duodenal ulcer with an antacid regimen. N. Engl. J. Med. 297:341–345.

Pryor, D. B., M. C. Hindman, G. S. Wagner, R. M. Califf, M. K. Rhoads, and R. A. Rosati. 1983. Early discharge after acute myocardial infarction. Ann. Intern. Med. 99:528–538.

The Rand Corporation. 1983. Submission to the Office of Management and Budget of Supporting Statement and Data Collection Instruments for Assessing the Effectiveness of the NIH Consensus Development Program (Contract No.: NO1-D-2-2128).

Ray, W. A., C. F. Federspiel, and W. Schaffner. 1977. Prescribing of tetracycline to children less than 8 years old: A two-year epidemiologic study among ambulatory Tennessee Medicaid recipients. J. Am. Med. Assoc. 237:2068–2074.

Rockette, H. E., C. K. Redmond, and B. Fisher. Participating NSABP investigators. 1982. Impact of randomized clinical trials on therapy of primary breast cancer: The NSABP overview. Controlled Clinical Trials 3:209–25.

Rogers, E. M., and F. F. Shoemaker. 1971. Communication of Innovations: A Cross-Cultural Approach. New York: The Free Press.

Russell, L. B. 1979. Technology in Hospitals: Medical Advances and Their Diffusion. Washington, D.C.: The Brookings Institution.

Schade, R. R., and R. M. Donaldson, Jr. 1981. How physicians use cimetidine: A survey of hospitalized patients and published cases. N. Engl. J. Med. 304:1281–1284.

Schaffner, W., W. A. Ray, C. F. Federspiel, and W. O. Miller. 1983. Improving antibiotic prescribing in office practice: A controlled trial of three educational methods. J. Am. Med. Assoc. 250:1728–1732.

Sherrington, A. M. 1965. An annotated bibliography of studies on the flow of medical information to practitioners. Method Inform. Med. 4:45–57.

Stern, B. J. 1927. Social Factors in Medical Progress. New York: Columbia University Press.

Stross, J. K., and W. R. Harlan. 1979. The dissemination of new medical information. J. Am. Med. Assoc. 241:2622–2624.

Stross, J. D., and W. R. Harlan. 1981. Dissemination of relevant information on hypertension. J. Am. Med. Assoc. 247:3231–3234.

Sussman, E. J., W. G. Tsiaras, and K. A. Soper. 1982. Diagnosis of diabetic eye disease. J. Am. Med. Assoc. 247:3231–3234.

Thomson, G. E., M. H. Alderman, S. Wassertheil-Smoller, J. F. Rafter, and R. Samet. 1981. High blood pressure diagnosis and treatment: Consensus recommendations vs. actual practice. Am. J. Public Health 71:413–16.

Wagner, E. H., R. A. Truesdale, and J. T. Warner. 1981. Compliance, treatment practices and blood pressure control: Community survey findings. J. Chronic Dis. 34:519–25.

Warner, K. 1975. A "desparation-reaction" model of medical diffusion. Health Service Res. 10:369–83.

Warner, R., S. M. Wolfe, and R. Rich. 1978. Off Diabetes Pills: A Diabetics Guide to Longer Life. Washington, D.C.: Public Citizen's Health Research Group.

Williamson, P. M. 1975. The adoption of new drugs by doctors practicing in group and solo practice. Social Sci. Med. 9:233–236.

Wilson, N. I. L., P. A. Wright, and C. S. McArdle. 1982. Survey of antibiotic prophylaxis in gastrointestinal surgery in Scotland. Br. Med. J. 285:871–873.

5 Reimbursement and Technology Assessment

Spending for health care in the United States rose from 6 percent of the gross national product in 1965, the year Medicare was created, to 10.8 percent in 1983, when it reached $355.4 billion. With public money being used for more than 40 percent of that spending for health care (Gibson et al., 1984), policymakers are searching for ways to reduce health care costs while maintaining quality care. Some analysts blame the use of new medical technologies and the overuse of existing technologies for up to 50 percent of the increases in expenditures for health care over recent years (Altman and Blendon 1979; Joskow, 1981). In that view, one way to reduce costs would be to reduce use of the technologies. Such an action, however, would be justifiable only if we could identify the technologies that are relatively ineffective, or even harmful, and discard them.

The primary purpose of technology assessment is to improve patient outcome. But it also is important to both private and public payers, receiving greater attention from policymakers as its potential for cutting costs of health care has become apparent.

This chapter traces the applications of medical technology assessment as they are evolving from a context of retrospective payment for health care to one of prospective payment. At first, when assessment was used largely to help make informed decisions about coverage of health care services by insurers and government, its application was only partially designed to control health care costs. But technology assessment now is seen as an aid to cost containment because it can help to determine relative cost-effectiveness of diagnostic and therapeutic procedures. The success of that application of assessment as an adjunct of economic policymaking will depend on many factors, including how to cover the costs of the assessment itself. This chapter also examines ways in which the reimbursement system could further technology assessment.

This chapter is based on materials drafted by Joanne Finley, Donald Young, and Lawrence Morris.

ASSESSMENT IN THE ERA OF RETROSPECTIVE PAYMENTS

The apparent intention of Congress at the time the Medicare amendments to the Social Security Act were passed was that the program generally should cover services ordinarily furnished by hospitals, skilled nursing facilities, and physicians. The law states:

> Notwithstanding any other provisions of this title, no payment may be made under Medicare for any expenses incurred for items or services . . . which are not reasonable and necessary for the diagnosis or treatment of illness or injury or to improve the functioning of a malformed body member. [Section 1862, Title XVII, Social Security Act Amendments of 1965.]

The program therefore does not explicitly include or exclude coverage for most medical devices, diagnostic and therapeutic services, or surgical procedures. The mechanisms for implementing the implied decisions about technologies that could be considered "reasonable and necessary" were left to regulations without further definition [42 CFRT 405.31(k)]. The clearest formal operating definition is contained in program instructions for the intermediaries contracted to process claims, prepared by the Health Care Financing Administration (HCFA), which directed that payment could be made only for health care procedures that were (1) generally accepted as safe and effective or were proved to be safe and effective, (2) not experimental, (3) medically necessary, and (4) furnished in accordance with accepted standards of practice in an appropriate setting.

When intermediaries processing claims for Medicare had questions about new technologies, they usually referred the more complex payment decisions back to HCFA. If medical consultation appeared necessary, that agency presented its questions to a panel of physicians. If a decision could not be reached by the panel, the matter was referred to the Public Health Service for further review.

In 1978, Congress created a National Center for Health Care Technology (NCHCT) to establish a more systematic approach to technology assessment and provide advice to HCFA on safety, efficacy, and cost-effectiveness. Although NCHCT recommendations were credited with saving millions of dollars for HCFA (Harvard Center for Analysis of Health Practices and University of California, Los Angeles [UCLA], School of Public Health, 1981), the NCHCT was opposed by the health care technology industry and some professional organizations. Appropriations for the center were halted in 1982. Since then the Office of Health Technology Assessment in the National Center for Health Services Research has had the responsibility for preparing assessments and recommendations regarding Medicare coverage questions referred to the Public Health Service by HCFA. Recent legislation (P.L. 98-551) changes the name of the National Center for Health Services Research to the National Center for Health Services Research and Health Care Technology Assessment (NCHSRHCTA) and establishes a National Advisory Council on Health Care Technology to assist in development of criteria and methods to be used by the center in making health care technology recommendations.

Most assessment decisions about paying for use of technologies remain with the contracting intermediaries who process Medicare claims. They generally accept for coverage technologies that are accepted by the local physicians and hospitals (Finkelstein et al., 1984). Specific technologies for which claims are paid by intermediaries vary across the country.

Increasing resistance to rising health care costs has led some of these contractors, whether making the decision for the federal government or for its plan's subscriber, to organize more formal procedures for assessing technologies. For example, a Medical Policy Committee of Blue Shield of California has been in existence for many years and evaluates safety, efficacy, cost, and cost-effectiveness of new technologies before making claims payment decisions. Similarly, the Interspecialty Medical Advisory Committee of Blue Shield of Massachusetts determines the general applicability of new medical technologies. The activities of the national Blue Cross and Blue Shield Association are a further example. This organization has encouraged support of the Clinical Efficacy Assessment Project of the American College of Physicians, discussed in Chapter 2, and also once commissioned the Institute of Medicine (1977) to examine the efficacy, utilization, and costs of computed tomography (CT) scanning.

Blue Cross and Blue Shield also established a Medical Necessity Project, which relies on assistance from specialty societies, and has issued respiratory therapy guidelines in association with the American College of Physicians, the American College of Surgeons, and the American Academy of Pediatrics. Additionally the project has developed guidelines for the coverage of 85 procedures, a policy on routine admission test batteries, and guidelines for diagnostic imaging.

The Blue Cross and Blue Shield Association also maintains a full-time staff that deals with technology issues, maintains a body to advise local plans, and otherwise supports member plans on these concerns. However, each policy statement is accompanied by a disclaimer indicating that it is a "guide to facilitate reasonable consistency among the medical judgments applied to claims . . . without unnecessary loss of plans' traditional sensitivity to local practices."

These examples illustrate the ability and interest of private health insurers to conduct technology assessment. But there are no national or regional standards. Medicare claims recommended for payment or subscribers' covered benefits vary across the nation. HCFA expects contractors to refer general coverage issues of national interest to the central office, but referral is not required either by statute or regulation. Nor does HCFA hold contractors accountable for adherence to the expectations (Banta et al., 1984). Unfortunately, information on a timely basis often is lacking for some new procedures; for example, total hip replacement was covered by most large third-party payers when it was still classified as experimental by the Food and Drug Administration (FDA) (Bunker et al., 1982a; Finkelstein et al., 1984).

Despite assessment activities by HCFA and others, spending for health care continued to rise. Some reasons that technology assessment has not restrained costs are legal matters (see Appendix 5-A). Societal and political factors such as those surrounding liver transplantation can impede cost-containment efforts. Antitrust challenges arise when insurers attempt to limit payments to certain providers. The authority to apply reimbursement sanctions to implement the findings of assessment, even if quality is at stake, must be clearly spelled out in the law. Unfortunately, even when states have passed legislation to protect against antitrust challenges payers efforts to limit reimbursement have been legally challenged on other grounds. Obstacles for private insurers also lie in market forces. Buyers of private programs want the widest array of benefits for the least outlay, and competition among various private insurers is fierce. Also, there are political considerations that blunt the effects of technology assessment; the system is an assessment of the validity of public expenditure, not of clinical usefulness in the specific case. Public programs have not regulated physicians' fees or rationed costly services such as hemodialysis. And private coverage is available to some groups to fill gaps in payment levels or benefit structures that occur in public programs.

Finally, even if these disincentives were removed, the data bases on which insurers have to depend to make informed coverage decisions are inadequate. Medicare cost reports and claim forms, the Medicaid management information system, and private insurance claims data have not included detailed information on patient characteristics, procedures used, and outcomes. Intermediaries submit 20 percent of the Medicare inpatient claims as samples to HCFA, which attempts to merge patient and financial data (the MEDPAR file). HCFA has attempted to extract enough information about patient characteristics, resources used, and costs to develop its Diagnosis-Related-Group (DRG)-based prospective payment system from this incomplete data base. The purpose of collecting these data has been to enable payers to pay claims. It is primarily financial data. There is a growing need by payers for more information that could be used for technology assessment as well as full analysis of the basis for differing costs for different kinds of patients. The routine claims-based data are not sufficient.

THE NEED FOR ASSESSMENT IN THE NEW ERA OF COST CONTAINMENT

Today the emphasis on cost containment in plans is on altering reimbursement (payment methods) to induce and even reward cost-saving behavior. Reimbursement can vary according to whether payments are based on costs or on charges, whether it is made retrospectively or by the terms of a prospectively fixed revenue budget, and whether it is able to control cost increases or not.

Radical change in federal reimbursement policy has occurred through amendments relating to Medicare. All of the above variables are touched by the new federal system, and responsibilities for some technology assessment as it may relate to the goal of cost containment as well as quality assurance for Medicare are written into the law. Because data requirements are also affected, chances may improve for technology assessment.

Until recently, major payers such as Medicare and Blue Cross reimbursed hospitals retrospectively on the basis of costs incurred. Under a system of cost-based reimbursement, the acquisition and use by hospitals of new technology and of all medical procedures (if the coverage decisions had already been made) could be fully covered regardless of their expense.

States were the first to experiment with mandatory prospective payment systems for hospital reimbursement. They established under various statutory provisions that reimbursement by state-regulated payers (Blue Cross, Medicaid) would be based on advance calculation of revenues needed to care for those patients. Payments would then be made on some timely basis so that by year's end they would add up to no more than the prospectively determined hospital revenue. When prospective reimbursement systems have been analyzed, they have been found to contain hospital charges to payers to whom the methods applied. If those payers represented a large enough proportion of hospital revenue sources, there also was a spillover effect so that hospitals' overall expenditures and expenditures per adjusted admission did not inflate as rapidly as the nation's (Biles et al., 1980).

On the premise that cost containment would be most effective if all sources of revenue were controlled, states experimenting with prospective payment systems sought waivers of Medicare's Principles of Reimbursement. These waivers enable all payers' reimbursements, including Medicare for inpatients, to be calculated in the same way. Maryland and New Jersey were the first states to be granted waivers as well as research and development funds to refine their cost-containment methods. New Jersey's system began with hospital cost containment for Blue Cross and Medicaid (Finley, 1983) and was expanded to all payers including Medicare in 1978.

Cost-based, retrospective reimbursement paid a per diem amount regardless of the patient's illness. This became seen as an incentive to increase reimbursement amounts by keeping patients longer than necessary. Cost-containment advocates devised a different way of calculating reimbursement. The Diagnosis-Related Group became the product definition for hospitals. The DRGs for each of hundreds of illnesses is the result of a distillation of patient discharge abstracts to find group characteristics that were clinically sensible and statistically clustered for cost, length of stay, and other measures of resource consumption (Office of Technology Assessment [OTA], 1983).

The relative success of New Jersey's experiment with DRGs interested the Department of Health and Human Services and the Congress, which in August 1982 passed the Tax Equity and Fiscal Responsibility Act (TEFRA; P.L. 97-248). It was aimed at relief for many classes of taxpayers, but it also dealt with cost containment for the Medicare program. A hospital's costs calculated on a case by case basis (Medicare discharges by DRGs) would be limited to a target rate of increase, and in no instance could a hospital's Medicare reimbursement exceed a mean per-case operating cost within its peer group.

In April 1983, the Social Security Reform Act (P.L. 98-21, Title VI) was enacted; Title VI moves Medicare payments over the next 3 years toward a prospective reimbursement system based on an average DRG-specific price. Medicare's calculation of average DRG prices (in 1984 there were 467 DRGs) is based on incomplete patient-specific data from a 20 percent sample of its claims (the MEDPAR file). The average cost for a DRG, calculated from financial elements required on Medicare cost reports related to direct patient care, is then weighted according to how much greater these costs are than the average for all Medicare discharges. The price for each DRG is adjusted by this weight. Adjustments are also made for differences in area wage rates, and a 0.25 percent factor (initially under TEFRA it was 1 percent), now said to be for technology, is added. Initially, only part of the hospital's Medicare reimbursement is based on this DRG price. The remainder, decreasing each year, will move from the regional average to a national average.

Under a reimbursement policy of presetting an institution's budget based on an average price within a group, decisions on the acquisition and use of new technologies must meet economic criteria. When a hospital begins to spend more money than it collects under a prospective per-case reimbursement system, administrators and finance directors may begin to analyze other technologies such as physician practice for cost-effectiveness. Therefore, the new reimbursement policy would appear to encourage the assessment of medical technologies for their safety and costs. But the strength of demand for technology assessment will depend on many factors. Six such factors are discussed below.

Leverage of the Reimbursement System over Institutions

If a hospital is not heavily dependent on Medicare revenues, the controls may not be sufficient to motivate technology assessment. "Under the new Medicare law about 32 percent of the revenues of nonfederal short-term hospitals will be subject to DRG payment" (OTA, 1983). Worse, as hospitals identify the most profitable patients and services, the access of some

Medicare patients may become limited. The political consequences from the first time Medicare patients are turned away may force some changes. Patients without insurance are already being transferred among institutions (Reinhardt, 1985). Changes also may be demanded because of the effect on other payers—not on Medicare—to whom costs can be shifted. These payers may have a large political voice. Cost shifting may become more difficult with the development of health maintenance organizations and preferred provider organizations and negotiations between industry and providers.

Capital Acquisition

At the outset the Medicare prospective payment system will add to the established DRG payment rate a cost-based factor for capital acquisition (depreciation and interest payments). However, the secretary of the Department of Health and Human Services (DHHS) must study the methods by which capital-related costs can be included in the prospective payment rate. The law stipulates a deadline of October 1, 1986, for a legislative proposal to deal with prospectively reimbursed capital costs also to be tied to patient mix. Many technologies that hospitals may wish to acquire can be classified as capital, such as a new linear accelerator or even expensive major movable equipment. For some hospitals that are not presently severely revenue constrained, this time gap in reimbursement policy may briefly propel them toward capital intensity without the desired technology assessment that should precede such decisions.

Some states with prospective reimbursement systems for all payers have built-in limits on capital acquisition that may make prepurchase assessment for cost-effectiveness more necessary. New Jersey has a method different from the federal government's for adding a capital facilities allowance to the DRG rate. Target occupancy levels based on regulation and current experience, rather than currently licensed capacity, are used to figure an annual prorated sum to be set aside for eventual replacement (Finley, 1983). Maryland attempts to limit new capital acquisition to that which is cost-effective. That state seldom grants increases for technologic additions, believing that approved technology, if cost-saving, should pay for itself within the prospective budget (from an interview with the Maryland Health Services Cost Review Commission, 1983). Both states lack sufficient data to distinguish a truly new way of diagnosing or treating an illness, for which a rate of increase might be granted, from a method that merely replaces the old.

State Certificate of Need (CoN) programs* regulate the establishment of major new health services and institutions and major capital expenditures for plant and equipment by legally requiring and controlling franchises or rights to add services and invest in physical capital. Historically, such programs have based their decisions on an assessment of whether population size, travel time, access, the lack of preexisting unused capacity, and other factors indicate a need for an investment or service. It was implicitly assumed that all or nearly all proposed investments were worthwhile in a technology assessment sense and therefore ought to be made available.

Recently, however, the state governmental leaders who run CoN programs have recognized that if health expenditures are to be limited to any significant degree, it will be necessary to advance from this all-or-nothing notion of effectiveness to a concept of *relative need*, a recognition that some investments are more desirable than

* Background materials provided by Jonathan Brown.

others. The principal way in which relative need has been proposed for application is a regional *capital cap*, an annual limit on the dollar commitments for new services and physical capital in a state or region. A cap forces investment and service proposals to compete for approval and requires the review agency and its governing board to rank the need for different proposals. Capital cap programs have been proposed or implemented in Massachusetts, Maine, New York, Michigan, Rhode Island, and New Jersey. Because the health of people is the presumed goal of most health care investments, a capital cap requires the CoN agency to assess the cost-effectiveness of each investment in terms of its impact on longevity and quality of life. To achieve these ends, new forms of concurrent information gathering and technology assessment must be combined with policies focusing on day-to-day provider decision making (rather than simply long-range regulation) if real increases in health system productivity are to be achieved with any consistency and reliability.

Stimulus for Technology Assessment in Reimbursement Policy

A reimbursement system may or may not incorporate incentives for cost-efficiency. Incentives can encourage the use of cost-saving technology, and even contribute funds for the acquisition of new technology and the conduct of assessment.

Private hospitals can generate funds to create clinical data bases to evaluate medical technologies. In the 1970s a group of Rochester, N.Y., hospitals banded together to develop a prospective payment plan that included Medicare, Medicaid, and Blue Cross patients. Once hospitals reduced their costs, they were allowed to share in the savings. By 1981 this program generated enough funds to maintain and expand a data base to test the cost-effectiveness of technologic innovation, and even to award $500,000 in research grants to study the efficiency of certain therapeutic practices (Rochester Area Hospitals' Corporation, 1980, 1982).

Another example of a reimbursement incentive for using information from technology assessment is offered by the New Jersey Hospital Rate-Setting Commission, which allowed a rate increase to a hospital that had been particularly effective in physician education, the goal of which was to alter expensive practices which were not of special benefit to patients. The increased revenue was time limited and earmarked for the development of a computer clinical management information system. This would then be made available to other New Jersey hospitals. It would signal to physicians writing patient orders what tests and procedures were and were not indicated (by DRGs) based on cost, yield, and therapeutic impact.

In contrast, federal law does not provide financial incentives for technology assessment. OTA has analyzed the stimulus for technology assessment of incentives built into the new laws. "Under the temporary provisions of TEFRA, the hospital reaps little reward for keeping its per-case costs low (maximum of 5 percent of its per-case rate) but bears the full penalty of exceeding the per-case limit. Under the new Medicare law, the hospital bears the full burden of a loss and reaps the full rewards of a surplus" (OTA, 1983). One is too restrictive to inspire technology assessment. The other may be too liberal, because use of the surplus is not restricted as to the kinds of technologies that might be acquired or to any proof that they have been assessed for cost-effectiveness.

DRG Price Development and Technology Assessment

The fact that hospital payment will now depend on the patient's illness rather than on the patient's occupancy of a room requires both the institution and the payer to keep accurate, complete, and timely medical charts. Proper DRG assignment cannot be made without charted detail on patient characteristics beyond diagnosis, for example, age and secondary diagnoses, procedures performed, complications, and hospital resources used or required.

These data have utility for technology assessment. Whether the payment system creates a greater perception of need for technology assessment may depend in part on how the DRG is priced and how much an institution knows about its dollar variances from some norm or standard. The more the institution's managers can visualize the cost centers (resources) involved in the generation of profit or financial loss, the more they can be motivated to analyze practices, equipment, and procedure utilization. In an ideal analysis these data should be linked to patient outcome, so that the motivation remains related to patients' benefit as well as price. However the DRG system provides a strong fiscal incentive to slant diagnostic and procedure data to a higher-paid DRG. Pricing methodology can also be so restrictive as to make technology assessment or acquisition impossible (Dickson, 1982).

DRG creep (the phenomenon in which coding is inappropriately altered to enhance payment) may have unintended downstream consequences for the weights assigned to similar DRG categories. HCFA has established a monitoring system that examines shifts in patterns on a hospital-by-hospital basis. Smits and Watson (1985) have shown that prospective payment based on DRGs will influence surgical practice both through the methods by which new procedures are assigned codes and through the monitoring systems designed to detect changes in DRG patterns. Within the field of coding the central problem is how to manage change and the ability of the coding system to respond to new events in clinical medicine. For example percutaneous transluminal coronary angioplasty has been assigned to a surgical DRG rather than a cardiac catheterization DRG and is therefore paid at a higher rate giving hospitals a bonus. Attention will need to be paid to these issues by HCFA and the Prospective Payment Assessment Commission (ProPAC).

The derivations of prices for DRGs in all the varying systems that use these patient classifications are quite different, but all depend on averages. Cost centers such as laboratory/operating room, physical medicine, intensive care unit, or radiology may differ in their cost performance. Therefore, the details of cost centers by which these costs are reported is also important. The DRG weights developed for TEFRA and the DRG prices under the new Medicare law are averaged from a 20 percent national sample of all Medicare hospital claims. Prices must also be derived from some given base year of hospitals grouped by similar characteristics and existing costs and billing data (bills have charges). Therefore, the use of ratios of costs to charges by DRG depends on averages among the peer groups of institutions. Higher costs of some DRGs in hospitals that use technology inefficiently will influence the average. This could lessen the motivation for technology assessment. Conversely lower-cost hospitals caring for complex DRGs may underutilize effective technology, and the average will pull down the appropriate price for other hospitals.

The Medicare program's pricing methodology works its way rapidly from a hospital-specific portion to a flat national average and will probably encourage technology assessment less than it will the tendency on the part of some hospitals to send expensive patients elsewhere. If this leads to an orderly plan for regionalization of care for complex and unusual cases, with a separate DRG price system, there might be a positive impact on quality and cost containment. If regulators furnish hospitals with sufficient data on their wide cost variances, by DRG, from regional and national standards, there is an opportunity to discover the reasons, including those which lie with technology.

Cost-Containment Information: Feedback for Change

Standard economic thinking suggests that purchasers will not buy a product they feel is too costly if they can get it elsewhere for less. But the users of hospital technologies are physicians. They have not been trained to think about patient care in economic terms, nor has there been any particular incentive for them to think that way. They may even feel that cost implications have no place in doing what they think is best for their patients. Therefore, effective cost containment is most apt to occur when it is structured so as to have an impact on physician practice patterns.

Doctors have desired information in the past about what may be useful or harmful to their patients, or what may expose the physician to liability. However physicians need the information in clinical terms relevant to their way of managing patients. Practice patterns are more likely to change if the use of the information by physicians' peers teaches that costlier behavior is not necessarily beneficial to patient outcomes.

The New Jersey prospective payment demonstration had two components to influence physician practice behavior: (1) a hospital cost factor for specific implementation of prospective payment was allowed as an add-on to the DRG rate; in addition to perfecting their computer data management and upgrading medical records capabilities, hospitals could seek education costs to help doctors understand and use the DRG information; (2) the New Jersey DRG system generated management reports to hospitals (including the medical director), showing cost performance by DRGs and by all ancillary cost centers compared with that of all other hospitals (the standard).

Using these annual management reports New Jersey hospitals have developed their own computer programs to itemize high-ranking, negative-variance DRGs (these produce dollar disincentives because some aspects of practice have made these DRGs more costly than the standard) into a performance track for each doctor admitting certain kinds of patients. The hospitals can now identify physicians in a total doctor cluster who are dealing with patients in a more costly way compared with that of their own peers, and can identify which technology cost centers (laboratory, operating room, intensive care unit, physical medicine, radiology, etc.) account for this.

An evaluation study of the impact of New Jersey's DRG system on hospital behavior found medical staffs much more involved in the organization of the hospitals. "The character and flow of information has changed. The quantity and type of information that is collected has expanded allowing for the development of more sophisticated management information decisions" (Boerma, 1982).

Medicare does not propose to feed back such information to hospitals as they enter the prospective payment system. The initial average DRG rates and the weights by urban/rural peers and regions have been published. Presumably a hospital using its own Medicare cost reports could analyze in what DRGs it has been paid less than under cost-based reimbursement. But they will not have management reports comparing them, cost center by cost center, to peer hospital or a regional standard unless they themselves develop such a comparative information system. Without such comparisons, data useful for making informed technology acquisition decisions and for influencing ineffective and costly physician patterns may be lost. Instead, hospitals may emphasize profitable lines, regardless of the needs of the community or the most effective ways to render care.

Mechanisms to Promote Appropriate Use of Technology

When a new technology becomes widely used, research and development costs will have been repaid, and volumes of services to which it is applied will increase. If there is a system in place for assessment, these forces should dictate a lower price for a technology. If a technology has a cost-beneficial effect on patient care, such as reducing the number of hospital days or preventing certain complications, that too should decrease the hospital price. But sporadic technology assessment applied to new equipment and procedures has not yet brought a reassessment and price decrease once widespread diffusion has occurred.

The primary objective of a DRG price adjustment process is to maintain equality across DRGs in the ratios of price to the cost of efficient care. This objective implies that as new cost-saving technology becomes available for use in certain DRGs, the relative price of these DRGs should be adjusted downward to reflect the new efficiencies. Alternatively, the development of new cost-raising technologies that improve patient outcomes enough to justify their use should be met with increases in the prices of relevant DRGs (OTA, 1983). In order to make price adjustments, an ample supply of data will be required.

In the 1983 Social Security Reform Act, Congress provided for an independent Prospective Payment Assessment Commission and charged it with tasks including the following: (1) to identify medically appropriate patterns of health resources use and to collect and assess information on medical and surgical services and procedures (including regional variations) "giving special attention to treatment patterns for conditions which appear to involve excessively costly or inappropriate services not adding to the quality of care"; (2) to assess the safety, efficacy, and cost-effectiveness of new and existing medical and surgical procedures; (3) to collect and assess the necessary factual data; (4) to attend to the appropriate updating of existing DRGs, or relative weighting factors so that "such groups reflect appropriate differences in resource consumption in delivering safe, efficacious, and cost-effective care."

Based on the commission's recommendations, the DHHS secretary must adjust the DRG prices and weights by fiscal year 1986 and at least every 4 years thereafter.

The commission is largely constrained by its limited funding (not by legislation) to the use of existing information, published and unpublished. This underscores the need for an organized, coherent, methodologically sound national system for technology assessment and for review of the adequacy of data which already exist. However, Congress also permitted the commission to award grants and contracts for "original research and experimentation, including clinical research, where existing information is inadequate . . ." [P.L. 98-21, (5)(E)(ii)].

"Reimbursement for the technology assessment indicated is authorized and the source specified: 85 percent from the Federal Hospital Insurance Trust Fund, and 15 percent from the Federal Supplementary Medical Insurance Trust Fund" [P.L. 98-21, section 601, (6)(A-1)].

The first appropriation for this commission was only $1.5 million, and the staff has been limited to no more than 25 persons. Thus, while cost containment and technology assessment are now explicitly linked, the commission must still depend largely on existing assessments, which may be inadequate, and the group will not have sufficient funds to assess a wide variety of high-cost technologies.

The law also provides for a continuation of peer review activities. The determination for Medicare, and sometimes for

Medicaid, of appropriate lengths of stay and the medical necessity for admission and for certain tests and procedures were the primary roles in the past of Professional Standards Review Organizations (PSROs). The Social Security Act Amendments re-created some of this process. Hospitals are required to contract with Peer Review Organizations (PROs) in order to retain eligibility for Medicare reimbursement. HCFA has drafted new scope of work requirements for PROs that have less of a focus on days of stay and will require that PROs have access to systems for medical technology assessment. Under the law, PROs must review the validity of diagnostic information provided by hospitals, because this is the basis on which proper patient assignment is made to a DRG.

PROs also are expected to watch over quality, for example, to develop methods to monitor unnecessary surgery and invasive procedures that may cause complications. All such questions of medical necessity and quality assurance call for methods of technology assessment, but because comprehensive discharge data are not required of providers PROs are left free to continue to use criteria based on typical patterns of practice in the geographic area. Norms of care vary greatly across the country. Often, these norms are averaged from reporting systems based on what doctors do, which may be based on good judgment and good physician education, but have not been assessed for efficacy, consistent patient benefit, or sometimes even for safety.

A serendipitous aspect of the Medicare prospective payment system may be the DRG data base itself. In New Jersey, the central agency has put into its computers a complete patient abstract based on Uniform Hospital Discharge Data Systems (UHDDS) and proposes to augment this with coded information needed to assess quality for every hospital discharge in the state since 1976. Linked with cost center data, this information has enabled a retrospective comparison of the outcomes and costs for patients in the same DRGs treated with different technologies.

Technology assessment does hold promise for containing costs while ensuring quality care for patients. Although the current federal reimbursement law potentially encourages the appropriate use of technology and could foster the accumulation of a useful data base, it can be improved further for technology assessment. For example, nothing in the law encourages technology assessment before wide diffusion of a technology. A technology factor has been added to the DRG price, but it has not been structured as a special opportunity for assessment. In addition, the incentives for technology assessment will have to be extended to cover other payment mechanisms.

PAYING FOR TECHNOLOGY ASSESSMENT

The growing portion of health care costs attributed to technologic interventions points to the need for assessment as a part of the national effort to contain these costs. Assessing technologies before and after introducing them into the health care system could result in better medical care and could decrease health care costs. It would provide physicians, third-party payers, and the public with an improved basis for decisions about the best uses of technologies and would facilitate appropriate utilization. Some interest in assessing technologies already in use also appears to have been revived in provisions of the amendments to the Social Security Act establishing the Medicare Prospective Payment System. A question remains as to who will pay for technology assessment.

Yarbro and Mortenson (1985) believe that under the DRG system institutions will be reluctant to carry out clinical trials because of cost considerations. They suggest a new DRG category to handle this. Davis (1985) believes this solution is unworkable and that the funding for trials must come from other sources.

As Appendix 5-A explains in detail and in more technical language, third-party payers would like to restrict their payments to claims for technologies that are clearly necessary and effective for the medical care of the patient. Therefore, they have a considerable stake in the availability of more research and research of high quality done by disinterested parties in technology assessment. This constraint is not merely self-serving; it makes the health care dollar more effective by applying resources where they are needed and where they work. Two main impediments to effective use of these ideas come from the courts. First, the third-party payers may find themselves accused of antitrust violations, for example, because similarity of exclusions by the several payers seems to be grounds for complaints of restraint of trade. Second, the insured may sue because of problems about the availability of coverage and disagreement about the provisions of the contract. Sometimes these claims about inappropriate lack of coverage can lead to large damages. Thus, it may turn out that the courts will not always accept good evidence about the ineffectiveness of certain technologies. And therefore third-party payers may not always be able to take proper advantage of improved knowledge about technologies. **The legal problems that pose such serious impediments to using information from technology assessment fall outside the committee's expertise and therefore are not fully addressed in this book. Nevertheless, it is believed that much more work needs to be done to resolve these issues.**

Many authors and conferees have addressed the question of reimbursement for technology assessment. Chalmers proposed that the federal government and the private sector "set up an evaluating body to organize and fund clinical trials." It is proposed they start with the most expensive procedures and decide which are worth paying for, traditional or not (Chalmers, 1982). Implicit in this recommendation is that all major public and private payers will reimburse for the costs of the trials and the care of the patients when the activities are part of a planned and approved clinical trial. However, conferees noted that there are antitrust impediments to such a recommendation.

A workshop on the role of third-party payers in clinical trials, sponsored by the Arthritis Foundation and the National Multiple Sclerosis Society (1983), recommended that HCFA undertake some funding of clinical trials of new and experimental procedures and that Congress make clear this authority and its underwriting by the Medicare trust funds. In addition, said the conferees, private insurers should reimburse the medical and treatment costs for patients participating in approved clinical trials in designated settings. This conference group also recommended a larger role in clinical trials for the National Institutes of Health (NIH) but only if additional funds for it were appropriated by Congress. NIH was also viewed as the entity into which private foundations, pharmaceutical firms, manufacturers, employers-payers, and third-party payers should channel funds.

Bunker et al. (1982a, b) analyzed the effects of coverage and reimbursement on biomedical innovation as well as the inadequacies and inconsistencies of funding new technologies and their evaluation. They recommend "a major shift in coverage policy" so that identified new therapies could be "selected for coverage contingent on the collection of appropriate evaluation data." The new money required for the process, they believed, should come from a joint fund established by all insurers. Furthermore, the establishment of an Institute of Health Care Evaluation (IHCE) is suggested. It would be supported by a voluntary per capita levy on all insurers plus HCFA grants and contracts for the research (Bunker et al., 1982a, b).

Relman (1980) once estimated that private and public third-party payers could contribute $100 million to $200 million to such a joint fund if each were assessed 0.2 percent of their total health care expenditures. There have been others who have suggested that even the life insurance industry should contribute to biomedical investigation, based on the speculation that the increased longevity that might result would be of direct benefit to these insurers. A 1 percent investment by the life insurance industry is estimated to provide $1 billion annually for medical research (Kahn, 1984).

An Institute of Medicine (IOM) committee issued a report, "Medical Technology Assessment: A Plan for a Public/Private Sector Consortium," in November 1983. It proposed that Congress appropriate start-up funds for such an entity, with an endowment to be raised thereafter by pooling the funds of interested parties—payers, professional associations, foundations, etc. Users' fees from those who would purchase the published results of assessments were hoped to bring in additional funds. Both Bunker and the IOM committee give examples of similar research consortia initiated with federal appropriations.

This chapter has emphasized the uses of technology assessment as a part of changing reimbursement policy. Reimbursement offered, or withheld, is a prime tool for the enforcement of socially necessary decisions. The consortia recommended by recent study groups and authors are advisory with no policymaking or regulating roles. Contracting fiscal intermediaries for Medicare recommend various coverage decisions, but HCFA may or may not follow them, nor are they codified into a uniform approach. The important Medicare Prospective Payment Assessment Commission is advisory to HCFA, but the law is not clear on any mandates to the Executive Branch for implementation of the findings of the commission, although the requirement that HCFA proposes amendments to the law by certain dates does appear as part of the intent of Congress. OTA does not make recommendations in its studies of various technologies, although its influence is obvious in the first decisions Medicare has ever made to restrict coverage for certain technologies to their use in a specific setting and by professionals with specific skills.

If the need for medical technology assessment couples so fully with the need for rational cost containment, a major policy issue is posed for lawmakers: Should reimbursement regulation be used to enforce scientific decisions about the safety, efficacy, and cost-effectiveness of technologies? The answer is not yet clear in law or in appropriation.

Chapter 2 discusses the scope of medical technology assessment in the United States and compares it with the cost of health care. There, it is estimated that in 1984 $384 billion was spent on health care while less than $1.3 billion was spent on medical technology assessment; a large portion of this was (roughly $800 million) spent by private industry.

It is strongly believed that additional support for medical technology assessment is needed and that it should come from the health care dollar. There are a number of ways this might be realized, whether by a per hospital bed assessment, provider contributions, third-party payer grants, or other mechanisms. Perhaps there is no single approach that will suffice; careful study will be needed by a specifically charged group to develop a specific plan. Technology assessment has the potential both to improve health care and to control costs. For this reason, a portion of the health care dollar should be allocated to its promulgation.

CONCLUSIONS AND RECOMMENDATIONS

Coverage and reimbursement policies can foster technology assessment. As seen in this chapter, technology assessment has limited use for containing costs in a system of making coverage decisions based on usual and accepted medical practice. If a technology could clearly be ruled obsolete, coverage could be denied. Similarly if a technology was experimental, coverage could be denied. Unfortunately while the FDA does have criteria for determining if a drug or device is experimental, there are no firm criteria for assigning a technology to the experimental or obsolete categories for Medicare. Market forces to sell insurance policies and provide the best coverage to clients make decisions about coverage of technologies on the basis of assessment difficult (even if information on which to base these decisions was available, which it often is not). The primary value of technology assessment in the reimbursement-based system is for determining safety and efficacy (Finkelstein et al., 1984).

Under a prospective payment system based on cost per case, such as DRGs, more powerful incentives appear to be present for technology assessment for cost-effectiveness, but much more can be achieved.

If physicians and hospitals can find more cost-effective ways for treating patients, larger profits can be gained from rendering health care, patients will get better care, and costs can be contained. Unfortunately, the information base for making such decisions does not exist nor is the system well structured to achieve more information.

In order to develop a coordinated system for technology assessment and to achieve cost savings through technology assessment, the assessment process and the reimbursement system must become more congruent. Some recommendations (in italics) affecting the reimbursement system follow.

- *Decisions about payment for medical care should be based on more than safety, efficacy, and research status of the care.* A beginning in expanding the criteria exists in the new prospective payment system, which encourages cost-effectiveness of care.
- *Data collected for claims purposes should be made more useful for technology assessment.* Again, the advent of prospective payment, which includes diagnosis and characteristics of care in the information needed for claims, seems likely to contribute to technology assessment.
- *Payment for medical technology assessment should be made through the system that pays for medical care.* The prospective payment system already includes a set-aside for technology, which could be earmarked for assessment. Another possibility is to pay for use of experimental technology if it collects data on safety, efficacy, and cost-effectiveness. Still another way is to set aside for assessment a percentage of the health care dollar, as handled by third-party payers or providers, both public and private.

APPENDIX 5-A: LEGAL CONSIDERATIONS IN PRIVATE HEALTH INSURER'S IDENTIFICATION AND EXCLUSION OF UNNECESSARY, INCOMPETENT, AND UNPROVED SERVICES

Proliferation of new medical and surgical procedures, devices, drugs, health care personnel, and facilities, and the related escalation in costs of care, have prompted public and private benefit programs to examine and reform their roles in the allocation of resources to health care. Long-standing public policy concern for protecting the ill from exploitation militates against providing health benefits for—and thus promoting—worthless treatments. This concern is increasingly joined by an economic imperative to spend limited health benefit funds only for care that discernibly benefits health.

In consequence, it is becoming commonplace for coverage to expressly exclude services that are medically unnecessary or inappropriate to diagnose or treat the patient's condition. Meaningful implementation of such an underwriting decision obviously depends heavily on the insurer's ability to identify and apply reasonable standards to distinguish effective care from that which is of uncertain or no value.

Given the very high cost of much care and the prevalence of health benefits in one or another form, these insurer efforts toward more-efficient application of benefit funds can significantly affect both their beneficiaries' access to desired care and the marketplace success of various providers and producers of health technologies. It is thus not surprising that such efforts by public and private benefit plans frequently result in legal challenges by affected beneficiaries, providers, or both. These challenges to private insurers have been of two principal types: (1) provider antitrust claims that insurer actions related to judgments about necessary and appropriate care unlawfully restrain trade in a product market in which they compete, and (2) program beneficiary contract and tort claims contesting both the threshold enforceability of benefit exclusions pertaining to unnecessary or unproved services and the reasonableness of the specific insurer determinations made in applying such exclusions to them.

Antitrust and insurance case law development during the past decade has significantly increased the private insurer's risk of both types of litigation and liability. During that period, a succession of court decisions has radically narrowed the exemptions that once shielded health care and insurance activities from antitrust law application. As a result, both the incidence and cost of health benefit antitrust litigation have multiplied. At the same time, insurers increasingly are exposed to beneficiary claims for compensatory and punitive damages for alleged misrepresentation of benefits, breach of contracts, bad faith, and similar evils. The plaintiff's health and financial circumstances often are dire and damage awards may be extremely large.

These contemporaneous developments in antitrust and insurance laws are relevant to private insurers' attempts to identify and avoid paying for unnecessary, incompetent, or unproved uses of health care "technology" because they tend to produce conflicting incentives for the insurer. On the one hand, recent insurance benefits litigation underscores the need for benefit contracts to provide clear and complete notice of all coverage limitations and exclusions as a condition of their enforceability. Similarly, the standards and procedures followed by the insurer in adjudicating individual claims for benefits must be reasonable and fairly accord the insured's interest at least as much consideration as the insurer gives to its own.

The insurer is thus propelled to search for increasingly precise and understandable descriptors for contract exclusions pertaining to unnecessary and unproved care and for defensible criteria for their application to specific cases. The search necessarily leads to the research findings and expert opinions of the scientific and medical communities and to the new drug and device evaluations of the FDA.

A countervailing pressure arises from the new phenomenon of provider antitrust suits against insurers and other providers in which it is alleged that insurance contract exclusions and denials of benefits for unnecessary or unproved services are the result of and means of effectuating agreements among competing providers to unreasonably restrain trade in a particular health service. Such cases are currently pending with regard to psychiatric care, chiropractic, treatment for arthritis with dimethyl sulfoxide (DMSO), bilateral carotid body resection for asthma and other respiratory disorders, radial keratotomy, Burton's immune augmentation therapy, and allergy treatment, among others. In addition, 2 years ago the U.S. Supreme Court held that an insured had antitrust standing to sue her insurer for treble damages that resulted from contract limitations on coverage of psychologists' services. Thus the contract beneficiary is now also a potential antitrust plaintiff.

In seeking reasonable standards of safe and effective use of the mushrooming array of health technology, the insurer (and medical consultants) must also be wary that their actions may later be construed as elements of a concerted refusal to deal by an aggrieved provider or patient. The insurer's development of reasonable benefit standards that courts will honor, and its avoidance of antitrust risk in the process, could be greatly enhanced by access to more and better-quality health technology assessment. Increased information from reliable evaluations performed by disinterested parties is needed to support benefit plan efforts toward more-efficient resource use.

REFERENCES

Altman, S. H., and R. Blendon (eds.). 1979. Medical Technologies: The Culprit Behind Health Care Costs? Proceedings of the 1977 Sun Valley Forum on National Health. Washington, D.C.: U.S. Government Printing Office.

Banta, H. D., G. Ruby, and A. K. Burns. 1984. Using Coverage to Contain Medical Costs. Proceedings of the Conference on the Future of Medicare. U.S. House of Representatives, February 1, 1984. Washington, D.C.: U.S. Government Printing Office.

Biles, B., C. J. Schramm, and J. G. Atkinson. 1980. Hospital cost inflation under state rate-setting programs. N. Engl. J. Med. 303:664–668.

Boerma, H. 1982. Organization Impact of Diagnostic Related Group Reimbursement in New Jersey. Trenton: Hospital Research and Educational Trust of New Jersey.

Bunker, J. P., J. Fowles, and J. Schaffarzick. 1982a. Evaluation of medical-technology strategies: effects of coverage and reimbursement (first of two parts). N. Engl. J. Med. 306:620–624.

Bunker, J. P., J. Fowles, and R. Schaffarzick. 1982b. Evaluation of medical-technology strategies: proposal for an institute for health care evaluation (second of two parts). N. Engl. J. Med. 306:687–692.

Chalmers, T. C. 1982. A potpourri of RCT topics. Controlled Clinical Trials 3:285–298.

Davis, C. K. 1985. The impact of prospective payment on clinical research. J. Am. Med. Assoc. 253:686–687.

Dickson, P. S. 1982. The DRG Appeals Process. New Jersey Hospital Rate Setting Commission. May. Memorandum.

Finkelstein, S. N., K. A. Issacson, and A. Frishkopf. 1984. The process of evaluating medical technologies for third-party coverage. J. Health Care Technol. 1:89–102.

Finley, J. E. 1983. Diagnosis Related Groups (DRGs) in Hospital Payment: The New Jersey Experience. U.S. Congress, Office of Technology Assessment. Washington, D.C.: U.S. Government Printing Office.

Gibson, R. M., K. R. Levit, H. Lanzenby, and D. R. Waldo. 1984. National health care expenditures 1983. Health Care Financing Review 6:1–29.

Harvard Center for the Analysis of Health Practice. 1981. Impact on Health Costs of NCHCT Recommendations for Nonreimbursement for Medical Procedures. Report produced under grant number HS 03314. Cambridge, Mass.

Institute of Medicine. 1977. Computed Tomographic Scanning. Washington, D.C.: National Academy of Sciences.

Institute of Medicine. 1983. Medical Technology Assessment: A Plan for a Public/Private Sector Consortium. Washington, D.C.: National Academy Press.

Joskow, P. L. 1981. Controlling Hospital Costs: The Role of Government Regulation. Cambridge, Mass.: MIT Press.

Kahn, C. R. 1984. A proposed new role for the insurance industry in biomedical research funding. Sounding Board. N. Engl. J. Med. January 26, 1984.

Maryland Health Services Cost Review Commission, Interview, 1983.

Office of Technology Assessment. 1983. Diagnosis Related Groups (DRGs) and the Medicare Program: Implications for Medical Technology. Superintendent of Documents. Washington, D.C.: U.S. Government Printing Office.

Reinhardt, U. E. 1985. Health care for America's poor. Princeton Alumni Weekly 27(February):23–29.

Relman, A. S. 1980. Assessment of Medical Practices: A Simple Proposal. N. Engl. J. Med. 303:153–154.

Rochester Area Hospitals' Corporation. 1980. RX for Hospitals. Annual Report of the Rochester Area Hospitals' Corporation, Rochester, N.Y.

Rochester Area Hospitals' Corporation. 1982. Midstream Assessment of HEP. Rochester, N.Y.

Smits, H. L., and R. E. Watson. 1985. DRGs and the future of surgical practice. N. Engl. J. Med. 311:1612–1615.

Yarbro, J. W., and L. E. Mortenson. 1985. The need for diagnosis-related group 471. J. Am. Med. Assoc. 253:684–685.

6 Medical Technology Assessment in Developed Countries: Trends and Opportunities for Collaboration

Health technology increasingly is the object of public concern not only in the United States but also in other industrialized countries. For years these governments have directed their health care expenditures toward safety, efficacy, and equitable access to care. But in the early 1970s health care costs increased steadily, approaching 7–10 percent of the gross national product (GNP) in many countries (Table 6-1) (Department of Health and Human Services [DHHS], 1982; Groot, 1982). For example, in 1970 West Germany spent 3.7* percent of its GNP on sickness funds (the insurance that covers 99 percent of the population with virtually full benefits) and 8.0 percent in 1980; costs in the Netherlands increased from 7.2 percent of GNP in 1971 to 8.6 percent in 1980 (Office of Technology Assessment [OTA], 1980; Shepard and Durch, 1984). As a result, a number of countries have begun cost-containment efforts that relate costs to effectiveness. These efforts have rekindled interest in international collaboration on technology assessment for new purposes.

The needs of industrialized and developing countries for medical technology assessment differ. Developing countries try to emphasize simple and effective technologies that the countries can afford, but industrialized countries ask whether the rapid development of highly sophisticated technology overshoots the target, serves the medical professions more than the patients, and drives health care costs too high. This latter concern, the interest of industrialized countries in technology assessment and how better to foster international collaboration, is the subject of this chapter.

This chapter begins by reviewing the approaches and policies of various developed countries for medical technology assessment. The trend is toward more efforts in medical technology assessment, and a few countries are trying to develop a coherent

---

This chapter was prepared by Enriqueta Bond, in part based on materials contributed by David Banta, Seymour Perry, and Duncan Neuhauser.

* There are other sources of data that estimate that Germany spends a far higher proportion of its GNP on health care than these data from sickness funds indicate. The important point is the percent difference in expenditures over the years.

TABLE 6-1 Health Care Costs in Selected Countries as Percentage of GNP, 1980

Countries	Health Care Costs as Percentage of GNP, 1980 (unless otherwise noted)
Belgium	7.5
Denmark	6.7 (1978)
Greece	3.7
West Germany	8.0
France	7.8
Ireland	8.4 (1978)
Italy	6.4
Luxembourg	10.4 (1977)
The Netherlands	8.6
United Kingdom	5.6
United States[a]	9.5[b]
Sweden	10.0 (1982–1983)

[a] U.S. data from U.S. DHHS (1982).
[b] United States in 1982: 10.5 percent GNP, according to Fall 1983 Health Care Financing Review.
SOURCE: Groot (1982).

system for such assessment. Next the chapter describes case studies of medical technology assessment for specific technologies in different countries. The case studies illustrate the differences in approaches to medical technology assessment and the needs of different countries. Finally, the efforts of international organizations to establish collaboration in technology assessment are examined for their applicability as models for an international system of technology assessment.

TRENDS IN ASSESSMENT AND REGULATION

A review of the current approaches and policies of different countries for assessing drugs and devices and controlling equipment purchases finds that there is increasing concern for safety, efficacy, costs, and social and ethical issues. This has catalyzed new institutional mechanisms for technology assessment. However, the institutional arrangements that exist to regulate medical technology and to carry out assessments vary substantially from country to country.

Most industrialized countries have consistent national policies and institutional arrangements for evaluating the safety and efficacy of drugs. These appear to have been strengthened in recent years, influenced to some extent by the United States Food and Drug Administration's example and assistance to other countries. The current World Health Organization program on effective drugs to assist countries that want to improve their drug regulatory systems reinforces this trend.

However, systematic regulation of devices has been established only in the United States, Sweden, Japan, and Canada; most assessment of devices elsewhere proceeds on an ad hoc basis. Even in countries with policies for assessment of devices, these mechanisms are of more recent origin and less systematic than for drugs.

Sweden is one of the few countries to develop a national policy or institutional arrangement for the assessment of devices, equipment, and procedures used in medical care. The Swedish Planning and Rationalization Institute of Health Services (SPRI) was established in 1968 by the Swedish government and the Federation of County Councils (the health care authorities), and has been involved in the conduct of technology assessment since 1980 (SPRI, 1981). The organization has a mandate to solve problems confronting those who work in the health care sectors and to promote better use of existing health services resources. Additional tasks include information dissemination, establishment of standard specifications for hospital equipment, and planning. In 1981 the SPRI budget was $8 million (total health service expenditures that year were $11 billion). A 15-member board oversees the work of the organization, whose central task is to provide advice that promotes a cost-effective health service. An example of one of their activities was the consensus conference on hip joint replacement discussed later in this report. In contrast to Sweden, professional organizations in other countries, i.e., private groups, have shouldered what assessment exists of medical practice.

RESEARCH AND DEVELOPMENT

All developed countries have policies toward scientific research and technologic development (R&D). Since World War II, governments of the industrialized world have become deeply involved in supporting R&D in many different fields. Increasingly, R&D for health has been seen as an appropriate investment. Across all industrialized countries, health R&D probably accounts for about 10 percent of all R&D expenditures by government (OTA, 1980). Nevertheless, different countries take very different approaches to planning and supporting biomedical research. They vary greatly in the total amount of support the government provides, in the proportions of that support given to different fields and kinds of research, in the role of the private sector in research support, in the mechanisms used to set priorities and choose research projects, and in the institutions and individuals that carry out the work (Shepard and Durch, 1984).

Table 6-2 shows the estimated spending of both public and private dollars in 1980 on biomedical research and development in 19 countries that are members of the Organization for Economic Cooperation and Development (OECD). Support for R&D is highly concentrated in only a few countries, with the United States accounting for nearly half of the total support for research among them. Japan, West Germany, France, and the United Kingdom, together with the United States, make up almost 85 percent (Shepard and Durch, 1984). Therefore, it is likely these countries will provide the bulk of the primary data information available for technology assessment or at least are potentially the major supporters of technology assessment. Establishment of technology assessment efforts are not necessarily dependent upon the generation of biomedical data by the country involved. Sweden and Canada, two of the leading countries engaged in technology assessment, are not among the highest supporters of biomedical research and development.

Other countries may provide special opportunities for technology assessment because of unique data collection systems or populations at high risk for the condition of study. For example, Sweden has a National Bureau of Statistics that assembles data concerning all Swedish patients, identified by their social security numbers. Because social security numbers are used for medical record identification, all medical services rendered to a given individual can

TABLE 6-2 Amount and Distribution of Total Biomedical Research and Development (BMRD) Funding, 1980 (in millions of 1975 U.S. dollars)[a]

Country	BMRD Funding	Percentage of Total BMRD in all Countries
United States	5,256	48.18
Japan	1,523	13.96
West Germany	1,271	11.65
France	712	6.53
United Kingdom	495	4.54
Italy	299	2.74
The Netherlands	257	2.37
Sweden	251	2.30
Switzerland	229	2.10
Canada	176	1.62
Belgium	122	1.13
Denmark	94	0.86
Australia	69	0.63
Spain	52	0.48
Norway	41	0.37
Finland	32	0.29
New Zealand	14	0.13
Portugal	10	0.09
Ireland	6	0.05

[a] Includes public and private funds.

SOURCE: Shepard and Durch (1984).

be accounted for and used in tabulating national health statistics. A country with a high prevalence of a particular disease, for example pertussis in England, may offer an opportunity for testing a new vaccine from somewhere else.

How much of the total amount of support for R&D is devoted to technology assessment in different countries is difficult to determine. The R&D system in most countries is largely decentralized, has a large private involvement, and often takes place in academic settings or in research centers. Academics in some countries, such as England and the United States, play a large role in shaping biomedical research priorities. However, since the 1960s more governmental efforts have gone into influencing research priorities in order to further social goals. The United States' "war on cancer" is one example.

Many countries now evaluate the benefits, risks, and costs of medical technology (Council of Science and Society, 1983; Groot, 1982; OTA, 1980; SPRI, 1979; U.S. DHHS, 1981). The Swedish program has been described. Canada has established a special activity in the federal government to develop guidelines for use of technology based on the best available scientific data. Australia has funded a special program to evaluate medical technology. Such programs are being discussed in France, West Germany, and the Netherlands, among others. These programs develop information as an aid to making decisions.

Governments increasingly want answers to such questions as which technologies should be covered by national health insurance. Although rising health care costs have fueled much of this increased interest, the improvement of medical practice still is an underlying rationale for technology assessment (U.S. DHHS, 1981). The international exchange of data would facilitate the assessment of programs of many countries, but only if some agreement on common methodology is reached.

Assessment of technologies can be divided into two broad categories:

1. assessment of safety, quality, efficacy, and effectiveness; and
2. assessment of the effects of technology on the organization, law, economics, and ethics of health care and on society.

Because most countries define safety similarly, the greatest benefits of sharing data probably would be gained in assessment of safety and efficacy of drugs, devices, or techniques. Cultural differences and differences among health care systems could make economic, ethical, and social considerations less comparable. Nevertheless, exchange of information on these matters of less commonality could provide new insights or approaches to problems and aid establishment of compatible policies for assessment.

Clinical Trials

Clinical trials often are the preferred method for assessment of safety and efficacy. Because their results are often used in countries other than the country of origin, controlled clinical trials have international implications. Britain invests more per capita than any other country in clinical trials because the total costs of patient care already are borne by the National Health Service (OTA, 1980). The apparent costs are low in comparison with the cost of trials in the United States, where some patient care costs must come from research funding. Smaller countries might have problems in carrying out clinical trials, particularly if they lacked an adequate research establishment or imported most of the technology to be assessed. They might make financial contributions to help ensure that technologies of interest to them are studied. However, mechanisms for such collaboration would have to be established before this could occur in a systematic manner. First, for example, the country would need to develop ways of identifying those technologies it wishes to have assessed and then find a way of supporting the appropriate studies. Alternatively, a group of countries could get together on a clinical trial and divide up the work.

Consensus Activities

In 1982 two consensus conferences on safety and efficacy issues related to hip joint replacement were held, one in the United States by the National Institutes of Health (NIH) Office for Medical Applications of Research (OMAR), the second by the Swedish Medical Research Council and SPRI (NIH, 1982; Rogers, 1982; SPRI, 1982). The two conferences were intended to be as similar as possible, employing the same formats and questions, but the Swedish conference went beyond the considerations of safety and efficacy by also considering the need for and the costs of hip joint replacement. While similar in their conclusions, the evaluation of safety and efficacy data in the NIH conference was more extensive in that more data were provided on indications, complications, etc. Furthermore, it is unlikely that results of economic and social considerations of the consensus conference in Sweden would be easily transferable for use by the United States because of the large differences in the financing and organization of health care. Despite these disparities, the similarities in the exercise open the way for further collaboration and indicate that information from such consensus conferences may be useful across countries. Perhaps more useful for exchange among countries would be the primary data used for such evaluations. The addition of economic and social considerations on the Swedish consensus exercise provides an interesting model for other countries.

More recently, Britain sponsored a consensus development conference on its coronary artery bypass surgery (Coronary Artery Bypass Surgery: A Consensus, 1984; Stocking and Jennett, 1984). Coronary artery bypass surgery is of great interest because of the wide difference in its frequency in different countries. If regular consensus programs develop in a number of different countries, a system for cross-national comparisons and data analysis may enhance their value in other countries. Since several countries in Europe are considering establishing consensus conferences, this option may be realizable.

Technology transfer often is aided by marketing efforts of the multinational companies or by organizations such as the U.S. Alliance for Engineering in Medicine and Biology. In 1973, a series of international workshops was held by the alliance, to aid governments, administrators, and executives in (1) formulating policies for planning, manufacturing, and medical and technical education and training; (2) coordinating the professional activities of physicians, life scientists, and biomedical engineers; and (3) developing facilities and personnel policies to open channels of communications among biomedical engineers and between biomedical engineers and health care professionals. Forums such as these provide opportunities for collaboration in the development of methodologies for appropriate assessment of technologies at the same time as assisting in technology transfer (American Institute of Biological Sciences, 1973). Since technology transfer and assessment is fostered by programs of this sort, consideration should be given to enlarging such assessment efforts, especially as related to technology transfer to developing countries.

USE OF TECHNOLOGY IN DIFFERENT COUNTRIES

Comparison of information on the use of medical technologies in different countries may indicate where costs may be saved by changing patterns of use. Rasmussen (1981) has collected information on pacemakers in 13 different countries. A closer look at pacemaker utilization in four English-speaking countries by Selzer (1983) reveals striking differences, with the United States leading by a substantial margin (Table 6-3). Such data suggest overuse of this technology in the United States or underutilization elsewhere.

Similarly, a survey carried out by Groot (1982) in countries of the European Common Market showed differences in numbers of coronary bypass operations, computed tomography (CT) scanners, kidney transplants, and radiation units (Table 6-4).

There appear to be substantial differences from country to country in both the numbers of operations and the numbers of diagnostic equipment. Explanations for the striking national differences in use of different technologies may lie in differences in economic capacities, differences in practice patterns, differences in health care delivery systems, and differences of need in the respective populations. Figure

TABLE 6-3 Use of Pacemakers in Selected Countries in 1978

	Number of Pacemakers per Million Population	
Country	All Uses	Use in Sinus-Node Disease
United States	309	125
Canada	145	42
Australia	82	20
United Kingdom	75	15

SOURCE: Selzer (1983).

TABLE 6-4 Use of Technologies in Selected Countries per Million Population in 1981[a]

	Heart Operations				Kidney	CT		Radiation	
Country	All		Coronary Bypass		Transplants	Scanners		Units	
Belgium	202	[355]	29		12.60	3.7	[3–4]	4.55	[6]
Denmark	160			[120]	27	2.4	[3.4]	5.50	
Germany									
Federal Republic					7.8				
North-Rhine Westphalia	190	[259]	106	[176]		3.4	[4]	1.76	[3.62]
Bremen						6.7	[5.7]		
Greece	72		18	[103]	4.2	1.23		3.08	[6.15]
France					8.19	0.98	[1.1–1.7]	7.37	[6.45]
Ireland	131	[348]	66	[174][b]	22.1	1.45		1.45	[2.91]
Italy	154	[210]			5.7	2.05			
Luxembourg					0	8.45	[2.97]	2.97	[8.91]
The Netherlands	397	[460]			15.3	2.8	[1.1–2.35]	3.47	[5.66]
United Kingdom	89		72	[90–100]	16.6	0.71		3.66	
United States	7,608		740		22.7	9.1[c]			

[a] Numbers in brackets indicate national planning/desirable guidelines. Data were not available for the spaces left blank.

[b] Taken as half the total number of heart operations.

[c] This value is for 1983.

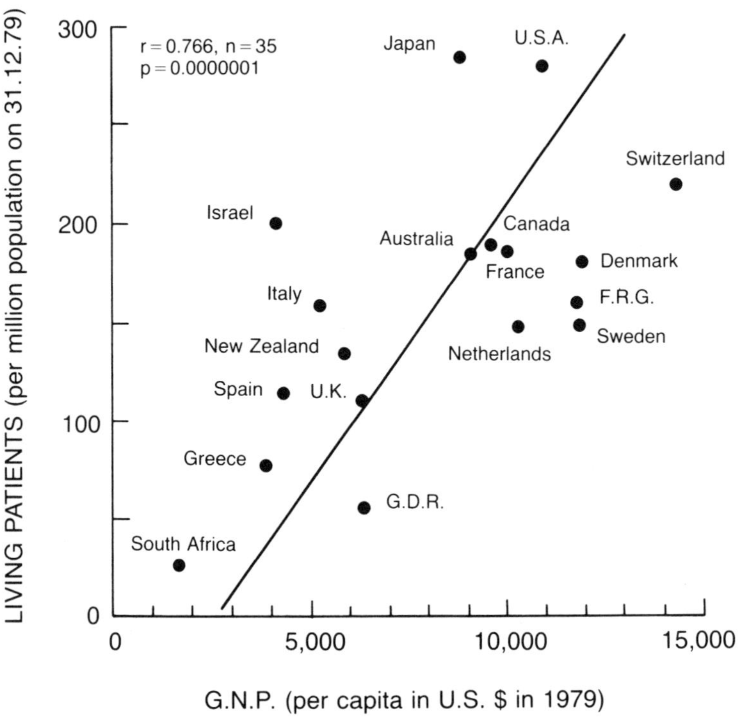

FIGURE 6-1 Correlation between number of patients treated for ESRD and GNP in 1979. SOURCE: Groot (1982).

6-1, from the report issued for the 11th Congress of the European Dialysis and Transplant Association, supports a hypothesis of economic capacity influencing use of technology by indicating that countries with larger GNPs treat a greater percentage of patients diagnosed as having end-stage renal disease (ESRD). Recent analysis of the treatment of ESRD in Britain shows that despite the fact that there are no special rules about which patients may or may not be treated, access to renal dialysis is limited (Aaron and Schwartz, 1984; Wing, 1983). Physicians functioning with a recognition of limited resources act as gatekeepers to limit dialysis.

ASSESSMENT OF DRUGS IN DIFFERENT COUNTRIES

Most European countries have regulations governing the safety and efficacy of drugs modeled on the Food, Drug, and Cosmetic Act of the United States, but the state of harmonization necessary for the acceptance by one country of a drug evaluated by another has not nearly been reached either among European countries or between the United States and any other developed country. For example, despite the desire in the United States for an improved pertussis vaccine such as the one made and accepted for use in Japan, the vaccine must undergo clinical trials with a possible delay of 4 years before licensure in the United States. Nevertheless, efforts are under way by the European Free Trade Association, the European Economic Community, and the World Health Organization (WHO) to establish uniform standards for drugs and biologicals, and it might be supported by governments to promote more international collaboration in the assessment of pharmaceuticals. As data developed in one country already are used for assessment of drugs by the relevant institution in another country, harmonization of requirements for regulatory purposes has the potential of saving costs and accelerating the marketing of useful drugs.

Barriers to collaboration are raised by factors such as differences in the drug regulatory agencies' organization and staff and differences in requirements for demonstrating safety and efficacy. Not only are the regulatory agencies different but also the industry differs from country to country. The German pharmaceutical industry was developed primarily from chemical companies, the British pharmaceutical industry has strong university roots, and the French pharmaceutical industry arose primarily from independent pharmacists working in the community compounding prescriptions. Furthermore, cultural differences in attitudes toward ill health, toward dying, and toward use of medication and differences in disease risks may affect the definition of safety and efficacy in different countries. Political differences in the developed countries are reflected in the regulation of drugs, the activities of national drug agencies, their communications with each other, and the consequences that decisions made in one country have for another. So far, there are few official contacts among the drug regulatory agencies of the member states of the European Economic Community, much less with the United States, nor is there mutual acceptance of drug applications, licensure, or a uniform policy on withdrawing drugs (Gross, 1980).

There are, however, many informal contacts and a few bilateral agreements between countries; for example, the United States has a memorandum of understanding with Sweden and Canada concerning inspection of foreign manufacturers. Bilateral agreement may offer special opportunities for collaboration between two similar countries, for example, the United States and Canada. Furthermore, there are informal contacts fostered largely by WHO and by the desire of countries to improve their regulatory processes. A closer look at some aspects of drug approval in France and in West Germany reveals some problems faced in information exchange. However, it also is apparent that similar information is required in both countries for determining safety and efficacy and that great benefits would occur from efforts to systematize collection and exchange of such data. Although decisions in one country may not be easily transferable, the information base for the decisions is transferable.

France

In 1978 the French Ministry of Health created the Commission d'Autorisation de Mise sur le Marché (CAMM) to advise it on drug marketing and authorization of new and old drugs (Weintraub, 1982). The commission considers safety and efficacy, therapeutic indications, and information about medications to be provided to physicians and patients. CAMM is staffed by the Office of Pharmacy and Medications in the Ministry of Health. Members of CAMM are of two types. The first group is composed of physicians and pharmacists; the second group includes academicians, medical practitioners, and a hospital pharmacist. Liaison members come from the National Institute of Health and Medical Research, the National Laboratory for Health, and the Office of Pharmacy and Medications. Observers from industry attend meetings and provide information.

In 1980 CAMM reviewed 400 applications of which 40 were for new drugs and 10 for new chemical entities (the rest were for combinations of already approved drugs). Decisions are based on reports provided to CAMM on biopharmaceutical, pharmacologic, toxicologic, and clinical data. Some U.S. companies submit their data for these reports with an addendum specifically prepared by a French expert.

In addition to considerations of safety and efficacy, the economic impact of drug approvals on the government, the pharmaceutical industry, and society comes into every debate, even though CAMM neither approves reimbursement through social security nor advises the government on setting prices.

Once a drug has been approved for sale in France, there are no restrictions on advertising or price. However, unless the drug is included on the reimbursable list of the social security system (which pays for medical care) there will not be a large market for it. In order to be placed on this list, the new drug must be shown to be more efficacious, have fewer side effects, or cost less than a similar drug already on the list. Once placed on the list, the drug's price is set by the ministry and advertising is restricted.

West Germany

Drug regulation in West Germany was strengthened with the implementation in 1978 of a law (enacted in 1976) requiring approval of drugs for marketing (Gross, 1980). The law gives more power to the Federal Health Office (Bundesgesundheitsamt) regarding acceptance, surveillance, quality control, distribution, and promotion of drugs. The new law also forces the agency to process drug applications within 4 months. From January 1978 to June 1980, about 850 applications for new drugs were submitted; 26 were rejected, 75 were withdrawn by manufacturers, and more data were requested for most of the rest.

Pharmacologic, toxicologic, and clinical data, and expert assessment of these, must be submitted to a special committee before the agency accepts a drug. This committee consists of representatives from the medical profession, dentistry, veterinary medicine, pharmacy, nonorthodox medicine, and the pharmaceutical industry. One major objection to the current law is its inadequate guarantee of efficacy. Comparative trials are not required. The agency may not refuse acceptance of a new drug if therapeutic results have been obtained in even a limited number of cases.

It is easy to see from these two descriptions that both France and West Germany require similar information when assessing the safety and efficacy of a drug. However, the regulations for licensing drugs in the two countries are not identical. For example, in West Germany a drug must be licensed if therapeutic results have been obtained in even a few cases. Therefore, the French authorities would not automatically accept a drug for marketing in France on the basis of its approval in West Germany. Efforts to collaborate on technology assessment then may need to be focused on the information-gathering level rather than on the policies for licensure resulting from the use of the information.

Because West Germany does not require permission from the drug regulatory agency before clinical trials can begin, manufacturers from other countries submit new drugs to first clinical studies in West Germany. However, language differences and differences in attitudes about aspects of the methodology or ethics of clinical trials may raise barriers to the conduct of trials in West Germany under protocols acceptable to France or other countries.

Despite efforts for harmonization, drug regulation in Europe is still far from being coordinated, and the auspices for mutual agreement regarding the acceptance of new drugs or the acknowledgment of data are still rather poor (Gross, 1980). Coordinative assessment and regulatory efforts could be enhanced if the national institutions for drug assessment worked toward mutually acceptable standards. WHO has organized yearly workshops in Europe on clinical pharmacologic evaluation in drug control. From 1972 to 1978, seven of these workshops have taken place with participation of agency representatives from 25

European countries. In the United States, recent revision of FDA regulations permits approval of drugs for domestic marketing solely on the basis of foreign data if certain criteria are met. However, acceptance of data from a country is not the same as accepting licensure by one country as licensure to market in a second. Gross (1980) suggests that supranational regulations will be composed of the strictest national regulations, and that these guidelines will not facilitate either preclinical or clinical studies.

HEALTH CARE SYSTEMS IN DIFFERENT COUNTRIES

Technology assessment needs vary among nations according to differences in organization and resources of the various health care systems. Some may see a larger role for technology assessment to control cost of care, while others use budget allocations as the main device for cost control. These variations do not alter the need for technology assessment but they will affect the nature of assessments, the responsible institutions, and the user of the assessment information. These variations have to be accommodated in international collaboration. Countries can nevertheless learn from one another and apply selected approaches and findings of others. The following examples illustrate how differing approaches to cost-containment affect the nature of technology assessment in different countries.

Britain

In Britain the National Health Service (NHS) operates on a budget set by Parliament (OTA, 1980). Health care is provided to patients without charge at the point of service delivery. The district management is responsible for all hospital and community services. In turn, the district is part of a larger area, overseen by regional authorities responsible to the Department of Health and Social Security (DHSS). While NHS funds are distributed to regions according to a complex formula based on population and modified by factors that indicate the need for health care, the regions and areas have the authority to allocate resources as they see fit.

Regional and area health authorities decide how money is to be spent, what equipment is needed, and which should be purchased. Therefore, funds for equipment are in direct competition with other health capital needs. There are no formal procedures for the evaluation of medical devices; assessments proceed on an ad hoc basis. Request for the evaluation of a particular procedure or piece of equipment may originate in a committee, unit, or council of the Medical Research Council, may be suggested independently by a researcher in a grant application, or may be requested by DHSS. Existing assessments are based almost entirely on clinical performance (safety and efficacy considerations) with little or no attention to general, social, or economic impacts of innovations. A recent report by the Council of Science and Society (1983) pointed out the haphazard manner in which expensive techniques are introduced into routine service. Criteria used for evaluation were deemed too narrow and too inattentive to patient reactions or to the social and psychological consequences of innovation. The report favored establishment of a national institute of health services research to coordinate and commission research on important technologies including clinical trials; the analysis of costs; and epidemiological, psychosocial, and policy studies. Another of the institute's functions would be to disseminate information.

The report urged the Secretary of State for Social Services to begin development of the institute by appointing an advisory group on expensive medical technologies responsible for ensuring that such technologies are properly evaluated clinically.

Because capital needs in Britain must compete with operating expenses for a total annual allocation of funds that is severely limited in virtually every region, costly technologies tend to spread there much more slowly than in the United States. For example, there was one computed tomographic scanner per 1,400,000 population in the United Kingdom in 1981 (Groot, 1982), in contrast to one per 110,000 population in the United States in 1980 (ECRI, 1983).

Japan

Medical care in Japan is delivered largely by solo general practitioners in clinic settings (OTA, 1980). The clinics generally possess 20 or fewer short-term (72 hours or less) beds. Hospitals are owned and managed by private physicians, unions, insurance plans, churches, and various levels of government. Traditional public health and environmental health programs—screening, immunization, physical exams for infants and school age children, etc.—are administered in local health centers.

Nearly all of the population is covered by health insurance that has evolved over 40 years from a broad law covering the working population. Patients in Japan have the right to seek care from any provider, and the provider in turn is able to bill any of the patient's appropriate health insurance plans for the services rendered. Fees for each service are negotiated on an annual basis within the Central Social Insurance Medical Council, an advisory body to the Ministry of Health and Welfare made up of representatives from medicine, dentistry, insurance plans, and other relevant groups.

Because of the rapid development and dissemination of new medical technology in Japan, evaluation has been ignored in many instances or set aside for future action. Drugs and medical devices are currently regulated in Japan under the Pharmaceutical Affairs Law passed in 1960. Whenever a new drug is proposed for marketing, data concerning its safety and efficacy must be submitted to the Bureau of Pharmaceutical Affairs. The Bureau of Pharmaceutical Affairs is assisted in implementing the Pharmaceutical Affairs Law by the Pharmaceutical Affairs Council, an advisory group with a number of committees. These committees deal with such matters as the approval of manufacture and import of new drugs, the establishment of quality standards for medical devices, measures to ensure the safety of drugs, and review of drugs already on the market for safety and effectiveness. The Pharmaceutical Affairs Council makes recommendations based on safety and efficacy, but final market approval is granted by the bureau. Evaluation of medical devices is based on an industrial standard law, largely focused on safety. However, escalating medical costs have led to greater interest in technology assessment for cost containment and cost-effectiveness.

Controls on investment in health care and use of technologies appear to be much greater in a country such as Britain with a national health care system and strict budgetary control than in countries such as Japan or the United States with a system of fee for service. Setting of fees and conditions of reimbursement would provide leverage for influencing technology diffusion in a country such as Japan, but not in the United Kingdom where few physicians or hospitals are paid fees. Technology assessment in Britain can be most useful in aiding the regions or areas to make good resource allocations, and in Japan assessments may be most useful for setting reimbursement schedules.

Differences among health care systems, perspectives, etc., would make it unlikely that decisions about or assessments for specific allocation purposes would be easily transferable; nevertheless, safety and efficacy assessments used by national bodies for marketing approval of drugs and devices would be transferable.

INTERNATIONAL ORGANIZATIONS

What roles can international organizations play in medical technology assessment? The following few categories give some indications of functions.

International Pharmaceutical Firms

Many companies have developed markets and production facilities for drugs and devices that are worldwide.

According to Fudenberg (1983) the major pharmaceutical firms in the United States spend about 5 to 10 percent of their total dollars on research. However current estimates range up to 12 percent (see Chapter 2). More than 15 percent of U.S. drug industry R&D expenditures are made abroad. The amount of R&D money that U.S. firms are spending abroad is increasing at 20 percent a year and will exceed $500 million in 1983 (Standard & Poor's Corporation, 1983).

SmithKline Beckman markets about 15 prescription pharmaceutical products, accounting in 1982 for $1.34 billion in sales. Its cimetidine was the world's largest-selling drug in 1983. Worldwide sales of cimetidine amounted to $857 million in 1982, when U.S. sales were about $450 million. SmithKline Beckman had to develop the information needed to get cimetidine licensed in the various countries. Such multinational pharmaceutical companies can become well positioned to foster international collaboration in assessing the safety and efficacy of drugs.

International Health Information

One of the largest repositories of biomedical information useful for technology assessment is the National Library of Medicine (NLM) of the U.S. National Institutes of Health. Since its inception in 1956, NLM activities have included acquiring and preserving information from around the world. Fully two-thirds of the journals cited in *Index Medicus* are published abroad. NLM currently has quid pro quo agreements with 13 countries and the Pan American Health Organization (Table 6-5) (OTA, 1982a). In exchange for indexing and other services, the foreign centers are allowed access to the MEDLARS (Medical Literature Analysis and Retrieval System, the NLM's computerized index of biomedical publications) data base.

Although MEDLARS provides a core of information useful for collaborative technology assessment efforts among countries, it is not sufficient. MEDLARS is primarily oriented toward the information needs of U.S. biomedical communities and makes no selection of the substantive literature for technology assessment as such. The ability to access MEDLARS in Europe is growing because of the expansion in specialized data telecommunications networks, but there may be price barriers to access for the diverse users represented by the technology assessment community. Perhaps, as part of the regional network being set up by WHO described below, consideration could be given to a literature collection valuable for these endeavors.

TABLE 6-5 Foreign Centers' Access to MEDLARS

Tapes	Tapes/Software	On-Line NLM
West Germany	Sweden	France
Japan	United Kingdom	South Africa
	Australia	Canada
	Pan American Health Organization	Mexico
		Colombia
		Kuwait
		Italy
		Switzerland

SOURCE: OTA, 1982a.

World Health Organization Network on Technology Assessment

Increased interest in technology assessment has led the World Health Organization to establish a network for information exchange on technology assessment (U.S. DHHS, 1981; WHO, 1977).

The European Regional Office of WHO has:

- a program on appropriate technology for health, including development of appropriate technology in laboratory services, radiology/radiotherapy/nuclear medicine, and biotechnology for health in member states;
- a program to promote the development of standard health technologies and identify, develop, and promote models for the systematic development of all major health care programs at the national level, including introduction of new health care technologies;
- a program to develop a health care technology assessment network, the hope being to link selected national institutes capable of ensuring technical and economic assessments of new equipment and technologies.

As information is gathered it will be disseminated to member states. Six European countries have provisionally agreed to participate in the first phase of the assessment network.

In November 1983 WHO held a meeting to permit member states to formulate guidelines for medical technology assessment and appropriate utilization (WHO, 1983). Principles for drafting national guidelines were drawn up outlining possible strategies such as research and development policies, assessment priorities and methodologies, market entry, and deployment and use. Future programs will be held on economic incentives for the appropriate and rational use of medical technologies in different member states; coordination of national standards for health care facilities, equipment and procedures; technology at the primary health care level; and geographic variation in use of health services.

The establishment in 1984 of a new journal, *The International Journal of Technology Assessment in Health Care* (Reiser, 1983), is evidence of the interest and ferment around this topic. The journal's scope of interest is in the generation, assessment, diffusion, and use of health care technology. It will examine the effects of technology as perceived by policymakers, different academic disciplines, and different countries, and examine methods to conduct studies and evaluations of technology. The journal will provide a vehicle for establishing ties with scholars, governments, and private institutions concerned with health care technology, and facilitating outreach and interaction on matters of technology assessment. The journal may also play a key role in identifying the most useful literature for purposes of technology assessment. Also, plans are developing for the creation of a New International Society for Technology Assessment in Health Care, which is designed to facilitate the exchange of ideas on technology assessment.

Postmarketing Surveillance of Drugs

Postmarketing surveillance* of drugs may offer a special opportunity for international collaboration. Postmarketing surveillance is generally used to determine a drug's beneficial and harmful effects, especially over longer periods of observation than are used in premarketing clinical trials. It would provide information that could be transferred across national boundaries for regulatory purposes. The

* The systematic collection and analysis of information from the normal therapeutic use of drugs, with the object of acquiring evidence on adverse effects or other phenomena associated with their use.

accelerated discovery and development of new drugs and the crippling consequences of thalidomide use during pregnancy have focused world attention on drug safety and the significance of shared information.

Benefits of such an international effort could be large (Finney, 1964). The public would gain in protection and physicians might gain in assurance if decisions could be based on experience in more than one country. Manufacturers might economize and expedite new testing if certified evidence on the efficacy and safety of a drug in one country can be used in support of its introduction into another.

Twenty-three countries participate in the World Health Organization's Program for International Monitoring of Adverse Reactions (OTA, 1982b). Each participating country provides to WHO reports summarizing adverse drug reactions that occurred during the past year. The purpose of the WHO program is to increase the probability of detecting effects that might be overlooked by individual countries. However, the program does not appear to be widely used for regulatory purposes. Problems exist with the timeliness, reliability, and completeness of the information available. The use of the information is still in a rudimentary phase, and a good conceptual framework for its application and development is lacking.

Nevertheless, the program could be developed into a useful component for international technology assessment of the safety and efficacy of drugs. New possibilities are opened by the capability of computerizing the system so that data can be entered promptly from one corner of the world and be accessible to others almost immediately.

CONCLUSIONS AND RECOMMENDATIONS

The information collected in the preparation of this chapter prompts the study committee to make the following recommendations (in italics).

- *International collaboration among the industrialized nations is necessary to the fullest establishment of a comprehensive system of medical technology assessment in any one of them. A first step should be collaboration in gathering data on such technologies and on research concerning their assessment.*

Developed countries increasingly are interested in technology assessment, particularly as related to devices, equipment, and medical practice. Such assessment typically is hoped to help in improving patient care, controlling costs, and diffusion of expensive technologies. As in the United States, many different groups and agencies in each country carry out and use the results of technology assessment. Most countries do not yet have a coordinated coherent system for medical technology assessment, with one possible exception being Sweden. Until coordinated systems are developed within countries, it will be very difficult if not impossible to develop any international system of medical technology assessment.

However, most countries do appear to have a system for determining the safety and efficacy of drugs. Therefore, it is not surprising that more progress appears to have been made toward international collaboration in the assessment of drugs than in the assessment of devices or medical practices. The presence of national organizations charged with drug evaluation provides a focus for these activities and facilitates international collaboration. The presence of formal mechanisms for assessment of drugs in the developed countries is evidence of international interest in technology assessment that may be extended to devices and procedures. This shared interest may prompt standardization of methods, data exchange, and other forms of collaboration especially if it leads to development of formal systems for such efforts.

Several international organizations, most particularly OECD and WHO, have made an important beginning to systematic approaches to the international assessment of drugs. These efforts must continue to be supported by the governments of different countries and by the pharmaceutical industry. Such programs may provide models for systematic collaborative efforts for assessing devices or medical procedures.

• *An international clearinghouse should be established to serve as an information pool of data gathered on medical technologies and research concerning their assessment.* Much can be done short of establishing an international system for technology assessment. An international clearinghouse for technology assessment would facilitate information dissemination, lessen duplicative efforts, and foster international collaboration. The WHO network is a beginning. In the United States the proposed Institute of Medicine (1983) consortium whose primary function could be to act as a clearinghouse would be part of an international clearinghouse for medical technology assessment.

Investigators from different countries already collaborate in developing information for technology assessment. More support should be made available to extend such research. For example, the Scandinavian countries have excellent routine data collection that could be used to gather information on safety and (in some cases) efficacy. Some of this is done at present, but much more could be done.

• *An international clearinghouse should be established for information about clinical trials.* A possible model is the British National Perinatal Epidemiology Unit at Oxford, which promotes clinical trials and conducts research on their effect on medical practice.

Much can be learned from other countries' experience with medical technology assessment. Although U.S. medical technology assessment is methodologically advanced, there is much to be learned about adoption of assessment findings by physicians and hospitals.

In this respect, a Swedish experience with a hip joint consensus meeting may be illuminating. The consensus format approach began in the United States at NIH, but it is was limited to considerations of safety and efficacy. In contrast, when the first European consensus meeting was held in 1982 in Sweden on hip surgery, costs and use were also on the agenda. In addition, there was extensive newspaper coverage throughout the country discussing the issues in lay terms, every medical opinion leader relevant to hip surgery attended the meeting (Sweden's population is eight million), and the jury panel included not only medical experts but politicians.

The immediate result was a major reorganization of hip surgery in the Stockholm area.

The U.S. Office for Medical Applications of Research responsible for the consensus conferences is currently funding research both to formalize and improve the consensus process and to find out how to enhance their impacts.

• *Industrialized nations with competence in medical technology assessment should work with less-developed countries to help them fill their special needs for information.* For example, fellowships to train individuals from less-developed countries in methods of technology assessment should be established in the United States and elsewhere.

REFERENCES

Aaron, H. J., and W. B. Schwartz. 1984. The Painful Prescription. Washington, D.C.: The Brookings Institution.

American Institute of Biological Sciences. 1973. International Prospective for Biomedical Engineering, Workshop VI. 6–10 August. Dubrovnik, Yugoslavia.

Coronary Artery Bypass Surgery: A Consensus. 1984. Lancet ii:1288.

Council of Science and Society. 1983. Expensive Medical Techniques: Report of a Working Party. London: Calvert's Press.

Department of Health and Human Services. 1982. Health-United States, 1982. Pub. No. (PHS) 83-1232. Washington, D.C.: Superintendent of Documents, U.S. Government Printing Office.

ECRI. 1983. The U.S. and Canada: Technology's role in the problems of two health care systems. ECRI, p. 1–6.

Finney, D. J. 1964. An international drug safeguard plan. J. Chronic Dis. 17:565–581.

Fudenberg, H. H. 1983. Basic biomedical research: A cost-benefit analysis. In Biomedical Institutions, Biomedical Funding, and Public Policy, H. H. Fudenberg, ed. New York: Plenum Press.

Groot, L. M. J. 1982. Advanced and Expensive Medical Technology in the Member States of the European Community, Legislation, Policy and Costs. Commissioned by the European Community.

Gross, F. 1980. Directions and Implications of Drug Legislation and Regulation in Europe and Constraints on Progress in Drug Development. Rochester, N.Y.: Center for the Study of Drug Development.

Institute of Medicine. 1983. Planning Study Report: A Consortium for Assessing Medical Technology. Washington, D.C.: National Academy Press.

National Institutes of Health. 1982. Total hip-joint replacement in Sweden. J. Am. Med. Assoc. 248:1822–1824.

Office of Technology Assessment. 1980. The Implications of Cost-Effectiveness Analysis of Medical Technology: The Management of Health Care Technology in Ten Countries. Stock No. 052-003-00783-5. Washington, D.C.: Superintendent of Documents, U.S. Government Printing Office.

Office of Technology Assessment. 1982a. Medlars and Health Information Policy. U.S. Congress. Stock No. 98-764. Washington, D.C.: Superintendent of Documents, U.S. Government Printing Office.

Office of Technology Assessment. 1982b. Postmarketing Surveillance of Prescription Drugs. Stock No. 052-003-00839-9. Washington, D.C.: Superintendent of Documents, U.S. Government Printing Office.

Rasmussen, K. 1981. Chronic sinus node disease: Natural course and indication for pacing. Eur. Heart J. 2:455–459.

Reiser, S. 1983. The International Journal of Technology Assessment in Health Care.

Rogers, E. V., J. K. Larsen, and C. V. Lowe. 1982. The consensus development process for medical technologies: A cross-cultural comparison of Sweden and the United States. J. Am. Med. Assoc. 248:1880–1882.

Selzer, Z. 1983. Too many pacemakers. N. Engl. J. Med. 307:183–184.

Shepard, D. S., and J. S. Durch. 1984. International comparison of resource allocation in health sciences: An analysis of expenditures on biomedical research in 19 industrialized countries. Final Report to the Fogarty Center, National Institutes of Health Contract No. 263-83-C-0244. Boston, Mass.: Harvard School of Public Health.

SPRI. 1981. What is SPRI? Stockholm, Sweden: SPRI, S-10254.

SPRI. 1979. International Workshop on Evaluation of Medical Technology held Stockholm, Sweden, September 18–19, 1979. Stockholm, Sweden: SPRI, Fack, S-10250.

SPRI. 1982. Consensus Development Statement: Total Hip Joint Replacement. Conference held May 12–14, 1982, Stockholm, Sweden.

Standard and Poor's Corporation. 1983. Industry surveys, health care. Basic Analysis 151:H13–H35.

Stocking, B., and B. Jennett. 1984. Consensus development conference: Coronary artery bypass surgery in Britain. Br. Med. J. 288:1712.

U.S. Department of Health and Human Services. 1981. Assessment of Biomedical Technology in the Health Care Field: International Perspectives in Methodology, S. Perry, ed. Proceedings for a Joint Symposium held in Copenhagen, September 7–9, 1981.

U.S. Department of Health and Human Services. 1982. Health United States, 1982. Washington, D.C.

Weintraub, M. 1982. The French drug approval process. J. Clin. Pharmacol. 22:213–222.

Wing, P. J. 1983. Why don't the British treat more patients with kidney failure? Br. Med. J. 287:1157–1158.

World Health Organization. 1977. Proceedings of the International Conference on the Role of the Individual and the Community in the Research, Development, and Use of Biologicals. Bull. W.H.O. 55(Suppl. 2):1–177.

World Health Organization. 1983. Summary Report: Consultation on National Guidelines for Medical Technology Assessment and Appropriate Utilization. Based on a meeting held in Brussels, November 2–4, 1983.

7 Conclusions and Recommendations

Over the years various organizations have developed assessments of medical technology in response to specific needs or demands. Many agencies and organizations conduct programs in assessment and dissemination of information about medical technology, each from its own perspective (see Chapter 2). Taken singly, each program fulfills a particular purpose. For example, the Food and Drug Administration's premarketing approval process protects the public from unsafe and inefficacious drugs; the Office of Technology Assessment (OTA) conducts assessments on a variety of other technologies. Taken in combination, however, these various responses do not constitute a coherent system for assessing all types of medical technologies.

Problems that result from the lack of a systematic approach can be readily identified.

- **The information base for technology assessment is often inadequate in depth and coverage.** The collection of relevant, valid, primary data about technologies has not kept pace with the development of new technologies for the prevention, detection, and treatment of disease. Many assessments, including those by the Office of Technology Assessment (Congress), the Office of Health Technology Assessment (Public Health Service), or the Office of Medical Applications of Research (National Institutes of Health) mention a lack of cogent evidence on which to base secure conclusions. Nor are there good scientific methods for interpolating or adjusting to compensate for missing data for assessments. These matters are well covered in Chapter 3.
- **Retrieval, collation, and dissemination of already available information is inadequate.** No organization comprehensively monitors, collects, indexes, and disseminates information on technologies. Medical technology assessment often may require information from many subject areas. Such information is developed in many different places by different investigators and is not easily available in appropriate form for decision making.
- **No systematic procedures exist for identifying major emerging technologies that may require special attention.** Tech-

nologies with major consequences for society—ethical or economic—may appear and urgently require assessment. Examples of such technologies are liver transplantation, the artificial heart, and magnetic resonance imaging. Use of technologies can become widespread before the necessary research is available on which to base policy decisions about use, reimbursement, or purchase. The required investigations may be extensive, diverse, and numerous for a new technology.

- **No organization is responsible for setting priorities for assessment of technologies.** No orderly system exists for identifying and setting priorities for studies of technologies that require assessment. The current system largely depends on the interest of many different organizations and agencies to sponsor research. These studies may not address society's most pressing questions about a technology.
- **Assessment of a technology may come too late—or never.** A systematic procedure exists for assessing the safety and efficacy of drugs and devices before widespread dissemination. But there are no such approaches for identifying and assessing medical and surgical procedures before they move into medical practice. Furthermore, cost considerations of new procedures are rarely studied.
- **New uses of established technologies may escape assessment altogether.** Drugs and devices receive rigorous evaluation for safety and efficacy before introduction into the market, but once on the market many drugs are used for purposes other than those for which they were evaluated and approved.
- **Underutilization of certain technologies may be wasteful.** A possible example of a useful and relatively neglected technology is percutaneous transluminal angioplasty as a treatment for peripheral vascular disease. Angioplasty alone is less costly but also less efficacious than surgery. A strategy that applies the two procedures stepwise (angioplasty first, then surgery if angioplasty is unsuccessful or if occlusion recurs) is uniformly superior to surgery alone in patients who have lesions for which angioplasty can be considered. If 40 percent of all patients in the United States with severe iliac or femoral artery disease were treated according to the stepwise strategy, there would be an estimated yearly savings (as compared with surgery alone) of 352 lives and $82 million, as well as an additional 5,006 functioning limbs (Doubilet and Abrams, 1984).
- **Assimilation of assessment findings into health care processes can be slow.** When new technologies are shown to be valuable—or obsolete—it may take a long time before clinical evaluation influences the adoption or abandonment of them. Obstacles can be as simple as the publication of studies in the wrong journal to have an impact on practice (Stross and Harlan, 1979). Diffusion of new methods is enhanced by the extent to which they are easy to use, require little effort to learn, impose little change in practice style, are highly remunerative and satisfying, and have no clinically worthy competitors. Also, some features of the setting in which physicians practice influence their use of medical technology; for example, physicians in group practices appear to adopt innovations more rapidly than physicians in solo practice. These and other determinants of diffusion of assessments are discussed in Chapter 4.

The principal objective in assessment of medical technology is the improved health of people. The primary costs of the lack of an adequate system for technology assessment are to human well-being—patients do not receive optimal care. But there also are economic costs when the most cost-effective technologies are not applied or when ineffective technologies are.

The worth of technology assessment in medicine reaches beyond its warranty to the patient and its utility to the health professional. The results of assessment also are needed by hospitals and other facilities that buy and apply technologies; by industries that develop technologies; by the professional societies that disseminate information to health care practitioners; and by the insurance companies, government agencies, and corporate health plans that pay for the use of technologies. A strategy for assessing medical technology, therefore, must take into account not only the methods of assessment but also the needs, demands, and resistances of the participants and beneficiaries in the process.

Medical technology assessment has developed piecemeal in response to specific demands rather than as a system designed to provide the information required to improve and protect the health of the public and inform national policy decisions. What is needed now is the creation of an overall system for the orderly conduct of medical technology assessment.

THE CHALLENGE

We believe that it is possible and desirable to establish a coherent system for technology assessment. As evident in Chapter 2, many elements of such a system already are in place and can be built on. Numerous agencies and organizations are supporting or conducting assessments. The committee endorses this pluralism, believing that it contributes to the richness and variety of assessment activities as well as serving as a system of checks and balances. Furthermore, as seen in Chapter 3, practical methods of inquiry into medical technology exist—methods that are well developed, widely accepted, and often reliable and that have a core of practitioners in place to apply them.

The challenge for the committee then was to devise one or more strategies for medical technology assessment that builds on current efforts, strengthening and supplementing them. First, the problems created by the lack of any coherent system were identified. This helped to identify and describe the key functions (described below) of an adequate system. Second, the institutional arrangements now available or that could be devised to achieve a rational approach for assessment were examined. Third, the recommendations concluding this chapter were developed, outlining a series of steps for achieving a coherent medical technology assessment system while taking advantage of the current multiple arrangements.

KEY FUNCTIONS NEEDING IMPROVEMENT

In preparation for reviewing options, the functions that must be well executed to ensure adequate medical technology assessment will be described briefly.

Information Monitoring and Acquisition

Any system for technology assessment must have the ability to identify, select, acquire, process, and sort documents and other materials and provide indexes to the collection. Because technology assessment draws on many fields, its information is in subject areas as diverse as law, finance, management, economics, biostatistics, epidemiology, and biomedicine. Further diversity is occasioned by the variety of organizations producing reports, tables, experiments, studies, and reviews. The extensive information needs for the assessment of medical technologies and the present lack of a central organization or agency make essential the creation of some systematic method for gathering information from multiple sources. In the committee's view, this monitoring function should extend beyond the United States to collect information from international efforts in medical technology assessment. As seen in Chapter

6, many developed countries are actively involved in technology assessment, but there is no clearinghouse for this information.

Combining Information from Different Sources

For maximum utility to health care professionals and policymakers, the information available on medical technologies has to be assembled and then combined in a systematic fashion. Individual research studies can easily be equivocal, but a clear view may be gained from a collection of studies, no one of which is strong enough to enable a conclusion. Thus the whole body of information needs to be examined so as to determine the appropriate differential weight to be given to studies of different scope and rigor. In addition, these studies pose multiple issues that must be addressed, such as safety, efficacy, costs, and social and ethical consequences of technologies. Information on these varied dimensions of concern also will turn out to be differentially valuable, and some further needs for information will be apparent merely from the assembly.

Dissemination of Information

Dissemination of information is a necessary component of any technology assessment system, because results must be promulgated both widely and through appropriate channels of communication if they are to influence patient care or provider reimbursement. The source of information or channel of communication can have varying degrees of influence on physician practice, as illustrated in Chapter 4. Research on dissemination practices should be part of a coherent approach to technology assessment.

Identification of Gaps in Knowledge That Require Research

In an orderly system, gaps in knowledge about medical technologies are identified and studies to acquire needed data are commissioned. As indicated, there are many gaps in knowledge that result from current efforts. For instance, drugs and devices are identified and evaluated for safety and efficacy as they emerge but not after dissemination. Some medical procedures and surgery may be widespread before they are ever studied; economic, ethical, and social effects of a technology are rarely studied. Therefore, any system for assessment must develop an approach for ascertaining what information is needed about what technology and when.

Data and Information Acquisition

When gaps in knowledge are identified, there must be the capability to acquire the necessary data or information. The most pressing problem of the current situation is the lack of valid, reliable primary data. Industry is now by far the largest investor in technology assessment research, mostly because of the regulations imposed by the Food and Drug Administration (FDA). But as indicated in Chapters 2 and 3, this leaves major gaps in knowledge for marketed drugs and devices and for medical procedures and surgery.

Priority Setting

The large number of technologies in clinical use means that resources must be allocated wisely to address important problems in technology assessment in some orderly way. At present dependence is largely on the interest of many different organizations and individuals, each approaching technology from the perspective of their own interest and need. Therefore, some system for developing a research agenda with a societal perspective is required.

Manpower for Technology Assessment

Technology assessment requires investigators with diverse backgrounds and diverse, specialized training (see Chapter 3). Vigorous research activity is the key to continual progress in most scientific and technical fields, and technology assessment is no exception. To maintain the quality and vitality of research conducted in these fields, any system must ensure an adequate supply of well-trained scientists.

The most comprehensive effort to estimate the number of active researchers in health services research, which overlaps the field of technology assessment, was a 1978 survey conducted by the then National Research Council of the National Academy of Sciences (NAS) Committee on National Needs for Biomedical and Behavioral Research Personnel. More than 1,370 persons were identified as once having received support from the National Center for Health Services Research (NCHSR) as principal investigators on research grants or contracts or as having received federal funds from the NCHSR or the Alcohol, Drug Abuse, and Mental Health Administration (ADAMHA) for training in health services research. As a point of comparison, in 1977 there were 31,000 biomedical science Ph.D.s (excluding postdoctoral appointees in academic employment) and about 9,800 M.D.s primarily engaged in research (NAS, 1983). Unfortunately, federal traineeships and fellowships for graduate students in health services research have essentially disappeared. NAS reports (1978, 1981) have consistently cited a lack of biostatisticians and epidemiologists.

Manpower development and education of individuals should go beyond educating only those scientists charged with conducting technology assessment, because a broader community of individuals need the results of these studies. They should be able to understand and take advantage of ongoing work; results should be diffused promptly and reliably to those who can act on the information.

Research and Development of Methods for Assessment

Any system for technology assessment must also foster the improvement of methods for technology assessment and the development of new approaches. Chapter 3 describes specific methods for evaluating technologies and also how these can be strengthened by further development through research. Each method has its strengths, weaknesses, and limitations for detecting favorable or unfavorable outcomes associated with a technology. Techniques for appraising the joint message of a set of related studies are in a flux of development; research in these methods—for meta-studies—is an important need. Some methods have not even been invented yet; for example, as pointed out in Chapter 3 there is limited ability to assess the social, legal, or ethical consequences of technologies. Other very weak methods, such as case studies, have been shown to have impacts far beyond their validity on clinical care; enhancing their reliability as guides to clinical action could produce large health benefits. The introduction of Diagnosis-Related Groups (DRGs) as a new payment mechanism suddenly brought a new dimension to technology assessment. Much research will be required to discover the changes needed to make the DRG system operate for cost-containment and technology assessment. If there were a system for technology assessment, it would be alert to such methodologic issues and would move promptly to develop the field.

Not only is knowledge limited about the characteristics of technologies, such as their safety, efficacy, costs, etc., but also little is known about how technology develops and diffuses into the health care system. Without such knowledge there is little hope of rationalizing health care services.

BUILDING A SYSTEM

As this analysis has revealed, existing institutional arrangements, and probably existing legislative authorities, are inadequate to support an orderly system for technology assessment. Ways must be found to organize and finance the functions described here. In addition, because some elements of an effective system already are in place, opportunities for building and strengthening existing functions may be as important as establishing new institutional arrangements when warranted.

ADVANTAGES AND DISADVANTAGES OF VARIOUS INSTITUTIONAL ARRANGEMENTS

Technology assessment now has multiple participants both in the private and public sectors. Therefore, the committee sought to understand the advantages and disadvantages of different kinds of entities—public or private or some combination of the two. Could one simply extend the functions of an existing body or is a new entity required? In its 1982 report, the OTA described various kinds of institutional arrangements (OTA, 1982): (1) congressional sponsorship of a private-public body or chartering of an organization to undertake medical technology assessment activities, (2) reinstatement of the authority or funding of the National Center for Health Care Technology (NCHCT), or (3) encouragement of the secretary of the Department of Health and Human Services (DHHS) to develop a coherent system of medical technology assessment under powers already vested by law. Another possible approach is creation of a new federal institution.

Private-Public Body

An organization could be chartered as a separate nonprofit organization or as part of an organization. Examples of such organizations include those in the proposal by Bunker and coworkers for an Institute for Health Care Evaluation (Bunker et al., 1982a,b) and in the Institute of Medicine (IOM) plan for a Consortium for Assessing Medical Technology (IOM, 1983).

One advantage of this approach would be the ability to capitalize on private sector initiative and interest and reliance on private as well as possible public funding. A combination of private and public sector involvement may be essential for any system of technology assessment to be acceptable to all parties concerned.

Apart from the very real possibility that such an arrangement could not be forged or not be effective, disadvantages of this approach include the difficulties of obtaining adequate levels of funding to be effective over time, lack of authority to enforce decisions, and possible bias toward marketing and profits for private sponsors. An additional limitation of the proposed Institute for Health Care Evaluation is the close relationship of medical technology assessment to the reimbursement system because of its proposed financing, which can be restrictive. For example funding might not be provided for examining social and ethical issues.

Existing private-public organizations have provided successful approaches to technical issues, such as building technology, health effects of vehicle emissions, and energy research and development. Examples include the National Institute of Building Sciences (NIBS), the Health Effects Institute, and the Electric Power Research Institute (EPRI) (Fox, 1981; EPRI Current Information, 1984). A new private-public Council on Health Care Technology, recently legislatively authorized, offers potential for coordinating technology assessment efforts (P.L. 98-551).

Whether a private-public organization could in fact develop a viable, effective system for medical technology assessment would depend in large measure on the securing of adequate resources to carry out the proposed functions and on maintaining a proper balance of all the vested interests.

Reestablish the NCHCT

The National Center for Health Care Technology had good enabling legislation that permitted it to meet many of the objectives of the proposed system. However, the levels of funding it attained were too modest for the goals and objectives envisioned here. In addition, presumably many of the same opposing interests that led to the demise of NCHCT would still be active. During its short life NCHCT provided a focal point for the Health Care Financing Administration (HCFA) to interact with the Public Health Service, and thus the bulk of its resources were committed to medical technology assessment as it related to the reimbursement system. Thus, while the legislative mandate of NCHCT was broadly drafted to permit it to develop a system for technology assessment, it never reached its full potential.

The research program of the NCHCT was transferred to the National Center for Health Services Research (NCHSR) as were the responsibilities for providing advice to the Health Care Financing Administration. Funding levels for the NCHSR have been falling steadily for a number of years, and current expenditures of approximately $14 million for technology assessment—primarily health services research—are meager in comparison with the tasks to be achieved. New legislation changes the name of NCHSR to the National Center for Health Services Research and Health Care Technology Assessment (NCHSRHCTA) and provides it with an Advisory Council on Health Care Technology to advise on technology assessment functions. Funding levels and functions still fall considerably short of what is envisioned in this report.

There are advantages to having a federal agency charged with developing a systematic approach to the assessment of medical technologies. Such an agency would be less encumbered by legal constraints, for example antitrust violations. Its interest would be the public interest, and it would be able to draw more easily on other government resources than would a private organization. In addition, a federal agency appears more likely than a private organization to obtain the necessary resources for such an endeavor.

Development of a System by the DHHS Secretary

Under powers vested by law, the secretary of the Department of Health and Human Services could proceed to develop a coherent system of medical technology assessment. In the committee's view, unless new sources of funds were infused, competing priorities of other department functions probably would never permit allocation of sufficient resources to develop an effective system. And if the function were placed in HCFA, the focus would primarily be limited to the reimbursement concerns of Medicare.

A Separate Federal Agency

Congress could establish an independent federal agency and charge it with developing a system for medical technology assessment. The 1983 amendments to the Social Security Act (P.L. 98-21) authorize the creation of a Prospective Payment Assessment Commission, appointed by the director of the congressional Office of Technology Assessment, and give it broad powers, including medical technology assessment and the evaluation of appropriateness of medical practice patterns. The commission is to collect and assess information on costs, productivity, technological advances, and cost-effectiveness of hospital services. The commission is expected to synthesize existing data in framing its recommendations and reimbursement rate setting, where those data are available, but it also is empowered to conduct research and to award grants and contracts for research. A major provision of this legislation allows the commission to obligate Medicare Trust Fund resources for external research activities, with the approval of the DHHS secretary.

Current levels of funding for this effort are too modest to accomplish the task set out by this committee. Furthermore, the focus of the activity is limited to Medicare prospective payment for inpatient hospital services. The commission cannot singlehandedly develop a system for medical technology assessment. Legal questions still remain about the use of trust fund monies to fund research. Nevertheless, because the commission can address the concerns of HCFA in a very focused way, if it does so vigorously, then fewer resources may be required to develop the system outlined in this chapter.

An independent federal agency would be advantageous in that it could be charged with setting priorities in technology assessment so as to reflect the needs of the nation.* It would likely be far more successful than an entity in the private sector in soliciting data and opinion from federal agencies involved in biomedical research, health care financing, or other areas relevant to medical technology. This would also probably hold true for obtaining information from organizations involved in technology assessment in the private sector. Prospects for adequate long-term financial support seem brighter for a federal agency than for a privately chartered institution. Finally, an independent federal agency, as contrasted with NCHCT or an agency in a cabinet department, would be less susceptible to the whims of a new administration or Congress. However, enormous barriers exist to establishing yet another independent federal agency, given pressures to decrease the number of or consolidate existing agencies.

NOT THE REGULATORY APPROACH

We notice that the fullest and most trustworthy health care technology assessment is to be found in the fields where regulatory authority and the profit motive are most operative: drugs and class III medical devices. The principal reason for this seems to be simply that the FDA requires substantial amounts of high-quality data as a part of its licensing process. Regulation can be used to demand the collection of missing data especially since the profits from marketing the drugs and devices can support the necessary research.

The committee would like to ensure new kinds of data acquisition by developing nonregulatory approaches, believing that cooperation may flow from an approach that offers incentives. One example is the development of reimbursement incentives for collection of data of prescribed scope and quality, for example, obtaining third-party contracts or grants for evaluating experimental technologies in exchange for data. But other ways of tapping the health care dollar might also be developed, e.g., a tax on each hospital bed or outpatient procedure, provider contributions, patient assessments. Another example is the independent, nonregulatory drug surveillance unit established at the University of Southampton, England (Inman, 1981; Drug Surveil-

* This is particularly important because recent imposition of the prospective payment system; information from technology assessment will be essential if there are to be sound decisions about which technologies to use when caring for patients.

lance Research Unit, 1983). The unit is jointly funded by the government and by industry to establish a national scheme for detecting adverse events occurring during drug therapy.

FINANCING

In Chapter 2, it was stated that $1.3 billion is a generous estimate for the amount spent on technology assessment. The drug industry, by far the largest investor, spends approximately $700 million–$750 million on technology assessment, the device industry, $30 million–$50 million; and the federal government contributes about $450 million if the amount spent by NIH on clinical trials is added to the vastly smaller amounts spent by the Office of Medical Applications of Research (NIH), National Center for Health Services Research and Health Care Technology Assessment, and other government agencies. This may appear to be a very large sum, until one realizes that it is about 0.3 percent of the nearly $400 billion spent on health care in 1984. Given the preponderance of money spent on health care and the comparatively vanishing amount spent on assessing medical technologies, the great need for primary data cited in many different studies and by different groups for making decisions about patient care, and the need to choose among technologies, the committee believes that the additional resources required to develop a coherent system should come from a larger share of the health care dollar.

Various proposals have been made for tapping this dollar as outlined in Chapters 2 and 5, but further study is needed to map out exactly how to do this. The Prospective Payment Assessment Commission is an example of a group established to undertake technology assessment funded from the health care dollar (U.S. Congress, House, 1983). As previously noted, the enabling legislation allows the commission to obligate Medicare Trust Fund resources for external research activities.

Relman (1982, 1980) has suggested that 0.2 percent of all third-party expenditures for medical care might be an appropriate allocation for additional technology assessment. Such an allocation would have amounted to $490 million in 1984.

Although it would be helpful to have more alternatives for additional funding of technology assessment, the actual solution will require political action. Whatever approach or combination of approaches is used for tapping the health care dollar, the committee believes that the modest sum of $30 million should promptly be set aside for improving some of the described functions. Though not adequate to support the system envisioned, this amount would permit valuable first steps to be taken in the development of a coherent system. But the committee also cautions that this support should grow in about 10 years to $300 million (in 1984 dollars) to finance the accumulation of primary data on which all assessment must depend. Chapter 2 suggests how such funds might be spent.

RECOMMENDATIONS

The committee wishes to promote the development of a coordinated system for medical technology assessment that would both capitalize on the strengths and resources of the free-market economy and meet societal needs to make available safe, effective medical care. We recommend an incremental approach to achieve this purpose. These recommendations (in italics), distinct from the very specific ones in the preceding chapters and the boldface contributions to a research agenda throughout the report, are intended to help in building an assessment system.

- *The monitoring, synthesizing, and disseminating functions of medical technology assessment should be established in some entity with a chartered mission and financing.* We put this first because it is not very intrusive or expensive, it is highly relevant in itself, and its success and products would illuminate wiser choices among further possible actions. A private-public organization seems the most appropriate setting for such a function because it is possible to coordinate both private and public activities, provide a neutral forum, elicit broad-based support, and impose on both sectors the responsibility to make the functions of the body useful.

• *The same entity should develop the research agenda for filling gaps in knowledge relevant to assessment.* One product of the entity might be state-of-the-art reports with clear recommendations for future research and some priority setting. This function flows quite directly from the task of monitoring and synthesis.

• *There should be a substantial increase in the accumulation of primary data for assessment.* We have proposed that funds to support this research come from the health care dollar. The crucial bridge of technology assessment between science, research, and development on the one side and patient care on the other receives too little attention. This circumstance may grow partly from the lack of an entity solely concerned with assessment. Inattention to assessment is prevalent in the private sector, where financial considerations are prominent. An initiative that does not directly produce revenues to cover outlays tends not to be well supported. A longer view would be hoped to reveal ample basis for a higher priority in the private sector if indeed use of more cost-effective technology proves to be advantageous for the health care industry.

• *A portion of the health care dollar should be allocated to existing Public Health Service components (such as NCHSRHCTA) that already have the task of supporting research on technology assessment.* A close link between their activity and the public-private sector entity is required both for programmatic and financial concerns. A natural vehicle for this could be obtained by commissioning the development of a research agenda from the public-private sector entity, which could guide funding priorities by the government components. The additional funds should be used to fill gaps in knowledge about technologies when the profit motive does not operate to catalyze the collection of primary data such as in the drug industry.

• *Those organizations that support research in technology assessment should engage in developing it as a scientific field, such as improving methodologies and supporting education and training of assessment personnel.* We have pointed out the need for supporting doctoral programs in epidemiology and biostatistics as well as quantitative training for physicians. The products of these research training programs are needed both to carry out technology assessments and to develop improvements in methodology. Improved quantitative training for physicians is required so that the need for careful technology assessment will be more widely appreciated in the medical community. Close links could be forged with the private-public sector entity by requesting this group to convene experts for advice and by using them as a forum for continuing education programs.

• *Support for medical technology assessment should rise over the next 10 years to reach an annual level $300 million greater (in 1984 dollars) than at present.* This should be phased in over a 10-year period. Funding continuity and stability should be emphasized to ensure a firm foundation for the enterprise.

CLOSING COMMENT

The committee believes that the functions identified for improvement should guide the strategy for developing a coherent technology assessment system.

Chapter 2 describes many different organizations and agencies doing technology assessment. This at once contributes to the richness and breadth of activities and to the need for some system. In a pluralistic society such as that of the United States, it would not be surprising to find functions for achieving a system of technology assessment distributed among several organizations or agencies. But to build on the strength of the current system, no single proposed option seems sufficient in itself to accomplish our objectives. Accordingly, different functions may need to be either strengthened or newly established in some combination of two or more organizations.

We have outlined the functions that are needed for a coherent technology assessment system and have suggested the division of these into two different organizations—one a private-public partnership and the other the strengthening of one or more existing government agencies. We acknowledge that there are other ways to achieve an overall strategy for assessment of medical technology, and we are not opposed to other approaches. What we are concerned about is that there be a system that deals with the total problem. Of one thing we are certain, technology assessment can help ensure that patients are getting the most appropriate and the highest-quality care available and that the money we spend on health care is spent wisely. Our study has convinced us that we now are doing far too little assessment, and not even doing that well. We urge policymakers to shore up the current assessment activities and build upon them a national system of technology assessment.

REFERENCES

Bunker, J. P., et al. 1982a. Evaluation of medical technology strategies: Effects of coverage and reimbursement. N. Engl. J. Med. 306:620–624.

Bunker, J. P., et al. 1982b. Evaluation of medical technology strategies: Proposal for an institute of health-care evaluation (second of two parts). N. Engl. J. Med. 306:687–692.

Doubilet, P., and H. L. Abrams. 1984. The cost of underutilization: Percutaneous transluminal angioplasty for peripheral vascular disease. N. Engl. J. Med. 310:95–102.

Drug Surveillance Research Unit, University of Southampton. 1983. PEM News 1:1–16.

EPRI Current Information. 1984. The Electric Power Research Institute, Palo Alto, California

Fox, J. R., Breaking the regulatory deadlock. 1981. Harvard Business Review 81506:97–105.

Inman, W. H. 1981. Postmarketing surveillance of adverse drug reactions in general practice. II. Prescription event monitoring at the University of Southampton. Br. Med. J. 282:1216–1217.

Institute of Medicine. 1983. Planning Study Report: A Consortium for Assessing Medical Technology. Washington, D.C.: National Academy Press.

National Academy of Sciences. 1978. Personnel Needs and Training for Biomedical and Behavioral Research. Washington, D.C.

National Academy of Sciences. 1981. Personnel Needs and Training for Biomedical and Behavioral Research. Washington, D.C.: National Academy Press.

National Academy of Sciences. 1983. Personnel Needs and Training for Biomedical and Behavioral Research. Washington, D.C.: National Academy Press.

Office of Technology Assessment. 1982. Strategies for Medical Technology. Washington, D.C.: Superintendent of Documents, U.S. Government Printing Office.

Relman, A. 1982. An institute for health-care evaluation. N. Engl. J. Med. 306:669–670.

Relman, A. 1980. Assessment of medical practice: A simple proposal. N. Engl. J. Med. 303:153–154.

Stross, J. K., and W. R. Harlan. 1979. The dissemination of new medical information. J. Am. Med. Assoc. 241:2622–2624.

U.S. Congress, House. 1983. Social Security Amendments of 1983, Conference Report. Report #98-47. 98th Cong., 1st sess.

APPENDIX A: Profiles of 20 Technology Assessment Programs

Clifford S. Goodman*

The profiles of 20 medical technology assessment programs in the United States contained in this appendix illustrate the great variety—in a common framework—of assessment activities in major sectors of the American health care system. The profiles represent selected assessment activities of medical societies, medical product makers, government assessment organizations, health care provider organizations, third-party payers, universities, and independent evaluators and policy research organizations. The information assembled for these profiles provided much of the basis for preparing Chapter 2, "The Scope of Medical Technology Assessment." The 20 profiled programs are the following:

Joint American College of Cardiology/American Heart Association Task Force on Assessment of Cardiovascular Procedures
American College of Physicians Clinical Efficacy Assessment Project
American Hospital Association Hospital Technology Series Program
American Medical Association Diagnostic and Therapeutic Technology Assessment Program
Battelle Memorial Institute Human Affairs Research Centers
Blue Cross and Blue Shield Association Medical Necessity Program
Blue Cross and Blue Shield Association Technology Evaluation and Coverage Program
ECRI
Institute of Society, Ethics and the Life Sciences (Hastings Center)
The Permanente Medical Group, Inc., Division of Health Services Research
Medtronic Inc.
National Center for Health Services Research and Health Care Technology Assessment Office of Health Technology Assessment
National Heart, Lung, and Blood Institute
National Institutes of Health Office of Medical Applications of Research Consensus Development Program
National Library of Medicine
Congressional Office of Technology Assessment Health Program
Prospective Payment Assessment Commission
Smith Kline & French Laboratories Cost-Benefit Studies Program
University of California at San Francisco Institute for Health Policy Studies

* National Research Council Fellow, National Academy of Sciences, Washington, D.C.

Veterans Administration Cooperative Studies Program

The profiles were prepared by assembling information from personnel of the profiled programs, program publications, reports in the literature, and other sources. In each case, at least two drafts were provided to program personnel to be reviewed for matters of fact, for updating since previous drafts, and for generating suggestions for content. The profiles could not have been written without the gracious assistance of the individuals shown at the end of this introductory section; however, any errors or inadequate representations are solely the responsibility of the preparer of this appendix.

Although the programs are profiled according to the same 16 information categories, the attempt was made to retain the perspective and flavor of the individual programs. Profile narratives are arranged as follows.

Introduction	Assessors
Purpose	Turnaround
Subjects of Assessment	Reporting
Stage of Diffusion	Impact
Concerns	Reassessment
Requests	Funding/Budget
Selection	Examples
Process	Sources

These profiles are a start at systematically characterizing current technology assessment activities in the United States. The profiles are intended to answer the who, what, where, why, how, and how much of technology assessment of the 20 selected programs. Profiles such as these may be useful for the type of technology assessment clearinghouse recommended in this report. They could be published or made available on-line and updated periodically. Organizations already profiled could make additions and modifications annually, or perhaps continuously, as might be the case with an on-line system. Organizations wishing to be included could work with clearinghouse staff to develop a new profile, much in the manner in which these were prepared. The sources of financial support for such an ongoing activity could include publication fees, subscriptions, or other types of access fees.

The possibilities for valuable cross-cuts of the profile data are many. Distributions of assessment programs such as those shown in Chapter 2 may be helpful in portraying gaps in and other characteristics of overall assessment activity. Listings of assessments by specific technologies would be useful for organizations contemplating their own assessments of these technologies, or seeking information concerning procurement or use of technologies.

Each profile begins with a summary section portraying the program's major concerns and technologies assessed in matrix form, and checklists summarizing the stage of technologies assessed, application of technologies, assessment methods, and approximate annual budget. The summary sections cannot substitute for the profile narratives. The summary sections necessarily make categorical distinctions where these may not be so clear in practice. The following discussion and definitions may be helpful in understanding the matrix and checklists of assessment activities in the summary sections of each profile.

TECHNOLOGY

As noted and discussed in Chapter 1, the usage of the terms medical technology and assessment are those of the congressional Office of Technology Assessment. For the purposes of the summary sheets, OTA's usage is expanded upon as follows.

Drug: any chemical or biological substance that may be applied to, ingested by, or injected in order to prevent, treat, or diagnose disease or other medical conditions. Included are biologicals such as vaccines and blood products, medicinals and botanicals, and pharmaceutical preparations.

Device: any physical item, excluding drugs, used in medical care. Included are diagnostic and therapeutic equipment, prostheses, surgical and medical instruments and supplies, dental equipment and supplies, ophthalmic goods, and in vitro diagnostic products—reagents, instruments, and systems used in the collection, preparation, and examination of specimens taken from the human body to determine the state of a patient's health.

Medical or surgical procedure: a practice of a health care provider that generally involves a combination, often quite complex, of special skills or abilities with drugs, devices, or both. In some cases, the drugs or devices involved are not predominant factors in a procedure. Instead, the technique of the provider performing the procedure is most important, such as in the performance of a surgical procedure facilitated by the use of scalpels, clamps, and drugs against infection. Psychotherapy or prescription of a special diet are examples of procedures which may not involve drugs or devices.

Support system: a system that provides the environment for and otherwise facilitates the provision of health care, but is not the focal technology in a medical regimen, surgical procedure, or other form of health care. Examples are laboratory and radiology services, medical information systems, blood banking services, hospital infection control programs, food services, laundry, hospital facilities, and physical plant. Many of these are often referred to as ancillary services, and some might be said to comprise the infrastructure of health care delivery.

Organizational/administrative system: used in management and administration to ensure that health care is delivered as effectively as possible. Included are alternative delivery modes or settings, e.g., health maintenance organizations (HMOs), area-wide emergency care systems, and home health delivery, and payment systems, e.g., prepayment using diagnosis-related groups.

The last two categories—support and organizational/administrative systems—are often considered to be subjects of health services research.

This classification of technologies recognizes that a given technology may be comprised of as well as part of other technologies. A drug may be a concoction of multiple chemical entities packaged in a capsule; a medical device may be made of valves, biomaterials, and microchips; a surgical procedure may involve drugs and medical devices as well as the surgeon's skilled hand. An area-wide emergency medical care system may encompass all of these, plus ambulances, helicopters, communications systems, and more. An organization such as the Prospective Payment Assessment Commission may have to evaluate aspects of drugs, devices, medical and surgical procedures, and support systems in order to adjust an administrative technology—prospective payment using diagnosis-related groups.

In portraying the technologies assessed by the programs, *X*s are placed across from drugs and medical devices/supplies/equipment when program assessments directly address the properties of the medical products themselves. Where a medical product is not the predominant factor in a procedure, or where the properties of the medical product are taken as given and the emphasis of the assessment is on the concerns of a product-embodied procedure relative to another, *X*s are placed across from medical/surgical procedure only. For instance, for the purpose of the summary section charts, an ECRI assessment of mechanical ventilators to measure and compare various technical properties of several brands of these devices would be considered an equipment assessment. On the other hand, an assessment by a third-party payer of the circumstances under which intermittent positive-pressure breathing using mechanical ventilators is medically necessary and therefore reimbursable would be shown as an assessment of a medical procedure.

The unusual type of assessment, e.g., where a third-party payer primarily assesses medical and surgical procedures but has in an instance assessed ambulance services (a support technology), may not be noted as a major emphasis in the summary section charts.

CONCERNS

An assessment may address one or more of many concerns, attributes, or properties of a technology. The summary section groups a number of these into four categories.

Safety: a judgment of the acceptability of risk in a specified situation, e.g., for a given medical problem, by a provider with specified training, at a specified type of facility.

Efficacy: benefit for a given medical problem under ideal conditions of use.

Effectiveness: benefit for a given medical problem under average conditions of use.

Cost/cost-effectiveness/cost-benefit: includes costs, charges, pricing, cost-benefit, cost-effectiveness, and related concerns. Specifically:

Cost-benefit: the costs of a project or technological application compared to the resultant benefits, with both costs and benefits expressed in the same units. This unit is nearly always monetary.

Cost-effectiveness: the costs of a project or of alternative projects compared to the resultant benefits, with cost and benefits/effectiveness not expressed by the same unit. Costs are usually expressed in dollars, but benefits/effectiveness are ordinarily expressed in terms such as lives saved, disability avoided, quality-adjusted life years saved, or other relevant objectives.

Ethical/legal/social: includes implications of technology for societal norms, morals, institutions, and relationships; and economic, medical, legal, and cultural values.

Effectiveness in the summary section charts refers not only to the absolute benefit of the technology taken alone, but also to the marginal benefits to be gained from use of a technology under particular circumstances, considering a given patient's status and the use of and information gained from other technologies. Thus, appropriateness, a primary concern of several of the profiled programs, is categorized in the summary sections under effectiveness and/or cost-effectiveness, where cost is an explicit consideration in determining appropriateness. Evaluations of the sensitivity, specificity, and other operating characteristics of diagnostic technologies are efficacy/effectiveness concerns.

Again, the summary section matrices cite the major program emphases. Thus, although many of the profiled programs have legal departments or various legal requirements in connection with their assessment activities, *X*s are placed under the ethical/legal/social concerns column only for those programs having these as central concerns of their assessments.

STAGE OF TECHNOLOGIES ASSESSED

Emerging: in the applied research stage, about the time of initial clinical testing, e.g., monoclonal antibodies for immunotherapy of cancer.

New: past the stage of clinical trials but not yet in widespread use, e.g., extracorporeal lithotripsy for treatment of kidney stones.

Established: considered by providers to be a standard approach to a particular condition and diffused into general use.

Obsolete/outmoded: superseded by another technology and/or demonstrated to be ineffective or harmful, e.g., gastric freezing for peptic ulcer.

Technologies may be assessed at different stages of diffusion. The point in a technology's life cycle at which it is assessed may depend upon the purposes of an assessment program, and the course of the life cycle may be affected by the assessment itself. For new drugs and certain devices, FDA regulatory requirements may mediate technological diffusion before, during, and after assessment benchmarks such as initiation of clinical trials, approval for marketing, and removal from the market in the case of a product found to pose an imminent health hazard. Indeed, as discussed in Chapter 2, technologies may be assessed for the very purpose of determining their stage of diffusion.

APPLICATION OF TECHNOLOGIES

Prevention: protects an individual from disease, e.g., vaccination.

Diagnosis: helps in determining what disease processes occur in a patient, e.g., upper gastrointestinal endoscopy.

Screening: detects disease or abnormality, or potential for these, often in asymptomatic patients, e.g., Pap smear for cervical cancer.

Treatment: relieves an individual from disease and its effects, including technologies that cure disease and those that give symptomatic relief but do not alter the underlying disease process, e.g., drug therapy for depression.

Rehabilitation: to restore to a condition of health or useful and constructive activity, e.g., assistive devices for severe speech impairment.

ASSESSMENT METHODS

Laboratory testing: nonclinical (in vitro) testing of medical technology, e.g., for drug, device, or equipment performance.

Clinical trials: prospective clinical experiments designed to test the safety and efficacy of a medical technology in which people are assigned to experimental or control groups and outcomes are compared. Includes randomized controlled clinical trials, in which people are randomly assigned to experimental and control groups.

Epidemiological and other observational methods: excludes the more rigorous experimental design studies such as randomized clinical trials. Included are such studies known as quasiexperiments; series; case studies; cohort studies; natural experiments; and certain cross-sectional, case control, and longitudinal methods.

Cost analyses: analyses, including cost-benefit and cost-effectiveness analyses, that enumerate, measure, and compare both the benefits and costs of medical technologies. Analyses may vary in terms of perspective (i.e., the parties to whom the benefits and costs accrue) and the choice and valuation of the benefits and costs considered.

Simulation/modeling: use of models—representations of real-world phenomena—to test or evaluate proposed interventions, often undertaken when evaluation of the actual intervention would be impractical. Simulations may involve manipulation of iconic, analog, or symbolic (often mathematical) models.

Group judgment: a process in which a group of experts interact in assessing a technology and formulate findings by vote or other process of reaching general agreement. The findings may note minority opinions; the group may determine that there is no consensus of opinion. The process may be informal, or it may be a formal one such as the nominal group or Delphi technique. Members of the group may be involved in drafting, editing, reviewing, and/or commenting upon the findings. To be categorized as a group judgment it is necessary that group members have the opportunity to interact in formulating and reviewing each other's and the group's observations and findings.

Expert opinion: consultation with individual experts who may be involved in drafting, editing, reviewing, or commenting upon assessments, but who do not interact as a group.

Literature syntheses: summarizing, integrating, and interpreting research findings reported in the literature. May include unstructured literature reviews as well as various systematic and quantitative procedures such as meta-analysis.

ACKNOWLEDGMENTS

I wish to thank the following individuals for providing source material, reviewing drafts of the profiles, and sharing important insights into the assessment programs of which they are a part.

John R. Ball, American College of Physicians

Clyde J. Behney, Congressional Office of Technology Assessment

Nancy E. Cahill, American Medical Association

Arthur L. Caplan, Hastings Center

Enrique D. Carter, National Center for Health Services Research

Susan M. Clark, National Institutes of Health Office of Medical Applications of Research

Morris F. Collen, Kaiser Permanente Medical Care Program

Dennis J. Cotter, Prospective Payment Assessment Commission

Martin Erlichman, National Center for Health Services Research

David J. Feild, American College of Cardiology
Robert C. Flink, Medtronic
Peter L. Frommer, National Heart, Lung, and Blood Institute
Susan Gleeson, Blue Cross and Blue Shield Association
Mark D. Goodhart, American Hospital Association
Jerome G. Green, National Heart, Lung, and Blood Institute
Ping Huang, Veterans Administration
Itzhak Jacoby, National Institutes of Health Office of Medical Applications of Research
Richard J. Jones, American Medical Association
Bryan R. Luce, Battelle Memorial Institute
Harold Margulies, National Center for Health Services Research
Judith D. Moore, Prospective Payment Assessment Commission
Lawrence C. Morris, Jr., Blue Cross and Blue Shield Association
Robert Mosenkis, ECRI
Jay Moskowitz, National Heart, Lung, and Blood Institute
Joel J. Nobel, ECRI
Thomas D. Overcast, Battelle Human Affairs Research Centers
Morton L. Paterson, Smith Kline & French Laboratories
Jonathan A. Showstack, University of California, San Francisco
Elliot Siegel, National Library of Medicine
Kent A. Smith, National Library of Medicine
David Tennenbaum, Blue Cross and Blue Shield Association
Malin VanAntwerp, ECRI
Linda Johnson White, American College of Physicians
Donald A. Young, Prospective Payment Assessment Commission

Joint American College of Cardiology/American Heart Association Task Force on Assessment of Cardiovascular Procedures

Heart House, 9111 Old Georgetown Road
Bethesda, MD 20814
(301) 897-5400

Major Emphases of Technology Assessment Activities

Technology	Concerns: Safety	Efficacy/ Effectiveness	Cost/Cost-Effect/ Cost-Benefit	Ethical/Legal/ Social
Drugs				
Medical Devices/Equipment/Supplies				
Medical/Surgical Procedures	X	X		
Support Systems				
Organizational/Administrative				

Stage of Technologies Assessed
- X Emerging/new
- X Accepted use
- ____ Possibly obsolete, outmoded

Application of Technologies
- ____ Prevention
- X Diagnosis/screening
- X Treatment
- ____ Rehabilitation

Assessment Methods
- ____ Laboratory testing
- ____ Clinical trials
- ____ Epidemiological and other observational methods
- ____ Cost analyses
- ____ Simulation/modeling
- X Group judgment
- X Expert opinion
- X Literature syntheses

Approximate 1985 budget for technology assessment: $12,000*

* This is a rough estimate of the joint ACC/AHA task force budget only, and does not include budgets for other ACC or AHA activities.

JOINT AMERICAN COLLEGE OF CARDIOLOGY/AMERICAN HEART ASSOCIATION TASK FORCE ON ASSESSMENT OF CARDIOVASCULAR PROCEDURES

Introduction

The Joint American College of Cardiology/American Heart Association Task Force on Assessment of Cardiovascular Procedures is a cooperative assessment effort of the two parent organizations, each of which conducts activities related to cardiovascular health.

The American Heart Association (AHA) is a voluntary health agency devoted to the reduction of premature death and disability caused by heart and blood vessel diseases. The association has 55 affiliates nationwide, and its headquarters are in Dallas. In 1984, AHA provided $43.7 million for biomedical research, $24.6 million for public health education, $14.8 million for professional education and training, and $22.6 million for community services.

The American College of Cardiology (ACC) is a 13,500-member, nonprofit professional medical society. The mission of the college is to ensure optimal care for persons with cardiovascular disease or the potential for developing it and, ultimately, through appropriate educational and socioeconomic activities, to contribute to the prevention of cardiovascular disease. Members are physicians and scientists concerned with clinical and basic science disciplines related to the cardiovascular system.

Among its major activities, the ACC conducts a comprehensive program of continuing education and establishes standards of cardiovascular care. The college has three mechanisms for the assessment of new medical knowledge and technology. Two of these, the Cardiovascular Procedures Committee and the Cardiovascular Norms Committee, are described briefly in this introductory section, along with other ACC activities related to assessment. The third, the Joint ACC/AHA Task Force on Assessment of Cardiovascular Procedures, is the main subject of this profile.

The ACC Cardiovascular Procedures Committee reviews requests from federal agencies as well as from the private sector (hospitals, clinics, third-party carriers) relative to standards, criteria, appropriateness, etc., of procedures normally performed in a hospital setting by physicians treating cardiovascular disease. Recommendations are forwarded from this committee to the president of the college. This committee consists of 12 members of the ACC.

The ACC Cardiovascular Norms Committee is a new activity begun in 1983. This committee reviews and assists the Executive Committee of ACC and the president in responding to requests concerning standards of care and in assessing proposed standards or norms of particular interest to the college membership. In addition, this committee obtains consensus on *dynamic norms*—defined by ACC as factors essential for quality care—for the diagnosis and management of the most common cardiac disorders, including considerations of the cost-effectiveness of alternative management plans or diagnostic techniques. This committee consists of eight members of the ACC.

Through these committees and related activities, the ACC has developed positions on such technologies as applicability of and indications for phonocardiography, cardiokymography, ergonovine testing, percutaneous transluminal coronary angioplasty, programmable pacemakers, transtelephonic pacemaker monitoring, and the training requirements for the safe handling of radioisotopes utilized for cardiovascular diagnostic testing. Opinions have been rendered on automated blood pressure monitoring, heparin infusion pumps, diagnostic endocardial electrical stimulation, intraoperative ventricular mapping, Doppler ultrasound, hyperbaric oxygen therapy, photoplethysmography, digital subtraction angiography, and rapid sequence pyelograms.

The ACC has initiated conferences to identify the state of the art on the relative sensitivity, specificity, and indications for diverse techniques in the assessment of ventricular functions. For instance, The Twelfth Bethesda Conference, held in 1981, on noninvasive technology in the assessment of ventricular function was a state-of-the-art conference to develop diagnostic strategies for using various types of echocardiography, nuclear cardiologic techniques, cardiac computed tomography, and digital subtraction angiography.

ACC has testified in support of the National Heart, Lung, and Blood Institute appropriations and authorizations and has supported increased warnings on cigarette packages, the desirability of sodium content labeling for prepared foods, special consideration for orphan drugs, and extension of patent protection time for drugs requiring prolonged clinical testing periods. ACC participates in the Medical Necessity Program of the Blue Cross and Blue Shield Association.

The Joint ACC/AHA Task Force on Assessment of Cardiovascular Procedures (joint task force) first met in November 1981.

Purpose

The purpose of the Joint ACC/AHA Task Force on Assessment of Cardiovascular Procedures (joint task force) is to define the role of noninvasive and invasive procedures in the diagnosis and management of cardiovascular disease. As opposed to the ACC Cardiovascular Procedures and Cardiovascular Norms Committees, which respond to inquiries made by outside parties, the joint task force initiates its own assessments.

Subjects of Assessment

The first assessment to be completed was of cardiac pacemaker implantation, in 1984. Assessments ongoing in 1985 were of exercise stress testing and nuclear imaging procedures. Among other procedures that are under consideration for assessment topics are angiography, Holter monitoring, echocardiography, and intracardiac electrophysiological studies for management of arrhythmias.

Stage of Diffusion

The program is primarily concerned with new and emerging technologies.

Concerns

The joint task force is most concerned with the safety and efficacy of cardiovascular procedures. Specifically, it may address the contribution, uniqueness, sensitivity, specificity, indications, and contraindications of cardiovascular procedures. Although the charge of the joint task force also includes cost-effectiveness as a potential concern, this has not yet been explicitly addressed in deliberations to date.

Requests

It is anticipated that the joint task force will develop most of its assessment topics, although suggestions may come from either the ACC or the AHA, for instance from the ACC Cardiovascular Procedures Committee via the president. The topic of the cardiac pacemaker implantation was generated by the ACC president, and the topics of exercise stress testing and nuclear imaging were generated by the joint task force.

Selection

The topics for assessment are chosen by consensus of joint task force members.

Process

Assessment reports are written by ad hoc subcommittees designated by the joint task force, e.g., the Subcommittee on Pacemaker Implantation. Portions of the reports are drafted first by individual subcommittee members. In addition to sharing the initial drafts with other subcommittee members, the subcommittee members may also seek advice and information from other experts. Subcommittee members then consolidate their section drafts into a single document, which is reviewed by all subcommittee members and which may be shared with other experts for their opinion. In the case of the cardiac pacemaker implantation report, the subcommittee met four times.

The final subcommittee draft is then forwarded to the joint task force for approval. The joint task force meets at least twice a year; its small size enables much of its work to be conducted by telephone and through the mail. Once approved by the joint task force, reports are forwarded to the presidents of ACC and AHA for approval by the organizations' respective ruling bodies. Final approval is given in a letter signed jointly by the presidents of the two organizations. This approval makes the report an official, jointly supported policy statement of the two organizations.

Assessors

The joint task force has a chairman and four other members, two representing ACC and two representing AHA and designated by their respective organizations. The chairperson of the joint task force is selected by agreement of the two organizations. Although it may not always be the case, the chairperson is likely to be a member of one or both organizations. No terms of office have been set for joint task force members. The joint task force selects the subcommittee chairpersons and other subcommittee members. Joint task force members may serve on the subcommittees. Subcommittee members are not necessarily members of either organization and are not necessarily physicians, although all subcommittee members appointed to date have been members of both the ACC and the AHA. Thus far, the number of members on the subcommittees has ranged from 6 to 11. Upon completion of their tasks, the ad hoc subcommittees are dissolved.

Turnaround

Turnaround time for joint task force reports will be variable, depending on the magnitude and complexity of the subject. It is anticipated that for most reports full turnaround time will be approximately 18 months. The time from adoption of cardiac pacemaker implantation as an assessment topic to publication of the report was 21 months. This included a year for appointment and work of the subcommittee and approval by the joint task force, 6 months for final approval by the two organizations, and publication 3 months thereafter.

Reporting

By agreement of ACC and AHA, final assessment reports are published simultaneously in the *Journal of the American College of Cardiology* and *Circulation*, which is published by the AHA. There are 20,000 worldwide individual and organizational subscribers to the *Journal of the American College of Cardiology*, including all ACC members. *Circulation* goes out to 13,000 U.S. and 10,000 overseas subscribers. The reports are also distributed to the other domestic and overseas journals and members of the press, policymakers, and other parties that may be interested in a given topic. Copies are also available on request from the ACC and the AHA.

Impact

There are currently no plans to study the impact of the assessment reports, other than through noting individual reactions to the reports and requests for reprints.

Reassessment

The joint task force will reassess a technology as warranted by new evidence regarding safety, efficacy, and appropriate use.

Funding/Budget

Expenses of the joint task force and staffing are shared equally by the two organizations. The annual budget of the joint task force is approximately $10,000 to $15,000. This amount covers direct costs only, and does not include estimates of indirect costs, the cost of staff time, the value of time provided by the committee members, or publication costs.

Example

On the following pages is the full text of the 1984 report of the Joint ACC/AHA Task Force on Assessment of Cardiovascular Procedures on guidelines for permanent cardiac pacemaker implantation, published in the *Journal of the American College of Cardiology*. It is reproduced here with permission.

Sources

American College of Cardiology. 1982. Twelfth Bethesda Conference: Noninvasive technology in the assessment of ventricular function. American Journal of Cardiology 49:1309–1374.

American College of Cardiology. 1985. Statements of charge: Joint ACC/AHA Task Force on Assessment of Cardiovascular Procedures (and Subcommittees), Cardiovascular Procedures Committee, and Cardiovascular Norms Committee.

American Heart Association. 1984. American Heart Association 1984 Annual Report. Dallas.

Feild, D. J., Director, Special Projects, American College of Cardiology. 1985. Personal communication.

Joint American College of Cardiology/American Heart Association Task Force on Assessment of Cardiovascular Procedures (Subcommittee on Pacemaker Implantation). 1984a. Guidelines for permanent cardiac pacemaker implantation, May 1984. Journal of the American College of Cardiology 4(2):434–442.

Joint American College of Cardiology/American Heart Association Task Force on Assessment of Cardiovascular Procedures (Subcommittee on Pacemaker Implantation). 1984b. Special report: Guidelines for permanent cardiac pacemaker implantation, May 1984. Circulation 70:331A–339A.

Knoebel, S. B. 1983a. President's page: The next challenge and balancing individual quality care with community resources. Journal of the American College of Cardiology 3:972–974.

Knoebel, S. B. 1983b. Presentation to the Department of Health and Human Services Technology Coordinating Committee.

SPECIAL REPORT

Guidelines for Permanent Cardiac Pacemaker Implantation, May 1984

A report of the Joint American College of Cardiology/American Heart Association Task Force on Assessment of Cardiovascular Procedures (Subcommittee on Pacemaker Implantation).

SUBCOMMITTEE MEMBERS

ROBERT L. FRYE, MD, FACC, Chairman
Rochester, Minnesota
JOHN J. COLLINS, MD, FACC
Boston, Massachusetts
ROMAN W. DESANCTIS, MD, FACC
Boston, Massachusetts
HAROLD T. DODGE, MD, FACC
Seattle, Washington
LEONARD S. DREIFUS, MD, FACC
Philadelphia, Pennsylvania
CHARLES FISCH, MD, FACC, Task Force Chairman
Indianapolis, Indiana
LEONARD S. GETTES, MD, FACC
Chapel Hill, North Carolina
PAUL C. GILLETTE, MD, FACC
Charleston, South Carolina
VICTOR PARSONNET, MD, FACC
Newark, New Jersey
T. JOSEPH REEVES, MD, FACC
Beaumont, Texas
SYLVAN LEE WEINBERG, MD, FACC
Dayton, Ohio

Background

It is becoming more apparent each day that despite a strong national commitment to excellence in health care, the resources and personnel are finite. It is, therefore, appropriate that the medical profession examine the impact of developing technology on the practice and cost of medical care. Such analysis, carefully conducted, could potentially impact on the cost of medical care without diminishing the effectiveness of that care.

To this end, the American College of Cardiology and the American Heart Association in 1980 established a Joint Task Force on Assessment of Cardiovascular Procedures with the following charge:

The Joint Task Force of the American College of Cardiology and the American Heart Association shall define the role of specific noninvasive and invasive procedures in the diagnosis and management of cardiovascular disease.
The Task Force shall address, when appropriate, the contribution, uniqueness, sensitivity, specificity, indications and contraindications and cost-effectiveness of such specific procedures.
The Task Force shall include a Chairman and four members, two representatives from the American Heart Association and two representatives from the American College of Cardiology. The Task Force may select ad hoc members as needed upon the approval of the Presidents of both organizations.
Recommendations of the Task Force are forwarded to the President of each organization.

The members of the Joint Task Force are: Roman W. DeSanctis, MD, Harold T. Dodge, MD, T. Joseph Reeves, MD, Sylvan L. Weinberg, MD and Charles Fisch, MD, Chairman.

The Subcommittee on Pacemaker Implantation was chaired by Robert L. Frye, MD and, in addition to the members of the Joint Task Force, included the following ad hoc members: John J. Collins, MD, Leonard S. Dreifus, MD, Leonard S. Gettes, MD, Paul C. Gillette, MD and Victor Parsonnet, MD.

This document was reviewed by the officers and other responsible individuals of the two organizations and received final approval on May 2, 1984. It is being published simultaneously in *Circulation* and *Journal of the American College of Cardiology*. The potential impact of this document on the practice of cardiology and some of its unavoidable shortcomings are clearly set out in the Introduction.

I. Introduction

The joint American College of Cardiology/American Heart Association Ad Hoc Task Force on Assessment of Cardio-

Address for reprints: Mr. David J. Feild, Director, Special Projects, American College of Cardiology, 9111 Old Georgetown Road, Bethesda, Maryland 20811.

0735-1097/84/$3.00

vascular Procedures was formed to make recommendations regarding the appropriate utilization of technology in the diagnosis and treatment of patients with cardiovascular disease. One such important technique is that of cardiac pacing. Rapid progress in a number of areas has led to extraordinary and still evolving advances in implantable cardiac pacemakers and in other devices which electrically stimulate the heart. For this reason, and also because of allegations of abuses of this technology, by the medical profession, the Task Force was assigned the task of defining current indications for permanent cardiac pacemakers. These recommendations are the subject of this report. Because of the multitude, complexity and initial cost of currently available pacing systems, the Subcommittee has included recommendations regarding selection of devices for specific clinical problems in which pacing is indicated. The Subcommittee recommendations are based on current evidence in relation to both knowledge of the natural history of disorders of cardiac rhythm as well as the characteristics of currently available pacemakers. Because of continuing research and development, some of these recommendations may be subject to modification in even the near future.

These recommendations apply to permanent pacing in the management of chronic, though sometimes intermittent, disorders of cardiac rhythm. For the most part, they do not pertain to identifiable factors which cause transient depression of cardiac impulse formation and conduction, such as drugs, electrolyte or endocrine imbalances, infection or the acute phase of myocardial infarction. The decision to implant a pacemaker must be reached by scrupulous adherence to a fundamental principle of clinical medicine which demands a careful, thoughtful analysis of each individual patient by the responsible physician. Attention must be given to the general medical, emotional and mental state of the patient as well as to the specifics of the cardiac rhythm disturbance before a proper decision with respect to pacing can be made.

The Subcommittee has not offered any recommendations regarding resources required to perform pacemaker insertions, training of individuals for this purpose or the appropriate follow-up and monitoring of patients with permanent pacemakers. These critically important topics have been addressed elsewhere (1). The Subcommittee unanimously urges careful review of the resource guidelines by all institutional administrators, physicians and surgeons who are responsible for pacemaker therapy. The clinical symptomatology associated with bradycardia needs definition at the outset since it recurs throughout the report as a major indication for permanent pacemaker therapy. In this report, the term "symptomatic bradycardia" is used to refer to the following clinical manifestations which are directly attributable to the slow heart rate: transient dizziness, light-headedness, near syncope or frank syncope as manifestations of transient cerebral ischemia, and more generalized symptoms such as marked exercise intolerance or frank congestive heart failure.

Indications for permanent pacemakers have been grouped according to the following classifications:

Class I: Conditions for which there is general agreement that permanent pacemakers should be implanted.

Class II: Conditions for which permanent pacemakers are frequently used but there is divergence of opinion with respect to the necessity of their insertion.

Class III: Conditions for which there is general agreement that pacemakers are unnecessary.

In those patients being considered for pacemakers, decision making may be influenced by the following additional factors:

1) overall physical and mental state of the patient, including the absence of associated diseases that may result in a limited prognosis for life;
2) presence of associated underlying cardiac disease that may be adversely affected by bradycardia;
3) desire of the patient to operate a motor vehicle;
4) remoteness of medical care, including patients who travel widely or live alone who therefore might be unable to seek medical help if serious symptoms arise;
5) necessity for administering medication that may depress escape heart rates or aggravate atrioventricular (AV) block;
6) slowing of the basic escape rates;
7) significant cerebrovascular disease that might result in a stroke if cerebral perfusion were to suddenly decrease; and
8) desires of the patient and family.

The format of this report consists of a brief definition and description of specific clinical situations in which pacing may be considered, and literature references to document the basis for the recommendations.

II. Pacing in Acquired Atrioventricular (AV) Block in Adults

Clinically, atrioventricular (AV) block is classified as first degree, second degree or third degree (complete) heart block; anatomically, it is defined as supra-His, intra-His and/or infra-His. Second degree heart block may be further classified as type I (progressive prolongation of PR interval before a blocked beat) or type II (no progressive prolongation of PR interval before blocked beats). "Advanced second degree block" refers to the block of two or more consecutive P waves. Patients with abnormalities of AV conduction may be asymptomatic or they may experience serious symptoms related to profound bradycardia and/or ventricular arrhythmias. Decisions regarding the need for a pacemaker are influenced most importantly by the presence or absence of symptoms that are directly attributable to bradycardia. It is clearly documented that patients with complete heart block and syncope have an improved survival with permanent pacing (2–5). There is no evidence to suggest that survival is prolonged with pacemakers in patients with isolated first degree AV block. The prognosis in type I second degree AV block, when due to AV nodal delay, tends to be benign (6–8). However, in patients with type II second degree AV block (either intra- or infra-His), symptoms are frequent, prognosis is compromised and progression to complete heart block is common (6,8,9).

Recommendations for insertion of permanent pacemakers in patients with AV block with acute myocardial infarction or congenital AV block are discussed in a separate section. AV block in the presence of supraventricular tachyarrhythmia does not constitute an indication for pacemaker insertion except as specifically defined in the recommendations that follow.

Indications for Permanent Pacing in Acquired AV Block in Adults

Class I.

A. Complete heart block, permanent or intermittent, at any anatomic level, associated with any one of the following complications:

1. Symptomatic bradycardia (discussed in the Introduction). In patients with these symptoms in the presence of complete heart block, the symptoms must be presumed to be due to the heart block unless proven to be otherwise.
2. Congestive heart failure.
3. Ventricular ectopy and other conditions that require treatment with drugs which suppress the automaticity of escape foci.
4. Documented periods of asystole of 3.0 seconds or longer, or any escape rate of less than 40 beats/min in symptom-free patients.
5. Confusional states which clear with temporary pacing.

B. Second degree AV block, permanent or intermittent, regardless of the type or the site of the block, with symptomatic bradycardia.

C. Atrial fibrillation, atrial flutter or rare cases of supraventricular tachycardia with complete heart block or advanced AV block, bradycardia and any of the conditions described under I-A. The bradycardia must be unrelated to digitalis or drugs known to impair AV conduction.

Class II.

A. Asymptomatic complete heart block, permanent or intermittent, at any anatomic site, with ventricular rates of 40 beats/min or faster.

B. Asymptomatic type II second degree AV block, permanent or intermittent.

C. Asymptomatic type I second degree AV block at intra-His or infra-His levels.

Class III.

A. First degree AV block (see section on bi-trifascicular block).

B. Asymptomatic type I second degree AV block at the supra-His (AV nodal) level.

III. Pacing in Atrioventricular (AV) Block Associated With Myocardial Infarction

Indications for permanent pacing after myocardial infarction in patients experiencing AV block are related in large measure to the presence of intraventricular conduction defects. The requirement for temporary pacing in acute myocardial infarction does not by itself constitute an indication for permanent pacing. The long-term prognosis in survivors of acute myocardial infarction who have had AV block is related primarily to the extent of myocardial injury and the character of intraventricular conduction disturbances, rather than to the AV block per se (10–14). Patients with acute myocardial infarction who have intraventricular conduction defects, with the exception of isolated left anterior hemiblock, have an unfavorable short- and long-term prognosis and increased incidence of sudden death (10–12). This unfavorable prognosis is not necessarily due to the development of high grade AV block, although the incidence of such block is higher in postinfarction patients with abnormal intraventricular conduction (12). Unlike some other indications for permanent pacing, the criteria in patients with myocardial infarction and AV block do not necessarily depend on the presence of symptoms.

Indications for Permanent Pacing After Myocardial Infarction

Class I.

A. Patients with persistent advanced second degree AV block or complete heart block after acute myocardial infarction (12,14). Decision for insertion of pacemaker should be made before discharge in this group of patients.

Class II.

A. Patients with persistent first degree AV block in the presence of bundle branch block not documented previously (13).

B. Patients with transient advanced AV block and associated bundle branch block.

Class III.

A. Patients in whom AV conduction disturbances are transient in the absence of intraventricular conduction defects (12).

B. Patients with transient AV block in the presence of isolated left anterior hemiblock (11).
C. Patients with acquired left anterior hemiblock in the absence of atrioventricular (AV) block.

IV. Pacing in Bifascicular and Trifascicular Block (Chronic)

Bifascicular and trifascicular block refer to electrocardiographic evidence of impaired conduction below the AV node in two or three of the fascicles of the right and left bundles. In patients with such electrocardiographic abnormalities, there is convincing evidence that advanced heart block with symptoms due to the block is associated with a high mortality and a significant incidence of sudden death (5,15).

Syncope is common in patients with bifascicular block. It is usually not recurrent, nor is it associated with an increased incidence of sudden death (16–18). It has been suggested that although pacing relieves the transient neurologic symptoms, it does not reduce mortaility from sudden death (19). There is convincing evidence, however, that in the presence of complete heart block, either permanent or transient, syncope is associated with an increased incidence of sudden death (5). Thus, being unable to define the cause of syncope in the presence of bifascicular or trifascicular block, it appears reasonable to assume that the syncope may be due to transient complete heart block and, thus, in the opinion of some investigators, prophylactic permanent pacing is indicated (20,21).

Although complete heart block is most often preceded by bifascicular block, the evidence is impressive that the rate of progression of bifascicular block to complete heart block is low. Furthermore, no single clinical or laboratory variable, including bifascicular block, identifies patients at high risk of death from a future bradyarrhythmia due to the bundle branch block (22).

Of the many laboratory variables, the PR and HV intervals have been singled out as possible predictors of complete heart block and sudden death. Evidence indicates that PR prolongation is common in patients with bifascicular block. However, the prolongation is most often at the level of the AV node. Furthermore, there is no correlation between the PR and HV intervals, nor is there a correlation between the length of the PR interval and progression to complete heart block and incidence of sudden death (23,24,28). Although most patients with chronic or intermittent complete heart block demonstrate prolongation of the HV interval during anterograde conduction, and some investigations (26,27) have suggested that asymptomatic patients with bifascicular block and a prolonged HV interval be considered for permanent pacing, the evidence indicates that while the prevalence of prolonged HV is high, the incidence of progression to complete heart block is low. HV prolongation accompanies advanced cardiac disease and is associated with an increased mortality; death is not sudden and is due to the underlying heart disease, and not to complete heart block (16,19, 23,28,29). The prolonged HV interval is, thus, not an independent marker for sudden death (22).

Atrial pacing as a means of identifying patients at increased risk of future complete heart block probably is not justified. The chance of induction of distal heart block with pacing is low (16,27,30,31). In fact, pacing often fails to induce distal His block in patients with documented abnormal conduction of the His-Purkinje system (16,26,27,32,33). Furthermore, failure to induce distal block cannot be taken as evidence that the patient will not develop complete heart block. However, if atrial pacing induces infra-His block, this may be considered an indication for pacing by some (34).

Indications for Permanent Pacing in Bifascicular and Trifascicular Block

Class I.

A. Bifascicular block with intermittent complete heart block associated with symptomatic bradycardia (as defined).
B. Bifascicular block with intermittent type II second degree AV block with symptoms attributable to the heart block.

Class II.

A. Bifascicular or trifascicular block with intermittent type II second degree AV block without symptoms.
B. Bifascicular or trifascicular block with syncope that is not proven to be due to complete heart block, but other possible causes for syncope are not identifiable.
C. Pacing-induced infra-His block.

Class III.

A. Fascicular blocks without AV block or symptoms.
B. Fascicular blocks with first degree AV block without symptoms.

V. Pacing in Sinus Node Dysfunction

Sinus node dysfunction (sick sinus syndrome) constitutes a spectrum of cardiac arrhythmias, including sinus bradycardia, sinus arrest, sinoatrial block and paroxysmal supraventricular tachycardia alternating with periods of bradycardia or even asystole. Patients with this condition may be symptomatic from paroxysmal tachycardia, bradycardia or both. Correlation of symptoms with the specific arrhythmias is essential. This may be difficult, however, because of the intermittent nature of the episodes. Sinus bradycardia is accepted as a physiologic finding in trained athletes, in whom awake resting heart rates of 40 to 50 beats/min are not uncommon and minimal heart rates during sleep may be as slow as 30 to 43 beats/min with sinus pauses as long as 1.6 to 2.8 seconds (35–37). This is due to increased vagal tone. Permanent pacing in patients with sinus node dysfunction may not necessarily result in an improvement in survival (38,39), but severe symptoms related to bradycardia may be relieved (40,41).

Indications for Permanent Pacing in Sinus Node Dysfunction

Class I.

A. Sinus node dysfunction with documented symptomatic bradycardia. In some patients, this will occur as a consequence of long-term essential drug therapy of a type and dose for which there is no acceptable alternative.

Class II.

A. Sinus node dysfunction, occurring spontaneously or as a result of necessary drug therapy, with heart rates below 40 beats/min when a clear association between significant symptoms consistent with bradycardia and the actual presence of bradycardia has not been documented.

Class III.

A. Sinus node dysfunction in asymptomatic patients, including those in whom substantial sinus bradycardia (heart rate <40 beats/min), is a consequence of long-term drug treatment.

B. Sinus node dysfunction in patients in whom symptoms suggestive of bradycardia are clearly documented *not* to be associated with a slow heart rate.

VI. Pacing in Hypersensitive Carotid Sinus Syndrome

The hypersensitive carotid sinus syndrome is defined as syncope resulting from an extreme reflex response to carotid sinus stimulation. It is an uncommon cause of syncope. There are two components to the reflex:

1) *Cardioinhibitory*, resulting from increased parasympathetic tone and manifested by slowing of the sinus rate and/or prolongation of the PR interval and advanced AV block; and
2) *Vasodepressor*, secondary to a reduction in sympathetic activity resulting in hypotension.

Before concluding that permanent pacing is clinically indicated, determination of the relative contribution of the two components of carotid sinus stimulation to the individual patient's symptom complex is essential. Hyperactive response to carotid sinus stimulation is defined as asystole due either to sinus arrest or AV block of more than 3 seconds and/or a substantial symptomatic decrease in systolic blood pressure. However, such heart rate and hemodynamic responses may occur in normal subjects and patients with coronary artery disease (42,43), and a conclusion of a cause and effect relation between the hypersensitive carotid sinus and the patient's symptoms must be made with great caution. Minimal pressure on the carotid sinus in the elderly or patients receiving digitalis may result in marked changes in heart rate and blood pressure, yet not be of clinical significance. Permanent pacing for patients with pure excessive cardioinhibitory response to carotid stimulation is effective in relieving symptoms (44–46). Since 10 to 20% of patients with this syndrome may have an important vasodepressor component, it is necessary to define this before concluding that all symptoms are related to asystole alone. In patients with both cardioinhibitory and vasodepressor components, attention to the latter in patients undergoing permanent pacing is essential for effective therapy.

Indications for Permanent Pacing in Hypertensive Carotid Sinus Syndrome

Class I.

A. Patients with *recurrent* syncope associated with clear, spontaneous events provoked by carotid sinus stimulation, in whom minimal carotid sinus pressure induces asystole of greater than 3 seconds in the absence of any medication that depresses the sinus node or AV conduction.

Class II.

A. Patients with *recurrent* syncope without clear, provocative events and with a hypersensitive cardioinhibitory response.

Class III.

A. Asymptomatic patients with a hyperactive cardioinhibitory response to carotid sinus stimulation.

B. Patients with vague symptoms, such as dizziness and/or light-headedness, and with hyperactive cardioinhibitory response to carotid sinus stimulation.

C. Patients with recurrent syncope, light-headedness or dizziness in whom the vasodepressor response is the cause for symptoms.

VII. The Use of Pacemakers in Children

Although the indications for pacemakers in children are similar to those in adults, there are some special considerations. The optimal indication for a pacemaker implantation in a child, as in an adult, is the concurrent observation of symptoms with bradycardia. For example, a patient with syncope who is observed electrocardiographically to have complete AV block or a patient with syncope who is noted on physical examination to have severe bradycardia such as a heart rate of 30 beats/min. Concurrence of symptoms and bradycardia can also be obtained by 24 hour ambulatory electrocardiography or by transtelephonic electrocardiography. Sometimes several 24 hour recordings are necessary.

Sinus node dysfunction (sick sinus syndrome), although becoming more frequently recognized in pediatric patients, is not in and of itself an indication for pacemaker implantation. In patients with sinus node dysfunction, even greater emphasis is placed on concurrence of sinus bradycardia or exit block with symptoms. Sinus node dysfunction is not likely to be a fatal arrhythmia in infants or children. Therefore, more time can be spent trying to document the presence of an arrhythmia during symptoms.

Symptomatic bradycardia (as defined in the Introduction) with sinus node dysfunction is considered to be an indication for a pacemaker, assuming that another etiology to account for such symptoms has been excluded. Such alternate etiologies to be considered include seizures resulting in hypoxia, breathholding or infantile apnea.

It is sometimes hard to differentiate whether apnea or bradycardia occurs first in symptomatic patients. The bradycardia-tachycardia syndrome is frequently an indication for pacemakers in children, particularly if an antiarrhythmic drug other than digitalis is necessary. It appears that the use of quinidine or other type I drugs is particularly dangerous in children with bradycardia-tachycardia syndrome. Propranolol and amiodarone also severely depress sinus node function and their use may require the use of a pacemaker in children with the bradycardia-tachycardia syndrome.

Indications for Permanent Pacing in Children

Class I.

A. Second or third degree AV block with symptomatic bradycardia as defined.
B. Advanced second or third degree AV block with moderate to marked exercise intolerance.
C. External ophthalmoplegia with bifascicular block (47).
D. Sinus node dysfunction with symptomatic bradycardia as defined.
E. Bradycardia-tachycardia syndrome in a child with a need for antiarrhythmic drugs other than digitalis.
F. Congenital AV block with wide QRS escape rhythm (48).
G. Asymptomatic patients after cardiac surgery with advanced second or third degree AV block persisting 10 to 14 days postoperatively (49).

Class II.

A. Second or third degree AV block within the bundle of His in an asymptomatic patient (49).
B. Prolonged subsidiary pacemaker recovery time (50).
C. Transient surgical second or third degree AV block, which reverts to bifasicular block.
D. Asymptomatic children with second or third degree AV block and a ventricular rate of less than 45 beats/min when awake (51).
E. Asymptomatic infra-His, second or third degree AV block (49).
F. An asymptomatic neonate with congenital complete heart block with bradycardia in relation to age (52).
G. Complex ventricular arrhythmias associated with second or third degree AV block or sinus bradycardia (53).

Class III.

A. Postoperative bifascicular block in the asymptomatic patient.
B. Postoperative bifascicular block with first degree AV block in the asymptomatic patient.
C. Transient surgical AV block that returns to normal conduction in less than 1 week.
D. Asymptomatic type I second degree AV block.
E. Asymptomatic congenital heart block without profound bradycardia in relation to age.

VIII. Pacing for Tachyarrhythmias

The use of implantable cardiac pacemakers to terminate supraventricular or ventricular tachycardias is just beginning. We will not discuss the use of overdrive pacemakers for the termination of ventricular tachycardia, since there is no clinically approved device for this indication and since the use of this device is still extremely controversial with risks perhaps outweighing benefits in some patients. The decision for chronic use of a pacemaker to control tachycardias should be made only after careful observation and electrophysiologic study by those experienced in this complex field.

Indications for Permanent Pacing for Tachyarrhythmias

Class I.

A. Patients with symptomatic supraventricular tachycardia which has not responded to a well planned medical regimen including documentation of adequate serum drug concentrations, or in whom the medical treatment causes major side effects or in whom the necessity for taking drugs seriously inhibits the patient's ability to carry out normal daily function. Before implantation of an antitachycardia pacemaker, an electrophysiologic study should be carried out and the various proposed modes of termination of tachycardia tested to determine which one is most appropriate for the particular patient. An external form of the implantable device should be available during electrophysiologic study to document the exact settings that will be used and will in fact terminate the patient's tachycardia. The physician who implants the pacemaker should be prepared to reprogram the pacemaker to new settings when the patient is again active.

Class II.

None.

Class III.

A. Patients with pre-excitation in whom atrial fibrillation with rapid ventricular response has occurred spontaneously or during electrophysiologic testing.

IX. Clinical Applications of Various Pacing Modes

This section lists the conditions for which various pacing modes might be selected. The acceptability of a given mode of pacing is divided into three classes according to the following definitions:

Class I: Conditions for which there is general agreement that such a mode of pacing is appropriate.

Class II: Conditions for which a given mode of pacing may be used, but there is divergence of opinion with respect to the necessity of that mode of pacing.

Class III: Conditions for which there is general agreement that such a mode of pacing is inappropriate.

Two varieties of pulse generators are available for permanent implantation:

1) single chamber pacemakers (SCP) for use in either atrium or ventricle; and
2) dual chamber pacemakers (DCP) for use in both chambers (usually programmable to SCP modes as well).

Virtually all modern pacemakers are multiprogrammable, which renders them more or less adaptable to changing clinical situations. Some pacing modes that were originally found as specific pacemaker models (such as VOO, VAT and VVT) are not discussed.* These modes are now optional settings of multiprogrammable pacemakers. Many new pacemakers also provide telemetry of stored and variable data that, on command, can provide information about pacemaker function and clinical performance. Both programmability and telemetry are helpful in optimizing pacemaker function, avoiding reoperation and extending pulse generator life. It is essential that the selection process be individualized to the needs of the patient, with appropriate consideration given to complication, complexity and cost.

Single Chamber Pacemakers

I. Atrial (AAI): Atrial pacing inhibited by sensed atrial activity.

Class I.

A. Symptomatic sinus node dysfunction (sick sinus syndrome), provided AV conduction is shown to be adequate by appropriate tests.

Class II.

A. Overdrive of supraventricular or ventricular arrhythmias.

B. Hemodynamic enhancement through rate adjustment in patients with bradycardia and symptoms of impaired cardiac output.

Class III.

A. Pre-existing AV conduction delay or block or if PR interval is inappropriately prolonged by atrial pacing.

B. Inadequate intracavitary atrial complexes.

II. Ventricular (VVI): The classic prototypical pacing mode; ventricular pacing inhibited by sensed spontaneous ventricular activity.

Class I.

A. Any symptomatic bradyarrhythmia, but particularly when there is:
   1) no significant atrial hemodynamic contribution (atrial flutter/fibrillation, giant atria), or
   2) no evidence of pacemaker syndrome due to loss of atrial contribution or negative atrial kick (a replacement pacemaker)†.

Class II.

A. Symptomatic bradycardia, where pacing simplicity is a prime concern, in cases of:
   1) senility (life-sustaining only),
   2) terminal disease,
   3) domicile remote from a follow-up center, or
   4) intact retrograde VA (ventriculoatrial) conduction.

Class III.

A. Known pacemaker syndrome (a replacement pacemaker) or symptoms produced by temporary ventricular pacing at the time of initial pacemaker implantation.

B. The need for maximal atrial contribution, because of:
   1. congestive heart failure, or
   2. special need for rate responsiveness.

Dual Chamber Pacemakers

I. VDD: Ventricular pacing in synchrony with sensed atrial activity, inhibited by sensed ventricular activity. (Although these units are rate-responsive, at a slow atrial rate below the set rate of the pacemaker only the ventricle is paced, in which case the pacemaker functions as a VVI unit.)

*The pacemaker mode is identified according to the Inter-Society Commission for Heart Disease Resources (ICHD) code (1).

†The pacemaker syndrome was first defined as the light-headedness or syncope related to long cycles of AV asynchrony that occurred at times during VVI or VOO pacing. The definition is now expanded to include: 1) episodic weakness or syncope associated with alternating AV synchrony and asynchrony; 2) inadequate cardiac output associated with continued absence of AV synchrony or with fixed asynchrony (persistent VA conduction); and 3) patient awareness of beat to beat variations in cardiac contractile sequence, often as a result of: a) cannon A waves; b) V waves transmitted to the atria or pulmonary veins; and c) bundle branch block patterns of ventricular contraction with a paced beat.

Class I.

A. Requirements for ventricular pacing when adequate atrial rates and adequate intracavitary atrial complexes are present. This includes the presence of complete AV block in patients:

1) requiring atrial contribution for hemodynamic benefit, or

2) with previous or anticipated pacemaker syndrome.

Class II.

A. Normal sinus rhythm and normal AV conduction in patients needing ventricular pacing intermittently.

Class III.

A. Frequent or persistent supraventricular tachyarrhythmias, including atrial fibrillation or flutter.

B. Inadequate intracavitary atrial complexes.

II. DVI: Pacing of both chambers at a preselected minimal rate, inhibited by ventricular but not atrial activity.

Class I.

A. The need for synchronous atrial-ventricular contraction in patients with symptomatic bradycardia and a slow atrial rate.

B. Patients with previously documented pacemaker syndrome.

Class II.

A. Overdrive of certain arrhythmias.

B. Frequent supraventricular arrhythmias in which combined pacing and drugs have been shown to be therapeutically effective.

C. Bradycardia-tachycardia syndrome, provided adjustment of atrial rate and AV interval terminates or prevents the emergence of supraventricular arrhythmias with or without concomitant drug administration.

Class III.

A. Frequent or persistent supraventricular tachyarrhythmias, including atrial fibrillation or flutter.

III. DDD: Pacing of both chambers, sensing of both chambers, inhibition of atrial or ventricular output by sensed atrial or ventricular activity; triggering of ventricular output by sensed atrial activity.

Class I.

A. Requirement for AV synchrony over a wide range of rates such as:

1. the active or young patient with atrial rates responsive to clinical need,
2. significant hemodynamic need, and
3. pacemaker syndrome during previous pacemaker experience, or a reduction in systolic blood pressure of more than 20 mm Hg during ventricular pacing at the time of pacemaker implantation (with or without evidence of VA conduction).

Class II.

A. Complete heart block or sick sinus syndrome and stable atrial rates.

B. Any patient in whom simultaneous control of atrial and ventricular rates inhibits tachyarrhythmias or in whom the pacemaker can be adjusted to a mode designed to interrupt the arrhythmia.

Class III.

A. Frequent or persistent supraventricular tachyarrhythmias, including atrial fibrillation or flutter.

B. Inadequate intracavitary atrial complexes.

References

1. Pacemaker study group, Parsonnet V, Furman S, Smyth PD, et al. Optimal resources for implantable cardiac pacemakers. Circulation 1983;68:225A–44A.
2. Friedberg CK, Donoso E, Stein WB. Nonsurgical acquired heart block. Ann NY Acad Sci 1964;111:833–47.
3. Gadboys HL, Wisoff BG, Litwak RS. Surgical treatment of complete heart block: an analysis of 36 cases. JAMA 1964;189:97–102.
4. Donmoyer TL, DeSanctis RW, Austen WG. Experience with implantable pacemakers using myocardial electrodes in the management of heart block. Ann Thorac Surg 1967;3:21[illegible]–27.
5. Edhag O, Swahn A. Prognosis of patients with complete heart block or arrhythmic syncope who were not treated with artificial pacemakers: a long-term follow-up study of 101 patients. Acta Med Scand 1976;200:457–63.
6. Dhingra RC, Denes P, Wu D, Chuquimia R, Rosen KM. The significance of second degree atrioventricular block and bundle branch block: observations regarding site and type of block. Circulation 1974;49:638–46.
7. Strasberg B, Amat-Y-Leon F, Dhingra RC, et al. Natural history of chronic second-degree atrioventricular nodal block. Circulation 1981;63:1043–9.
8. Donoso E, Adler LN, Friedberg CK. Unusual forms of second-degree atrioventricular block, including Mobitz type II block, associated with the Morgagni-Adams-Stokes syndrome. Am Heart J 1964;67:150–7.
9. Ranganathan N, Dhurandhar R, Phillips JH, Wigle ED. His bundle electrogram in bundle-branch block. Circulation 1972;45:282–94.
10. Ginks WR, Sutton R, Oh W, Leatham A. Long-term prognosis after acute anterior infarction with atrioventricular block. Br Heart J 1977;39:186–9.
11. Col JJ, Weinberg SL. The incidence and mortality of intraventricular conduction defects in acute myocardial infarction. Am J Cardiol 1972;29:344–50.
12. Hindman MC, Wagner GS, JoRo M, et al. The clinical significance of bundle branch block complicating acute myocardial infarction. 2. Indications for temporary and permanent pacemaker insertion. Circulation 1978;58:689–99.
13. Ritter WS, Atkins JM, Blomqvist CG, Mullins CB. Permanent pacing in patients with transient trifascicular block during acute myocardial infarction. Am J Cardiol 1976;38:205–8.
14. Domenighetti G, Perret C. Intraventricular conduction disturbances in acute myocardial infarction: short- and long-term prognosis. Eur J Cardiol 1980;11:51–9.
15. Penton GB, Miller H, Levine SA. Some clinical features of complete heart block. Circulation 1956;13:801–24.
16. Fisch GR, Zipes DP, Fisch C. Bundle branch block and sudden death. Prog Cardiovasc Dis 1980;23:187–224.
17. Dhingra RC, Denes P, Wu D, et al. Syncope in patients with chronic bifascicular block. Significance, causative mechanisms, and clinical implications. Ann Intern Med 1974;81:302–6.
18. DePasquale NP, Bruno MS. Natural history of combined right bundle branch block and left anterior hemiblock (bilateral bundle branch block). Am J Med 1973;54:297–303.

19. Peters RW, Scheinman MM, Modin G, O'Young J, Somelofski CA, Miles C. Prophylactic permanent pacemakers for patients with chronic bundle branch block. Am J Med 1979;66:978–85.

20. Spurrell RAJ, Smithen CS, Sowton E. Study of right bundle-branch block in association with either left anterior hemiblock or left posterior hemiblock using His bundle electrograms. Br Heart J 1972;34:800–6.

21. Kulbertus H, Collignon P. Association of right bundle-branch block with left superior or inferior intraventricular block: its relation to complete heart block and Adams-Stokes syndrome. Br Heart J 1969;31:435–40.

22. McAnulty JH, Rahimtoola SH, Murphy ES, et al. Natural history of "high risk" bundle-branch block: final report of a prospective study. N Engl J Med 1982;307:137–43.

23. Scheinman MM, Peters RW, Modin G, Brennan M, Mies C, O'Young J. Prognostic value of infranodal conduction time in patients with chronic bundle branch block. Circulation 1977;56:240–4.

24. McAnulty JH, Kauffman S, Murphy E, Kassebaum DG, Rahimtoola SH. Survival in patients with intraventricular conduction defects. Arch Intern Med 1978;138:30–5.

25. Denes P, Dhingra RC, Wu D, Wyndham CR, Anat-y-Lean F, Rosen KM. Sudden death in patients with chronic bifascicular block. Arch Intern Med 1977;137:1005–10.

26. Vera Z, Mason DT, Fletcher RD, Awan NA, Massumi RA. Prolonged His-Q interval in chronic bifascicular block: relation to impending complete heart block. Circulation 1976;53:46–55.

27. Narula OS, Gann D, Samet P. Prognostic value of H-V intervals. In: Narula OS, ed. His Bundle Electrocardiography and Clinical Electrophysiology. Philadelphia: FA Davis, 1975:437–49.

28. Denes P, Dhingra RC, Wu D, et al. H-V interval in patients with bifascicular block (right bundle branch block and left anterior hemiblock): clinical, electrocardiographic and electrophysiologic correlations. Am J Cardiol 1975;35:23–9.

29. Probst P, Pachinger O, Murad AA, Leisch F, Kandl F. The HQ time in congestive cardiomyopathies. Am Heart J 1979;97:436–41.

30. Rosen K, Dhingra R, Wyndham C, Bauernfeind R, Sirym S, Denes P. Significance of atrial pacing induced block in the His-Purkinje system in patients with chronic bifascicular block (abstr). Am J Cardiol 1979;43:400.

31. Cheng TO. Atrial pacing: its diagnostic and therapeutic applications. Prog Cardiovasc Dis 1971;14:230–47.

32. Gupta PK, Lichstein E, Chadda KD. Intraventricular conduction time (H-V interval) during antegrade conduction in patients with heart block. Am J Cardiol 1973;32:27–31.

33. Altschuler H, Fisher JD, Furman S. Significance of isolated H-V interval prolongation in symptomatic patients without documented heart block. Am Heart J 1979;97:19–26.

34. Dhingra RC, Palileo E, Strasberg B, et al. Significance of the H-V interval in 517 patients with chronic bifascicular block. Circulation 1981;64:1265–71.

35. Meytes I, Kaplinsky E, Yahini JH, Hanne-Papara N, Neufeld HN. Wenckebach A-V block: a frequent feature following heavy physical training. Am Heart J 1975;90:426–30.

36. Talan DA, Bauernfeind RA, Ashley WW, Kanakis C Jr, Rosen KM. Twenty-four hour continuous ECG recordings in long-distance runners. Chest 1982;82:19–24.

37. Dreifus LS, Michelson EL, Kaplinsky E. Bradyarrhythmias: clinical significance and management. J Am Coll Cardiol 1983;1:327–38.

38. Rasmussen K. Chronic sinus node disease: natural course and indications for pacing. Eur Heart J 1981;2:455–9.

39. Shaw DB, Holman RR, Gowers JI. Survival in sinoatrial disorder (sick-sinus syndrome). Br Med J 1980;280:139–41.

40. Rubenstein JJ, Schulman CL, Yurchak PM, DeSanctis RW. Clinical spectrum of the sick sinus syndrome. Circulation 1972;46:5–13.

41. Kay R, Estiok M, Wiener I. Primary sick sinus syndrome as an indication for chronic pacemaker therapy in young adults: incidence, clinical features, and long-term evaluation. Am Heart J 1982;103:338–42.

42. Heidorn GH, McNamara AP. Effect of carotid sinus stimulation on the electrocardiograms of clinically normal individuals. Circulation 1956;14:1104–13.

43. Brown KA, Maloney JD, Smith HC, Hartzler GO, Ilstrup DM. Carotid sinus reflex in patients undergoing coronary angiography: relationship to degree and location of coronary artery disease in response to carotid sinus massage. Circulation 1980;62:697–703.

44. Walter PF, Crawley IS, Dorney ER. Carotid sinus hypersensitivity and syncope. Am J Cardiol 1978;42:396–403.

45. Peretz DI, Gerein AN, Miyagishima RT. Permanent demand pacing for hypersensitive carotid sinus syndrome. Can Med Assoc J 1973;108:1131–4.

46. Chughtai AL, Yans J, Kwatra M. Carotid sinus syncope: report of two cases. JAMA 1977;237:2320–1.

47. Morriss JH, Eugster GS, Nora JJ, Pryor R. His bundle recording in progressive external ophthalmoplegia. J Pediatr 1972;81:1167–70.

48. Pinsky WW, Gillette PC, Garson A Jr, McNamara DG. Diagnosis, management, and long-term results of patients with congenital complete atrioventricular block. Pediatrics 1982;69:728–33.

49. Gillette PC. Recent advances in mechanisms, evaluation, and pacemaker treatment of chronic bradydysrhythmias in children. Am Heart J 1981;102:920–9.

50. Benson DW Jr, Spach MS, Edwards SB, et al. Heart block in children. Evaluation of subsidiary ventricular pacemaker recover times and ECG tape recordings. Pediatr Cardiol 1982;2:39–45.

51. Karpawich PP, Gillette PC, Garson A Jr, Hesslein PS, Porter C, McNamara DG. Congenital complete atrioventricular block: clinical and electrophysiologic predictors of need for pacemaker insertion. Am J Cardiol 1981;48:1098–102.

52. Michaëlsson M, Engle MA. Congenital complete heart block: an international study of the natural history. Cardiovasc Clin 1972;4:85–101.

53. Winkler RB, Freed MD, Nadas AS. Exercise-induced ventricular ectopy in children and young adults with complete heart block. Am Heart J 1980;99:87–92.

Clinical Efficacy Assessment Project

American College of Physicians
Department of Health and Public Policy
4200 Pine Street
Philadelphia, PA 19104
(215) 243-1200

Major Emphases of Technology Assessment Activities

Technology	Concerns			
	Safety	Efficacy/ Effectiveness	Cost/Cost-Effect/ Cost-Benefit	Ethical/Legal/ Social
Drugs				
Medical Devices/Equipment/Supplies				
Medical/Surgical Procedures	X	X	*	
Support Systems				
Organizational/Administrative				

Stage of Technologies Assessed
_X_ Emerging/new
_X_ Accepted use
____ Possibly obsolete, outmoded

Application of Technologies
_X_ Prevention
_X_ Diagnosis/screening
_X_ Treatment
____ Rehabilitation

Assessment Methods
____ Laboratory testing
____ Clinical trials
____ Epidemiological and other observational methods
____ Cost analyses
____ Simulation/modeling
_X_ Group judgment
_X_ Expert opinion
_X_ Literature syntheses

Approximate 1985 budget for technology assessment: $160,000

* Some CEAP evaluations note comparative costs of procedures, but cost analyses are not conducted.

AMERICAN COLLEGE OF PHYSICIANS CLINICAL EFFICACY ASSESSMENT PROJECT

Introduction

The Clinical Efficacy Assessment Project (CEAP) is a medical technology evaluation program of the American College of Physicians (ACP). The ACP is a 60,000-member national medical specialty society for internists and related subspecialists.

CEAP is an expansion of the college's participation in the Blue Cross and Blue Shield Association's Medical Necessity Project for evaluating the appropriateness of medical procedures, begun in 1976. In early 1981 the project was renamed the Clinical Efficacy Assessment Project and expanded with the assistance of a 3-year grant from the John A. Hartford Foundation. The Hartford Foundation support ended in July 1984. CEAP is now fully supported by the ACP.

Since 1976, ACP has conducted approximately 100 evaluations through the Medical Necessity Project (jointly with Blue Cross and Blue Shield) and CEAP (beginning in 1981).

From 1981 through 1984, CEAP activities have included evaluation, approval, and dissemination of recommendations of over 60 procedures and tests.

Purpose

The purpose of CEAP is to help physicians practice high-quality, more-efficient, and cost-effective medicine. CEAP recommendations provide physicians with current information and guidelines regarding the use of tests, procedures, and therapies and the rationale for such recommendations founded on both the literature and broad-based expert opinion. CEAP's specific objectives are to

1. expand and refine the methods of investigation used under the (Blue Cross and Blue Shield Association) Medical Necessity Project;
2. coordinate the collection, analysis, and dissemination of expert opinion and information obtained from analyses of data to the ACP membership and other interested organizations;
3. utilize an explicit and scientific data-based method for assessing the safety, efficacy, and clinical effectiveness of medical tests and procedures;
4. develop new methods for assessing the safety, efficacy, and clinical effectiveness of medical tests and procedures;
5. study the work of other organizations engaged in similar pursuits throughout the world; and
6. evaluate the impact of CEAP recommendations on costs and use of these medical tests, procedures, and therapies.

Subjects of Assessment

CEAP evaluates medical tests, procedures, and therapeutic interventions within the purview of internal medicine and/or its certified subspecialties, e.g., gastroenterology, cardiology, and oncology.

Stage of Diffusion

CEAP evaluates established technologies, particularly when newly available information indicates that changes in patterns of use might be appropriate. CEAP evaluates new technologies only where data adequate for evaluation are available. It may, however, recommend that appropriate studies be conducted.

Concerns

CEAP evaluates the safety, efficacy, effectiveness, appropriate use, and relative costs of technologies. Where appropriate and possible, the project also considers broader societal implications of technologies. Evaluations may include comparisons of procedures or tests, and some evaluations include cost information where it may affect use of procedures. CEAP findings do not include reimbursement recommendations.

Requests

The CEA Subcommittee will identify technologies that are potential candidates for CEAP evaluations through one or more of the following sources:

1. Internally generated by the CEA Subcommittee by reviewing policy needs, practitioner opinion, academic opinion, recent journal articles, and professional meetings.
2. Recommendations and requests from other ACP committees.
3. Requests by outside organizations.

ACP has considered requests for technology assessment from government agencies, Blue Cross and Blue Shield, other private insurance companies, the Council of Medical Specialty Societies, other medical specialty societies, ACP committees, and ACP members and fellows.

Selection

Assessment topic selection decisions are made by the CEA Subcommittee, following screening by the CEAP staff. The major criteria for CEAP selection of technologies are the following:

1. Degree of interest to practitioners of internal medicine, whether or not internists are directly responsible for its application.

2. Potential for wide application or existing high prevalence of use.
3. Potential for significant benefit if widely applied.
4. Potential for risk if widely applied, particularly in relation to potential for benefit.

In addition, the CEA Subcommittee will consider the feasibility of undertaking an evaluation based on staff capabilities and ACP resources and whether sufficient data are available for evaluation.

CEAP indicates that these selection criteria should be viewed as guidelines only; there may be instances in which the CEA Subcommittee will elect to undertake an assessment for other reasons, such as the request of an agency of government or of another professional body.

Process

The evaluation process is as follows (CEAP Procedural Manual, 1983):

1. *Evaluation is announced, comments invited.* Notices of an impending CEAP evaluation are published in the *Annals of Internal Medicine*, the *New England Journal of Medicine*, and the *ACP Observer*. The notices invite interested parties to send in comments. For special or major evaluations, other specialty journals may be asked to publish notices of CEAP evaluations.

2. *Staff conducts literature review.* The CEAP staff, in consultation with the CEA Subcommittee, selects the appropriate member societies of the Council of Subspecialty Societies (CSS) and the Council of Medical Societies (CMS) (these are advisory councils to the College's Board of Regents) to review the technology in question. These societies are asked to provide opinion and data on the safety, efficacy, effectiveness, and cost of the technology, as well as to identify other experts (proponents, opponents, and those who are neutral on the topic) to provide information on the technology. Data and expert opinion may be solicited from experts recommended by the CSS and CMS societies, the CEA Subcommittee, and the CEAP staff.

3. *Consultants and/or physician staff draft statement.* CEAP staff or outside consultants analyze the literature, review assessments of other organizations, and obtain the opinions of the CSS/CMS members and other experts. CEAP staff or consultants synthesize this information into a draft statement. The draft statement includes a description of the technology and its intended purpose; summaries of the clinical efficacy and effectiveness of the technology; and its safety, appropriate use, and relative costs. Areas requiring further research are also summarized. When necessary, a detailed background paper documenting the conclusions in the summary statement is developed.

4. *Draft statement reviewed by outside experts, including pro, con, and neutral.* The draft statement (including background papers, if any) is submitted to the CEA Subcommittee for its initial review. Following this, the draft statement is sent back to the representatives of CSS, CMS, and the consulting societies and experts for review. In addition, experts from among those who review *Annals of Internal Medicine* manuscripts as well as other identified experts may be asked to review the proposed statement. Attempts are made in each case to identify and ask the opinions of both proponents and opponents of the technology.

5. *Statement amended.* CEAP staff or outside consultants amend the draft based upon review by the CEA Subcommittee and outside experts.

6. *Statement reviewed/approved by CEA Subcommittee.* The draft statement is represented to the CEA Subcommittee along with the following information:

> a. the name of the requesting agency, date of request, dates for the approval to evaluate and for the completion of the evaluation, and the name of the principal author of the statement;
> b. the names of the consulting organizations and experts;
> c. the consultants' statements;
> d. identification of differences of opinion and justification of the proposed CEAP statement when consensus has not been achieved.

7. *Statement reviewed/approved by ACP Health and Public Policy Committee.* Fol-

lowing CEA Subcommittee approval, the draft statement is presented to the ACP Health and Public Policy Committee (HPPC) for approval.

8. *Statement reviewed/approved by ACP Board of Regents.* Following HPPC approval, the draft statement is presented to the Executive Committee of the Board of Regents for approval. The HPPC and the Executive Committee also receive a summary of the process used in formulating the CEAP statement.

CEAP statements range from one paragraph to 10 pages in length. CEAP statements do not have a set format or explicit categories for evaluation findings or recommendations. Statement format depends on the nature of the particular technology evaluated. Generally, however, CEAP evaluation statements include guidelines directed to the clinician which specify the circumstances for which the tests or procedures are indicated, not indicated, or contraindicated. Guidelines usually identify areas where data are inadequate to permit any authoritative recommendation, and recommendations generally specify the nature of research necessary to resolve controversial issues. ACP does not itself sponsor or undertake clinical trials/research.

Assessors

CEAP evaluations are conducted in a cooperative effort of the CEA Subcommittee, outside experts, and CEAP staff, as described above under Process. The six-member CEA Subcommittee that governs CEAP has experience in medicine, clinical epidemiology, statistics, decision analysis, technology assessment, economics, and public policy. CEA Subcommittee members are appointed by the Chairman of the ACP Board of Regents, subject to approval by the board, for 1-year terms, and they may be reappointed.

From 1978 to 1980, the ACP Medical Practice Committee responded to Blue Cross and Blue Shield Medical Necessity requests regarding appropriateness of procedures. In 1981, that committee coordinated CEAP activities. Beginning in 1982, the ACP established the CEA Subcommittee.

Turnaround

Most CEAP evaluations are completed within 6 to 9 months of selection for evaluation.

Reporting

Approved CEAP statements appear in press releases. All CEAP statements are summarized in the *ACP Observer*, and some are published in full in the *Annals of Internal Medicine*. Statements and background papers are disseminated to the medical community (ACP membership, medical organizations, practicing physicians, medical journals, and the medical educational system), reimbursers, and other policymakers. Statements are also available to the public. Private letters are sent to the original questioner. Table A-1 lists the CEAP evaluation statements issued since 1981.

Impact

The CEAP grant from the Hartford Foundation included an agreement with the Blue Cross and Blue Shield Association to evaluate the impact of CEAP recommendations. The purposes of this study are to discover the impact of CEAP on other organizations and how the recommendations affect physician behavior and health care costs. The results of the organizational survey show that all 50 CEAP statements issued between 1981 and 1983 were used for educational and/or policy-setting purposes. None of the 238 respondents stated disagreement with the recommendations or found them to be unhelpful. The protocol for measuring the impact of CEAP statements on health care costs is currently being designed.

In its final report to the Hartford Foundation, ACP concluded that CEAP enabled the College to (1) design a workable and credible system for evaluating technologies; (2) demonstrate that a professional society can assess the practices of its members and achieve their acceptance of the assessments; (3) stimulate other organizations' involvement in CEAP and in the development of their own assessment projects; and (4) develop the protocol

TABLE A-1 Approved CEAP Recommendations, 1981 through early 1985

1981

1. Ultrasonic arteriography
2. Use of ultrasonic arteriography in distinguishing diseases of the carotid artery system
3. Gastric analysis by the capsule method (Heidelberg)
4. Intracutaneous titration
5. Estrogen pellet implantation
6. Management of histapenia
7. Activated prothrombin complex concentrate in patients with hemophilia A and inhibitor antibodies to factor VIII
8. Human tumor cell drug sensitivity assay in the treatment of solid tumors
9. 24-hour sphygmomanometry
10. Ergonovine provocative testing (reconsidered in 1983)
11. Percutaneous transluminal coronary angioplasty (reconsidered in 1983)
12. 25 hydroxyvitamin D level test
13. Intravenous histamine therapy
14. Hyperbaric oxygen therapy in the treatment of arthritis
15. Pneumococcal vaccine

1982

16. Phonocardiography
17. Cardiokymography
18. Antilymphocyte and antithymocyte globulin in renal transplantation
19. Hyperbaric oxygen therapy in the treatment of actinomycosis
20. Hyperbaric oxygen therapy in the treatment of chronic osteomyelitis
21. Immunotherapy of cancer
22. Bentonite flocculation test
23. DNA antibody test
24. Kunkel test (total serum gamma globulin)

Respiratory therapy modalities:

25. Intermittent positive pressure breathing
26. Incentive spirometry
27. Postural drainage with or without chest wall manipulation
28. Aerosol therapy
29. Oxygen therapy

1983

Breath tests for diagnosing digestive disorders:

30. Breath hydrogen lactose intolerance test for diagnosing lactose
31. Lactulose breath test for small intestinal transit time and small intestinal overgrowth
32. $^{13}CO_2$ breath test for diagnosing fat maldigestion and malabsorption
33. $^{13}CO_2$ breath test for diagnosing bile acid malabsorption

34. Hyperbaric oxygen therapy of chronic and acute peripheral vascular insufficiency
35. Hyperbaric oxygen therapy in treatment of acute, traumatic peripheral ischemia
36. Hyperbaric oxygen therapy in the treatment of senility

Selected methods for the management of diabetes mellitus:

37. Computerized blood glucose insulin infusion devices
38. External infusion pump for treatment of diabetes
39. Home blood glucose monitoring
40. Pancreas transplantation for treatment of diabetes mellitus

41. Automated ambulatory blood pressure monitoring
42. Hepatitis B vaccine
43. Topical oxygen therapy for the treatment of decubitus ulcers
44. Ergonovine provocative testing for coronary artery spasm (supersedes 1981 recommendation)
45. Dexamethasone suppression test for the detection, diagnosis, and management of depression
46. Implantable and external infusion pumps for the treatment of thromboembolic disease in outpatients

TABLE A-1 *Continued*

Percutaneous transluminal angioplasty:
47. Coronary arteries (supersedes 1981 recommendation)
48. Iliac, femoral, popliteal arteries
49. Renal arteries
50. Carotid, vertebral, subclavian arteries

1984
51. Apheresis in the treatment of chronic, severe rheumatoid arthritis (supersedes 1980 recommendation)
52. Diagnostic endocardial electrical recording and stimulation
53. Endoscopic sclerotherapy of esophageal varices
54. Radiologic methods to evaluate bone mineral content
55. Endoscopic retrograde cholangiopancreatography (ERCP)
56. Glycosylated hemoglobin assays in the management of diabetes mellitus
57. Biofeedback for gastrointestinal disorders
58. Biofeedback for headaches
59. The use of diagnostic tests for screening and evaluating breast lesions
60. Endoscopy in the evaluation of dyspepsia

1985
61. Biofeedback for hypertension
62. Biofeedback for neuromuscular disorders
63. Colonoscopy: management of colorectal neoplasia
64. The safety and efficacy of ambulatory cardiac catheterization in the hospital and free-standing setting (supersedes 1980 recommendation)
65. Lithotripsy
66. Pneumococcal vaccine (supersedes 1981 recommendation)
67. Diagnostic spinal tap
68. Diagnostic thoracentesis and pleural biopsy
69. Apheresis for chronic inflammatory demyelinating polyneuropathy and renal transplantation
70. Automated ambulatory blood-pressure monitoring
71. Cardiokymography (supersedes 1982 recommendation)

for a network of physicians to collect data on their actual use of tests, procedures, and therapies.

Reassessment

At intervals following approval of a CEAP statement, staff members accept comments and solicit advice from the relevant CSS/CMS members and/or other experts as to the availability of any important new information on the technology previously reviewed. If substantive new information is available, the CEA Subcommittee will consider re-evaluating the topic. The CEA Subcommittee also considers requests from ACP members and others for re-evaluation of a statement when the request is accompanied by compelling documentation. Re-evaluation is subject to the process described above. The following are examples of technologies reassessed by CEAP.

- *Cytotoxic food testing* was determined in a 1979 CEAP statement to have no scientific basis. In 1981 CEAP found it to be as yet unproven and requiring further testing.
- *Ergonovine provocative test* was considered in 1981 to be standard and efficacious clinically when performed in a cardiac catheterization laboratory in patients who do not have documented fixed coronary obstructive lesions at angiography. In 1983 the CEAP statement notes that while the procedure involves serious potential risks and thus is generally performed in a cardiac catheterization

laboratory, it may also be safely done in a critical care unit in carefully selected patients who are treated strictly according to a well-tested protocol.

• *Percutaneous transluminal angioplasty for coronary arteries* (PTCA) was found in 1980 to be an investigative procedure. In a 1983 statement, CEAP suggests that PTCA is an alternative to coronary artery bypass graft surgery in patients with high-grade stenosis (greater than 50 to 70 percent) confined to a single coronary artery and limiting anginal symptoms despite an adequate trial of medical treatment.

• *Plasmapheresis in the management of rheumatoid arthritis* did not meet the standards of clinical efficacy according to a 1980 CEAP statement that indicated it should be performed only as part of a disciplined clinical investigative effort. In 1984 CEAP again found apheresis for rheumatoid arthritis to be investigational, though patients with life-threatening rheumatoid vasculitis may be candidates for a trial course of plasmapheresis.

Funding/Budget

The John A. Hartford Foundation grant for the support of the CEAP demonstration project was $650,412 over 3.5 years, from January 1981 through July 1984. The approximate 1985 budget for the program is $160,000. Regardless of further foundation support, ACP is committed to continuing CEAP. No charges are made for CEAP evaluations.

Example

On the following pages is the 1984 CEAP recommendation on endoscopy in the evaluation of dyspepsia. The recommendation was published in the *Annals of Internal Medicine*, 102:266–269, 1985, and is reproduced here with permission.

Sources

American College of Physicians. 1983a. Fact Sheet: Clinical Efficacy Assessment Project (CEAP). Philadelphia.

American College of Physicians. 1983b. Clinical Efficacy Assessment Project Procedural Manual. Philadelphia.

American College of Physicians. 1983c. Clinical Efficacy Assessment Project Final Report. December 31. Philadelphia.

Ball, J. R., and L. J. White. American College of Physicians. 1985. Personal communications.

Health and Public Policy Committee, American College of Physicians. 1985. Endoscopy in the Evaluation of Dyspepsia. Annals of Internal Medicine 102:266–269.

Reprinted from ANNALS OF INTERNAL MEDICINE Vol. 102; No. 2 February 1985
Reprinted in USA

Endoscopy in the Evaluation of Dyspepsia

HEALTH AND PUBLIC POLICY COMMITTEE,* AMERICAN COLLEGE OF PHYSICIANS; Philadelphia, Pennsylvania

DYSPEPSIA, frequently seen in the general population by primary care physicians and gastroenterologists, has been a common indication for esophagogastroduodenoscopy. Any recommendations regarding the use of this technique in patients with dyspepsia depend on a precise definition of the symptom. The term "dyspepsia," however, represents a vague grouping of upper abdominal symptoms that may be manifested by various underlying illnesses and pathophysiologic findings. The basic element of dyspepsia is epigastric pain or discomfort, accompanied by fullness, burning, belching, bloating, nausea, vomiting, fatty food intolerance, or difficulty completing a meal; bowel habits generally remain unaltered. Despite the difficulties in precisely defining dyspepsia, most studies agree that the pathologic finding common in dyspeptic patients may be classified as either gastric ulcer, duodenal ulcer, gastric cancer, or non-ulcer non-cancer dyspepsia (1-15).

Heartburn, a hot or burning sensation located in the substernal region, is often related to position and is generally distinguishable from dyspepsia by researchers, clinicians, and patients. The symptoms of biliary colic, visceral pain characterized by a severe, steady ache, are usually distinguishable from the epigastric discomfort identified as dyspepsia. In fact, cholecystitis has been included as a cause of dyspepsia in only a few studies, usually in referred patients. Because the literature and the clinical research describing the evaluation of heartburn and biliary colic are generally distinct from that describing dyspepsia, they will not be considered in this review. This statement addresses the clinical efficacy of esophagogastroduodenoscopy in the evaluation of patients with dyspepsia as an isolated symptom. These patients will be distinguished from patients who have dyspepsia in addition to weight loss, severe systemic illness, obstruction, perforation, or multisystem disease.

Esophagogastroduodenoscopy is a diagnostic technique that offers clinical information regarding the patient's gastrointestinal symptoms by allowing visual inspection of the mucosal surfaces of the esophagus, stomach, and duodenum. Most fiberoptic endoscopes are approximately 1 metre in length, have a visual field width of 85 to 105 deg, and a shaft that contains channels for passage of biopsy forceps, cytology brushes, and washing or suction catheters (16, 17). The technique generally requires 15 to 30 minutes, including the time for premedicating the patient (18, 19). The examination may be done in the hospital, ambulatory clinic, or physician's office.

Safety

Upper gastrointestinal endoscopy has a small but definite risk of complications. Any estimate of the complication rate in a patient with dyspepsia is limited, because indications for endoscopy are only rarely mentioned in reports. A 1974 survey by the American Society for Gastrointestinal Endoscopy of 211 410 procedures showed an overall complication rate of 0.13% (20). The major complications were perforation (0.03%), bleeding (0.03%), cardiopulmonary problems (0.06%), and infection (0.008%). It seems reasonable to assume that the already low complication rate for esophagogastroduodenoscopy in general is even lower when considering the rate of complication in the dyspeptic patient who will usually be less sick than the patient with gastrointestinal bleeding.

Costs

Standard texts of gastroenterology, as well as the American Society for Gastrointestinal Endoscopy, have ascribed to financial considerations the usual sequence of an upper gastrointestinal barium study preceding esophagogastroduodenoscopy in the evaluation of the dyspeptic patient (21-23). However, the advent of newer endoscopes, the training of more endoscopists, the reduction in the time to do a complete esophagogastroendoscopic examination, in conjunction with the high predictive value of this technique, have led some to suggest a need to reevaluate its costs. Although not generally mentioned, other costs must also be considered (18). When endoscopy is done in a hospital rather than a physician's office, a hospital room fee is also charged. Charges submitted for diagnostic esophagogastroduodenoscopy by individual physicians in 1983 for Medicare patients in six geographic regions averaged $325 with a range from $145 to $900. The initial cost of an endoscope and light source ranges from $10 000 to $20 000. The charges for upper gastrointestinal series generally do not exceed $150 including both physician and procedure charges. The cost

*This paper was authored by Katherine Kahn, M.D., and Sheldon Greenfield, M.D., and was developed for the Health and Public Policy Committee by the Clinical Efficacy Assessment Subcommittee: Donald E. Olson, M.D., *Chairman*; David Banta, M.D.; Howard S. Frazier, M.D.; Richard B. Hornick, M.D.; Seymour Perry, M.D.; and Willis C. Maddrey, M.D. Members of the Health and Public Policy Committee for the 1984-85 term include Edwin P. Maynard III, M.D., *Chairman*; John H. Eisenberg, M.D.; Richard G. Farmer, M.D.; Daniel D. Federman, M.D.; John R. Hogness, M.D.; Leo E. Hollister, M.D.; Charles E. Lewis, M.D.; Donald E. Olson, M.D.; Malcolm L. Peterson, M.D.; Theodore B. Schwartz, M.D.; and Helen L. Smits, M.D. This paper was adopted by The Executive Committee of the Board of Regents on 16 November 1984.

of medical therapy with either liquid antacids, cimetidine, or both, ranges from $35 to $60 per month (24).

Efficacy

Evaluation of the efficacy of esophagogastroduodenoscopy depends on the prevalence of the disease conditions underlying the symptom, the cost and effectiveness of diagnostic modalities, and the effect this technique will have on patient outcome. Diagnostic options include prescribing an immediate upper gastrointestinal barium series, immediate esophagogastroduodenoscopy, or empiric treatment with a subsequent diagnostic investigation. Most reports have described the diagnostic sequence of upper gastrointestinal barium series for patients with dyspepsia followed by esophagogastroduodenoscopy for suspicious lesions (1, 21, 22).This strategy is based on the perceived need for early diagnosis and the low cost of upper gastrointestinal series compared to that of esophagogastroduodenoscopy.

In order to further conserve costs while maintaining benefits, alternative strategies must be considered. One strategy is to treat empirically all patients with dyspepsia who do not have clinically obvious serious disease by withdrawing offending agents (ethyl alcohol, ulcerogenic medications, and cigarettes) and by prescribing antacids or H_2 blockers. Patients with clinically obvious serious conditions such as weight loss, severe systemic illness, bleeding, perforation, symptoms of upper gastrointestinal obstruction, or other evidence for cancer should have prompt diagnostic investigation.

The following five reasons support the initial use of clinical appraisal followed by response to an empiric course of therapy in patients with uncomplicated dyspepsia. Esophagogastroduodenoscopy would be reserved for patients who remain symptomatic or have a relapse.

First, only 20% of patients with dyspepsia have an ulcer disease: either duodenal ulcer (range, 7% to 34%), or gastric ulcer (range, 2% to 20%) (1-15). Fewer than 1% of patients with dyspepsia will have cancer (2, 4, 5, 11, 12). The prevalence of gastritis, duodenitis, or erosions (non-ulcer dyspepsia) is difficult to quantify, but the range reported in the literature is from 5% to 40%. The remainder of patients have dyspepsia without apparent pathologic characteristics despite endoscopic or radiographic evaluation. These estimates for specific disease entities may be high because information about the prevalence of associated diseases is closely linked to the setting in which the information was obtained (5, 12). In fact, the changing practices of some segments of the American population toward visiting the physician after a shorter duration of symptoms may dramatically lower the prevalence rates of dyspepsia-associated diseases (25). Although esophagogastroduodenoscopy as an initial diagnostic approach might offer additional diagnostic information, the marginal value of such information must be assessed. Initial therapy for patients with dyspepsia as an isolated symptom remains the same whether the diagnosis is duodenal ulcer, gastric ulcer, gastroduodenitis, or even normal mucosa. Although a visual image of the gastrointestinal mucosa allows a more precise diagnosis, the value of such information is minimal if it does not change patient management or outcome.

Second, if gastric cancer occurred frequently, for example, in greater than 5% of patients with dyspepsia, endoscopic diagnosis in all dyspeptic patients might be appropriate. However, in primary care practice the prevalence will be lower, probably less than 1%. No physician wants to overlook a case of highly curable cancer. But in this country, the detection rate of early gastric cancer has not increased to more than approximately 6% of those stomach cancers found (26-32). Using a prevalence of 1% of dyspeptic patients having cancer, and 6% of those cancer patients having early gastric cancer, 6 per 10 000 dyspeptic patients will have early gastric cancer. Although the 5-year survival rate for gastric cancer detected early is 95%, the infrequency of early detection leaves the overall 5-year survival for gastric cancer in this country at 10% with an occasional 5-year survival rate at 30% (33). It is not known precisely how many of the patients with potentially curable early gastric cancer will progress to higher, less curable stages if esophagogastroduodenoscopy is delayed 6 to 8 weeks in favor of empiric treatment, but there is no evidence to suggest that it is more than a few. It is difficult to justify performing immediate esophagogastroduodenoscopy or upper gastrointestinal series on all patients with dyspepsia in the expectation of curing cancer.

Third, the history of treated ulcer disease must be considered. Fifteen percent of patients with gastric ulcer will have a persistent ulcer crater after 8 weeks of therapy despite having complete resolution of symptoms (34). Of these asymptomatic patients with persistent gastric ulcer, it is safe to assume that most will heal even without therapy, because the healing rate for patients with gastric ulcers treated with placebo is up to 68% at 12 weeks. For patients who become asymptomatic while being treated, many will have recurrence of symptoms after therapy is discontinued and at that time may receive esophagogastroduodenoscopy. Of patients whose gastric ulcer requires more than 9 weeks to heal, between 55% and 89% may have a recurrent ulcer within the year (35-37). Many of these patients would then be endoscopically examined for symptom recurrence. The same is true for patients with duodenal ulcer in whom approximately 50% to 85% recur within the year (38). Virtually all patients with refractory ulcers will be identified by the recurrence of symptoms after therapy is withdrawn. There is no evidence that the complication rate among patients treated initially with empiric therapy and endoscopically examined later for recurrent or persistent symptoms should be any higher than in those patients diagnosed initially by esophagogastroduodenoscopy.

Fourth, approximately 70% of patients with gastric (or duodenal) ulcer or mucosal disease will become asymptomatic within several weeks after institution of therapy (34, 38). In the absence of symptom recurrence, they will require no further diagnostic evaluation. In addition, patients who have symptom recurrence after therapy will require further diagnostic evaluation.

Fifth, the effect of an empiric trial of therapy on patients who do not have an ulcer or gastroduodenitis must be considered. Studies have shown that some patients with normal findings on radiography and endoscopy have histologic evidence for acute or chronic gastroduodenitis (39-41). Some fraction of patients with dyspeptic symptoms, who do not have peptic disease by any criteria, will have symptom resolution with empiric treatment. Limiting the treatment period to 6 to 8 weeks will avoid chronic usage of unnecessary medication. The persistence of symptoms despite 6 to 8 weeks of therapy or the exacerbation of symptoms during therapy, must result in further diagnostic evaluation.

Use of the proposed strategy would provide empiric therapy as the initial approach to patients with dyspepsia as an isolated symptom. Endoscopy will be reserved for two subsets of patients: those who have no or minimal response to therapy after 7 to 10 days; and the approximately 30% of patients whose symptoms persist, improved but not resolved, after a 6- to 8-week period. If all dyspeptic patients are treated empirically, considerable diagnostic resources will be saved.

After selecting this group of patients with refractory symptoms, the question must be asked whether the usual pattern of upper gastrointestinal series tests followed by esophagogastroduodenoscopy is still the appropriate sequence. It can be argued that the higher false-negative rate of greater than 18% and the false-positive rate of between 13% and 35% for the upper gastrointestinal series is unacceptable for this small group of patients who are refractory to treatment or at higher risk of cancer (42-56). Further, the use of double contrast reduces the false-negative rate only to between 9% and 17% and the false-positive rate to between 8% and 11% (46, 51, 53, 54). In addition, barium studies do not allow the opportunity for biopsy or cytologic examination that is indicated in patients with radiographic lesions considered to be suspicious. To detect cancer or to decide on long-term or modified therapy, the more accurate diagnostic modality of esophagogastroduodenoscopy is preferable.

Recommendation

Considering the available data on costs and benefits, as well as the relationships between diagnoses, treatments, and patient outcomes, it seems prudent to adopt strategies that reduce financial costs, yet retain the potential for appropriate patient management. Reserving the use of diagnostic esophagogastroduodenoscopy for those patients with symptoms despite 6 to 8 weeks of therapy provides a strategy for cost reduction while maintaining prudent patient care. Those patients who have no response to therapy after 7 to 10 days, those who develop complications of peptic disease, those who show signs of a severe systemic illness, and those with symptom recurrence should receive diagnostic evaluation earlier in the course of their illness. Adoption of this recommendation must be modified in the light of each patient's clinical presentation, including patients at high risk or with multisystem problems.

ACKNOWLEDGMENTS: The Clinical Efficacy Assessment Project (CEAP) of the American College of Physicians is designed to evaluate and inform College members and others about the safety and efficacy of diagnostic and therapeutic modalities. Evaluation of technologies begins with a notice in *Annals of Internal Medicine* and the *ACP Observer* inviting comments. Appropriate members of the Council of Medical Societies and the Council of Subspecialty Societies as well as other experts are asked to review technologies. The CEAP statements thus represent a synthesis of the literature and expert opinion and are intended to reflect the current state-of-the-art knowledge concerning a technology. Statements may be reconsidered as new information becomes available.

Grant support: The development of this paper by the Clinical Efficacy Assessment Project was funded by the John A. Hartford Foundation.

▶ Requests for reprints should be addressed to Linda Johnson White; Clinical Efficacy Assessment Project, Department of Health and Public Policy, American College of Physicians, 4200 Pine Street; Philadelphia, PA 19104.

References

1. Data base on dyspepsia [Editorial]. *Br Med J.* 1978;**6121**:1163-4.
2. MOLLMANN KM, BONNEVIE O, GUDBRAND HOYER E, WULFF HR. A diagnostic study of patients with upper abdominal pain. *Scand J Gastroenterol.* 1975;**10**:105-9.
3. BARNES RJ, GEAR MWL, NICOL A, DEW AB. Study of dyspepsia in a general practice as assessed by endoscopy and radiology. *Br Med J.* 1974;**4**:214-6.
4. KIIL J, ANDERSON D. X-ray examination and/or endoscopy in the diagnosis of gastroduodenal ulcer and cancer. *Scand J Gastroenterol.* 1979;**15**:39-43.
5. READ L, PASS TM, KOMAROFF AL. Diagnosis and treatment of dyspepsia, a cost effectiveness analysis. *Med Decis Making.* 1982;**2**:416-38.
6. HORROCKS JC, DE DOMBAL FT. Clinical presentation of patients with dyspepsia, detailed symptomatic study of 360 patients. *Gut.* 1978;**19**:19-26.
7. RINALDO JA JR, SCHEINOK P, RUPE CE. Symptoms diagnosis: a mathematical analysis of epigastric pain. *Ann Intern Med.* 1963;**59**:145-54.
8. ROSS P, DUTTON AM. Computer analysis of symptom complexes in patients having upper gastrointestinal examinations. *Dig Dis Sci.* 1972;**17**:248-54.
9. SCHEINOK PA, RINALDO JA JR. Symptom diagnosis: optimal subsets for upper abdominal pain. *Comput Biomed Res.* 1967;**1**:221-36.
10. COLCHER H. Current concepts, gastrointestinal endoscopy. *N Engl J Med.* 1975;**293**:1129-31.
11. MARTON KI, SOX HC, WASSON J, DUISENBERG CE. The clinical value of the upper gastrointestinal tract roentgenogram series. *Arch Intern Med.* 1980;**140**:191-5.
12. MEAD GM, MORRIS A, WEBSTER GK, LANGMAN MJS. Uses of barium meal examination in dyspeptic patients under 50. *Br Med J.* 1977;**1**:1460-1.
13. LIEBLING PO. The use and abuse of barium meals. *Practitioner.* 1966;**196**:695-702.
14. GEAR MWL, BARNES RJ. Endoscopic studies of dyspepsia in a general practice. *Br Med J.* 1980;**280**:1136-7.
15. FISHER JA, SURRIDGE JG, VARTAN CP, LOEHRY CA. Upper gastrointestinal endoscopy—a GP service. *Br Med J.* 1977;**2**:1199-1201.
16. VENNES JA, SILVERSTEIN FE. UGI fiberoptic endoscopy. In: SLEISENGER MH, FORDTRAN JS, eds. *Gastrointestinal Disease.* Philadelphia: W.B. Saunders; 1983:1599-1615.
17. HIRSCHOWITZ BI. Endoscopic examination of the stomach and duodenal cap with the fiberscope. *Lancet.* 1961;**1**:1074.
18. SHOWSTACK JA, SCHROEDER SA, STEINBERG HR. Evaluating the costs and benefits of a diagnostic technology. *Med Care.* 1981;**19**:498-509.
19. TEDESCO FJ, GRIFFIN JW, CRISP WL, ANTHONY HF JR. Skinny upper gastrointestinal endoscopy—the initial diagnostic tool: a prospective comparison of upper gastrointestinal endoscopy and radiology. *J Clin Gastroenterol.* 1980;**2**:27-30.
20. SILVIS SE, NEBEL O, ROGERS G. Endoscopic complications: results of the 1974 American Society for Gastroenterology Survey. *JAMA.* 1976;**235**:928-30.
21. AMERICAN SOCIETY FOR GASTROINTESTINAL ENDOSCOPY. *The Role of Endoscopy in the Management of Patients with Duodenal Disease, Guidelines for Clinical Application.* The Standards of Training and Practice Committee. American Society for Gastrointestinal Endoscopy; 1978.
22. RICHARDSON CT. Gastric ulcer. *Gastrointestinal Disease.* In: SLEISENGER MH, FORDTRAN JS, eds. Philadelphia: W.B. Saunders; 1983:672-93.
23. SPIRO H. *Clinical Gastroenterology.* New York: Macmillan Publishing Co., Inc; 1983:304-54.
24. *The Redbook Drug Topic.* Oradell, New Jersey: Medical Economics Co., Inc.; 1984:68, 311.
25. NEWHOUSE J, MANNING W, MORRIS C, et al. Some interim results

from a controlled trial of cost sharing in health insurance. *N Engl J Med.* 1981;**305:**1501-7.
26. Cady B, Ramdsen D, Stein A, Haggitt RC. Gastric cancer: contemporary aspects. *Am J Surg.* 1977;**133:**423-9.
27. Morrissey JF. The diagnosis of early gastric cancer: a survey of experience in the United States. *Gastrointest Endoscopy.* 1976;**23:**13-5.
28. Adashek K, Sanger J, Longmire WP. Cancer of the stomach: review of consecutive ten year intervals. *Ann Surg.* 1979;**189:**6-10.
29. Dupont JB, Rillens Lee J, Burton GR, Cohn I Jr. Adenocarcinoma of the stomach: review of 1,497 cases. *Cancer.* 1978;**41:**941-7.
30. Olearchyk AS. Gastric carcinoma: a critical review of 243 cases. *Am J Gastroenterol.* 1978;**70:**25-45.
31. Evans DMD, Craven JL, Murphy F, Cleary BK. Comparison of early gastric cancer in Britain and Japan. *Gut.* 1978;**19:**1-9.
32. Sugawa C, Schuman BM. *Primer of Gastrointestinal Fiberoptic Endoscopy.* Boston: Little Brown & Co; 1981.
33. Kasuagi T; Kobayashi S. Evaluation of biopsy and cytology in the diagnosis of gastric cancer. *Am J Gastroenterol.* 1974;**62:**199.
34. Isenberg JI, Peterson WL, Elashoff JD, et al. Healing of benign gastric ulcer with low-dose antacid or cimetidine: a double-blind randomized placebo-controlled trial. *N Engl J Med.* 1983;**308:**1319-24.
35. Pipe DW, Shinners J, Greig M, Thomas J, Waller SL. Effect of ulcer healing on the prognosis of chronic gastric ulcer. *Gut.* 1978;**19:**419-24.
36. Jensen KB, Mollmann KM, Rahbek I, Madsen JR, Rune SJ, Wulff HR. Prophylactic effect of cimetidine in gastric ulcer patients. *Scand J Gastroenterol.* 1979;**14:**175-6.
37. Machell RJ, Ciclitira PJ, Farthing MJG, Dick AP, Hunter JO. Cimetidine in the prevention of gastric ulcer relapse. *Postgrad Med J.* 1979;**55:**393-5.
38. Ippoliti AF, Sturdevant RA, Isenberg JI, et al. Cimetidine versus intensive antacid therapy for duodenal ulcer. *Gastroenterology.* 1978;**74:**393-5.
39. Greenlaw R, Sheahan DC, DeLuca VA, Miller D, Myerson D, Myerson P. Gastroduodenitis—a broader concept of peptic ulcer disease. *Dig Dis Sci.* 1980;**25:**660-72.
40. DeLuca VA, Winnan G, Sheahan DC, et al. Is gastroduodenitis part of the spectrum of peptic ulcer disease? *J Clin Gastroenterol.* 1981;**3:**17-22.
41. Lagarde S, Spiro H. Non-ulcer dyspepsia. *Clin Gastroenterol.* 1984;**13:**437-46.
42. Waye JD. The current state of esophagoscopy, gastroscopy, and duodenoscopy. *Mt Sinai J Med.* 1975;**42:**57-80.
43. Knutson CO, Max MH, Ahmad W, Polk HC Jr. Should flexible fiberoptic endoscopy replace barium contrast study of the upper gastrointestinal tract? *Surgery.* 1978;**84:**609-15.
44. Martin TR, Vennes JA, Silvis SE, Ansel HJ. A comparison of upper gastrointestinal endoscopy and radiography. *J Clin Gastroenterol.* 1980;**2:**21-5.
45. Martin TR, Vennes JA, Silvis SE, Ansel HJ. UGI endoscopy vs. radiography: is radiography obsolete? *J Clin Gastroenterol.* 1980;**2:**27-30.
46. Montagne J, Moss AA, Margulis AR. Double-blind study of single and double contrast upper gastrointestinal examinations using endoscopy as a control. *Am J Roentgenol.* 1978;**130:**1041-5.
47. Tedesco FJ, Best WR, Littman A, et al. Role of gastroscopy in gastric ulcer patients: planning a prospective study. *Gastroenterology.* 1977;**73:**170-3.
48. Weinstein WM. Gastroscopy for gastric ulcer. *Gastroenterology.* 1977;**73:**1160-2.
49. Cumberland DC. Fibre-optic endoscopy and radiology in the investigation of the upper gastrointestinal tract. *Clin Radiol.* 1975;**26:**223-36.
50. Dekker W, Tytgat GN. Diagnostic accuracy of fiber-endoscopy in the detection of upper intestinal malignancy, a follow-up analysis. *Gastroenterology.* 1977;**73:**710-4.
51. Herlinger H, Glanville JN, Kreel L. An evaluation of the double contrast barium meal (DCBM) against endoscopy. *Br Med J.* 1977;**28:**307-14.
52. Laufer I, Mullens JE, Hamilton J. The diagnostic accuracy of barium studies of the stomach and duodenum—correlation with endoscopy. *Radiology.* 1975;**115:**569-73.
53. Laufer I. Assessment of the accuracy of double contrast gastroduodenal radiology. *Gastroenterology.* 1976;**71:**874-8.
54. Rogers IM, Sokhi GS, Moule B, Joffe SN, Blumgart LH. Endoscopy and routine and double-contrast barium meal in diagnosis of gastric and duodenal disorders. *Lancet.* 1976;**1:**901-2.
55. Salter RH. Upper-gastrointestinal endoscopy in perspective. *Lancet.* 1975;**2:**863-4.
56. Schuman BM. The gastroscopic yield from the negative upper gastrointestinal series. *Gastroenterol Endosc.* 1972;**19:**79-82.

Hospital Technology Series Program
American Hospital Association
Division of Technology Management and Policy
840 North Shore Drive
Chicago, IL 60611
(312) 280-6026

Major Emphases of Technology Assessment Activities

Technology	Concerns: Safety	Efficacy/ Effectiveness	Cost/Cost-Effect/ Cost-Benefit	Ethical/Legal/ Social
Drugs				
Medical Devices/Equipment/Supplies		X	X	
Medical/Surgical Procedures				
Support Systems		X	X	
Organizational/Administrative				

Stage of Technologies Assessed
_X_ Emerging/new
_X_ Accepted use
____ Possibly obsolete, outmoded

Application of Technologies
____ Prevention
_X_ Diagnosis/screening
_X_ Treatment
____ Rehabilitation

Assessment Methods
____ Laboratory testing
____ Clinical trials
____ Epidemiological and other observational methods
_X_ Cost analyses
____ Simulation/modeling
____ Group judgment
_X_ Expert opinion
_X_ Literature syntheses

Approximate 1985 budget for technology assessment: $250,000

AMERICAN HOSPITAL ASSOCIATION HOSPITAL TECHNOLOGY SERIES PROGRAM

Introduction

The American Hospital Association (AHA) initiated the Hospital Technology Series program in 1982. This program is a health care technology evaluation and information dissemination program targeted to the hospital administrator. It is coordinated by the AHA Division of Technology Management and Policy. The Hospital Technology Series provides three publications (described below under Reporting), including *Guideline Reports*, which features AHA technology evaluations.

Purpose

The primary purpose of the AHA Hospital Technology Series program is to assist hospital administrators in making prudent and informed management and investment decisions regarding new and existing technologies.

Subjects of Assessment

The Hospital Technology Series program evaluates diagnostic, therapeutic, and support systems and technologies. The program deals primarily with service implications of technological advances from the hospital's perspective. The program generally does not evaluate procedures, although they are discussed insofar as they bear upon strategic equipment and service choices.

Stage of Diffusion

The program is concerned with new and existing technologies.

Concerns

AHA evaluations are primarily concerned with the cost and service implications of technologies that are entering clinical practice. They also consider manufacturer issues, such as vendor stability, the capacity for technologies to be upgraded, and other compared attributes of competing technologies. Evaluations published in *Guideline Reports* emphasize what to look for in acquiring and managing technologies. Although evaluations do not include brand name ratings, they sometimes provide brand-specific information on commercially available equipment, such as cost and installation information, service support arrangements, etc. Specifically, AHA evaluations are most concerned with the following:

1. cost and organizational implications;
2. installation costs;
3. staffing and training requirements;
4. probable number of patients affected;
5. effects on other hospital resources, e.g., the extent to which a technology will enable the replacement of existing resources, or the extent to which it will necessitate the addition of new resources; and
6. clinical effectiveness: not patient outcomes per se, but effects on the use of hospital resources, such as inpatient versus outpatient stay, average length of stay, etc.

Requests

Topics originate with program staff.

Selection

Subjects for assessment are selected on the basis of a staff review of their importance to hospital management, especially their impact on costs.

Process

The evaluations are syntheses of the literature, focused interviews with manufacturers and users, and compilations of reported user-based experience in such matters as negotiating purchase contracts, common mistakes made in implementation, etc. Outside consultants are frequently used in these evaluations.

Assessors

Evaluations are conducted by staff of the AHA Division of Technology Management and Policy, with the assistance of outside consultants.

Turnaround

Evaluations generally require about 6 months from the time of selection to the finished report.

Reporting

Evaluation findings are reported in *Guideline Reports* issued as the evaluations are completed. This is one of three publications of the AHA Hospital Technology Series, which includes the following:

- *Guideline Reports*: evaluations of specific hospital technologies; approximately eight distributed per year to member hospitals. By 1984, AHA had completed approximately 20 guideline reports.
- *Executive Briefing*: an overview of major developments affecting hospitals' use of technology in the delivery of patient care. Directed to hospital chief executive officers (CEOs); distributed monthly.
- *Technology Scanner*: a collection of categorized summaries of articles relevant to hospital technology, drawn from 70 medical and technical journals. Directed to hospital administrators; distributed monthly.

Guideline Reports include annual compilations of the technology assessments conducted by the Office of Health Technology Assessment of the Public Health Service for the Health Care Financing Administration

(HCFA) to assist HCFA in making Medicare coverage decisions. A listing of *Guideline Reports* issued by AHA is shown in Table A-2. Selected *Guideline Reports* and other program reports are summarized in *Hospitals* magazine.

TABLE A-2 Guideline Reports Issued by the AHA Hospital Technology Series, 1982–1985

Diagnostic Systems and Technologies
Nuclear Magnetic Resonance (NMR)
Computerized Tomographic Scanners
Digital Subtraction Angiography
Echocardiography
Computerized Arrhythmia Monitoring Systems
Automated Indirect Blood Pressure Measurement Devices
Trends in Nuclear Medicine
NMR—Issues for 1985 and Beyond
Therapeutic Systems and Technologies
Evaluation Methods for Intensive Care Unit Systems
Automated Infusion Devices
Autotransfusion Units
Adult Volume Ventilators
Lithotripters
Computer Technologies
Clinical Laboratory Information Systems
Materials Management Information Systems
Microcomputers in Hospitals
Other Technology-Related Reports
Medicare Technology Assessments: 1981
Medicare Technology Assessments: 1982
Medicare Technology Assessments: 1983
Ethylene Oxide Sterilization
Buying and Selling Used Medical Equipment
Purchasing a Satellite Receiving Earth Terminal
Equipment Acquisition Under Prospective Payment
A Medical Device Recall and Reporting System
Bar Code Technology—Applications in Health Care

The AHA Hospital Technology Series, including *Guideline Reports*, is available at a yearly subscription cost of $150; individual issues of *Guideline Reports* can also be ordered separately at a nominal fee.

Impact

Approximately 1,250 U.S. hospitals subscribe to the Hospital Technology Series.

Reassessment

Technologies will be reassessed subject to perceived need of hospitals and new information. Reassessments will follow the same format as the original assessments.

Funding/Budget

The annual budget of the Hospital Technology Series program is approximately $250,000. Program support is derived from subscription fees.

Example

On the following pages is a technology briefing excerpted by AHA from its February 1985 *Guideline Report* "NMR—Issues for 1985 and Beyond." The full 235-page report is available from AHA.

Sources

American Hospital Association. 1983. Hospital Technology Series (pamphlet). Chicago.

American Hospital Association. 1985. AHA Hospital Technology Series Guideline Report: NMR—Issues for 1985 and Beyond (technology briefing excerpt). Chicago.

Goodhart, M., Manager, Technology Policy, American Hospital Association. 1985. Personal communications.

NUCLEAR MAGNETIC RESONANCE

A technology briefing excerpted from NMR--Issues for 1985 and Beyond, a Hospital Technology Series guideline report.

Nuclear magnetic resonance, (NMR) is a diagnostic imaging modality that uses magnetic and radio-frequency fields to image body tissue and monitor body chemistry non-invasively. It uses no ionizing radiation or contrast agents, and is unimpeded by bone. Because it is so highly sensitive and safe, it is becoming a replacement for some CT as well as an array of invasive, often risky procedures such as myelography and angiography.

Yet the rate of diffusion of this technology may not be proportional to its clinical superiority because NMR is reaching the health care marketplace at a time when the economic climate is volatile. The hospital that purchases prematurely without carefully weighing the options, risks, and benefits associated with NMR could find itself in severe financial difficulties. At the same time the hospital that fails to provide access to the modality could find itself at a considerable competitive disadvantage, particularly if neurology, cardiology, and/or oncology account for a substantial percentage of admissions. Once today's better educated, better informed health care consumers, and their referring physicians truly understand the technology and the advantages it can offer in terms of cost avoidance and reduced patient risk and suffering, they are likely to demand NMR services and seek them elsewhere if the hospital can't provide them. Conversely, the hospital that competes in these areas and does offer NMR could enjoy a competitive edge. Because of the recent wide availability of mobile systems NMR has become an important issue for smaller hospitals as well as larger ones. These and other factors make the decision to invest in NMR a difficult one.

Determining the need for NMR

Some clinical applications save money

By eliminating the need for many other exams, biopsies, and exploratory surgical procedures, NMR could eventually save health care dollars and substantially reduce risk and discomfort to the patient. For example, today contrast enhanced CT and myelograms are used to diagnose tumors in the posterior fossa of the brain or on the spinal column. Abdominal aortic aneurysms often require angiography. Examining the prostate gland to determine the cause of an enlargement usually requires biopsy or exploratory surgery. NMR has already demonstrated its ability to minimize the need for some of these procedures or to displace them entirely as well as to shorten the hospital stay usually associated with them.

AHA has identified some 40 cost saving applications, 19 of which are essentially here now and would clearly save money if employed. Based on clinical experience with only 7 of the 19 currently available cost saving applications, we estimate (we believe conservatively) that NMR should eliminate at least 20% of CT head, 7.5% of body, 28% of major vessel angiography, and 50% of kidney angiography. We also believe that targeting research efforts intensively in these specific areas could do much to encouage more universal reimbursement.

Projecting utilization

Key to assuring that your financial projections are accurate, and to securing CON approval, is a reliable utilization projection. Seven methodologies are currently in use, the most popular of which was developed by NMR Inc., a joint venture of three community hospitals in Omaha. It scores the percentage of patients for whom NMR would be indicated in each of over 250 ICD-9-CM categories. To project utilization for any individual hospital or group of hospitals, the number of patients discharged in each category can be multiplied by the percentage figure for that category, and the total of all categories computed.

Factors that may distort your projections

A number of planners have argued that this and other similar methodologies now in use are inherently conservative for several reasons. First of all, they are based on inpatient data, even though most of the NMR exams will probably be performed on outpatients. This is misleading, however, because many of those who are screened for serious conditions by NMR on an outpatient basis, and who may even be treated in ambulatory surgery facilities or receive radiation therapy on an outpatient basis, are eventually treated as inpatients. Only primary diagnoses are used to calculate percentages even though secondary diagnoses could also trigger use of NMR; only one NMR scan per patient is assumed when scans may be multiple, especially for cancer patients; and only current clinical applications are used to calculate the patient base.

Two additional factors could lead to inaccurate projections. Although the radiologists who determined the weighting percentages obviously have some knowledge of NMR's progress from attending professional meetings and reading the literature, few, if any, have had direct clinical experience with NMR. This could lead them to embrace more or fewer applications than would radiologists who have direct experience. Also the degree of superiority of NMR to various other less expensive tests has yet to be fully explored. In many cases a sophisticated, and expensive modality such as NMR may not be needed, and if so, NMR should not be substituted for the lower cost technique, even if that technique is somewhat cruder. Thus listing NMR as appropriate for treating certain disease categories when lower-cost options already exist could result in counting duplicative tests that will eventually be eliminated, and which for the moment would only serve to inflate the percentages.

To respond to these and other issues raised, AHA developed its own model. We subjected 321 ICD-9-CM categories to a panel of NMR experts, each of whom has had access to an NMR unit for a couple of years, and some of whom are published authorities in the field of NMR. We solicited an independent judgment from each panelist as to the percentage of NMR use in each of the ICD-9-CM categories. That disagreement as to what constitutes accepted use for NMR surfaced is hardly surprising. We eliminated those categories where disagreement was substantial.

The result is a conservative model for projecting utilization based on current clinical applications. Using this model, we forecast 1.8 million patients annually would need scans. When followup procedures on these patients are added the total number of scans becomes 2.9 million annually. Followup procedures were calculated by using an accepted methodology for computing followup procedures for CT. By interfacing our NMR model with the CT model, we estimated that overall NMR will replace 34% of CT. The greatest area of impact on CT is projected to be in the area of nervous system disease (94% replacement), circulatory system disease (75% replacement) and neoplasms (30% replacement).

Selecting the magnet

High field strength or low field strength - which is best?

No issue is more hotly debated than that of the relative superiority of high field strength to low field strength systems. Unfortunately, the heat of this debate has exaggerated the differences. In most NMR applications, the hydrogen atom is resonated to produce the images. This is called proton-imaging and it can be performed at high or low field strengths. The difference (if it exists at all) between proton images produced at high field strengths and those produced at low field strengths, in terms of throughput or quality, appears to be small.

The debate obscures the basic difference between high and low field strength systems which is that only high field strength systems will be useful for non-proton imaging applications (where atoms other than hydrogen atoms are resonated to produce the image) and spectroscopy. As far as proton imaging is concerned, the better low field systems always seem to be able to match and, in some cases and for certain applications, exceed the performance capabilities of the higher field strength systems, producing very high quality images within reasonable time frames. We predict most of the improvements that will come in proton imaging will probably be due to improvements in coil technology (particularly surface coils) and not to increases in the strength of the magnetic field. The significant contribution of high field strength is likely to be in spectroscopy applications.

The future of spectroscopy

Spectroscopy is a non-invasive technique for measuring biochemical changes in tissue that signal the onset of disease long before other symptoms appear. If it succeeds, it could eventually replace invasive biopsy. Spectroscopy, however, is still very much in the experimental stage. It is possible only on the higher field strength systems, and is often cited as a reason for purchasing a higher field strength system. We contend that potential purchasers should not tell themselves that "high field strength will allow us to do spectroscopy", but rather ask the question "What kind of spectroscopy will be possible with the 1.5T or 2T units available today, and what can we use it for?" A number of recent developments show that the 1.5T to 2T systems can produce phosphorus spectra that yield some useful information. However, the high resolution phosphorus spectra of small, well localized tissue masses that physicians predict will be useful have not yet been produced on current high field strength systems. Some researchers think this kind of spectra can be generated at 1.5T; others believe it possible only at much higher field strengths of 4T or 8T. It will be a few years before the clinical significance of spectroscopy can be determined. Because the field strength debate is far from being resolved, we conclude that the decision to purchase a higher field strength system should be based on careful monitoring and assessment of whether or not high resolution spectra of small, well localized tissue masses can eventually be produced at fields of 1.5T to 2T. Current high field strength systems cost nearly twice as much as the lower field strength systems when the additional architectural costs are included, and the number of applications of low field strength systems is already large.

The progress of reimbursement

Much of the optimism about the progress of reimbursement is based on encouraging results of surveys taken of private commercial insurance carriers who are exhibiting a growing willingness to pay. One of these surveys, recently conducted by Mobile Technology Inc., showed that 71% of the top 30 private insurance carriers now pay for NMR services according to company policy guidelines or on a case-by-case basis. This represents an increase of 50% in just four months according to survey researchers.

However, most Blue Cross/Blue Shield plans, and HCFA do not yet pay for NMR. If they decide to continue to refuse payment for NMR, or if they establish criteria that are highly specific, the encouraging trend could shift dramatically. Given the wide applicability of NMR technology, and the mounting pressure to contain costs, we find it likely that the reimbursement authorities will be more restrictive and/or indication-specific with respect to NMR than they were with respect to CT. Near term, this is likely to alter projected revenue streams from NMR services. The Hospital Technology Series will continue to monitor developments in the national reimbursement policy for NMR.

Staffing

Radiologists will need about a year and a half of training in order to fully understand the technology and be able to use it most effectively although some diagnostic skills can be learned in about three months. While NMR images look much like the images produced by CT scanning, the technology that underlies the composition of those images is vastly different. The radiologist unfamiliar with NMR will see structures that look familiar but won't understand why something shows up or fails to show up, and will have to learn how to select a pulse sequence appropriate for detecting the suspected disease. Who will pay for this training looms as a major issue. Introduction of NMR technology can also be expected to raise some turf and staffing issues. These are discussed in a special section of the report to help you better anticipate the length of time you need to allocate for personnel training, and to alert you to political problems you may need to resolve.

Choosing your manufacturer

It pays to select both your architect and your manufacturer carefully.

Manufacturers have varying degrees of expertise in site design and the cost of installing the same magnet can vary as much as $100,000 from one manufacturer to another. Improvements in shielding systems and availability of self-shielding superconducting systems even for the higher field strength units have brought construction costs down.

Fifteen manufacturers now produce NMR units, and the number of available magnet types is now eight. An NMR unit can cost from $600,000 to $2.5 million. Some magnet systems are mobile and can be installed in trailers and moved from site to site. These can make the technology available to the smaller institutions on a shared basis, and to institutions in remote locations. In the future, smaller, special purpose, less expensive units for imaging specific areas of the body can be expected. Clinical trials are supposed to begin shortly for one such head-only permanent magnet system, which is expected to sell for only $600,000. With so many options, and so many manufacturers competing for your business you will need to know the strengths and weaknesses of each to decide which one will be most able to support both your present and projected needs.

To assist you in choosing an appropriate manufacturer, we have compiled a list of 243 hospital and nonhospital installations of NMR systems worldwide through 1985, by manufacturer. It is published in NMR--Issues for 1985 and Beyond, copies of which can be purchased from AHA Services, Inc., 4444 W. Ferdinand, Chicago, IL 60624. The cost is $35 for AHA members; $45 for nonmembers. Quantity discounts are available, and an order form is attached for your convenience.

Diagnostic and Therapeutic Technology Assessment Program
American Medical Association
535 North Dearborn Street
Chicago, Illinois 60610
(312) 645-5000

Major Emphases of Technology Assessment Activities

Technology	Concerns: Safety	Efficacy/ Effectiveness	Cost/Cost-Effect/ Cost-Benefit	Ethical/Legal/ Social
Drugs	X*	X*		
Medical Devices/Equipment/Supplies	X*	X*		
Medical/Surgical Procedures	X	X		
Support Systems				
Organizational/Administrative				

Stage of Technologies Assessed
X Emerging/new
X Accepted use
___ Possibly obsolete, outmoded

Application of Technologies
___ Prevention
X Diagnosis/screening
X Treatment
___ Rehabilitation

Assessment Methods
___ Laboratory testing
___ Clinical trials
___ Epidemiological and other observational methods
___ Cost analyses
___ Simulation/modeling
___ Group judgment
X† Expert opinion
X Literature syntheses

Approximate 1985 budget for technology assessment: $380,000

* Drugs and medical devices involved in DATTA assessments are addressed insofar as they are applied in medical and surgical procedures, e.g., chelation therapy or application of implantable infusion pump. Particular brand-name products are not compared or assessed as such.

† The program polls a panel of experts regarding their rating of a technology, but panel members do not interact as a group in formulating the DATTA opinion.

AMERICAN MEDICAL ASSOCIATION DIAGNOSTIC AND THERAPEUTIC TECHNOLOGY ASSESSMENT PROGRAM

Introduction

The American Medical Association (AMA) is a national organization of 260,000 member physicians. The AMA provides technology assessment information in several ways. This profile is devoted primarily to the AMA Diagnostic and Therapeutic Technology Assessment Program (DATTA).

AMA's primary channel of evaluative information is its 27 scientific publications, especially the *Journal of the American Medical Association* (*JAMA*). The AMA also provides assessment information through the reports of the Council on Scientific Affairs. Since its creation in 1976, the council has published over 100 reports developed with the assistance of staff, often supported by ad hoc expert panels, dealing with advances or controversies in diagnostic, therapeutic, and other medical technologies. Many council reports have been published in *JAMA*. Since 1979, the Council on Scientific Affairs has issued reports such as the following:

- The Indications for Aortocoronary Bypass Graft Surgery
- Exercise Programs in Rehabilitation of Patients with Coronary Heart Disease
- Indications and Contraindications for Exercise Testing
- Organ Donation and Transplantation
- The Importance of Diagnostic Computerized Tomographic Scanning
- Maternal Serum Alpha-Fetoprotein Screening
- Acupuncture
- Electronic Fetal Monitoring
- Continuous Ambulatory Peritoneal Dialysis
- Cochlear Implants
- Percutaneous Transluminal Angioplasty

In each case the Council appoints medical expert panels who are knowledgeable in the procedure and can address the issue in detail. These panels are usually comprised of 6 to 10 physicians.

DATTA was instituted by the American Medical Association in 1982. All DATTA opinions appear in *JAMA*. The first DATTA reports were published in *JAMA* in 1983. The service is under the aegis of the AMA Council on Scientific Affairs.

Purpose

DATTA was developed for establishing a mechanism within AMA to briefly and promptly answer questions that might arise on the safety, effectiveness, and level of acceptance in clinical practice of medical technologies.

Subjects of Assessment

DATTA primarily assesses diagnostic and therapeutic procedures and technologies. Preventive and rehabilitative technologies may also be assessed by DATTA, but they have not yet been subject to full assessments.

Stage of Diffusion

DATTA assesses new and existing technologies. Possibly obsolete or outmoded technologies also have been dealt with by DATTA, but they have not yet been subject to full assessments.

Concerns

DATTA assessments are concerned with the safety and effectiveness of diagnostic and therapeutic procedures and technologies, consonant with available peer-reviewed information.

Requests

DATTA considers requests for assessment from any source as long as they are clearly stated in writing and focused so that a clear opinion can be rendered. Questions generally present matters of controversy in the clinical community. The AMA prefers that requests be accompanied by appropriate bibliographic references or suitable documentation that will help to justify the question.

Selection

The AMA responds to thousands of inquiries annually regarding information on assessment of diagnostic and therapeutic procedures and technologies, particularly established technologies. Inquiries are handled by AMA staff, principally those in the two science divisions and the medical library. Those not appropriate for DATTA may be referred elsewhere within AMA for response. In addition to DATTA, inquiries may be referred to the AMA library, the "Questions and Answers" section of *JAMA*, the Council on Scientific Affairs, or other AMA councils and departments.

The selection of questions for DATTA is made by staff under the direction of the DATTA Subcommittee of the Council of Scientific Affairs, which reserves the right to accept, reject, or revise the wording of ques-

TABLE A-3 DATTA Assessments and Technology Ratings, 1983–1985

Assessment Topic (*JAMA* volume:page)	Panel Rating
1983	
Quantitative EEG [Fast Fourier Transform Analysis] Monitoring (250:420)	No consensus
Radial Keratotomy[a] (250:420)	Investigational
Diathermy (250:540)	Established
Mandatory ECG Before Elective Surgery (250:540)	Established
Carbon Dioxide Laser Treatment of Gynecologic Malignant Neoplasms (250:672)	Established
Chelation Therapy for Atherosclerotic Disease (250:672)	Unacceptable
Implantable Infusion Pump[a] (250:1906)	Investigational
Biofeedback (250:2381)	Established
24-Hour Ambulatory EEG Monitoring (250:3340)	Established
1984	
Whole-Body Hyperthermia Treatment of Cancer[a] (251:272)	Investigational
Apnea Monitoring for Newborns at Risk of Sudden Death Syndrome (251:531)	No consensus
Cranial Electrostimulation (251:1094)	Investigational/ unacceptable
Cardiokymography for Noninvasive Cardiological Diagnosis (251:1094)	Investigational/ indeterminate, not acceptable
Diaphonography [Transillumination of the Breast] for Cancer Screening (251:1902)	Investigational
Bone Marrow Transplantation in Childhood Leukemia (251:2155)	Established (majority), investigational (minority)
Implanted Electrospinal Stimulator for Scoliosis (251:2723)	Investigational
Gastric Restrictive Surgery for Morbid Obesity (251:3011)	No consensus
Noninvasive Extracorporeal Lithotripsy[a] (252:3301)	Investigational (78%)[b], other (22%)
Percutaneous Nephrolithotomy (252:3301–3302)	Established (74%)[b], investigational or indeterminate (26%)
Endoscopic Transurethral Nephrolithotomy (252:3302)	Investigational (78%)[b], established (22%)
1985	
Continuous Arteriovenous Hemofiltration (253:1325–1326)	
—for fluid removal in refractory fluid overload or acute renal failure	Established (60%)[b], other (40%)
—for uremia in acute renal failure	Established (53%), other (47%)
Endoscopic Management of Gastrointestinal Tract Hemorrhage (253:2732–2735)	
—laser photocoagulation —thermal coagulation —electrocoagulation —topical therapy	[Published DATTA report cites panelists' ratings by number and percentage of each of these four types of endoscopic treatments, as applied for each of three or four anatomic sites, respectively: esophagus, stomach-duodenum, small intestine, and colon.][b]
Diagnostic Intraoperative Ultrasound (254:285–287)	Established (44%)[b], investigational (42%), indeterminate (12%), unacceptable (2%)

TABLE A-3 *Continued on next page*

NOTE: The DATTA reports and panel ratings in this table were published in the *Journal of the American Medical Association*. See *JAMA* for full wording of DATTA topic questions and complete report narratives. The manner in which panel ratings are reported by DATTA has evolved since the program's inception. Panel ratings cited here do not fully reflect the discussions of DATTA opinions provided in the published DATTA reports.
[a] Panel ratings have been suspended and assessments reopened for these technologies. The panel rating for whole-body hyperthermia treatment for cancer was updated in September 1984 to *established* for certain indications.
[b] Percentages cited for panel ratings reflect only those panelists offering opinions. For some assessments, more than half of the panelists surveyed offered no opinion.

tions. DATTA will not undertake assessment of the safety and efficacy of a drug or medical device for a use that is included in FDA-approved labeling. It may, however, evaluate the safety, efficacy, and indications for use of a drug or device that are not included in FDA-approved labeling.

Process

Questions approved for DATTA are prepared by staff for evaluation by panelists. This includes stating the question so that it can be answered according to a standardized format. DATTA staff researches questions for background information in the peer-reviewed literature and seeks information on existing assessments (completed or in preparation) from other organizations, including appropriate medical specialty societies. Where appropriate, information regarding regulatory status of drugs and medical devices is obtained from the FDA. Information on the subject of a question is made available to panelists on request to the AMA library, but otherwise does not accompany the DATTA questionnaire that is sent to panelists.

DATTA panels comprise at least 40 physicians selected by DATTA staff from a large reference panel. Procedures or therapies which are the subject of DATTA questions are rated by the panelists as

- established (limitations explained for general use, if appropriate);
- investigational (limited to use under research protocol);
- unacceptable;
- indeterminate/no consensus to date (evidence insufficient for decision); or
- no opinion (panelist has insufficient experience with the technology).

Panelists are also asked to comment on specific knowledge of controlled trials, their experience with the technology, overall benefits and risks associated with the technology, and special populations or patients for whom different ratings may be appropriate. Panelists do not review each other's opinions as a group. DATTA assessments are based upon the extent of agreement of the individual panelists. As is evident from Table A-3, published DATTA panel ratings have become more descriptive since the program's inception. Since mid-1984, published DATTA assessment panel ratings have reflected divisions of opinion, and now do so in quantitative terms, including the number of panelists offering no opinion.

In addition to the ratings of established, investigational, unacceptable, or indeterminate, DATTA opinions as published in *JAMA* include a narrative explanation of literature reports and panel findings. All DATTA opinions are reviewed and approved by the DATTA Subcommittee of the Council on Scientific Affairs. When a consensus cannot be reached on an especially important question, a special study, conference, or report may be called for by the Council on Scientific Affairs. DATTA opinions are sent to the questioner, to the panelists queried, and to *JAMA* and other AMA publications as appropriate (see Reporting below).

Assessors

DATTA is operated by AMA staff under the direction of a subcommittee of four members of the Council on Scientific Affairs. Staff selects panelists for each DATTA assessment from a reference panel which comprises more than 600 physicians. The reference panel, representing a broad spectrum of major specialties and subspecialties, is appointed by the Council on Scientific Affairs. Panel members include those in practice, medical education, and biomedical research. Nominees are solicited from all segments of medicine, including state medical societies, medical specialty societies, the AMA Section on Medical Schools, and other groups represented in the AMA House of Delegates and the AMA Councils. Panel composition is reviewed annually, and additional nominees are sought as specialty or geographic needs arise. Membership in the reference panel is published as a matter of record, but the identity of individual panelists responding to a particular inquiry is not disclosed by the AMA except with the express permission of the panelists and at the request of the Council on Scientific Affairs.

Turnaround

The time from selection of a question to the completion of a DATTA assessment is approximately 4 to 6 months. DATTA panelists are asked to return their completed questionnaires within 2 weeks of receiving them. Turnaround time is expected to be 3 to 4 months in 1985.

Reporting

Upon approval by the Subcommittee of the Council on Scientific Affairs, a final DATTA opinion on the technology in question is sent to the original questioner and to each panelist queried. DATTA opinions are also submitted to *JAMA* and other AMA publications for dissemination to the medical community. Publication in the "Questions and Answers" section of *JAMA* makes DATTA findings directly available to 343,000 U.S. subscribers, including AMA's 260,000 members, to 5,000 foreign subscribers, and to the indexed medical literature. In addition, the Council on Scientific Affairs publishes DATTA opinions in its annual reports. Each DATTA opinion is prefaced by the statement: "This report is not intended to be construed or to serve as a standard of medical care. It reflects the views of DATTA panelists and reports in the scientific literature as of [date of the report]."

Table A-3 lists the DATTA technology assessments and ratings published since the program's inception.

Impact

Given the size of the *JAMA* readership and the journal's inclusion in the indexed medical literature, opinions are available to a large readership. Although no assessment of DATTA's impact is planned, *JAMA* has received numerous letters to the editor commenting on DATTA findings. Many of these letters cite new or previously uncited studies which are germane to DATTA topics addressed in previous issues of *JAMA*.

DATTA opinions are submitted to the AMA Board of Trustees and House of Delegates, which includes representatives from major U.S. medical societies. Membership may vote on accepting DATTA findings as official AMA policy, although none have come up as such as of this writing.

Reassessment

DATTA will reassess technologies, especially those found to be investigational, based upon the publication or submission of significant new evidence. DATTA obtains monthly updates of major peer-reviewed journals and other reports to track the status of investigational technologies.

When the FDA approves a new device or a new indication for a device already in use on the basis of well-controlled clinical trials that demonstrate safety and efficacy, DATTA will reopen the assessment of any previously published DATTA opinion regarding that device or a related procedure to determine whether the conclusions remain valid. In those instances where the data and regulatory judgment regarding device safety and efficacy bear directly on the safety and efficacy of the clinical procedure involved, DATTA will publish an update notice reflecting current professional opinion and the basis for that opinion. Such a reassessment occurred following FDA approval (in January 1984) of labeling claims for specified palliative use of a hyperthermia system. An earlier DATTA opinion (published by AMA in October 1983 and appearing in *JAMA* 251:272, 1984) that found adjunctive use of whole-body hyperthermia in the treatment of solid neoplasms to be investigational was reassessed in light of clinical trials data submitted to the FDA, and it was updated in September 1984 to reflect the FDA decision. DATTA has also reopened assessments of the implantable infusion pump, noninvasive extracorporeal lithotripsy, and radial keratotomy.

Funding/Budget

The AMA budget includes approximately $380,000 for DATTA in 1985.

Example

On the following pages is the DATTA report on continuous arteriovenous hemofiltration. The report was published in the *Journal of the American Medical Association*, 253:1325–1326, 1985, and is reproduced here with permission.

Sources

American Medical Association. 1983. Reports of the Council on Scientific Affairs of the American Medical Association. 1982. Chicago.

American Medical Association. 1984. DATTA Update on Hyperthermia Treatment for Cancer. Chicago.

American Medical Association. 1985. Diagnostic and Therapeutic Technology Assessment (DATTA): An AMA Program of Medical Technology Assessment (program description). Chicago.

Cahill, N., and J. Beljan. 1984. Technology assessment: Differing perspectives. Journal of the American Medical Association 252:3294–3295.

Cahill, N. E., Director, Technology Assessment, American Medical Association. 1985. Personal communication.

Jones, R. J., Acting Director, DATTA. 1983. Personal communication. August 2.

Jones, R. J. 1983. The American Medical Association's Diagnostic and Therapeutic Technology Assessment Program. Journal of the American Medical Association 250:387–388.

Questions and Answers

Diagnostic and Therapeutic Technology Assessment (DATTA)

DATTA consultant physicians are asked to address controversial and timely questions relative to the safety, efficacy, and level of acceptance in medical practice of particular drugs, medical devices, and procedures. The consultants selected represent (1) persons in major teaching centers who are considered to be knowledgeable of the state-of-the-art as it pertains to the question; (2) areas of medicine where the drug, device, or procedure is used in practice; and (3) primary care specialties wherein daily decisions must be made about referring patients for the type of service in question. An effort is made to reflect a national geographic spectrum of diverse practice environments.

This report is not intended to be construed or to serve as a standard of medical care. It reflects the views of DATTA panelists and reports in the scientific literature as of Oct 24, 1984. DATTA-related inquiries should be submitted to Nancy E. Cahill, Director, Technology Assessment, American Medical Association, 535 N Dearborn St, Chicago, IL 60610.

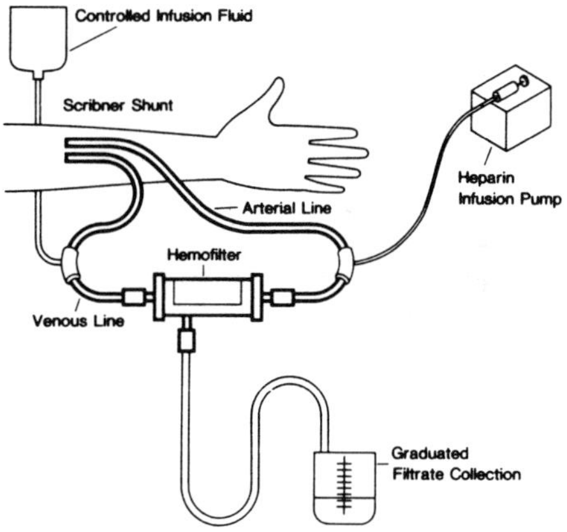

Extracorporeal circuit for continuous arteriovenous hemofiltration. Reproduced with permission from the Amicon Corporation, Danvers, Mass.

Continuous Arteriovenous Hemofiltration

Q Is continuous arteriovenous hemofiltration (CAVH) safe and effective therapy for the removal of fluid and uremic toxins from patients with refractory fluid overload or acute renal failure?

A This question was submitted to 80 DATTA panelists; 30 offered an opinion. A majority (18/30) considered CAVH safe and effective ("established") therapy for fluid removal in either of the stated conditions. Sixteen of these same panelists regarded this technique as established for the treatment of uremia in acute renal failure. The remaining panelists offered no opinion because of insufficient knowledge or experience with the technology.

Continuous arteriovenous hemofiltration is an extracorporeal process in which fluids, electrolytes, and other low-molecular weight substances are removed from blood by filtration at low pressure through hollow artificial fiber membranes.[1-3] The membrane allows passage of molecules smaller than albumin, producing an ultrafiltrate. This continuous process approximates the function of the renal glomerulus by using the patient's own arterial pressure to transport substances across a semipermeable membrane.

The principles of this process differ from that of hemodialysis, which depends on diffusion of substances (plasma solutes) along a concentration gradient into a large dialysis volume. The rate of diffusion is proportional to the concentration of the solute and inversely proportional to its molecular size. Water (volume overload) is not removed by this process.[4] Hemodialysis is more efficient than hemofiltration in clearing low-molecular weight substances such as urea, potassium, and creatinine but less efficient in removal of the medium-range substances.[4]

Blood flow is established by placing a Quinton-Scribner or other arteriovenous shunt in the patient or by cannulation of the femoral artery and vein. The hemofilter cartridge is placed on-line. This unit contains thousands of hollow fiber filters made of polysulfone or polyamide. Blood entering the cartridge passes through the interior of the hollow fibers, where all substances less than a certain molecular size (water, urea, creatinine, and middle-molecular weight substances) pass through the filter.[5] The cellular components and species of the size of albumin or greater continue on to the venous exit port. Those substances that cross the filter make up the ultrafiltrate, and this is collected and drained into a calibrated urine bag via the ultrafiltrate port (technical data provided by Gambro Inc, Barrington, Ill, and by Amicon Corporation, Danvers, Mass). Heparin solution is infused into the arterial line, usually at the rate of 10 IU/kg of body weight per hour. Replacement fluid is infused into the venous line at a rate determined by the clinical setting.

Edited by Hilda L. Slive, Assistant Editor.
Every letter must contain the writer's name and address, but these will be omitted on request. Submitted questions are published as space permits and at the discretion of the editor. All inquiries receive a direct mail reply.

The DATTA panelists emphasized that special groups of patients are candidates for CAVH, including those not suitable for hemodialysis because of hemodynamic instability and those who require treatment of volume overload.[5,6] In CAVH therapy, the filtration rate decreases as the patient's blood pressure goes down. Therefore, hypotensive episodes are avoided. The dysequilibrium syndrome is also avoided because there are no sudden shifts in body fluid compartments. Typical patients are those with multiple organ failure, including acute renal failure following surgery or severe trauma.[7,8] Complications are those that may be encountered with any extracorporeal circuit: need for vascular access, heparinization, and infection. The prefilter infusion of heparin does not significantly affect the patient's partial thromboplastin time or prothrombin time if there is no preexisting coagulopathy.[9] However, in the patient with normal platelet counts and coagulopathy, even this small amount of heparin may induce bleeding.[5]

No studies have been reported that assess the relative merits of CAVH, hemodialysis, and peritoneal dialysis. The DATTA panelists found CAVH safe and effective. Clinical judgment must determine which patients would benefit from this therapy.

1. Henderson LW, Besarab A, Michaels A, et al: Blood purification by ultrafiltration and fluid replacement (diafiltration). *Trans Am Soc Artif Intern Organs* 1967;13:216-226.

2. Bixler HJ, Nelsen LM, Bluemle LW: The development of diafiltration system for blood purification. *Trans Am Soc Artif Intern Organs* 1968; 14:99-108.

3. Kramer P, Seegers A, DeVivie R, et al: Therapeutic potential of hemofiltration. *Clin Nephrol* 1979;11:145-149.

4. Henderson LW, Silverstein ME, Ford CA, et al: Clinical response to maintenance hemodiafiltration. *Kidney Int* 1975;2(suppl):58-63.

5. Kaplan A, Longnecker RE, Folkert VW: Continuous arteriovenous hemofiltration. *Ann Intern Med* 1984;100:358-367.

6. Lauer A, Saccaggi A, Belledonne M, et al: Continuous arteriovenous hemofiltration in the critically ill patient. *Ann Intern Med* 1983;99:455-460.

7. Olbricht C, Mueller C, Schurek HJ, et al: Treatment of acute renal failure in patients with multiple organ failure by continuous spontaneous hemofiltration. *Trans Am Soc Artif Intern Organs* 1982;28:33-37.

8. Paganini EP, Nakamoto S: Continuous slow ultrafiltration in oliguric acute renal failure. *Trans Am Soc Artif Intern Organs* 1980;26:201-204.

9. Kramer P, Bohler J, Kehr A, et al: Intensive care potential of continuous arteriovenous hemofiltration. *Trans Am Soc Artif Intern Organs* 1982;28:28-32.

Battelle Memorial Institute
Human Affairs Research Centers
4000 N.E. 41st Street
Seattle, WA 98105
(206) 525-3130

Major Emphases of Technology Assessment Activities

Technology	Concerns: Safety	Efficacy/ Effectiveness	Cost/Cost-Effect/ Cost-Benefit	Ethical/Legal/ Social
Drugs		X	X	X
Medical Devices/Equipment/Supplies	X	X	X	X
Medical/Surgical Procedures	X	X	X	X
Support Systems				
Organizational/Administrative				

Stage of Technologies Assessed
- _X_ Emerging/new
- _X_ Accepted use
- ____ Possibly obsolete, outmoded

Application of Technologies
- _X_ Prevention
- _X_ Diagnosis/screening
- _X_ Treatment
- ____ Rehabilitation

Assessment Methods
- ____ Laboratory testing
- _*_ Clinical trials
- _X_ Epidemiological and other observational methods
- _X_ Cost analyses
- _X_ Simulation/modeling
- ____ Group judgment
- _X_ Expert opinion
- _X_ Literature syntheses

Approximate 1985 budget for technology assessment: $900,000

* Battelle participates in expanded clinical studies and trials by developing research protocols and collecting and analyzing safety, efficacy, and cost-effectiveness data. However, Battelle does not conduct its own clinical trials.

BATTELLE MEMORIAL INSTITUTE HUMAN AFFAIRS RESEARCH CENTERS

Introduction

Established in 1929, Battelle Memorial Institute is an independent, nonprofit organization devoted to the advancement and use of science and technology. In addition to research and development in the physical, life, engineering, behavioral, and social sciences, Battelle manages programs and facilities and conducts educational activities and encourages the utilization of new inventions and discoveries.

Battelle has a staff of some 7,200 scientists, engineers, and support personnel at major research centers in its Columbus, Ohio, headquarters and in Richland, Washington; Frankfurt, West Germany; and Geneva, Switzerland. Sites for specialized research and educational programs are located in Duxbury, Massachusetts; Houston, Texas; Seattle and Sequim, Washington; Washington, D.C., and other sites around the world. The Battelle Human Affairs Research Centers (HARC) is a component of the Pacific Northwest Division of Battelle Memorial Institute.

Assessments of health care technologies are

undertaken by the Health and Population Study Center in Seattle. The Health and Population Study Center also has programs in health care financing; policy planning and evaluation; chronic disease, disability, and long-term care; epidemiology and environmental health; physician behavior and medical manpower; life-cycle transitions; work and the family; and social inequity.

Purpose

The purpose of Battelle technology assessments is to promote the advancement and appropriate use of medical technology. Specific objectives vary with assessments conducted for sponsoring agencies. For instance, the primary purpose of the National Heart Transplantation Study for the Health Care Financing Administration (HCFA) is to assist the agency to determine whether heart transplantations should be covered and reimbursed under the Medicare program.

Subjects of Assessment

The primary emphasis of assessments thus far has been on medical/surgical procedures, although assessment activities focusing on drugs and medical devices have been initiated in Battelle's Washington, D.C., office. Battelle's major recent health care efforts have been the broad assessments of heart transplantation and kidney dialysis and transplantation. As a part of these projects, Battelle has examined the government and private third-party payment mechanisms used for these expensive technologies. The role of the physician has been studied, including factors influencing physician productivity, need for physician manpower, and physician distribution issues. Table A-4 lists selected active and recent Battelle projects in health care.

Other studies have examined the economic and psychosocial consequences of chronic and catastrophic disease. For example, a recently completed project investigated the incidence and characteristics of pain associated with various types of cancer. A series of studies have also been completed on the provision of long-term care in the nursing home industry. Battelle has recently prepared a manual for the medical device industry to guide firms in conducting cost-effectiveness analyses of their products.

TABLE A-4 Battelle Health and Population Study Center: Selected Active and Recent Projects in Health Care

Project Title (sponsor and end date)
Cost-Effectiveness of Cyclosporine as Primary Immunosuppressive Therapy for Kidney Transplant Recipients (Health Care Financing Administration, 1987)
Performing Cost-Effectiveness Analysis: A Practical Guide for the Health Care Industry (1985)
Survey to Identify Active Bone Banks (Naval Research and Development Command, 1985)
National Kidney Dialysis and Kidney Transplantation Study (Health Care Financing Administration, 1984)
National Heart Transplantation Study (Health Care Financing Administration, 1984)
Analysis of University of Southern California Data on Family and General Practitioners (University of Washington/Robert Wood Johnson Foundation, 1982)
Estimate 1990 Manpower Requirements for Six Medical Specialties (Health Resources Administration, 1982)
An Analysis of the Impact of Physician Practice Arrangement on the Use of Drugs and Laboratory Tests (Health Resources Administration, 1981)
Evaluation of the Process and Outcome of a Prospective Management Team Approach to the Control of Pain in Cancer Patients (National Cancer Institute, 1981)
Assist in Development of a Comprehensive Health Care Financing Plan for Alaska (State of Alaska, 1981)
Implement Necessary Protocols for Estimation of Manpower Requirements for Eight Surgical Specialties (Health Resources Administration, 1980)
Examination of Rates of Return on Equity Capital and Risks in Nursing Homes under Medicare and Various State Medicaid Reimbursement Systems (Health Care Financing Administration, 1980)
Analysis of the Content of Specialty Practices and Their Service Capacities (Health Resources Administration, 1980)
Study of the Relationships Between Case Mix and Facility Staff Time and Costs for Direct Care of Nursing Home Patients (Health Resources Administration, 1979)

Stage of Diffusion

New and emerging technologies (e.g., heart transplantation) and existing technologies (e.g., kidney transplantation and dialysis) have been assessed thus far, although technologies at any stage of diffusion would be considered for assessment.

Concerns

The concerns of Battelle technology assessments vary among projects, but are generally those of the broader types of assessment. Technology need, availability, safety, effectiveness, cost, cost-effectiveness, and ethical and legal issues are explicit concerns of these assessments. Battelle is currently expanding its efforts in cost analyses of medical technologies by encouraging the collection of cost data in clinical trials and developing industry guides for performing cost-effectiveness and cost-benefit evaluations of new and existing technologies.

The National Kidney Dialysis and Kidney Transplantation Study is concerned with the quality of life, level of disability, quality of care, and cost of treatment associated with kidney dialysis and kidney transplantation. The National Heart Transplantation Study has been undertaken to determine the need for heart transplantation in the United States, the survival of heart transplant recipients, the availability of donor hearts, the cost of performing a heart transplantation procedure, the rehabilitation and quality of life of heart transplant recipients, and the legal and ethical issues surrounding heart transplantation. The Table A-5 listing of Update Series reports for the Battelle studies on heart transplantation and kidney transplantation and dialysis illustrates the range of concerns involved in these major assessments.

Requests

Much of Battelle's sponsored research is initiated from proposals of its own multidisciplinary teams. Other study topics come from organizations requesting Battelle's assistance for addressing specific problems, primarily federal agencies, foundations, and medical device and drug manufacturers and their trade and professional associations.

Selection

Assessment topics are agreed upon by Battelle and its sponsoring organizations.

Process

The procedures used by Battelle for conducting assessments of heart transplantation, kidney transplantation and dialysis, and other technologies are the following:

1. Identify technology to be assessed and prepare brief research protocol.
2. Establish a technical advisory panel made up of individuals who are familiar with the technology to provide assistance, on a consulting basis, in the evaluation effort.
3. Contact appropriate professional associations for representatives to provide input as needed.
4. Prepare a detailed research protocol, including background information on each technology, list of institutions or sources from which primary data are to be collected, a brief description of the data analysis plans, and schedule for project activities.
5. Collect data.
6. Analyze data.
7. Prepare final report.

The assessments include the following elements:

- an estimation of the need for the technology;
- an analysis of the survival rates (if applicable) of the recipients of the technology;
- consideration of the availability of the technology;
- a complete analysis of the cost of the technology including a detailed analysis of the cost of alternative treatments for the disease or condition in question;
- a full assessment of the purported benefits of the technology including both objective and subjective parameters;
- a review and evaluation of any legal issues surrounding the technology, including regulation of use and distribution, selection

TABLE A-5 Battelle Update Series for National Heart Transplantation Study and National Kidney Dialysis and Kidney Transplantation Study

National Heart Transplantation Study
Economic and Social Costs of Heart Transplantation (#3)
Defining the Need for Heart Transplantation (#5)
Patient Selection for Heart Transplantation (#6)
Dimensions of Family Impact Pertinent to Heart Transplantation (#8)
Title VI and Heart Transplantation: Discrimination in Patient Selection (#12)
Survey of Hospitals with Open-Heart Surgery Facilities (#20)
An Outline of Legal Issues in the Assessment of Health Care Technology: The Case of Heart Transplantation (#23)
Fundamental Legal Rights and Governmental Regulation of Heart Transplantation (#26)
Donor Organ Procurement Policies and Procedures Throughout the United States: A State-by-State Analysis (#31)
The Present and Future Needs for and Supply of Organs for Transplantation (#33)
Estimating the Costs of Organ Procurement for Heart Transplantation (#38)
National Kidney Dialysis and Kidney Transplantation Study
The Conceptualization and Measurement of the Social Costs of End-Stage Renal Disease (#11)
Case-Mix, Treatment Modalities, and Patient Outcomes: Results from the National Kidney Dialysis and Kidney Transplantation Study (#14)
Complexities in the Treatment of End-Stage Renal Disease: Economic Efficiency and Treatment Modality Prescription (#20)
The Demographic Characteristics of the National Kidney Dialysis and Kidney Transplantation Study: A Comparison with the End-Stage Renal Disease Population (#21)
Peritonitis, Hospital Admissions, and Days Hospitalized Among Patients on Continuous Ambulatory Peritoneal Dialysis (CAPD) and Continuous Cycling Peritoneal Dialysis (CCPD): A Comparative Assessment (#24)
A Comparative Assessment of the Quality of Life of End-Stage Renal Disease Patients on Four Treatment Modalities: Results from the National Kidney Dialysis and Kidney Transplantation Study (#26)
Travel Costs and End-Stage Renal Disease (#30)

NOTE: Battelle has printed about 80 reports in the Update Series' for the National Heart Transplantation Study and the National Kidney Dialysis and Kidney Transplantation Study, respectively. All are available from Battelle; a few have been published. The selected report titles listed here illustrate the range of concerns involved in these major studies. The respective Update Series report numbers are shown in parentheses.

of recipients, risk imposed on recipients, and so forth;

• an analysis of the ethical concerns associated with the use of the technology, including patient selection, imposition of risk, distributional concerns, etc.

Assessors

Battelle has a core staff of scientists from a variety of disciplines, including medical sociology, psychology, computer sciences, law, and health services, that are primarily responsible for the conduct of studies. In addition, Battelle has established working relationships with outside individuals who serve primarily on advisory committees and technical review panels, and who, in certain cases, are responsible for selected portions of the research. Staff assigned to assessments varies for each study. Major projects such as the heart transplantation study may involve as many as five full-time and eight part-time staff, plus 15 consultants and a review/advisory panel.

Turnaround

Turnaround time for studies varies. Battelle has undertaken numerous short studies, requiring a few months, at the request of HCFA and others which consist primarily of literature reviews and statistical compilations. Other studies take longer, such as the heart transplantation study (42 months) and the kidney dialysis and transplantation study

(32 months). During the course of these longer studies, interim status reports (the Update Series) are made available.

Reporting

In addition to the final reports of assessments delivered to sponsoring agencies, Battelle publishes numerous interim reports in its Update Series. For example, about 50 update reports were made available for the heart transplantation study, and about 40 update reports were made available for the 3-year kidney study. HCFA has encouraged Battelle to disseminate widely reports on studies being carried out for that agency. Organizations such as HCFA publish Battelle study summaries and reports conducted for those agencies in their publications. Battelle researchers also publish their findings in journals such as *Contemporary Dialysis*, *Heart Transplantation*, *Journal of the American Medical Association*, *Journal of Health Politics, Policy & Law*, *Lancet*, *New England Journal of Medicine*, and *Science*.

Impact

Although there is no tangible evidence for direct impact of studies, there are other indications that the Battelle projects are of interest. Study personnel are often asked to participate and make presentations at conferences (e.g., NIH Consensus Development Conferences) and before congressional committees and subcommittees, state governments, and other policymaking bodies.

Funding/Budget

The total annual research budget for the Health and Population Study Centers has been approximately \$2 million–\$2.5 million in recent years. Funding for technology assessment activities has been approximately \$900,000 annually in recent years, most of which has been for the heart transplantation and kidney studies funding by HCFA.

Example

The following is a summary description of the National Heart Transplantation Study undertaken by Battelle Human Affairs Research Centers. This summary is the full text of "Update Series #1, The National Heart Transplantation Study" (February 22, 1982), available from Battelle, Seattle.

NATIONAL HEART TRANSPLANTATION STUDY

Overview

The National Heart Transplantation Study is a cooperative study involving several major heart transplant programs across the United States. The major objective of the study, more completely delineated below, is to examine all aspects of heart transplants, including the scientific, social, economic, and ethical issues, and, in particular, the impact of a possible Medicare decision to pay for heart transplants on the Medicare program, Medicare beneficiaries, and providers of health care. In particular, the study will focus on seven major areas. These are: (1) the estimation of the potential need for heart transplants, (2) the survival of heart transplant recipients, (3) the potential availability of donor hearts, (4) the cost of performing heart transplants, (5) the rehabilitation and quality of life of heart transplant recipients, (6) the legal, and (7) the ethical aspects of heart transplantation. It is expected that the study results will have implications for the promulgation of Medicare policy with respect to heart transplantation.

The National Heart Transplantation Study is to be conducted over an 18 month period beginning in October, 1981 and ending in April, 1983, is funded by the Office of Research and Demonstrations of the Health Care Financing Administration (HCFA). The study is being directed by Dr. Roger Evans of the Health and Population Study Center at the Battelle Human Affairs Research Centers in Seattle, Washington.

Background

In November, 1979, the Health Care Financing Administration authorized Medicare payments for heart transplantation procedures performed for Medicare beneficiaries at Stanford University Medical Center. This was an interim decision, based on preliminary findings by the Public Health Service (PHS) regarding the safety and efficacy of heart transplants performed at that center. HCFA anticipated when reimbursement was tentatively authorized, that it soon would be able to reach a final decision not only about coverage at that center, but also on generally applicable, broadly based criteria for approving Medicare coverage of heart transplantation at other facilities.

As HCFA proceeded to review Medicare coverage of heart transplants, it was determined that the issues were much more complex than originally thought and that many of them could not be immediately resolved because adequate data did not exist. There were numerous questions, for example, concerning the patient selection process, the basis for assessing safety and efficacy, the long-term social and economic consequences of the procedure, broad ethical considerations, the cost-effectiveness of the procedure, and the potential, if any, for substantial expansion in the availability of heart transplantations. It was concluded that HCFA did not have sufficient information at this time to support the development of generally applicable coverage criteria.

On June 12, 1980, Patricia Roberts Harris, then Secretary of the U.S. Department of Health and Human Services (DHHS), announced a decision to exclude heart transplants from Medicare coverage, with the exception of a very few patients previously selected for and awaiting transplants. This announcement was published in the *Federal Register* on August 6, 1980 (Volume 45, No. 153, Pages 52296–52297). At this time, Harris announced that all new technologies must be evaluated not only on the basis of their medical efficacy but also on the basis of their "social consequences" before "financing their wide distribution." The approach being suggested by Harris was even more comprehensive than that used by, for example, the Environmental Protection Agency (EPA) in dealing with pesticides, the Food and Drug Administration (FDA) in its treatment of pharmaceuticals, and the Occupational Safety and Health Administration's (OSHA) approach to carcinogens in the workplace. New health technology was to be evaluated concerning its cost-effectiveness, cost-benefit ratios, and its "long-term effects on society."

The decision to exclude heart transplants from Medicare coverage was accompanied by an announcement that HCFA, in close cooperation with the Public Health Service's National Center for Health Care Technology (NCHCT) would conduct a broad study of the sort described by Harris. This study, now referred to as the National Heart Transplantation Study, was to address all of the issues identified above including the scientific, social, ethical, legal, and economic issues. As already stated, the study was also to examine the impact of a potential coverage decision on beneficiaries, the Medicare program, and health care providers.

The institutions or clinical centers chosen to participate in this study have been selected very carefully. In reviewing the applications submitted by the clinical centers, it was, a priori, determined that cardiac transplantation could not be considered as simply a surgical procedure. It was further decided that clinical effectiveness and usefulness are dependent upon careful and appropriate patient selection, expert surgery, post-operative care, immunosuppression, evaluation for incipient rejection of the donor heart, management of complications associated with immunosuppression, patient education, and liaison with the patient's permanent physicians for subsequent lifelong care. Criteria for the selection of participating clinical centers were developed by the National Heart, Lung and Blood Institute, with the advice of an advisory group of experts in cardiology, cardiovascular surgery, organ transplantation, and immunology. Three major criteria were specified for the selection of clinical centers. They were: (1) the institution must have had experience with a clinical heart transplant program within the past five years, (2) the institution must have adequate patient selection criteria, and (3) the institution must have adequate patient management plans and protocols.

All participating clinical centers (i.e., heart transplant programs) will be expected to furnish, or facilitate access to, a wide variety of data regarding heart transplants previously performed at their facilities during a period starting no later than January 1, 1975, and continuing over the 18 month period of the study. This will include data on each institution's facility and personnel resources, heart donor program, patient selection criteria, transplant and patient care protocols, patient follow-up care, patient survival, costs of establishing and maintaining a heart transplant program, patient charge information, and other similar and related information.

Sources

Battelle. 1983. Battelle: Seeking Solutions to Significant Social Problems. Seattle.

Battelle Human Affairs Research Centers. 1982. The National Heart Transplantation Study (Update Series #1). Seattle.

Evans, R. W. 1983. Organ transplantation. Science 222:232.

Luce, B., Senior Research Scientist, Battelle, Washington, D.C. 1985. Personal communication.

Overcast, T. D., Senior Research Scientist, Battelle. 1985. Personal communications.

Introduction to Blue Cross and Blue Shield Association

Blue Cross and Blue Shield are the names and symbols used by the 87 local, nonprofit plans that contract with hospitals, physicians, and other health care providers and facilities to provide prepaid health care services to their subscribers. The Blue Cross plans primarily cover hospital expenses, though they have expanded coverage into outpatient care. The Blue Shield plans primarily cover physicians' services, though they have expanded into such benefits as dental, vision, and outpatient services. Some local Blue Cross and Blue Shield plans are jointly operated. The Blue Cross and Blue Shield organization is not a single company; rather, it is a nationwide federation of locally governed, autonomous corporations, each operating under state law as a nonprofit service organization.

There are about 80 million regular Blue Cross and/or Blue Shield plan subscribers, including subscribers under the Federal Employee Program and coverage supplementing Medicare. Approximately 29 million people are served by plans in their roles as intermediaries for Medicare Part A, and as carriers for Medicare Part B, Medicaid, and CHAMPUS (Civilian Health and Medical Program of the Uniformed Services). Eliminating duplication between the programs, the total number of people served is about 100 million. In 1983, Blue Cross and Blue Shield plans paid $34.6 billion for care received by plan subscribers, and another $38.2 billion was paid for persons in federal programs.

The local Blue Cross and Blue Shield plans have medical departments and engage in varying levels of technology review activities. The California Blue Shield Medical Policy Committee assesses for coverage purposes new diagnostic and therapeutic technologies, and initiated the review of obsolete procedures that grew into the Medical Necessity Program of the Association. Beginning in 1982 with percutaneous transluminal coronary angioplasty, California Blue Shield became the first private third-party payer to institute selective reimbursement—i.e., payment for certain procedures at designated institutions only—and currently reimburses selectively for heart transplants and liver transplants.

The Blue Cross and Blue Shield Association is a coordinating agency of the plans. The Association speaks on behalf of the plans on matters of national concern and operates programs of public education and professional relations. It also works with plans on cost-containment efforts and provides research, statistical, actuarial, marketing, and other services to the plans. The Association administers plan membership standards and maintains a computerized telecommunications system linking all the plans. The Association helps to coordinate the uniform administration of health care coverage for large national employers with plants and offices in more than one region, and is the prime contractor for the organization's administration of Medicare Part A. Notwithstanding the national coordinating role of the Association, local plans are responsible for making their own administrative and coverage policy.

In addition to the Medical Necessity Program and the Technology Evaluation and Coverage Program described in the following profiles, the Blue Cross and Blue Shield Association supports other organizations in their technology evaluation efforts. For example, it commissioned an Institute of Medicine study of the effectiveness of computed tomography (CT) scanning, and provided funding for a Conference of Medical Specialty Societies on technology assessment in 1981. The Blue Cross and Blue Shield Association does not conduct its own original clinical research. Blue Cross of Massachusetts has obligated over $5 million in matching funds to the Massachusetts Fund for Cooperative Innovation, a grant program for hospital cost-containment experiments administered jointly with the Massachusetts Hospital Association.

Medical Necessity Program
Blue Cross and Blue Shield Association
Technology Management Department
676 North St. Clair Street
Chicago, IL 60611
(312) 440-6155

Major Emphases of Technology Assessment Activities

Technology	Concerns: Safety	Efficacy/ Effectiveness	Cost/Cost-Effect/ Cost-Benefit	Ethical/Legal/ Social
Drugs				
Medical Devices/Equipment/Supplies				
Medical/Surgical Procedures		X		
Support Systems				
Organizational/Administrative				

Stage of Technologies Assessed
____ Emerging/new
_X_ Accepted use
_X_ Possibly obsolete, outmoded

Application of Technologies
____ Prevention
_X_ Diagnosis/screening
_X_ Treatment
____ Rehabilitation

Assessment Methods
____ Laboratory testing
____ Clinical trials
____ Epidemiological and other observational methods
____ Cost analyses
____ Simulation/modeling
_X_ Group judgment
_X_ Expert opinion
_X_ Literature syntheses

Approximate 1985 budget for technology assessment: $350,000*

* This amount represents the Association's expenditures for technology management and coding processes, and related activities. Included are significant portions devoted to implementing the Medical Necessity Program and the Technology Evaluation and Coverage Program.

MEDICAL NECESSITY PROGRAM BLUE CROSS AND BLUE SHIELD ASSOCIATION

Introduction

Most Blue Cross and Blue Shield plan benefit contracts contain a medical necessity clause which provides that services are covered when they are medically necessary. When a technology is properly used and is covered by the contract, it will be paid. The plans view as medically unnecessary certain technologies used inappropriately or simply due to routine.

The Medical Necessity Program (MNP) rests on the assumption that physicians prefer to practice good medicine, but not all are aware of more recent clinical developments. The program recognizes the difficulty in establishing rules for clinical treatment to which there are no exceptions, and provides that technologies addressed in the program will be paid for if their use is justified by a physician.

The identification of obsolete procedures by Blue Cross and Blue Shield plans began in 1975 with the California Blue Shield's Medical Policy Committee. The Blue Cross and Blue Shield Association Medical Necessity Program was begun in 1977 as one of the first national private initiatives to assess medical technology for coverage purposes, in cooperation with the American College of Physicians, the American College of Surgeons, and the American College of Radiology. An outgrowth of the Medical Necessity Program is the Clinical Efficacy Assessment Project of the American College of Physicians.

Purpose

The purpose of MNP is to provide information to member plans to assist them in determining their subscriber contractual obligations which require reimbursement only for necessary medical care. Plans will pay for any recognized procedure found necessary by the admitting physician, but view as medically unnecessary certain clinical practices performed simply out of routine or habit. For plans that adopt the Medical Necessity Program guidelines, the program "shifts the burden of proof" from payer to provider in that providers must justify their use of procedures and services falling outside of MNP guidelines. MNP guidelines are not statements of Blue Cross and Blue Shield coverage; terms of individual plan contracts govern such coverage.

Subjects of Assessment

The Medical Necessity Program deals primarily with medical and surgical procedures. Many of these entail the use of drugs and medical devices, but the emphasis of the assessments is on the indications for use of the drug- or device-embodied procedures, rather than on the attributes of the medical products as such. With the initiation of the program in 1977, 42 diagnostic and surgical procedures were identified as outmoded or of unproven value. The second phase of the program called for the elimination of routine laboratory and x-ray testing at the time of hospital admission. As of 1985 there were nearly 90 procedures on the outmoded procedures list. With the development in 1982 of MNP guidelines for respiratory therapy, the scope of the program was expanded to deal with procedures that may be overutilized or inappropriately used.

The Medical Necessity Program has developed guidelines on the following clinical issues:

- outmoded procedures list (1977)—updated periodically
- routine admission testing policy (1979)
- respiratory care guidelines (1982)
- diagnostic imaging guidelines (1984)
- cardiac care guidelines (1985)

The program is currently developing guidelines on clinical laboratory and pathology services and on the use of chest x ray and electrocardiogram in hospital admission and preoperative evaluation.

Stage of Diffusion

The Medical Necessity Program originally focused on technologies that were outmoded or unproven. The program has since expanded its focus to include procedures and services that are standard practice, but are utilized in inappropriate circumstances or more often than warranted by good medical practice.

Concerns

Of primary concern are the clinical effectiveness and specific indications for use of a technology for physician education and coverage purposes. The Medical Necessity Program is intended to curtail the unnecessary use of certain procedures. Although cost and cost-effectiveness of technologies have not been explicit concerns of the program, it has recently begun to consider cost-effectiveness for selected procedures such as chest x rays.

Requests

The MNP addresses questions that are raised directly by local plans, and may independently initiate a review of topics which have implications for all plans.

Selection

Issues having highest priority are those that may have the greatest impact on all plans and those that may require immediate attention by the plans. Plans are advised of issues that will be considered by the program.

Process

The Association commissions critical evaluations of existing medical literature by recognized experts and seeks clinical opinions of recognized medical specialty societies. The medical specialty societies are responsible for supplying the clinical expertise on various procedures and services; the Association's responsibility is to disseminate this medical consensus. The Association convenes periodic national conferences and invites national medical specialty society representatives for the purpose of soliciting clinical opinions. In all cases, the Association's position or guidelines consider its evaluation of existing medical literature and the opinions of the Association's Medical Advisory Panel. The guidelines are reviewed by the Medical Advisory Panel and are approved by the Association's board. The Association does not conduct original clinical research to determine clinical efficacy and indications.

Sensitivity in administration of MNP guidelines is used. For example, plans will view hospital regulations that call for admission batteries as meeting the MNP hospital admission tests battery requirement, provided that the hospital staff has studied the needs of its patient population and has limited the battery to those tests required by a significant majority of admitted patients.

An important aspect of the MNP is the education of health professionals regarding new guidelines. In the case of the MNP guidelines for diagnostic imaging issued in 1984, information regarding the new guidelines was to be made available to health care providers for a period of 6 to 12 months, after which several plans may start disallowing payments for procedures not meeting the guidelines.

Assessors

The Medical Advisory Panel consists of about 10 members and is selected by the senior staff of the Association. Most members are plan medical directors, primarily of the larger plans, and represent a mixture of specialties, geographic locations, and backgrounds in clinical practice, academe, and administration.

The Association has cooperated with a number of medical societies in the Medical Necessity Program. These have included the following:

American Academy of Dermatology
American Academy of Family Physicians
American Academy of Neurology
American Academy of Pediatrics
American Association of Neurological Surgeons
American College of Nuclear Physicians
American College of Obstetricians and Gynecologists
American College of Physicians
American College of Radiology
American College of Surgeons
American Psychiatric Association
College of American Pathologists
Society of Nuclear Medicine

The medical societies that participated in writing MNP guidelines are generally cited in the respective guidelines or in accompanying press releases.

Turnaround

It takes approximately 1 year from the time of designating a subject for consideration by the program to the time that the MNP guidelines are formally approved and distributed.

Reporting

The guidelines developed by the MNP often are announced in national press conferences. Guidelines generally include the following:

1. brief description of the technology;
2. policies regarding specific clinical indi-

cations for use and nonuse of the technology; and

3. further policy considerations or rationale supporting policies.

Medical Necessity Program guidelines are transmitted directly to plans by the Association's *TEC Newsletter* and various plan bulletins. The guidelines are provided by many plans to area physicians who provide care to subscribers and to other requesting parties.

Reassessment

The Association will reassess MNP guidelines when it is apparent that new clinical evidence exists and clinical opinions have changed sufficiently to warrant revised guidelines. This could be the case for procedures once considered to be standard practice later found to be obsolete, or for procedures first determined to be obsolete which are later found to be rarely yet appropriately used. An example is radical hemorrhoidectomy (whitehead type), which was cited in the MNP procedures list in 1977 and deleted in 1980.

Impact

The Association does not systematically track the impact of MNP guidelines. Because of contract variations, hold harmless provisions (i.e., where a subscriber is not held financially responsible for care provided outside of MNP guidelines), state-legislated mandates, and local practice variations, the impact of the MNP guidelines probably varies among plans.

When introducing new MNP guidelines, the Association has cited the overall magnitude of expenditures devoted to the general area of health care involved, e.g., $10 billion devoted annually for diagnostic radiology (Blue Cross and Blue Shield Association, 1984b) and $2 billion–$4 billion spent annually for hospital respiratory care services (Blue Cross and Blue Shield Association, 1982). All plans are advised to seek justification before denying payment for services that fall outside the MNP guidelines.

In 1977, the Medical Necessity Program announced that 42 outmoded diagnostic tests and surgical procedures should no longer be performed. According to early analyses, if the program's policies regarding these outmoded procedures were fully implemented through 1981, they could have resulted in an estimated $300 million annual savings (see Greenberg and Derzon, 1981). These estimates have not been followed up by broad-based studies of actual savings, however. A review of a sample of insurance claims for portions of the Federal Employee Health Benefits Program administered by Blue Cross and Blue Shield plans in 1975 and 1978 showed a decline in claims for listed surgical procedures of 26 percent and a decline in diagnostic test claims of 85 percent (Blue Cross and Blue Shield Association, 1982). However, without earlier points of reference, it is difficult to attribute the decline in tests in surgery to the issuance of the MNP guidelines.

The impact of the MNP was cited in a 1980 report of the General Accounting Office (GAO). Upon studying the MNP, the GAO concluded that medical necessity programs can reduce health care costs, and the agency recommended that the federal government's Office of Personnel Management adopt similar policies throughout its Federal Health Benefits Program.

Using data from eight local hospitals, Blue Cross and Blue Shield of Oregon estimated that implementation of the Medical Necessity Program routine hospital admission testing policy resulted in a savings of $22 per admission, and that full implementation on an area-wide basis would result in a projected savings of $8 million.

Funding/Budget

The Association devotes approximately $350,000 annually to its technology management and coding processes, including the MNP and the Technology Evaluation and Coverage Program. The Association offers this technical assistance as part of its ongoing support to plans, and does not charge plans a user fee.

Examples

On the following pages are excerpts from three types of Medical Necessity Program guidelines. The first is a page out of the Medical Necessity Procedures List, showing 10 diagnostic procedures requiring satisfactory justification (for payment, as recommended by the Association) and the specific reason for their inclusion in the list. The inclusion of these particular 10 procedures was endorsed by the College of American Pathologists (CAP) and the American College of Physicians (ACP). The second example is the Medical Necessity Program statement regarding hospital admission test batteries. The third example is excerpted from the 1985 MNP guidelines on cardiac care, and includes the cover sheet, table of contents, and guidelines on echocardiograms, 1 of 13 procedures addressed in that set of guidelines.

Sources

Blue Cross and Blue Shield Association. October 12, 1982. Press release: Blue Cross and Blue Shield Association Issues Guidelines on Respiratory Care. Chicago.

Blue Cross and Blue Shield Association. Medical Necessity Procedures List. Revised according to BCBSA 81 coding and nomenclature. Revised June 1983. Chicago.

Blue Cross and Blue Shield Association. 1984a. Questions and Answers about the Blue Cross and Blue Shield Organization. Chicago.

Blue Cross and Blue Shield Association. 1984b. Press release: Blue Cross and Blue Shield Association Issues Guidelines to Reduce Diagnostic Imaging Procedures. Chicago.

Blue Cross and Blue Shield Association. 1985. Medical Necessity Guidelines on Cardiac Care. Chicago.

Blue Cross of Massachusetts/Massachusetts Hospital Association Fund. 1985. Blue Cross/MHA Fund for Cooperative Innovation: Report for 1984.

General Accounting Office, U.S. Congress. 1980. The OPM Should Promote Medical Necessity Programs for Federal Employees' Health Insurance. Washington, D.C.: U.S. Government Printing Office.

Greenberg, B., and R. A. Derzon. 1981. Determining health insurance coverage of technology: Problems and options. Medical Care 19:967-978.

Morris, L. C., Senior Vice President, Health Benefits Management, Blue Cross and Blue Shield Association. 1985. Personal communications.

Schaffarzick, R., Senior Vice President and Medical Director, Blue Shield of California. 1985. Personal communication.

Tennenbaum, D., Manager, Medical Necessity Program, Blue Cross and Blue Shield Association. 1985. Personal communications.

BLUE CROSS AND BLUE SHIELD ASSOCIATION
MEDICAL NECESSITY PROCEDURES LIST
REVISED ACCORDING TO BCBSA 81 CODING AND NOMENCLATURE

BCBSA 1981 PROCEDURE CODES ANNOUNCED 1979	UMP	DESCRIPTION	SPECIFIC REASON	ENDORSED
		Procedures Requiring Satisfactory Justification		
82155		Amylase, blood isozymes, electrophorectic	Not clinically useful	CAP/ACP
82345		Calcium, feces, quantitative, timed specimen	Obsolete; replaced by quantitive stool for fat	CAP/ACP
+ 82387		Cephalin flocculation, blood	Obsolete; liver enzyme determinations more accurate	CAP/ACP
82490		Chromium, blood	No clinical indication	CAP/ACP
82505		Chymotrypsin, duodenal contents	Unreliable; replaced by secretin test	CAP/ACP
+ 82510		Congo red, blood	Obsolete; replaced by rectal or gingival biopsy	CAP/ACP
82939		Gastric analysis, tubeless, (Diagnex blue)	Not reliable	CAP/ACP
82997		Gonadotropin, chorionic, bioassay, quantative	Obsolete; radiommunossy more accurate and specific	CAP/ACP
+ 82999		Gonadotropin, chorionic pregnancy test, small animal	Obsolete; radioimmunoassay more accurate and specific	CAP/ACP
83005		Guanase, blood	Obsolete; liver enzyme determinations more useful	CAP/ACP

Revision Number: 1
Revision Date: 6/83

Date of Issue: 1977, 1979, 1980

+ = BCBSA '81 code only; no CPT-4.

Section: 2-MNP
Page: 1 of 1

BLUE CROSS AND BLUE SHIELD ASSOCIATION
MEDICAL NECESSITY PROGRAM
HOSPITAL ADMISSION BATTERIES

I. Hospital Admission Batteries

In February, 1979 the Blue Cross and Blue Shield Association, based upon advice from the American College of Physicians, recommended to Plans that routine hospital diagnostic batteries for medical admission be added to the Medical Necessity Project. Two months later, upon the advice of the American College of Surgeons, that recommendation was extended to include surgical admissions.

A. Medical Admissions

1. The American College of Physicians recommends that diagnostic tests should not be required as routine procedures for patients admitted to a hospital. Examples of routine diagnostic admission tests may include the following:

- blood hemoglobin
- urine analysis
- biochemical blood screens
- chest x-ray
- electrocardiogram

2. Given the American College of Physicians' policy concerning diagnostic tests, the Blue Cross and Blue Shield Association recommends that Plans:

Continue to provide benefits for tests performed for a patient admitted to a hospital for medical treatment but only upon evidence that the tests were ordered by an attending or admitting physician specifically for that patient.

B. Surgical Admissions

1. The American College of Surgeons stated that the routine use of batteries of tests without specific orders on admission should apply to surgical as well as medical cases. Diagnostic admission tests ordered for the pre-operative patient require discrimination by the physician.

2. Based on this advice from the American College of Surgeons, the Blue Cross and Blue Shield Association recommends that Plans:

Continue to provide benefits for tests performed for a patient admitted to a hospital for surgical treatment but only upon evidence that the tests were ordered by an attending or admitting physician specifically for that patient.

Revision number: 1
Revision Date: 6/83 Date of issue: 1979

MEDICAL NECESSITY GUIDELINES

SUBJECT	SECTION 5-MNP-85
CARDIAC CARE	PAGE 1 of 15

MEDICAL NECESSITY GUIDELINES

ON

CARDIAC CARE

BLUE CROSS AND BLUE SHIELD ASSOCIATION

These Guidelines have been issued as part of the Blue Cross and Blue Shield Association's Medical Necessity Program. They have been developed in cooperation with medical specialty societies and the Blue Cross and Blue Shield Association for use by the Blue Cross and Blue Shield Plans.

REVISION NO.
REVISION DATE

Date of Issue: 2-1-85

MEDICAL NECESSITY GUIDELINES

SUBJECT CARDIAC CARE	SECTION 5-MNP-85 PAGE 2 of 15

TABLE OF CONTENTS

Most health benefits coverage excludes procedures used to screen asymptomatic persons for evidence of disease. The omission of any such screening procedures from these Guidelines does not reflect any judgment about the appropriateness or desirability of such public health measures. Similarly, these Guidelines are not and should not be construed as a statement of Blue Cross and Blue Shield coverage for the procedures and services discussed herein. The terms of individual Plan contracts govern such coverage.

REVISION NO.
REVISION DATE

Date of Issue: 2-1-85

MEDICAL NECESSITY GUIDELINES

SUBJECT	SECTION 5-MNP-85
CARDIAC CARE	PAGE 12 of 15

(Cardiac Catheterization Continued)

2. Appropriate Length of Hospital Stay for an Uncomplicated Cardiac Catheterization or Angiography

The maximum length of hospital stay for an uncomplicated cardiac catheterization or angiography is two nights and three days.

VI ECHOCARDIOGRAM

A. DESCRIPTION:

An echocardiogram is a non-invasive ultrasound imaging procedure of the heart.

B. POLICY:

A combined two-dimensional (2-D) and M-mode echocardiogram is the format of choice for most echocardiographic examinations. Both 2-D and M-mode echocardiograms should be done at the same time and should be considered integral parts of a single examination.

1. Indications for 2-D Echocardiogram

An initial 2-D echocardiogram may be indicated in patients with suspected or known heart disease for the noninvasive evaluation of cardiovascular anatomy and function and documentation of structural or functional derangements.

Changes in clinical or cardiac status may be an indication for a repeat study. In a stable patient with heart disease, repeat 2-D echocardiograms may be indicated if there is a change in clinical status or to monitor suspected subclinical progression of the disease that may require a change in clinical management. Repeat echocardiograms to monitor subclinical progression of the disease are not indicated more often than once a year.

2. Indications for M-mode Echocardiogram

The indications for M-mode echocardiogram are the same as those for a 2-D examination, both for initial and repeat studies. However, M-mode echocardiogram alone is indicated only if equipment to perform a 2-D echocardiogram is not available.

Technology Evaluation and Coverage Program
Blue Cross and Blue Shield Association
Technology Management Department
676 North St. Clair Street
Chicago, IL 60611
(312) 440-5529

Major Emphases of Technology Assessment Activities

Technology	Concerns: Safety	Efficacy/Effectiveness	Cost/Cost-Effect/Cost-Benefit	Ethical/Legal/Social
Drugs				
Medical Devices/Equipment/Supplies	X	X		
Medical/Surgical Procedures	X	X		
Support Systems				
Organizational/Administrative				

Stage of Technologies Assessed
X Emerging/new
X Accepted use
___ Possibly obsolete, outmoded

Application of Technologies
___ Prevention
X Diagnosis/screening
X Treatment
___ Rehabilitation

Assessment Methods
___ Laboratory testing
___ Clinical trials
___ Epidemiological and other observational methods
X Cost analyses
___ Simulation/modeling
X Group judgment
X Expert opinion
X Literature syntheses

Approximate 1985 budget for technology assessment: $350,000*

* This amount represents the Association's expenditures for technology policy, coding, and related activities. Included are significant portions devoted to implementing the Technology Evaluation and Coverage Program and the Medical Necessity Program.

TECHNOLOGY EVALUATION AND COVERAGE PROGRAM BLUE CROSS AND BLUE SHIELD ASSOCIATION

Introduction

The Technology Evaluation and Coverage Program of the Blue Cross and Blue Shield Association develops medical policies for the Association's *Uniform Medical Policy Manual*. Uniform Medical Policies are provided to Blue Cross and Blue Shield plans primarily for advisory purposes; however, their implementation is stipulated for certain national account contracts. National account contracts generally are made with large corporations, such as General Motors and AT&T, that operate in more than one state or region and are served by more than one local Blue Cross or Blue Shield plan. In these cases, a model Matrix Contract for national accounts may be adopted so as to provide uniform benefits to a corporation's beneficiaries. As agreed to in such a contract, the administration of these benefits is subject to the *Uniform Medical Policy Manual*, as revised.

Purpose

The purpose of the Technology Evaluation and Coverage Program (TEC) is to help the Blue Cross and Blue Shield plans fulfill their responsibility to uniformly pay for care of good quality at reasonable cost. The role of the Association in evaluating technologies is primarily advisory. The program is intended to help plans to deal quickly and equitably with specific questions of efficacy and coverage. While Association advice is often accepted, plans generally make their own determinations.

Subjects of Assessment

TEC primarily assesses medical and surgical procedures which relate directly to issues of coverage. Drugs and medical devices generally are evaluated insofar as they are embodied in procedures and billed as such, e.g., in the case of surgery to implant a particular device. In a few cases, support systems have been evaluated, e.g., ambulance services. New diagnostic procedures are given particular scrutiny. TEC addressed 90 issues in 1983 and 63 issues in 1984. The following are examples of issues addressed in 1984.

- in vitro fertilization
- magnetic resonance imaging
- major organ transplants
- medical foods—amino acid based foods
- extraoperative electrocorticography
- local hyperthermia
- intraoperative sensory evoked potentials (SEP)
- portable nocturnal hypoglycemia detectors
- automatic implantable defibrillators
- automatic external defibrillators
- suction assisted lipectomy
- bone marrow transplants
- diagnostic endocardial electrical recording and stimulation
- neutron beam therapy
- proton beam therapy
- percutaneous transluminal angioplasty
- biofeedback
- sudden infant death syndrome (SIDS) monitoring
- physician assistants
- ambulance services

Stage of Diffusion

TEC is primarily concerned with new and emerging technologies and with certain existing technologies that are not in widespread use. Determining a technology's level of development is one of the program's concerns, as described below.

Concerns

The main concerns of TEC are the safety and effectiveness of technologies, and their level of development. TEC has recently begun to consider the cost-effectiveness of a few technologies. Most Blue Cross and Blue Shield plan contracts, including the national account contracts, exclude benefit payments for technologies which are termed *experimental* or *investigative*. Uniform Medical Policies are used in administering such contract exclusions. Thus TEC is concerned with determining whether technologies are experimental, investigative, or standard, and if appropriate, identifying clinical indications for their use. Experimental technologies are those that have been largely confined to laboratory and/or animal research. Investigative technologies are those that have progressed to limited human applications but lack wide recognition as proven and effective procedures in clinical medicine. Standard technologies are those that are widely accepted as clinically effective procedures; however, such technologies may need to be qualified as standard only under certain specified circumstances.

TEC increasingly seeks information from medical societies and the medical literature documenting the safety and effectiveness of technologies. TEC may also provide plans with information regarding coverage matters that should be considered when determining reimbursement, such as costs of acquisition, facilities, training, and depreciation.

Requests

Topics for assessment originate through the claims process. Most, though not all, new procedures are first seen by the plans through claims from individual practitioners. Because of contract variations, state-legislated mandates, and local practice variations, inquiries regarding local Blue Cross and Blue Shield policy normally are directed first to the individual plans. Increasingly, inquiries about the coverage of procedures and particular medical products are being made prior to claims submission, as the system is better known. Association staff work with plans on a day-to-day basis in responding to inquiries regarding medical policies and related matters.

Selection

The need for involvement of the Association is determined by plans' ability to resolve coverage matters locally. Before considering coverage for drug- or device-embodied procedures, plans generally require that the drug or medical device have FDA premarket approval, though FDA approval is not sufficient for plan coverage. Likewise, although HCFA decisions are carefully considered by the plans, HCFA approval of a technology as "reasonable and necessary" for Medicare beneficiaries is not sufficient for plan coverage.

A claim for an unrecognized procedure will be forwarded to the medical director of the receiving plan. Medical directors have varying resources for resolving claims. At California Blue Shield, for example, there is a Medical Policy Committee representing most specialties and the research establishment. If the medical staff of the plan is unable to dispose of the procedure, the Medical Policy Committee will be called upon for advice. Blue Shield of Massachusetts convenes an Interdisciplinary Medical Advisory Committee to assist it in making coverage decisions for new technologies. Other plans may conduct their own assessments or surveys of available information on new technologies. The many plans that serve as Medicare fiscal intermediaries (i.e., administer Medicare claims for HCFA) may closely observe or participate in the HCFA assessment process.

Process

If a claim is not resolved locally, it may be referred to the Blue Cross and Blue Shield Association. The Association's response may consist of advice to the inquiring plan, advice to all plans, or development of a Uniform Medical Policy or a new procedure code.

Upon receiving a request from the plan, the Association will first attempt to determine if the procedure is really new, since "new" procedures may simply be minor variations of existing procedures. If the variation is not significant for the purposes of reimbursement, the plan will be advised to code the procedure as the recognized procedure. This has the advantage of minimizing fragmentation, and of using established data bases for pricing and utilization review.

If the procedure appears to be new, the Association will poll plans to determine if any have dealt with it. If the issue has already been resolved by one or more plans, and if the resolution appears to be reasonable, the information will simply be transmitted to the requesting plan. If the issue has not been resolved among polled plans, inquiry may be made to yet other plans, HCFA, or the Office of CHAMPUS.

If the issue remains unresolved, TEC staff gathers information on the issue from a number of other sources. Staff may conduct a literature search and may seek opinions from among the Association's registry of consultants in various specialties. In addition, the staff may contact appropriate medical specialty organizations for any experience in addressing the issue. The Association does not conduct original clinical research to determine clinical efficacy and indications. Information derived from the literature search and consultation is forwarded to the Association's Medical Advisory Panel. This panel, which generally meets quarterly, considers the available information in an interactive though not formalized group setting.

Depending upon the issue, the panel may circulate its draft findings to all or a sample of plan medical directors for comment before reaching a final opinion.

The Medical Advisory Panel has several possible courses. It may simply issue advisory opinions to plans. Advice to plans may consist of noting a technology's stage of development and level of acceptance; recommendations or guidelines clarifying technical and clinical details regarding safety, effectiveness, or appropriate use; and important issues for plans to consider in their coverage decisions. When formulating advice on new technologies, the Association may consider cost-effectiveness information. This information does not affect the recommendations directly, but is transmitted to the plans. The Association does not recommend an amount for reimbursement. However, as noted above, it may provide information which plans may use in determining appropriate reimbursement. Plans are free to weigh the information in their respective coverage policy decisions.

The Medical Advisory Panel may also elect to assign a code to the procedure. This code establishes the procedure's identity for purposes of reimbursement and utilization review. Ordinarily, new codes will be assigned only where significant differences from existing technology are perceived.

Frequently, the Association incorporates its recommendations in the *Blue Cross and Blue Shield Uniform Medical Policy Manual*. This manual became effective January 1982 and governs the administration of contracts in which it is incorporated, as described above. Of the issues reviewed by the Medical Advisory Panel, approximately one-half become Uniform Medical Policy.

The panel reports its recommendations to Association staff, and for selected issues, to the Association's committees and board. A separate but entirely parallel process is used for the assessment of dental technology, involving a Dental Advisory Panel.

Assessors

The Medical Advisory Panel consists of about 10 members and is selected by the senior staff of the Association. Most members are plan medical directors, primarily of the larger plans, and represent a mixture of specialties, geographic locations, and backgrounds in clinical practice, academe, and administration.

Turnaround

The length of time required to review an issue varies considerably. Some issues can be resolved by TEC staff within 48 hours. Uniform Medical Policies generally require about 6 months to be made final, and most issues are disposed of within 1 year. Factors influencing turnaround include the complexity of the issue and whether it is necessary to seek the clinical opinions of medical specialty societies.

Reporting

The dissemination of information varies. Medical policy advice and information is transmitted directly to plans by the Association's *TEC Newsletter* and various plan bulletins. Uniform Medical Policies are transmitted as inserts to the *Uniform Medical Policy Manual*.

The information is normally presented as medical policy which includes the following components:

1. applicable procedure code(s);
2. brief description of the technology;
3. status of service, i.e., experimental, investigative, or standard (generally accepted) practice;
4. the specific clinical indications which apply to the coverage of services (if appropriate); and
5. further policy considerations, exceptions.

Impact

In addition to those plans that are obliged to comply with Uniform Medical Policies as per their national account contracts, most other plans voluntarily adopt the Uniform Medical Policies in the administration of local accounts. However, the Association does not track changes in reimbursement patterns that may have resulted from the implementation of Uniform Medical Policies.

Reassessment

Uniform Medical Policies are reviewed at least every 2 years to determine if revisions are necessary. Existing policies may be reassessed sooner if it is apparent that new evidence exists and clinical opinions have changed sufficiently to warrant a revised policy, e.g., the reassessment of chemonucleolysis following FDA approval of chymopapain.

Funding/Budget

The Association offers this technical assistance as part of its ongoing support to plans. The Association does not charge plans a user fee. In its annual budget the Association devotes approximately $350,000 to technology management and coding, and related activities, with significant portions devoted to implementing TEC and the Medical Necessity Program.

Example

On the following pages are Uniform Medical Policies on sensory evoked potential (SEP) response studies (revised December 1984) and chemonucleolysis (revised December 1984).

Sources

Blue Cross and Blue Shield Association. Uniform Medical Policy Manual. Sensory Evoked Potential (SEP) Response Studies. Section I. Page 92280.0-2. Revised December 1984.

Blue Cross and Blue Shield Association. Uniform Medical Policy Manual. Chemonucleolysis. Section III. Page 62292.0. Revised December 1984.

Gleeson, S., Executive Director, Technology Management, Blue Cross and Blue Shield Association. 1985. Personal communications.

Morris, L. C., Senior Vice President, Health Benefits Management, Blue Cross and Blue Shield Association. 1985. Personal communications.

Office of Technology Assessment. 1984. Health Technology Case Study 27: Nuclear Magnetic Resonance Imaging: A Clinical, Industrial, and Policy Analysis (Chapter 8: Third Party Payment Policies). Washington, D.C.: U.S. Government Printing Office.

Tennenbaum, D., Manager, Medical Necessity Program, Blue Cross and Blue Shield Association. 1985. Personal communications. Assistance was also provided by K. Smith, Manager, Technology Evaluation and Coverage Program, Blue Cross and Blue Shield Association.

UNIFORM MEDICAL POLICY MANUAL

SUBJECT SENSORY EVOKED POTENTIAL (SEP) RESPONSE STUDIES — SECTION I, PAGE 92280.0

PROCEDURE CODE RANGE 92280 **
92585
95925

DESCRIPTION A noninvasive* technique in which evoked responses are measured and recorded through electrodes, and averaged by computer. An assessment is then made of the integrity of specific neurologic and auditory functions.

POLICY The following three types of EVOKED RESPONSE STUDIES are generally accepted ** medical practice*: **

1. VISUALLY EVOKED POTENTIAL (VEP) RESPONSE STUDY **

   This procedure is considered generally ** accepted medical practice in ** detecting delays in the conduction of the visual pathways as may result from the demyelination process, especially as they relate to:

   - o detection of possible multiple sclerosis;
   - o monitoring changes related to treatment or spontaneous remission of the disease process; and
   - o establishing past visual involvement in suspected mul-

CONTINUED

REVISION NUMBER 5
REVISION DATE 12/84

tiple sclerosis patients who have no visual problems at the present.

2. BRAINSTEM AUDITORY EVOKED RESPONSE (BAER/BSER) STUDY: **

This procedure is considered generally accepted medical practice* when used for the following:

- o to differentiate metabolic from structural lesions of the brainstem and to define the location and nature of the latter;
- o to localize brainstem tumors, particularly those which can not be revealed by CT scanning;
- o to assess recovery of function in cases of brainstem lesions due to demyelination or trauma. Such potentially irreversible lesions include multiple sclerosis, central pontine myelinolysis, brainstem contusions, vertebrobasilar insufficiency, postremoval of space occupying lesions compressing the brainstem;
- o to supplement the EEG in evaluating the irreversibility of coma or "brain death"; and
- o to measure the type and extent of hearing impairment and to determine the degree of neural maturation in children and neonates.

CONTINUED

UNIFORM MEDICAL POLICY MANUAL

SUBJECT	SENSORY EVOKED POTENTIAL (SEP) RESPONSE STUDIES	SECTION I PAGE 92280.2

3. SOMATOSENSORY EVOKED POTENTIAL (SSEP) RESPONSE STUDY (CEREBRAL EVOKED POTENTIALS) **

   This procedure is considered generally accepted medical practice* in evaluating the following: **

   - o spinal cord injuries;
   - o severe head injuries; and
   - o specific neurologic deficits.

EFFECTIVE DATE 7/82
6/83 Reevaluated **
6/84 Reevaluated **

EXCEPTIONS INTRAOPERATIVE SENSORY EVOKED POTENTIAL (SEP) MONITORING

DESCRIPTION Noninvasive* monitoring techniques used during surgery to assess the neurological function of the anesthetized patient or to minimize postoperative morbidity.

POLICY The INTRAOPERATIVE use of SENSORY EVOKED POTENTIALS (SEP) is EXPERIMENTAL/INVESTIGATIVE*, including:

1. visually evoked potentials;

2. brainstem auditory evoked response;

3. somatosensory evoked potentials (SSEP) during spinal and orthopedic surgery; and

4. SEP monitoring of the sciatic nerve during total hip replacement.

EFFECTIVE DATE 1/85

REVISION NUMBER 5
REVISION DATE 12/84

UNIFORM MEDICAL POLICY MANUAL

SUBJECT CHEMONUCLEOLYSIS

SECTION III
PAGE 62292.0

PROCEDURE CODE	62292	**
DESCRIPTION	Chymopapain, a proteolytic enzyme, is injected into a herniated disc to cause breakdown of the chondromucoprotein within the disc.	**
POLICY	CHEMONUCLEOLYSIS utilizing chymopapain (Chymodiactin) is generally accepted medical practice* only for herniated intervertebral lumbar discs unresponsive to conservative treatment.	**
EFFECTIVE DATE	4/81 3/83 Reevaluated 6/84 Reevaluated	 ** **
POLICY CONSIDERATIONS	CHEMONUCLEOLYSIS is approximately one-half, or fifty percent as difficult as a laminectomy, or approximately three times as difficult as a discogram. A discogram is an integral part of CHEMONUCLEOLYSIS. When a radiologist performs the discogram, his efforts constitute approximately one-third of the CHEMONUCLEOLYSIS procedure.	**

REVISION NUMBER 5
REVISION DATE 12/84

ECRI
5200 Butler Pike
Plymouth Meeting, PA 19462
(215) 825-6000

Major Emphases of Technology Assessment Activities

Technology	Concerns: Safety	Efficacy/ Effectiveness	Cost/Cost-Effect/ Cost-Benefit	Ethical/Legal/ Social
Drugs				
Medical Devices/Equipment/Supplies	X	X	X	X
Medical/Surgical Procedures				
Support Systems	X	X	X	X
Organizational/Administrative				

Stage of Technologies Assessed
X Emerging/new
X Accepted use
X Possibly obsolete, outmoded

Application of Technologies
X Prevention
X Diagnosis/screening
X Treatment
X Rehabilitation

Assessment Methods
X Laboratory testing
X Clinical trials
X Epidemiological and other observational methods
X Cost analyses
X Simulation/modeling
___ Group judgment
X Expert opinion
X Literature syntheses

Approximate 1985 budget for technology assessment: $5,000,000

ECRI

Introduction

ECRI (formerly the Emergency Care Research Institute) is an independent, nonprofit corporation that evaluates and assesses medical devices and equipment. ECRI also provides publication, information, education, and consultation services to assist hospitals, health care professionals, and governmental and voluntary sector agencies in improving the safety, efficacy, and cost-effectiveness of health care technologies.

This discussion of ECRI evaluation activities is devoted primarily to the Health Devices Program (ECRI/HDP), an evaluation and information dissemination service provided to over 2,500 member hospitals. Member hospitals receive comparative medical device evaluations conducted by ECRI and published in the ECRI journal *Health Devices*, which is similar in purpose and format to the popular *Consumer Reports*. ECRI provides other publications addressing medical devices, hospital risk control, and related issues, which are described below under Reporting.

In addition to its Health Devices Program, ECRI provides a wide variety of technology-related consulting services to health care facilities, including assistance with codes, standards and accreditation, equipment planning, acquisition and testing, chemical and gas monitoring, accident investigation, and risk control services. In a program initiated in 1984, an interdisciplinary staff of analysts conducts comprehensive assessments focusing on diagnostic imaging and clinical laboratory technologies for publication in ECRI's new peer-reviewed *Journal of Health Care Technology: Assessment, Planning, and Value Analysis.*

The National Implant Registry is a pilot program established as a nonprofit organization by ECRI. This registry maintains a perpetual, central record of medical device implants (e.g., pacemakers and prostheses such as heart valves and artificial hip joints) and patients, and automatically notifies hospitals and physicians of implant recalls or deficiencies, identifying patients and addresses when action may be indicated. The National Implant Registry is supported primarily by member hospitals and physicians.

Purpose

The purpose of ECRI is to assist hospitals, health care professionals, and governmental and voluntary sector agencies in improving the safety, efficacy, and cost-effectiveness of health care technologies. In particular, the purposes of ECRI/HDP are to

1. conduct assessments of medical devices and other technologies
2. provide independent, objective judgment for selection, purchase, and use of medical instruments, equipment, and systems
3. function as a clearinghouse and investigate and resolve hazards and deficiencies in medical devices
4. encourage the improvement of medical devices through an informed marketplace

Subjects of Assessment

ECRI/HDP evaluates many types of diagnostic and therapeutic medical devices, equipment, and support systems, as well as some preventive and rehabilitative technologies. These range from disposables such as hypodermic syringes and nasal oxygen cannulas to electric beds, x-ray units, and patient monitoring systems. Comparative evaluations are usually conducted within a product category. Table A-6 shows technologies evaluated in the journals *Health Devices* and the new *Journal of Health Care Technology.*

Stage of Diffusion

ECRI/HDP evaluates new and existing technologies that are being actively marketed by industry and purchased by hospitals. Some technologies may be evaluated as obsolete or outmoded.

Concerns

ECRI/HDP conducts comparative evaluations of the efficacy, performance, safety, ease of use, and cost-effectiveness of technologies. The comparative evaluations are used to provide brand name ratings of specific products. In addition to these concerns, the publication *Issues in Health Care Technology* addresses legal, ethical, economic, and social issues of medical technologies; and the publication *Health Devices Alerts* provides weekly notification of hazardous devices and recommendations that require corrective action.

Requests

Topics for ECRI/HDP evaluation are staff initiated or originate from inquiries made to ECRI by hospital members of the Health Devices Program that are considering technologies for purchase. These inquiries provide indications to ECRI that its hospital membership may be especially interested in evaluative information for certain product categories.

ECRI operates two formal networks to handle requests, inquiries, and reports of user experience. The Problem Reporting Network receives reports of adverse experiences with medical devices from hospitals, health professionals, government agencies, and manufacturers, and reviews and abstracts the relevant clinical, engineering, and legal literature. These reports are evaluated by ECRI engineers and, when appropriate, are reported in ECRI/HDP publications to in-

TABLE A-6 Evaluations Published in *Health Devices*, 1981–1985, and *Journal of Health Care Technology*, 1984–1985

Health Devices (volume:page)
Anesthesia unit gas scavengers (12:267)
Arrhythmia monitoring systems (11:211)
Batteries, medical device (14:209)
Blood gas/pH analyzers (12:59)
Blood warmers (13:191)
Breathing circuits (12:183)
Defibrillators, line-powered (12:291)
Disposable pressure transducers (13:268)
Electrocardiographs, three-channel (13:235)
Electrode monitoring systems, electrosurgical, return (14:115)
Electronic intermittent thermometers (12:3)
Electrosurgical electrodes, active, hand-switched (11:69)
Enteral feeding pumps (14:9)
Ethylene oxide sterilizers (11:287)
External transcutaneous pacemakers, Pace*Aid Model 50C (13:3)
Fetal monitors (11:123)
Heat and moisture exchangers (12:108)
Incontinent pads (12:108)
Infant incubators (11:47)
Infant radiant warmers (13:119)
Infant transport incubators (11:179)
Infusion controllers (11:75; 14:219)
Infusion pumps (13:31)
Operating room ECG monitors (11:155)
Oxygen analyzers (12:183)
Oxygen monitors, transcutaneous (12:213)
Patient bed scales (13:75)
Physiologic monitoring systems (11:211; 14:143)
Pneumatic tourniquets (13:299)
Suction canisters (12:127)
Surgical case carts (11:311)
Surgical gloves (12:83)
Volume ventilators (11:264)
Wall vacuum regulators (14:191)
X-ray film processors (11:99)
Journal of Health Care Technology (volume:page)
Automated leukocyte differential counters (2:51)
Automated microbiology systems (1:213)
Deaths during general anesthesia (1:155)
Digital imaging storage and retrieval (1:13)
Digital subtraction angiography (DSA) (1:177)
Freestanding imaging centers (1:257)
Magnetic resonance imaging (MRI) (2:23)
Therapeutic apheresis (1:279)
Therapeutic drug monitoring (TDM) (1:39)

form users of the problems and recommended solutions. A number of ECRI's sources of information about medical devices have been consolidated into the User Experience Network, a data base of user experience with specific device brands and models. It includes reports from the Problem Reporting Network, results of regular surveys and questionnaires directed to device users, and interviews about user experience that are a regular part of ECRI/McGraw-Hill Product Comparison Systems (a series of information services about specialized technologies). Other reports are based on ECRI's extensive accident investigation and forensic engineering studies. Reports derived from the User Experience Network appear in ECRI publications and electronic data bases (e.g., National Clinical Engineering Computer Network). Approximately 40,000 reports were on ECRI's computer data base as of January 1985.

To avoid conflict of interest, neither ECRI nor its staff members provide medical device evaluation services to inventors, manufacturers, or distributors of medical devices, or accept financial support from these parties.

Selection

Topics for evaluations are selected based on the volume of inquiries from ECRI/HDP member hospitals and the experience of ECRI's senior staff about their importance to hospitals and to safe, efficacious, and cost-effective patient care.

Process

The comparative evaluations conducted by ECRI/HDP and reported in *Health Devices* are based on ECRI laboratory, clinical, and field (i.e., in-hospital) evaluations. Laboratory evaluations are conducted in ECRI's 45,000-square-foot facility, and clinical studies (in vivo evaluations of device performance) are conducted in selected member hospitals. Evaluations follow appropriately reviewed medical/scientific protocols developed by ECRI for device evaluation.

Assessors

Evaluations are conducted by ECRI's full-time interdisciplinary staff of more than 120, representing medical, engineering, and analytical sciences. There is an extensive review process involving both in-house and independent reviewers, typically including clinicians with special expertise in the subject area. No staff member may consult for or own stock in medical device companies.

Turnaround

The usual time between the selection of an evaluation topic and the publication of the evaluation in *Health Devices* is 6 to 9 months.

Reporting

ECRI has 15 publications addressing medical device evaluation, hospital risk control, and related issues. Three of these publications are included in the ECRI/HDP: *Health Devices*, *Health Devices Alerts*, and *Issues in Health Care Technology*.

- *Health Devices* is published monthly by ECRI. In addition to comparative evaluations, *Health Devices* includes editorials and hazard reports of deficiencies and hazards reported to ECRI by equipment users and manufacturers. (Manufacturers are made aware of hazard reports related to their equipment as soon as deficiencies are found, and they are invited to respond.) Approximately 170 comparative evaluations have been published in *Health Devices* since 1973. Subscriptions to *Health Devices* are available only through membership in the ECRI/HDP.
- *Health Devices Alerts* is a weekly abstracting service which summarizes articles, letters, recalls, and problems with medical devices from the medical, engineering, and legal literature, calling out action items that require immediate response.
- *Issues in Health Care Technology* is a bimonthly publication provided in loose-leaf form which addresses emerging technologies, economics, ethics, reimbursement, and government regulations and policies. The "New Technology Briefs" section of this publication contains miniassessments of a broad range of new clinical technologies.

Members of ECRI/HDP receive a full volume of 12 issues of *Health Devices*, 52 issues of *Health Devices Alerts*, and 6 mailings of *Issues in Health Care Technology* annually, in addition to telephone consultation and other services. In 1985, an annual membership in the Health Devices Program cost $875, and single copies of *Health Devices* cost $50.

Additional ECRI publications include the following:

- *Technology for Health Care* is a set of monthly specialty newsletters on anesthesia, cardiology, emergency medicine, materials management, respiratory therapy, and surgery.
- *Health Devices Sourcebook* is an annual directory of 6,000 categories of medical devices, equipment, and manufacturers, based on a continually updated computerized data base. It provides a widely used standard nomenclature and computer coding.
- *Hospital Risk Control* is a four-volume, loose-leaf, monthly publication on issues of hospital risk management.
- *Journal of Health Care Technology* is a journal begun in 1984 that includes assessments performed by ECRI staff on clinical laboratory and radiography/imaging technologies, and submitted papers on a broad range of health technology issues.

Because ECRI depends on publication revenue to support its assessment activities and the policy of the National Library of Medicine (NLM) is to index only those publications that they may freely reproduce, ECRI publications are not included in NLM indexes. However, indexes and data base searches are available from ECRI.

ECRI has three technology comparison services in loose-leaf binder formats marketed by McGraw-Hill. These address the selection and purchase of capital equipment for hospitals, clinical laboratory equipment and supplies, and diagnostic imaging and radiology products. Other information services in similar formats for surgery, emergency medicine, anesthesia-critical care, materials management, supplies and disposables, and home health care products will be introduced in the near future.

Impact

ECRI provides the Health Devices Program to over 2,500 member hospitals, representing about 70 percent of all acute-care hospital beds in the United States. (Many Canadian hospitals and overseas health care organizations also are members.) The Health Devices Program membership renewal rate has exceeded 95 percent since its inception.

Periodic surveys of Health Devices Program members have indicated a high degree of satisfaction with the program. According to ECRI, a majority of the hospital CEOs reading *Issues in Health Care Technology* rated it as more useful and valuable than other hospital publications that they read.

Insofar as the impact of the Health Devices Program on safety of patient care is concerned, numerous specific product improvements have been directly attributed to product evaluations published in *Health Devices*, thus benefiting all hospitals, not just those that are program members. For instance, ECRI reports that following an extensive 1973 study of electrosurgical machines, most manufacturers undertook major redesign to improve safety. With an estimated 90 percent replacement of the U.S. nationwide inventory with improved equipment over the past decade, the impact has been significant; many fewer electrosurgical burns are currently reported to ECRI. ECRI attributes cost savings in the hundreds of millions of dollars to ECRI/HDP evaluations and other technology-related efforts on behalf of member hospitals (e.g., the National Electrical Code controversy over isolated power requirements in anesthetizing locations).

Reassessment

Product categories are reassessed based upon member hospital inquiries for more current information than is available from previous evaluations. These normally occur when a significant number of new product models appear on the market in a given product category.

Funding/Budget

The 1985 budget for ECRI's total technology assessment activities is approximately $5.0 million. ECRI is supported through earned income, grants, and contributions. Most of its operating budget comes from publication sales, information program membership, and fees from consulting, laboratory, and technical services. ECRI does not accept financial support from inventors, manufacturers, or distributors of medical devices.

Example

The following is the first page of an ECRI comparative evaluation of critical care ventilators published in *Health Devices* (August 1982, Vol. 11, No. 10) and is reproduced with permission here. Due to its length (20 pages) and copyright limitations, the balance is not included here.

Sources

ECRI. 1982. Critical care ventilators. Health Devices 11:264–283.

ECRI. 1983. ECRI: Information and Consultation Services for the Health Community. Plymouth Meeting, Pa.

ECRI. Undated. National Implant Registry. Plymouth Meeting, Pa.

Mosenkis, R., Vice President, Publications, ECRI. 1984. Personal communications.

Nobel, J., President, ECRI. 1984. Personal communication.

VanAntwerp, M., Director of Policy Analysis, ECRI. 1985. Personal communications.

Evaluation

Health Devices Sourcebook
1982-83 Reference

Ventilators, Volume
[14-362]

Critical Care Ventilators

Positive pressure ventilation is the insufflation of the lungs by the forceful delivery of gas. Although known and practiced for more than a century, the technique was not widely used until the late 1950s, when it superseded negative pressure ventilation. Negative pressure ventilators (*e.g.*, the "iron lung," the cuirass shell) were popular because they imitated natural breathing (by exerting negative pressure on the chest as the diaphragm does) but were eventually recognized as less effective, convenient, and versatile than devices that provide positive pressure ventilation. Technical advances in positive pressure ventilation and the ability to quickly and accurately determine the effectiveness of ventilation (through the measurement of arterial blood gases) have allowed rapid development of the modern critical care ventilator.

As the figure illustrates, these devices are connected to a source of breathing gases (usually oxygen and ambient or compressed air) and deliver breaths to the patient via an airway, or breathing circuit. Breathing circuits currently used by most ventilators have both inhalation and exhalation lines. [The breathing circuit may also include accessories, such as a humidifier and a nebulizer.] During inhalation, the exhalation valve must remain closed to prevent loss of gases intended for the patient. The valve opens to permit the exhaled breath to exit through the exhalation port until the airway pressure has been reduced to the desired level.

SUMMARY

We evaluated six critical care ventilators. Five are equipped to deliver PEEP and IMV; the sixth unit is not equipped for these functions and, therefore, is not appropriate for use on patients with complex respiratory problems. Most of the units exhibit an improvement over critical care ventilators of the past in that they detect various kinds of disconnects; the one exception is rated Conditionally Acceptable. Another unit was rated Conditionally Acceptable because its breathing circuit may be occluded when electrical power fails.

On the cover: The evaluated ventilators (from left): the Puritan-Bennett MA-1 and MA 2+2, the Monaghan 225/SIMV, the Siemens-Elema 900C and 900B, and the Bourns BEAR 1.

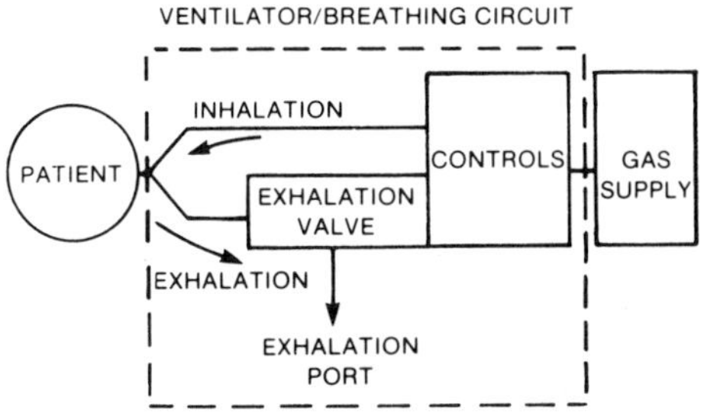

Typical Ventilator System

The ventilator provides direct control of the patient's ventilation variables (see *A Primer on Ventilation*, p. 265), as well as other variables (*e.g.*, the concentration of inspired oxygen) and the limits on certain variables for safe operation. All these controls allow the clinician to provide better patient management, even for patients with serious respiratory impairments.

The ventilator can be adjusted to suit the needs of a particular patient and his current phase of treatment. For example, the ventilator can sense inspiratory efforts of a patient who is regaining his capacity to breathe and immediately deliver an assisting breath. If the mode of treatment or the patient's condition changes, the operating mode of some ventilators can be changed, via panel controls, to provide special functions (*e.g.*, positive end expiratory pressure, or PEEP; see *Primer*) without requiring the addition or reconnection of various pieces of equipment (*e.g.*, a PEEP valve).

The greater the complexity of the ventilator equipped for multiple therapies, the greater the chance for malfunction and operator error (see the table on p. 268, constructed from literature reports of both simple and complex ventilators). Therefore, the devices are equipped to monitor variables such as pressure, exhaled volume,

Hastings Center
Institute of Society, Ethics and the Life Sciences
360 Broadway
Hastings-on-the-Hudson, NY 10706
(914) 478-0500

Major Emphases of Technology Assessment Activities

Technology	Concerns: Safety	Efficacy/ Effectiveness	Cost/Cost-Effect/ Cost-Benefit	Ethical/Legal/ Social
Drugs				
Medical Devices/Equipment/Supplies				
Medical/Surgical Procedures				X
Support Systems				X
Organizational/Administrative				X

Stage of Technologies Assessed
- X Emerging/new
- ___ Accepted use
- ___ Possibly obsolete, outmoded

Application of Technologies
- ___ Prevention
- X Diagnosis/screening
- X Treatment
- ___ Rehabilitation

Assessment Methods
- ___ Laboratory testing
- ___ Clinical trials
- ___ Epidemiological and other observational methods
- ___ Cost analyses
- ___ Simulation/modeling
- X Group judgment
- X Expert opinion
- X Literature syntheses

Approximate 1985 budget for technology assessment: $250,000

HASTINGS CENTER INSTITUTE OF SOCIETY, ETHICS AND THE LIFE SCIENCES

Introduction

The Hastings Center is a nonprofit corporation formally known as the Institute of Society, Ethics and the Life Sciences. Since its founding in 1969, Hastings has addressed ethical issues arising from advances in health and medicine, the natural sciences, and the social and behavioral sciences. In addition, Hastings conducts studies in natural science, the humanities, behavioral science, and professional ethics. Other services include an educational program; fellowships, scholarships, and internships; consultation; and publications.

The Hastings Center is one of few organizations which systematically examines ethical issues arising from medical technologies. Bioethicists at the Kennedy Institute of Ethics at Georgetown University are primarily concerned with teaching and individual research. The Battelle Institute addresses ethical issues for certain projects, and the Congressional Office of Technology Assessment cites ethical, social, and legal issues in certain of its medical technology assessments.

The Center has about 9,000 individual

members, including 1,600 libraries. Membership fees range from $22 for students to $35 for institutions and libraries.

Purpose

The Hastings Center seeks to carry out nonpartisan research on pressing ethical issues; to develop educational programs and literature; and to assist universities, legislators, and professional organizations in coping with moral problems.

Subjects of Assessment

Technologies assessed have included drug- and medical device-embodied technologies, medical and surgical procedures, and support systems used in screening, diagnosis, and treatment, as well as organizational/administrative technologies. Examples of particular technological areas addressed in Hastings research projects have included recombinant DNA research, organ transplantation, prenatal diagnosis of genetic disease and genetic counseling, human experimentation, life-extending technologies, and health cost-containment policies.

Most Hastings Center work is conducted by research groups that address certain technological areas. Among those currently active are groups on health policy research, chronic illness, neonatology, occupational health, and organ transplantation. Others have been groups on genetics research; ethical, social, and legal issues in genetic counseling and genetic engineering; death and dying; and alternative forms of care for the terminally ill.

The death and dying research group, established in 1970, has examined the moral, social, and legal issues of the care of the dying engendered by advanced medical technology. Subjects included organ transplantation and the definition of death, the termination of treatment of dying patients, and the allocation of scarce resources to the dying. A successor group examines the goals of medicine and their relationship to death, suffering, and well-being. It has examined changing social attitudes and practices toward childbirth; the difficulties of treating pain that appears to be psychological in origin; and the nature of suffering in a life-threatening illness, including the role of hospices.

The Health Policy Research Group is concerned about the quality, cost, and distribution of health care in the United States. This group is studying the ethical issues raised by the increasing rate of technological innovation in medicine. By examining technologies already in use—such as dialysis and heart transplants—and those currently under development, its members aim to arrive at some consensus that may prove useful to researchers and policymakers who face difficult decisions about the appropriate direction for financing and distributing new medical technologies.

Another study being conducted by the health policy group is addressing the ethical, social, and political problems raised by efforts on the part of government to encourage those forms of behavior considered advantageous for the preservation of health, and to discourage personal behavior deemed hazardous to health.

The program on ethical problems of research on human subjects monitors government regulations regarding human subjects research, develops educational and training programs and related activities, and serves as a resource for institutional review boards.

Stage of Diffusion

Most of the technologies that have been subjects of Hastings assessments have been new and emerging technologies, while some have been widely used technologies.

Concerns

Hastings is concerned with ethical, social, and legal issues of technologies. The Center is especially interested in highlighting the role played by regulatory agencies and committees—such as institutional review boards (IRBs) and hospital ethics committees—in monitoring new technologies.

Requests

Subjects for assessments may originate from many sources, including Center staff, fellows of the Center, medical societies and professional organizations, government agencies, foundations, and subscribing members of the Center.

Selection

The selection of topics for Hastings projects is generally made by Center staff, as approved by the board of directors. In some cases, final selection is made by foundation approval of project grant proposals made by the Center.

Process

Hastings works primarily through small, multidisciplinary study groups of about 10–12 outside specialists. Each group is set up to address a particular set of problems, and may meet four or five times over 12 months or more. Groups usually first meet for informal planning in response to staff suggestions. Work plans are finalized and approved by groups, then approved by the Center director or associate director. Groups often discuss relevant case studies or case histories, and may use a consensus development format. Reports and guidelines go through numerous drafts by Center staff and subgroups. In addition to the study group, Hastings conducts other activities related to technology assessment. Staff members have served as consultants to state and federal officials and congressional committees. Staff members have also served as consultants to organizations such as Blue Cross and Blue Shield of Massachusetts, the Massachusetts Hospital Association, the Battelle Institute, the Congressional Office of Technology Assessment, the Office of Protection from Research Risks at NIH, the President's Commission for the Study of Ethical Problems in Medicine and Biomedical and Behavioral Research, the New York State Department of Health, the Labor Resources Committee of the United States Senate, and the House Committee on Science and Technology. Center staff publish papers on ethical issues in medical technology, speak at medical conferences, and respond to inquiries from attorneys and journalists.

The Hastings education program conducts workshops for teachers and other professionals throughout the country, and sponsors internships for graduate and undergraduate students and fellowships for visiting scholars. The Hastings Center holds workshops on problems in the ethical and legal assessment of new technologies, e.g., a 1-day workshop held in 1983, "Which Babies Shall Live?," and week-long seminars on medical ethics.

Assessors

Hastings has a full-time staff of about 23. The research staff members have backgrounds in such disciplines as philosophy, medicine, political science, law, and psychology.

The multidisciplinary study groups generally include physicians, lawyers, ethicists, and economists. Other participants have come from the fields of literature, history, religious studies, philosophy, and sociology. The selection/appointment of research groups is made by the staff, the director, and the president and occasionally through inquiries made to Hastings Center fellows, of which there are currently approximately 150.

The Center has a 23-member board of directors comprising persons in medicine, law, ethics, education, industry, and biomedical, social, and behavioral research. New board members are nominated by Center fellows and are approved by the sitting board.

Turnaround

Turnaround time varies among types of projects. Most studies range from 6 to 12 months, although some have taken 2 years. The Center must also respond quickly to certain types of requests, such as for presenting testimony at congressional hearings and for state and local government agencies.

Reporting

The bimonthly *Hastings Center Report*, which reaches an audience of nearly 10,000, is devoted to case studies, court decisions, and other news and articles regarding ethical problems of the biomedical, behavioral, and social sciences and issues in professional and applied ethics. Published since 1971, this is the Center's primary means of communication with its members and the general public. Many of the publication's topics deal with ethical questions arising from the development of new medical technologies. Articles of the *Report* are frequently reprinted in books, other journals, newsletters, and for classroom use.

IRB: A Review of Human Subjects Research has been published since 1979 and appears 10 times a year. Other publications include monographs and books arising out of project work. Also, members of the Center staff act as consultants to communications media and to academia on ethical issues of medical technologies.

The Center also offers reading packets for teaching and public information in such categories as ethics and the life sciences; death, dying, and euthanasia; experimentation and informed consent; genetic engineering; and health policy and the allocation of scarce resources.

The Hasting Center Series in Ethics (published by Plenum Press) includes books such as *Which Babies Shall Live* (1985), *Ethics, the Social Sciences, and Policy Analysis* (1983), *In Search of Equity: Health Needs and the Health Care System* (1983), *Ethics and Hard Times* (1983), and *Violence and the Politics of Research* (1981).

Reassessment

The health policy project has reassessed implications of dialysis technologies.

Impact

Because Hastings does not set policy, it is especially difficult to measure its impact. A 1981 Hastings report listed a variety of activities in which it had participated to indicate both the scope of its work and range of possible impact. Cited were numerous instances of testimony before federal and state legislative committees, over 20 instances of assistance to other public bodies, membership on committees and commissions (e.g., NIH consensus development conferences), organization of national conferences, and assistance to a wide variety of public and private associations and societies. Also cited were publication of proposed guidelines on mass screening for genetic diseases, the definition of death and prenatal diagnosis, and participation in drafting legislation on hereditary diseases and the definition of death adopted in a number of states. Over 300 universities and professional schools have received Hastings Center assistance in the development of teaching programs in ethics. The New Jersey State attorney general, concerned about the implications of the Karen Ann Quinlan case—in which a young woman became comatose and was being kept alive by life-support systems—sought the Center's advice in establishing a definition of death.

Funding/Budget

The annual budget of the Center is about \$1.4 million. Of this amount, about \$250,000 is devoted to studies in health and medicine. About 54 percent of Center funding is derived from grants (both for specific projects and for the general fund) and contributions from individuals, foundations, and corporations (including drug and medical device companies and insurers); 18 percent is from government agencies (e.g., NIH and the National Center for Health Services Research); and the remainder is from membership dues, publications, workshops, and other sources.

Technology assessment activities are supported directly by foundations such as The Henry J. Kaiser Family Foundation, the Pew Memorial Trust, and the Charles C. Culpeper Foundation and by general funds from the Hastings Center's budget. The ongoing project on ethical issues of neonatology, for example, is supported by the National Foundation-March of Dimes, Squibb, and the Upjohn Company, among others.

Example

On the following pages is the full text of the Hastings Center report "The Care of the Terminally Ill: Mortality and Economics," published in 1983 in the *New England Journal of Medicine* (309:1490–1494) and is reproduced here with permission.

Sources

Caplan, A. L., Associate Director, Hastings Center. 1985. Personal communication.

Goodman, W. June 18, 1984. Medical Ethics are Fare at Hastings Center Party. New York Times.

Hastings Center. 1981. The Hastings Center: Ethics in the 80s.

Hastings Center. 1983. Financial statements for the year ended December 31, 1982.

Otten, A. L. November 23, 1983. As Medicine Advances, Hastings Center Tries to Solve Ethical Issues. Wall Street Journal.

SPECIAL ARTICLE

THE CARE OF THE TERMINALLY ILL: MORALITY AND ECONOMICS

RONALD BAYER, PH.D., DANIEL CALLAHAN, PH.D., JOHN FLETCHER, PH.D.*, THOMAS HODGSON, PH.D.†, BRUCE JENNINGS, M.A., DAVID MONSEES, PH.D.‡, STEVEN SIEVERTS, M.S.§, AND ROBERT VEATCH, PH.D.¶

Abstract Are current expenditures on dying patients disproportionate, unreasonable, or unjust? Although a review of empirical data reveals that care for the terminally ill is very costly, it is not appropriate to conclude that such expenditures represent a morally troubling misallocation of societal resources. Moreover, though efforts to reduce the costs of caring for the dying are not unreasonable, they must be undertaken with great caution. At present, such efforts should concentrate on three basic goals: development of better criteria for admission to intensive- and critical-care units; promotion of patient and family autonomy with regard to decisions to stop or refuse certain kinds of treatment; and promotion of alternative forms of institutional care, such as hospice care.

The most difficult moral problems will arise when patients and their physicians seek access to therapies judged only marginally useful. There may be conflict between administrators with broad institutional responsibilities and clinicians committed to particular patients. (N Engl J Med 1983; 309:1490-4.)

DURING the past decade, the care of the terminally ill has become a topic of sharpened debate. The conditions under which people die, the attitudes and practices of the medical profession toward them, and the ability of dying patients to control or modify the circumstances of their death have attracted wide attention. These concerns raise some exceedingly difficult practical and ethical questions for those who care for the terminally ill.

From the Hastings Center, 360 Broadway, Hastings-on-Hudson, NY 10706, where reprint requests should be addressed to Dr. Bayer.

Supported by a grant from the Health Services Improvement Fund of Blue Cross/Blue Shield of Greater New York.

*National Institutes of Health, Bethesda, Md.
†National Center for Health Statistics, Bethesda, Md.
‡National Institute of Child Health and Development, Bethesda, Md.
§Blue Cross/Blue Shield of Greater New York, New York, N.Y.
¶Kennedy Institute of Ethics, Washington, D.C.

Yet, as perplexing as these questions are, they become even more complex because of a growing, if ill-defined, economic concern that often lurks just below the surface of recent discussions. Terminal care often involves intensive and expensive treatment, and questions have been raised about its value. Is the cost too high? Is it "wasteful"?

Many recoil when such questions are raised. Indeed, a repugnance at the implications of a more "sensible," calculating approach to the care of the dying may lead one to repress the problem altogether. We believe, however, that the relation between the economic and the moral dimensions of care for the terminally ill is a subject that can be addressed openly, without embracing a crude calculus that trades life for dollars. It is ultimately neither possible nor desirable simply to ignore matters of costs and economics. If such issues are not brought out into the open, deci-

Reprinted from *The New England Journal of Medicine*
309:1490-1494 (December 15), 1983

sions may be made in a way that is beyond the pale of public scrutiny or accountability and on the basis of criteria that are capricious, unreasonable, or dangerous. Equally important, only a direct, careful discussion of the issues will prevent unexamined economic suppositions from artificially restricting full consideration of the moral and clinical aspects of terminal care.

The purpose of this paper is to stimulate responsible public discussion of the pertinent moral problems, and to do so by identifying some of the moral, conceptual, economic, and clinical issues that arise in the care of the terminally ill. After reviewing the evidence and attempting to specify the relevant moral considerations, we propose some general moral principles that may serve as a prolegomenon to more specific moral rules. We also suggest some strategies of cost containment that may lower expenses, but in ways that are responsible and humane from both a medical and a moral viewpoint.

The Costs of Caring for the Terminally Ill: Are There Moral Issues?

Is a disproportionate, unreasonable, and unjust amount of money being spent on the care of the terminally ill? In essence, that is the moral question that haunts current discussions about the care of dying patients. Since the medical needs of the terminally ill are often more acute than those of most other patients and their care is often more labor- and capital-intensive, it should hardly be surprising that such care is very costly. But are the costs disproportionate relative to the needs? Is it unreasonable to allocate expensive care to the terminally ill if that care is therapeutically warranted by reasonable standards of clinical judgment? And is it unjust to expend resources on the patients most in need of them rather than on those who will otherwise survive?

Furthermore, what does "terminal illness" mean? Though widely used, it is not a standard technical term with clear and precise criteria. The difficulties of prognosis, the occasional surprise recovery, and a combination of aspiration and hope can make such a determination problematic in many cases. No wonder many if not most physicians are often reluctant to declare formally that a patient is terminally ill.

The label "terminal illness" must therefore be used with caution. For the purpose of this paper, we define it as an illness in which, on the basis of the best available diagnostic criteria and in the light of available therapies, a reasonable estimation can be made prospectively and with a high probability that a person will die within a relatively short time. This definition is both specific enough to allow some focused discussion and general enough to take into account the difficulties of making precise predictions about the trajectory of dying.

Many of the moral and economic questions with which we are concerned in this paper also pertain to a consideration of the problems in caring for the critically ill — i.e., patients with poor prognoses whose death is possible but not highly probable, or those who *may* die. However, our discussion is restricted to patients for whom it is possible to make a prospective determination of terminal illness — i.e., those *known* to be dying.

Despite the importance of this distinction for a careful analysis of the moral issues surrounding the care of the dying, empirical research has been primarily retrospective and has tended to focus on the cost of care in the last months of life. Thus, the data available tend to conflate the costs of caring for the terminally ill and the critically ill. Nevertheless, a strong inference can be derived from the literature that the terminally ill receive proportionately much more expensive care than do other patients. Two kinds of data based primarily on retrospective analyses are available on the cost of caring for the terminally ill; for convenience, they may be called "macrolevel" and "microlevel" data.

In 1974 Selma Mushkin estimated that over 20 per cent of all nonpsychiatric hospital and nursing-home expenditures in nongovernment facilities were spent on the care of the terminally ill.[1] Although only 5 per cent of all Medicare enrollees died in 1967, 22 per cent of all reimbursements from that program were made on their behalf. The 1968 figures are similar,[2] and the proportions have remained relatively stable over the years. The Health Care Financing Administration reported that the cost of such care ranged from 19 to 22 per cent of all reimbursed Medicare charges from 1974 through 1976.

Of course, these data are only suggestive and reflect only the costs of care for patients covered by Medicare. Nonetheless, they are compatible with other microlevel data — that is, with the costs of caring for patients who are terminally ill with cancer and for those who do not survive after treatment in critical- or intensive-care units.

Scotto and Chiazze found that total hospitalizations and payments for patients with cancer who died within the 24-month period of data collection from 1969 to 1970 averaged almost twice those for patients who survived longer than 24 months.[3] This ratio of decedent-to-survivor costs echoes the average Medicare decedent-to-survivor ratio,[2] which is over 2:1. Detsky et al. studied an intensive-care unit and reported that "the care of nonsurvivors involved a significantly higher mean expenditure than did the care of survivors. . . ."[4] In an earlier study of 17 acute-care hospitals, the same researchers stated, "the data indicate that use of resources for dying patients exceeds resource use for other high-cost patients."[5] In a 1970 study of the Surgical Intensive-Care Unit at Massachusetts General Hospital, Civetta noted that "overall, the intensive care costs generated by prolonged utilization of this type of facility seem to be inversely related to the probability of patient survival."[6]

Some of the possible implications of these data have not gone unnoticed. For example, in his study of the treatment of patients who were acutely ill with cancer,

Silverman concluded, "a disproportionate amount of intervention was employed on patients who eventually expired. It seems evident that efforts directed at reducing cost and increasing efficiency must be focused on this high-risk, high-cost, low-yield group."[7] However, Detsky and his colleagues have sounded a note of caution:

> the relations between prognosis, expenditure, and outcome are more complex than can be appreciated when a study focuses only on nonsurvivors or on subsets of patients with the poorest prognosis or the highest costs. Among nonsurvivors, the highest charges were due to caring for patients who were perceived at the time of admission as having the greatest chance of recovery. Among survivors, the highest charges were incurred by those thought to have the least chance of recovery. Patients with unexpected outcomes . . . incurred the greatest costs. . . . For the clinician, the problem may seem hopelessly complex. Simple cost-saving solutions, such as withholding resources from the hopelessly ill or earlier transfer of those requiring only anticipatory care, are difficult to apply to an individual patient because prognosis is always uncertain.[4]

Where does that leave us? The available data do not allow us to conclude that the care is disproportionate, unreasonable, or unjust. Nonetheless, as new medical technologies lengthen the time span between the onset of the terminal phase of an illness and death, and as the number of persons over 65 years of age (the largest age group of terminally ill patients) increases, the cost of care for the terminally ill will surely rise above its present level. Hence, the belief in the need for cost-containment policies in terminal-care medicine will undoubtedly persist and may even gain intensity. An intelligent response to this belief requires a more complete and careful discussion of the general moral issues raised by cost-conscious decision making in the care of the terminally ill.

Defining the Moral Issues

There is no need here to repeat the many moral arguments that have been made to justify different forms of care for the terminally ill than for other patients. Their needs are different, and thus their care should be different — not less but different.

But can the special features of terminal illness support a moral case that less money should be spent on the care of the dying solely on the grounds that they are known to be dying? Or that more money should be spent on their care solely on the grounds that they are dying? Either general proposition, on its face, is hard to defend. To deny care to the terminally ill solely on the grounds that such care does not return the economic investment would be to stigmatize the dying as second-class persons, treating them with less than the respect deserved by all patients. The position that the dying have a greater right to economic resources runs the double risk of doing an injustice to other patients and using scarce resources without reflection. The real problem is to determine when and in what way a consideration of costs is reasonable either in clinical or administrative decision making, and then to devise acceptable criteria for making cost-conscious decisions.

The central dilemma here arises from the uncertainty regarding therapies that are only "marginally useful." It is unlikely, at one extreme, that anyone — administrator, clinician, family, or patient — would in principle be prepared either to justify diagnostic tests and therapies that promise no benefits whatsoever or to dismiss procedures that hold the possibility of substantial benefits. The important differences of opinion will focus on the use of marginally useful therapies, which can be defined as those that provide a slight but real contribution (physical or psychological) to the welfare of all or most patients or that make a moderately valuable contribution to the welfare of some but not most patients (with no certain foreknowledge of which patients are in the minority that will benefit).

Given the wide range of possible variations in the notion of "marginally useful" — from physical to psychological benefits, from moderate benefits for some to none for others, and so forth — it is hardly surprising to discover a wide array of attitudes toward them. For some, a benefit is a benefit, marginal or not. For others, a pursuit of marginal benefits has to be justified vigorously. What the administrator may view as a pattern of unjust or wasteful expenses for statistically minuscule benefits the clinician whose practices are being examined may consider a pattern of justified expenses for a series of individual treatments, each undertaken in the best interests of the particular patient.

The potential for conflict between administrators and clinicians is likely to be most pronounced in any attempt on the part of the former to set limits on the availability of diagnostic procedures and therapies. Administrators have obligations that are broader than those that confront clinicians. Whether responsible for the functioning of hospitals, concerned about the fiscal integrity of health-insurance programs, or involved in the planning of health services for a community, administrators must attempt to balance competing interests. At times, financial constraints will force decisions that are justified in terms of institutional or program survival rather than equity. Not infrequently, administrators at different levels of responsibility will confront each other with claims about the consequences for patients of efforts to limit health-care expenditures. In the end, the clinician's duty to individual patients may exist in a state of tension with the duties and commitments of the administrator. Given the likelihood of conflict, clinicians, patients, and the families of patients will benefit if they have a clear understanding of administrative policies, the constraints these policies impose, and the reasons for them.

Strategies of Cost Control

We believe that the attempt to find ways of reducing the costs of the care given to the dying is a reasonable one, since at least some of the current costs are a consequence of practices that are of little value to the patients and may in fact be harmful to their interests. But great caution is necessary in trying to reduce costs. Any such attempt cannot begin by assuming, as if demonstrated, that a large-scale socioeconomic problem exists or that there is a widespread and irresponsible indifference to costs.

We believe that at present, cost-containment policies for terminal care should concentrate on three basic goals: developing better criteria for admitting patients to intensive- or critical-care units, promoting the autonomy of patients and their families, and promoting alternative forms of institutional care.

Developing Better Criteria for Admission to Intensive- and Critical-Care Units

Considerable evidence suggests that a prime ingredient in the costs of caring for the terminally ill is the high cost associated with intensive- and critical-care units. However, the difficulties of prognosis stand in the way of any simple standards for deciding which patients should not receive such (expensive) care. The Massachusetts General Hospital's patient-classification system and the Therapeutic Intervention Scoring System represent efforts to address such difficulties.[8,9] Our point here is not to recommend these particular approaches, which suffer from a failure to take into account patient and family perspectives, but to underscore the need for further efforts of this kind.

Promoting Patient and Family Autonomy

A major focus in recent years has been the promotion of greater patient and family participation in decision making and the provision of a wider range of options for patients. In the case of the terminally ill, such efforts have centered on their right to withdraw from treatment or to refuse certain kinds of treatment and to have a larger number of choices concerning where they spend the remainder of their lives.

If patients and their families had greater decision-making powers, the cost of their care might be reduced, and their welfare enhanced. Our working assumption is that at least some terminally ill patients receive expensive care of a kind they would not, if better informed, desire.

Finally, every effort should be made at the policy level to maximize the participation of lay people — of eventual patients — in decisions to place limits on the kinds of care that will be made available to the terminally ill or on the services for the terminally ill that will be reimbursable under insurance plans.

Promoting Alternative Forms of Institutional Care

The hospice movement stands as the primary symbol of efforts to promote alternative institutional forms of care for the dying. Its premises are that many of the terminally ill prefer to die at home or in facilities other than those of a hospital, that more appropriate care may be provided in institutions designed primarily for palliation and caring rather than curing, and that patient autonomy and dignity are enhanced by the existence of alternative institutions among which patients can choose. Enough information has begun to accumulate to suggest that for those who seek such care — both the dying and their families — there are benefits. The terminal illness is made more bearable for the patients, and their families seem to adjust to the illness and to the bereavement afterward with greater psychological strength. Yet, to what extent the hospice movement will lead to a decrease in the costs of dying is far less clear. Considerably more experience and data will be necessary to reach any final judgment on the long-term economic benefits of hospice care.[10-12]

In 1982 the Congress moved to bring hospice care within the framework of Medicare, marking a shift in the reluctance of third-party payers to cover such services. We believe that though there are some risks to this new course, they ought to be run. No evidence exists to show that the net costs of such coverage will exceed those of hospital care for the dying, nor is there evidence that the extension of coverage will be subject to any special abuse or financial mismanagement. Most important, without a serious and much more widespread effort to test the hospice concept, there will be no way to judge the potential economic savings or the benefits to patients.

Developing Guidelines for the Future

Despite the existence of some anxiety about the misallocation of resources in the care of the dying, there is no solid evidence that the health-care system has reached a "tragic choice situation" requiring painful decisions to withhold medical care. Nonetheless, some tentative steps can certainly be taken to minimize the possibility of a wasteful or inappropriate allocation of resources for the care of the terminally ill. It is premature to propose a detailed set of moral rules for allocating resources to the dying, but it is not premature to suggest some broad guidelines that can at least help focus the issues. The general statements that follow are meant to summarize our analysis and findings and to suggest procedures for the future.

The Determination of Terminal Illness

Even though it may be difficult in many cases, clinicians should be prepared to make a determination that an illness is terminal and to propose changes in care when such a determination has been made.

Services for Terminally Ill Patients

When the consequence of a determination that a patient is terminally ill is to change the nature of services that the patient will receive, the clinician should ensure that no services that can considerably prolong the patient's life or reduce physical or psychological suffering are withheld (unless the patient refuses them).

In ordering services for the terminally ill, clinicians should request no diagnostic tests that do not promise to provide useful information for patient care. Therapeutic or rehabilitative services should be proposed only to increase the patient's comfort and the quality of his or her remaining life. Responsiveness to the patient's expressed needs and wishes should remain an important norm.

The Settings for Care of the Terminally Ill

Policy makers and health planners should accelerate current efforts to develop reimbursement plans for the care of dying patients in various settings. At a minimum, all communities should have care available in short-term inpatient hospital facilities, in institutional outpatient settings, and in patients' homes or surrogate homes.

Services for terminally ill patients in all alternative settings should be planned and managed to meet the special medical, psychological, spiritual, and human-support needs of each patient. The hospice concept provides the ingredients for this kind of care. Families that provide services needed by the terminally ill should receive appropriate support and, when necessary, special training.

Government and private insurance plans should be designed to encourage voluntary efforts. For example, policies that fail to support training programs for home care should be changed. However, government at all levels should accept the responsibility to ensure that terminally ill patients who lack funds from other sources are given the necessary support through the public welfare system.

Future Research Needs

The lack of good data on the costs of caring for the terminally ill both fuels anxiety about the issue and prevents any useful judgment about whether there is a genuine issue. Despite our skepticism that a serious problem exists, further studies can be helpful. Past efforts to collect good data have been hampered by the difficulties inherent in defining terminal illness, by the fact that the studies have been retrospective, and by the fact that available records typically show only that a patient died, not whether the patient was declared terminally ill at some point and, if so, how he or she was subsequently treated. The need for prospective studies, perhaps even participant-observer investigations, is obvious. Such studies will have to make clear the distinct patterns of care required for patients affected by different diseases and the variations in care given to patients in different age groups. The concept of marginally useful therapy also requires further investigation.

A number of studies under way at present may provide better data on the costs of cancer, catastrophic illness, and terminal illness. Some of the studies bear directly on the costs of terminal illness or illness in the last year of life, whereas others have an indirect bearing, in the sense that they focus on the total cost of illness. Much more, however, needs to be done.

We are indebted to the following participants in the Hastings Center Project on Terminal Illness: Dorothy Rice, Richard Rettig, Ph.D., David Willis, M.P.H., Ida Martinson, R.N., Ph.D., Carol Farkas, Stanley Jones, Charles Goulet, Norman Walter, M.D., and Jerome Yates, M.D.

References

1. Mushkin SJ, ed. Consumer incentives for health care. New York: Prodist, 1974:183-216.
2. Piro PA, Lutins T. Utilization and reimbursement under Medicare for persons who died in 1967 and 1968. Washington, D.C.: Social Security Administration, 1973. (DHEW publication no. (SSA)74-11702).
3. Scotto J, Chiazze L. Third national cancer survey: hospitalizations and payments to hospitals. Part A: Summary. Bethesda, Md.: National Institutes of Health, 1974. (DHEW publication no. (NIH)76-1094).
4. Detsky AS, Stricker SC, Mulley AG, Thibault GE. Prognosis, survival, and the expenditure of hospital resources for patients in an intensive-care unit. N Engl J Med 1981; 305:667-72.
5. Schroeder SA, Showstack JA, Roberts HE. Frequency and clinical description of high-cost patients in 17 acute-care hospitals. N Engl J Med 1979; 300:1306-9.
6. Civetta JM. The inverse relationship between cost and survival. J Surg Res 1973; 14:265-9.
7. Silverman DG, Goldiner PL, Kaye BA, Howland WS, Turnbull AD. The therapeutic intervention scoring system: an application to acutely ill cancer patients. Crit Care Med 1975; 3:222-5.
8. Optimum care for hopelessly ill patients: a report of the Clinical Care Committee of the Massachusetts General Hospital. N Engl J Med 1976; 295:362-4.
9. Cullen DJ, Civetta JM, Briggs BA, Ferrara LC. Therapeutic intervention scoring system: a method for quantitative comparison of patient care. Crit Care Med 1974; 2:57-60.
10. Bloom BS, Kissick PD. Home and hospital cost of terminal illness. Med Care 1980; 18:560-4.
11. Kassakian MG, Bailey LR, Rinker M, Stewart CA, Yates JW. The cost and quality of dying: a comparison of home and hospital. Nurse Pract 1979; 4(1):18-23.
12. Comptroller General of the United States. Report to Congress. Hospice care — a growing concept in the United States (March 6, 1979). Washington, D.C.: Government Printing Office, 1979:25.

Division of Health Services Research
Department of Medical Methods Research
The Permanente Medical Group, Inc.
3451 Piedmont Avenue
Oakland, CA 94611
(415) 428-6700

Major Emphases of Technology Assessment Activities

	Concerns			
Technology	Safety	Efficacy/ Effectiveness	Cost/Cost-Effect/ Cost-Benefit	Ethical/Legal/ Social
Drugs				
Medical Devices/Equipment/Supplies		X	X	
Medical/Surgical Procedures		X	X	
Support Systems		X	X	
Organizational/Administrative		X	X	

Stage of Technologies Assessed
X Emerging/new
X Accepted use
X Possibly obsolete, outmoded

Application of Technologies
X Prevention
X Diagnosis/screening
X Treatment
___ Rehabilitation

Assessment Methods
___ Laboratory testing
X Clinical trials
X Epidemiological and other observational methods
X Cost analyses
X Simulation/modeling
X Group judgment
X Expert opinion
X Literature syntheses

Approximate 1985 budget for technology assessment: $50,000*

* This is the average amount spent for technology assessments since 1979.

DEPARTMENT OF MEDICAL METHODS RESEARCH THE PERMANENTE MEDICAL GROUP, INC. DIVISION OF HEALTH SERVICES RESEARCH

Introduction

The Kaiser-Permanente Medical Care Program (KPMCP) in Northern California is a group practice prepayment plan providing comprehensive medical and hospital services to about 1.9 million members with 13 hospitals, 19 outpatient medical offices, and 1,800 physicians. KPMCP established in 1961 its Department of Medical Methods Research (MMR) for the purpose of conducting health services research directed toward utilizing modern technology for improved delivery of medical care with the KPMCP.

MMR is administered professionally by its director under The Permanente Medical Group (TPMG) and has a total staff of about 70 persons. All MMR grants and contracts funded from sources outside KPMCP are administered by the Kaiser Foundation Research Institute, a nonprofit, tax-exempt corporation.

MMR's main divisions of activity include Epidemiology and Biostatistics, and Health Services Research. The Health Services Research Division now includes the activities of the former Technology Assessment Division, which was established in 1979 in response to increased interest of KPMCP in medical and surgical procedures, equipment, and systems.

Purpose

The primary purpose of the technology assessments carried out by the Division of Health Services Research is to aid in the consideration of alternative choices of technology-based services.

Subjects of Assessment

The Division has carried out assessments of procedures, equipment, and systems used in diagnostic, therapeutic, and coordinating patient care services.

Stage of Diffusion

The Division considers for assessment emerging, new, existing, and potentially outmoded technologies.

Concerns

The primary concerns of assessments are costs, effectiveness, and the impact on the organization as to technical personnel, equipment, facilities, and financing. The assessments generally are not made in order to arrive at a single decision or recommendation; rather, they present the important consequences—intended and unintended—of appropriate alternative technologies so that management can make more rational decisions; thus the assessments are made to decrease the uncertainty of decision making.

Requests

Technologies suitable for assessment have been identified within KPMCP at all organizational levels; these have included the executive director (for biofeedback), professional service chiefs (alternative treatment modes of end-stage renal disease [ESRD]), and pediatric geneticists (alpha-fetoprotein screening). The Division also has conducted periodic surveys of about 300 KPMCP professional services chiefs to identify substantial capital-investment equipment needs that might be candidates for assessment.

Selection

The primary selection criterion for assessments have been total annual costs. A procedure may be selected for assessment if it has a low unit cost but a very large case load (e.g., chest x rays) or a large unit cost but a small case load (e.g., renal dialysis). Also selected for assessment have been procedures with insufficient information for a decision to include them as Health Plan benefits (e.g., biofeedback). Studies comparing alternative programs (e.g., multiphasic checkups versus traditional health checkups, primary care by team versus by traditional mode, and computer versus manual hospital information systems) have been conducted by the Division of Health Services Research.

Process

Assessments consider the characteristics of the population utilizing the technology, the work loads for its utilization, and its total annual costs. Alternative technologies used for the same specified objectives are evaluated as to important intended and unintended consequences, with consideration of the alternative competing technologies per million people. These studies all have used epidemiologic methods, medical record studies, and literature reviews; consensus development was used for the alpha-fetoprotein study, sensitivity analysis for the ESRD study, and controlled studies for the multiphasic and primary care team studies.

Assessors

Assessments are coordinated by the director of the Division who works with the project chief, who assembles a team of 4-10 experts from the KPMCP.

Turnaround

The average time for an assessment is approximately 6 months. The shortest time to complete an assessment was 3 months for the biofeedback study; the longest was 18 months for the end-stage renal disease study.

Reporting

In the past 5 years, four assessments have been presented to the executive director of TPMG and its board of directors; these are briefly summarized below under Examples.

Impact

The TPMG board of directors selected one of the alternatives proposed in the biofeedback study. The alpha-fetoprotein study was accepted by the board but action was deferred pending the State of California's initiation of its mandated alpha-fetoprotein screening program. The end-stage renal disease study resulted in the executive director of The Permanente Medical Group appointing a special team to develop a long term plan for ESRD care in the Northern California KPMCP.

Reassessment

No technology has been reassessed thus far. It is possible that a reassessment of biofeedback may be requested if new data would become available suggesting improved cost-effectiveness.

Funding/Budget

Approximately $50,000 per year was expended by the Kaiser-Permanente Department of Medical Methods Research for technology assessments in the period 1979–1983. The study on utilization of diagnostic x rays was supported in part by the Bureau of Radiological Health.

Examples

Four assessments conducted by MMR (specifically by the former Division of Technology Assessment) are summarized below. The first, on end-stage renal disease, is discussed in greater detail than the others on biofeedback, utilization of diagnostic x rays, and serum alpha-fetoprotein.

A Technology Assessment of Care for End-Stage Renal Disease The purpose of this study was to assess the effects on costs to the Northern California Kaiser Foundation Health Plan (KFHP) of alternative treatment technologies for end-stage renal disease (ESRD) and of various economic and case load factors.

ESRD is a unique disease category for KFHP in that it is primarily treated by other than the Permanente Medical Group (TPMG) physicians in outside facilities and Medicare is the primary payer. As a result, KFHP is in a vulnerable financial situation when either Medicare alters its reimbursement schedule or when non-TPMG providers use treatment technologies which could be more economically provided by TPMG physicians in Kaiser-Permanente (K-P) facilities. At the beginning of 1982, KFHP was paying in part for the care of 457 ESRD patients (compared to 300 in 1978), and the number of new ESRD cases entering the program for care was about 100 a year. The total payments for care of these ESRD members was estimated to be $12 million, of which Medicare paid about 65 percent and KFHP paid about 35 percent or roughly $2 per member for the year.

For this study, a computer model was employed to generate 5- and 10-year cost projections for 16 scenarios. The model used data from 1978-1981 KFHP experience, and from estimates arrived at by consensus of a group of K-P nephrologists. Due to the uncertainty of both past and future economic data, the study involved a sensitivity analysis in which a variety of assumptions were made for important variables, and cost projections were calculated for each assumption using the computer model. The model used several important variables, including the following:

1. the mix of ESRD technologies used (institutional, center self-care, home care, continuous ambulatory peritoneal dialysis, and kidney transplants from live or cadaver donors)
2. the ESRD patient case load
3. the proportion of ESRD patients cared for within K-P facilities
4. the general economic inflation rate
5. the Medicare reimbursement schedule

The study recognized that, of these five important variables, K-P can only influence significantly 1 and 2.

The study showed how relatively less sensitive are KFHP's total payments to changes in inflation, case load growth rates, and the percentage of patients treated in K-P facilities. The study indicated that when KFHP becomes the primary payer, then the cost-effective use of alternative treatments and the care of ESRD patients by TPMG physicians will become very important. The scenarios tested showed that KFHP could protect itself by

1. more aggressive region-wide negotiations with non-TPMG providers for lower payment schedules
2. monitoring payments by a centralized computer-based registry
3. lobbying for continuing Medicare support
4. phasing in additional dialysis centers while attempting to decrease internal dialysis costs and initiating programs to employ more lower-cost dialysis treatment modes
5. limiting ESRD benefits to patients cared for by TPMG physicians within K-P facilities

The study concluded that it would be prudent to consider the probability of a serious decrease in Medicare support of ESRD care by 1986, and K-P could benefit by obtaining more actual in-house experience from establishing pilot programs to develop cost-effective methods for certain modes of treatment. Such action could save KFHP $1 million in 1986 and as much as $18 million over 10 years.

Biofeedback A new treatment modality was advocated by some TPMG physicians for chronically recurring headaches and other conditions. An assessment was completed using data from three Kaiser-Permanente medical centers and from the literature. The consequences were assessed as they would relate to three alternative organizational decisions for providing biofeedback as a Health Plan benefit, namely, full biofeedback benefits, partial benefits for treatment of chronic headaches only, and no biofeedback benefits. Included was a sensitivity analysis of effects from a variety of biofeedback treatment schedules.

Utilization of Diagnostic X Rays Skull, chest, and upper gastrointestinal tract diagnostic x-ray procedures are the leading radiological expenditures for ambulatory care services. An assessment was completed analyzing clinical indications (i.e., referral criteria) for ordering these x-ray examinations and the effects of the radiologists' reports on the diagnosis, treatment, and outcome of patients. (This study was supported in part by a grant from the FDA's Bureau of Radiological Health.)

Serum Alpha-Fetoprotein Increasing California State legislative interest in this procedure could require KPMCP to provide serum alpha-fetoprotein screening tests to 30,000 pregnant women each year, followed by a series of costly technical procedures (including ultrasonography and amniocentesis) when positive. An assessment compared the consequences of screening versus no screening of this subpopulation.

Sources

Collen, M. F., Director, Technology Assessment, Department of Medical Methods Research, The Permanente Medical Group, Inc. 1982. Technology Assessment in Prepaid Group Practice (see Appendix B).

Collen, M. F., Consultant in Technology Assessment, Department of Medical Methods Research, The Permanente Group, Inc. 1985. Personal communications.

The Permanente Medical Group, Inc., Department of Medical Methods Research. 1983. A Technology Assessment of Care for End-Stage Renal Disease (ESRD) for the Kaiser-Permanente Medical Care Program Northern California Region.

Medtronic, Inc.
3055 Old Highway Eight
P.O. Box 1453
Minneapolis, MN 55440
(612) 574-4000

Major Emphases of Technology Assessment Activities

Technology	Concerns: Safety	Efficacy/ Effectiveness	Cost/Cost-Effect/ Cost-Benefit	Ethical/Legal/ Social
Drugs				
Medical Devices/Equipment/Supplies	X	X	X	
Medical/Surgical Procedures				
Support Systems				
Organizational/Administrative				

Stage of Technologies Assessed
- X Emerging/new
- X Accepted use
- ___ Possibly obsolete, outmoded

Application of Technologies
- ___ Prevention
- X Diagnosis/screening
- X Treatment
- ___ Rehabilitation

Assessment Methods
- X Laboratory testing
- X Clinical trials
- X Epidemiological and other observational methods
- X Cost analyses
- X Simulation/modeling
- ___ Group judgment
- X Expert opinion
- X Literature syntheses

Approximate 1985 budget for technology assessment: $38,000,000*

* This is an estimate of total 1985 research and development (R&D) expenditures, about 9 percent of the company's annual sales. No line item exists for technology assessment, for which expenditures are considerably less than this amount. Clinical trials expenditures vary according to stage of development of major products; e.g., Medtronic spent roughly 7 percent of its 1983 heart pacing product R&D budget on clinical trials.

MEDTRONIC, INC.

Introduction

Medtronic, Inc., designs, manufactures, and markets heart pacemaker systems, neurological systems, mechanical heart valves, and instrumentation for medical diagnosis and monitoring. The company's service operations include patient monitoring (e.g., ambulatory heart monitoring) and physician education. Medtronic is the world's leading producer of implantable medical devices, both in terms of sales and number of units sold. As of 1983, one million Medtronic pacemakers and ten thousand Medtronic mechanical heart valves had been implanted in humans. Cardiac pacing products and services accounted for 83 percent of Medtronic's

$422.7 million in fiscal 1984 sales. Medtronic accounted for an estimated 40 percent of the total 1982 pacemaker market in the United States, where 130,000 implantations are performed annually (Standard & Poor's, 1983).

Medtronic employs approximately 5,000 people around the world and does business in over 75 countries. From 25 to 30 percent of Medtronic's 1983 sales were to overseas markets. International production facilities are located in Brazil, Canada, France, and The Netherlands. U.S. plants are located in Arizona, Colorado, Massachusetts, Michigan, Minnesota, and Puerto Rico. World headquarters are in Minneapolis. Medtronic was incorporated in Minnesota in 1957.

Purpose

The purpose of Medtronic's evaluation activities is to produce products of high quality and reliability, and to build the knowledge and expertise on which future products are based.

Subjects of Assessment

Medtronic evaluates its medical devices, materials (e.g., polymers, metals, and ceramics), components (e.g., microelectronic circuits), fabrication methods, and application/implantation methods used for its products.

In 1984, Medtronic was evaluating a variety of new products in various stages of development. These included a cystic fibrosis screening system, a portable blood pressure monitor, several cardioversion-defibrillation products, vascular prostheses, sensors for rate-responsive pacing, blood gas monitors, computer-enhanced imaging systems for diagnosis and stress testing, and a microprocessor-based artificial heart valve monitor. Also under evaluation were electrode gels, electrochemical sensors, drug administration (implanted pump and reservoir) devices, rate-responsive pacing systems (which alter pacing rate in response to changes in patient activity), external and implantable devices for treating scoliosis, spinal cord stimulation systems for treatment of chronic intractable pain, and a synthetic speech source device.

Assessment of the medical procedures in which Medtronic devices play a key role is an important element of evaluation. For example, assessments of procedures for device implantation are used to provide instructions for the use of pacemaker leads.

Medtronic also works with materials and component suppliers to improve the function, reliability, and quality of the technological elements which make up devices.

Stage of Diffusion

In addition to evaluating the emerging and new technologies it develops, Medtronic evaluates existing technologies for product improvement and quality control purposes.

Concerns

Technology evaluation is concerned with safety, efficacy, cost-benefit, cost-effectiveness, and quality of life. Comparisons are made among Medtronic products, as well as those of other manufacturers, particularly for the purpose of improving durability, design features, manufacturing methods, and longevity. For example, new and existing pacemaker power sources undergo comparative testing.

Requests

The primary source of the technologies developed and evaluated by Medtronic is clinical practice. A number of major Medtronic products originated from the ideas of clinicians, and were developed in collaboration with Medtronic. Some ideas for products have resulted from reconsideration of technologies which had been evaluated earlier, without further action at the time.

Medtronic has assembled medical panels to discuss the capabilities of current products and to explore clinical need and directions for new product development. Other sources for product development and improvement efforts include reports of clinical engineers studying Medtronic products and detailed analyses of returned devices. These sources are particularly useful for development and improvement of device components, fabrication methods, and manufacturing controls.

Selection

There is no formal process for selecting technologies to be evaluated; technologies which are designed to meet clinical needs and which show promise are those which are allocated resources for development and further evaluation.

Process

The evaluation process varies according to the product, e.g., entirely new products usually undergo different evaluations than do modifications of existing products. Evaluations generally begin with a literature review and extend through preclinical testing and clinical trials with review points where it is determined whether adequate promise exists to begin subsequent stages of the assessment. Thus, satisfactory results of preclinical testing must precede the support of clinical evaluation in humans. Computer modeling is used in some circumstances. Food and Drug Administration (FDA) study requirements are followed wherever applicable. Medtronic has various sources of data for follow-up study of pacemakers and other of its products. Medtronic conducts so-called phase IV follow-up studies as a condition of FDA approval for marketing certain devices. Medtronic maintains a registry of device implantation data and implant experience. (When Medtronic pacemakers are implanted, physicians complete implant data reports which are collected and compiled by Medtronic). Implant physicians are kept apprised of experience related to the lots of devices that they have implanted and are encouraged to report to the company any further information regarding implant experience. Medtronic also conducts telephonic monitoring of pacemakers, and expects to reach 150,000 patients through this service by 1988.

Assessors

Each Medtronic business group (these are the Components and Instruments Group, Pacing Systems Group, International Group, and New Businesses Group) is responsible for the evaluation of its products along with its other business operations. Evaluations are undertaken by a wide range of experts in technology, science, and medicine. Examples include biochemists, physicists, polymer chemists, electrical engineers, clinical engineers, cardiologists, and orthopedic surgeons.

Consisting of the executives of the business groups, The Corporate Research and Technology Committee coordinates work across business groups based on corporate strategies and provides a channel for sharing evaluation findings and other developments. A major role of the committee is to review major proposed and new technologies which represent significant departures from those being used currently. Corporate research expenditures are based on the committee's findings.

Turnaround

Complete evaluation of a major new product, including clinical studies and FDA review, generally requires several years. Some products require more time for development and evaluation. The time from initial research to marketing of the single-channel scoliosis system (discussed under Example below) was 12 years, followed by several years of postmarketing study and reporting required by the FDA. An improvement in an existing product, the heart valve, required 5 years from conception to marketing. Minor changes, such as modification of a lead conductor or a software change in a programmable pacemaker, take less time. Due to differing regulatory requirements for evaluation, marketing outside the United States may occur several years earlier than U.S. marketing for a given product.

Reporting

Medtronic provides appropriate reports to the FDA to obtain premarket approval for its products. Medtronic also prepares reports for clinicians who will use Medtronic devices, showing the results of evaluations, particularly those conducted in a clinical setting. Clinicians involved in Medtronic studies frequently report clinical findings to their peers through published literature and at conferences and symposia. Company technical specialists and scientists also report through these forums.

In addition to Medtronic's own reporting, considerable independent evaluation of Medtronic products and similar products manufactured by other companies is undertaken and reported in the literature. Reprints of these independent reports are often distributed with Medtronic reports. Among recent examples, the Pacemaker Center, University of Southern California School of Medicine, reported on the long-term performance of pulse generators used in cardiac pacemakers manufactured by Medtronic and other manufacturers (Bilitch et al., 1984). Butrous et al. (1983) compared the effect of power frequency high intensity electric fields on 16 different pacemaker models from six manufacturers, including Medtronic. Hanson and Grant (1984) examined the 9-year experience during 1972-1982 of over 1,000 pacemakers in over 800 patients for such concerns as changing indications for pacing, patient survival, and experience with different pacemaker types, including 10 Medtronic models. Herbert (1983) reported on three treatments of scoliosis using electrical stimulation of muscle, including the Electro Spinal Orthosis (ESO) treatment developed by Medtronic and described below under Example.

Impact

FDA reviews of evaluations usually allow for the next phases of evaluation, or marketing, in the United States. The choices clinicians make are likely based on their own assessment of the clinical performance of the device, peer information, the literature, and/or other sources.

Reassessment

The performance of currently used technologies is continuously reassessed, based on experience in the field, analysis of returned products, and in-house bench testing of production samples.

Funding/Budget

In fiscal year 1984, Medtronic invested approximately 9 percent of sales, i.e., $37.6 million, in research and development. In 1984, Medtronic predicted that over $250 million would be devoted to research and development over the next 5 years.

Example

On the following pages is the table of contents and introduction only to a 15-page report of the clinical evaluation of the "Medtronic Scoliosis System Electro Spinal Orthosis (ESO) for the Treatment of Scoliosis" (Medtronic, May 1983), which are reproduced here with permission. The full report is a summary of current ESO clinical study results.

Sources

Bilitch, M., R. G. Hauser, B. S. Goldman, S. Furman, and V. Parsonnet. 1984. Performance of cardiac pacemaker pulse generators. PACE 7:157-161.

Butrous, G. S., J. C. Male, R. S. Webber, D. G. Barton, S. J. Meldrum, J. A. Bonnell, and A. J. Camm. 1983. The effect of power frequency high intensity electric fields on implanted cardiac pacemakers. PACE 6:1282-1292.

Flink, R. C., Director of Corporate Standards, Medtronic. 1985. Personal communication.

Hanson, J. S., and M. E. Grant. 1984. Nine-year experience during 1972-1982 with 1,060 pacemakers in 805 patients. PACE 7:51-62.

Herbert, M. A. 1983. The treatment of scoliosis using electrical stimulation of muscle. Engineering in Medicine and Biology. September:43–49.

Medtronic, Inc. 1983. Medtronic Scoliosis System® Electro Spinal Orthosis (ESO) for the Treatment of Scoliosis: Clinical Study Results. Minneapolis.

Medtronic, Inc. 1985. Annual Report, 1984. Minneapolis.

Standard & Poor's Corporation. 1983. Industry Surveys. Health Care: Basic Analysis 151:H13-H35.

Medtronic Scoliosis System™ Electro Spinal Orthosis (ESO) For the Treatment of Scoliosis

CLINICAL STUDY RESULTS

May 1983

NOTE: This report is only a summary of current ESO clinical study results. The ESO study will continue until sufficient data have been collected to confirm safety and efficacy of the ESO system, pursuant to U.S. requirements. More specific information is available if required by contacting Medtronic, Attention: Scoliosis Marketing, at the address on the back cover. Your comments on this report will be most appreciated.

Table of Contents

Illustrations

I. Introduction

Medtronic first became involved in the area of scoliosis in 1971 when approached by Dr. Newton McCollough, University of Miami, who was interested in the concept of stimulating the muscles of the back to treat scoliosis. In 1972-73, Medtronic worked with Dr. McCollough in designing a stimulation unit. In 1974, a pilot study was initiated to investigate the possibility of using such surface stimulation. As the study progressed, a national study group was formed in 1977 under Dr. McCollough's directorship. This study group is the foundation of the data collected and presented in this report.

The MEDTRONIC® ESO (Electro Spinal Orthosis) system consists of a stimulator, electrical cables, and electrodes. The stimulator contains the power source and the electronic circuitry of the system. The cables and electrodes transfer intermittent pulses to the patient.

Objectives

The primary objectives of the clinical investigation have been to demonstrate the safety, efficacy, and reliability of Medtronic scoliosis stimulation devices (single and dual channel models). Specifically, the objectives are:

1. To evaluate the effectiveness of this treatment in stabilizing single lumbar, thoracolumbar, thoracic, or double major idiopathic scoliotic curves by comparing curve measurement before treatment and at appropriate times during and following the conclusion of treatment.

2. To evaluate patient acceptance and compliance to this form of treatment.

3. To verify the effectiveness of alternative electrode placement sites in relation to the apex and length of the curve.

4. To evaluate the success of the treatment in relation to a series of interdependent variables, including bone age maturity, initial curve size, and rates of progression.

5. To evaluate the safety of this treatment and potential side effects and complications.

The following report outlines the results to date using the MEDTRONIC® ESO system. (Note that there are separate sections for single- and dual-channel results.)

Protocol

A protocol was established for the ESO study to differentiate patients on the basis of specific variables. In a study such as this, we cannot, of course, look at every possible application; lines must be drawn somewhere. However, we chose to study patients we felt were most likely to progress—i.e., the "worst case" group. And, within our guidelines, patients were differentiated on the basis of their likelihood of progression.

It should be pointed out, though, that these patients are *not* the only group that can potentially be treated. Additional clinical studies are now underway to evaluate other indications, such as kyphosis.

The protocol for using the Electro Spinal Orthosis required that only patients between 20° and 40° curve measurement (using the Cobb measurement technique) be included in the study. In addition, for patients with curves between 20° and 29°, 5° of documented progression during the previous 12-month period was required. The patients had to have at least one year of bone growth remaining, documented by either Risser sign (excursion and fusion of the iliac crest), bone age as defined by Greulich and Pyle Atlas using distal radial epiphysis, or vertebral body maturation.

Curve location was defined using the guidelines of the Scoliosis Research Society. Thoracic curves included those with apex above T12. Thoracolumbar curves included those with apex at T12 or L1, and lumbar curves included those with apex below L1.

Electrode Sites

Electrodes were placed using three general locations. Physicians selected the electrode site that provided the best acute curve correction, defined as best muscle contraction. The three electrode sites were:

1. *Paraspinal placement:* approximately 2.5 - 4 cm from the spine and surrounding the curve apex.

2. *Intermediate placement:* approximately midway between the paraspinal and lateral position.

3. *Lateral placement:* at or slightly posterior to the midaxillary line and surrounding the apical rib.

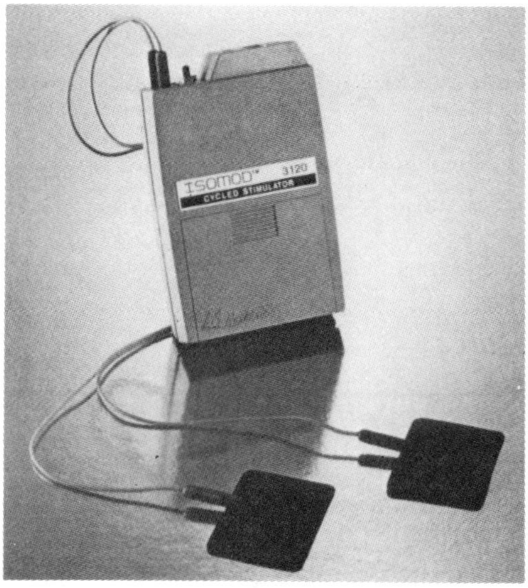

Figure 1. MEDTRONIC® Single-Channel ESO System

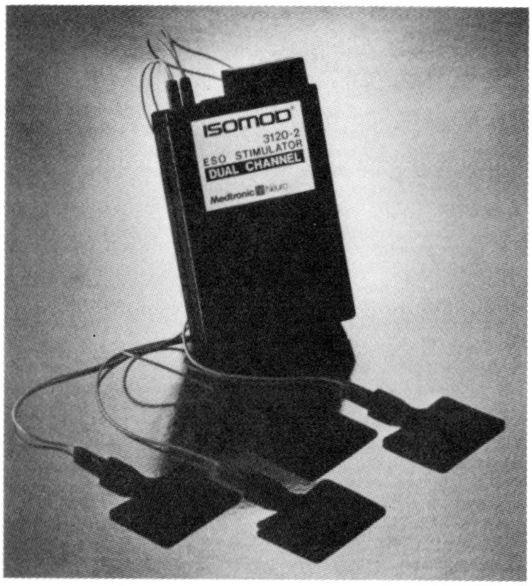

Figure 2. MEDTRONIC® Dual-Channel ESO System

Following the initial application of the ESO system, patients returned one week later for a check of electrode positions, and to obtain answers to any questions either they or their parents had concerning the device. Patients then returned after one month for an x-ray and electrode placement check. They returned every four months during the course of treatment for x-rays and curve measurements. If any adverse effects occurred between treatment follow-up visits, they were documented at the time of the visit and corrective measures were taken. Patient compliance was measured either by the use of patient diaries, interrogation of the patient and parents by the physician or physical therapist or, in the case of the dual-channel device, by a 1,000-hour patient compliance meter, which operated while the device was operating.

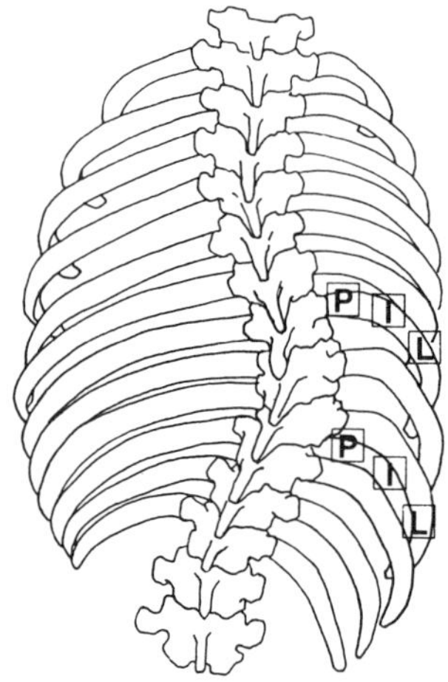

Figure 3. Electrode Placement Sites

Office of Health Technology Assessment
National Center for Health Services Research and Health Care Technology Assessment

5600 Fishers Lane, 3-10 Park Building
Rockville, MD 20857
(301) 443-4990

Major Emphases of Technology Assessment Activities

Technology	Concerns: Safety	Efficacy/ Effectiveness	Cost/Cost-Effect/ Cost-Benefit	Ethical/Legal/ Social
Drugs				
Medical Devices/Equipment/Supplies	X	X		
Medical/Surgical Procedures	X	X		
Support Systems				
Organizational/Administrative				

Stage of Technologies Assessed
X* Emerging/new
X Accepted use
X Possibly obsolete, outmoded

Application of Technologies
___ Prevention
X Diagnosis/screening
X Treatment
___ Rehabilitation

Assessment Methods
___ Laboratory testing
___ Clinical trials
___ Epidemiological and other observational methods
___ Cost analyses
___ Simulation/modeling
___ Group judgment
X Expert opinion
X Literature syntheses

Approximate 1985 budget for technology assessment: $700,000

* The great majority of assessments have dealt with new technologies or new applications for existing technologies.

OFFICE OF HEALTH TECHNOLOGY ASSESSMENT NATIONAL CENTER FOR HEALTH SERVICES RESEARCH AND HEALTH CARE TECHNOLOGY ASSESSMENT

Introduction

The Public Health Service (PHS) has been responding to requests for assessments from the Social Security Administration, and to the Health Care Financing Administration (HCFA), since the late 1960s. The Office of Health Technology Assessment (OHTA), of the National Center for Health Services Research and Health Care Technology Assessment (NCHSRHCTA), under the Office of the Assistant Secretary for Health, has the direct responsibility for conducting technology evaluations and making recommendations in response to HCFA requests. OHTA (originally as the Office of Health Research, Statistics, and Technology) assumed these responsibilities following the dissolution of the National Center for Health Care Technology

(NCHCT) in 1981. Other assessment activities of the NCHSRHCTA are discussed elsewhere in this report.

Among the technology assessment and information dissemination duties of OHTA/NCHSR described in the *Federal Register* (January 19, 1983; Vol. 48, No. 13, p. 2444) are

- administer a program of assessments of health care technologies which take into account their safety; efficacy; cost-effectiveness; and social, ethical, and economic impacts, and
- make recommendations on health care technology issues in the administration of the laws under the Assistant Secretary for Health's jurisdiction, including preparation of the PHS position regarding appropriateness of Medicare coverage of health care technology.

In late 1984, Congress (in P.L. 98-551) renamed the National Center for Health Services Research (NCHSR) the National Center for Health Services Research and Health Care Technology Assessment, and set aside $3 million of its FY 1985 budget (and $3.5 million in FY 1986 and $4 million in FY 1987) specifically for technology assessment. This increased support is primarily intended to strengthen the agency's ability to make recommendations regarding Medicare coverage issues.

Purpose

The objective of the OHTA evaluation is to provide HCFA with the most current information on health care technology to support coverage decisions. To assist HCFA in deciding what diagnostic and therapeutic techniques and procedures ought to be covered by Medicare, OHTA carries out evaluations of selected technologies. The final decisions on coverage are made by HCFA; the PHS has neither statutory nor regulatory authority to decide such matters. (See Department of Health and Human Services, Office of the Assistant Secretary for Planning and Evaluation [1984] for a detailed description of the HCFA coverage decision process.)

The basis for HCFA requests for information was originally outlined in an administrative agreement between HCFA and PHS. Under the agreement HCFA sought recommendations regarding

> . . . the safety and clinical effectiveness of medical products or procedures identified by HCFA for which a coverage determination cannot be made by HCFA on the basis of existing policies and rules, prior coverage determinations, or prior advice from PHS (OHTA, 1983).

Subjects of Assessment

Technologies to be assessed may include any discrete and identifiable techniques or procedures used to diagnose or treat illness, prevent disease, maintain patient well-being, or facilitate the provision of health care services. Table A-9 shows the OHTA Assessment Report Series and coverage recommendations made to HCFA.

Stage of Diffusion

Subjects for OHTA assessment may range from practices that are obsolete or of questionable effectiveness to new technologies, either those recently introduced into medical practice or those still in an investigational stage. Thus far, the majority of assessments have dealt with new technologies or new applications for existing technologies.

Concerns

Although the duties prescribed for OHTA/NCHSR by Congress include assessments that take into account cost-effectiveness and social, ethical, and economic impacts, the primary concerns to date of OHTA in making its coverage recommendations are the safety and clinical effectiveness of the technology. In addition, appropriateness (as an adjunct or alternative to conventional practice or standard accepted practice) and desirable skills, facilities, and support systems may be addressed. Cost is not an explicit concern for purposes of HCFA coverage decisions. OHTA may recommend that the technology not be covered by Medicare, that it be covered with certain restrictions, or that it be covered without restriction.

In making coverage determinations for

TABLE A-9 OHTA Assessment Report Series and Coverage Recommendations

Volume	Recommendation
Volume 1, 1981	
1. Alcohol Aversion Therapy	Covered
2. Hydrotherapy (Whirlpool) Baths for Treatment of Decubitus Ulcers	Not covered
3. Ultraviolet Light for Treatment of Decubitus Ulcers	Not covered
4. Transsexual Surgery	Not covered
5. Urine Autoinjection (Autogenous Urine Immunization)	Not covered
6. Apheresis in the Treatment of Rheumatoid Arthritis	Not covered
7. Stereotaxic Depth Electrode Implantation	Covered
8. Cytoxic Leukocyte Test for the Diagnosis of Food Allergies	Not covered
9. Sublingual Provocative and Neutralization Therapy for Food Allergies	Not covered
10. Intracutaneous (Intradermal) and Subcutaneous Provocative and Neutralization Testing and Neutralization Therapy for Food Allergies	Not covered
11. Intracranial Pressure Measurement	Covered
12. B-Scan of Peripheral Vessels	Covered
13. Tinnitus Masker	Not covered
14. Percutaneous Transluminal Angioplasty for Treatment of Arteriosclerotic Obstructions in the Lower Extremities	Covered
15. Transcutaneous Electrical Nerve Stimulation for Treatment of Post-Operative Incision Pain	Covered
16. Shortwave Diathermy	Covered
17. Human Tumor Stem Cell Drug Sensitivity Assays for Predicting Anticancer Drug Effects	Not covered
18. EDTA Chelation Therapy for Atherosclerosis	Not covered
19. Ultraviolet Absorbing Lenses for Aphakic and Pseudophakic Patients	Covered
20. Bentonite Flocculation Test in Rheumatoid Arthritis	Covered
21. Desoxyribonucleic Acid-Bentonite Flocculation Test in Rheumatoid Arthritis	Covered
22. Mycoplasma Complement Fixation Test in Rheumatoid Arthritis	Not covered
23. Kunkel Test in Rheumatoid Arthritis	Not covered
24. Technetium-99m Pertechnetate Joint Scans in Arthritis	Covered
25. Anti-Inhibitor Coagulant Complex in Hemophilia A with Inhibitor Antibodies to Factor VIII	Covered
Volume 2, 1982	
1. Electrotherapy for Treatment of Facial Nerve Paralysis (Bell's Palsy)	Covered
2. Hyperbaric Oxygen Therapy for Treatment of Organic Brain Syndrome (Senility)	Covered
3. Hyperbaric Oxygen Therapy for Treatment of Multiple Sclerosis	Not covered
4. Gastric Freezing for Peptic Ulcer Disease	Not covered
5. Bolen's Test for Cancer	Not covered
6. Bendien's Test for Cancer and Tuberculosis	Not covered
7. Rehfuss Test for Gastric Acidity	Not covered
8. Rheumatoid Vasculitis Therapeutic Apheresis	Covered
9. Home Blood Glucose Monitors	Not covered
10. Ambulatory Blood Pressure Monitoring in Hypertensive (Semiautomatic)	Not covered
11. Apheresis for Multiple Sclerosis	Not covered
12. Hyperbaric Oxygen Therapy for Treatment of Arthritic Diseases	Not covered
13. Plasmapheresis and Plasma Exchange for Treatment of Thrombotic Thrombocytopenic Purpura	Covered
14. Obesity and Protein-Supplemented Fasting	Not covered
15. Serum Seromucoid Assay	Not covered
16. Percutaneous Transluminal Coronary Angioplasty for Treatment of Stenotic Lesions of a Single Coronary Artery	Covered
17. Melodic Intonation Therapy	Covered
18. Photodensitometry	Not covered
19. Bone Biopsy for Mineral Analysis or Bone Histology	Covered

TABLE A-9 *Continued*

20. Photon Absorptiometric Procedure for Bone Mineral Analysis	Covered
21. Hyperbaric Oxygen for Treatment of Soft Tissue Radionecrosis and Osteoradionecrosis	Covered
22. Hyperbaric Oxygen for Treatment of Chronic Refractory Osteomyelitis	Covered
23. Carbon Dioxide Laser Surgery	Covered
24. Percutaneous Transluminal Angioplasty for Treatment of Stenotic Lesions of the Renal Arteries	Covered
25. Endothelial Cell Photography	Covered
26. Photoplethysmography	Not covered
Volume 3, 1983	
1. EEG Monitoring During Open Heart Surgery	Not covered
2. Apheresis for the Treatment of Goodpasture's Syndrome	Covered
3. Apheresis for the Treatment of Membranous Proliferative Glomerulonephritides	Covered
4. Electroversion Therapy for the Treatment of Alcoholism	Not covered
5. Anti-Gastroesophageal Reflux Implantation	Not covered
6. Closed-loop Blood Glucose Control Device	Covered
7. Plasma Perfusion of Charcoal Filters for Treatment of Pruritis of Cholestatic Liver Disease	Covered
8. Topical Oxygen Therapy in the Treatment of Decubitus Ulcers and Persistent Skin Lesions	Not covered
9. Fully Automated Ambulatory Blood Pressure Monitoring of Hypertension	Not covered
10. Hyperbaric Oxygen for Treatment of Actinomycosis	Covered
11. Displacement Cardiography—Photomography	Not covered
12. Displacement Cardiography—Cardiokymography	Not covered
13. Negative Pressure Respirators	Covered
14. Diathermy as a Physical Therapy Modality	Covered
15. Hyperbaric Oxygen Therapy for Treatment of Crush Injury and Acute Traumatic Peripheral Ischemia	Covered
16. Transplantation of the Liver	Covered with guidelines
17. Computer Enhanced Perimetry	Covered
18. Lactose Breath Hydrogen Test for the Diagnosis of Lactose Malabsorption	Covered
19. Implantable Chemotherapy Infusion Pump for the Treatment of Liver Cancer	Covered
20. External Infusion Pump for Heparin	Covered
21. Lactulose Breath Hydrogen Test for Diagnosing Small Bowel Bacterial Overgrowth and Measuring Small Bowel Transit Time	Not covered
22. Thermography for Breast Cancer Detection	Not covered
Volume 4, 1984	
1. Transillumination Light Scanning for the Diagnosis of Breast Cancer	Not covered
2. Implantable Pump for Chronic Heparin Therapy	Not covered
3. Electrotherapy for Treatment of Facial Nerve Paralysis	Not covered
4. $^{13}CO_2$ Breath Test for Diagnosing Bile Acid Malabsorption	Not covered
5. Noninvasive Method of Monitoring Cardiac Output by Doppler Ultrasound	Not covered
6. Ambulatory Electroencephalographic (EEG) Monitoring	Covered
7. $^{13}CO_2$ Breath Test for Diagnosing Fat Malabsorption	Not covered
8. Transcutaneous Electrical Nerve Stimulation for Acute Pain Treatment for Ambulatory Patients	Covered
9. Apheresis Used in Preparation for Kidney Transplant	Not covered
10. Carbon Dioxide Lasers in Head and Neck Surgery	Covered
11. Hyperbaric Oxygen Therapy for Acute Cerebral Edema	Not covered
12. Intraoperative Ventricular Mapping	Covered
13. Apheresis in the Treatment of Chronic Relapsing Polyneuropathy	Covered
14. Diagnostic Endocardial Electrical Stimulation (Pacing)	Covered
15. Neuromuscular Electrical Stimulation in the Treatment of Disuse Atrophy in the Absence of Nervous System Involvement	Covered

TABLE A-9 *Continued*

16. Hyperbaric Oxygen for Treatment of Chronic Peripheral Vascular Insufficiency	Not covered
17. Hyperbaric Oxygen in Treatment of Severed Limbs	Covered
18. External Counterpulsation	Not covered
19. Transplantation of the Pancreas	Not covered
20. Streptokinase Infusion for Acute Myocardial Infarction	Not covered
21. Nd:YAG Laser for Posterior Capsulotomies	Covered
22. External Open-Loop Pump for the Subcutaneous Infusion of Insulin in Diabetics	Not covered
23. Laser Trabeculoplasty for Open-Angle Glaucoma	Covered
24. Local Hyperthermia for Treatment of Superficial and Subcutaneous Malignancies	Covered with guidelines
25. Percutaneous Transluminal Angioplasty for Obstructive Lesions of the Aortic Arch Vessels	Not covered
26. Percutaneous Transluminal Angioplasty for Obstructive Lesions of Arteriovenous Dialysis Fistulas	Not covered
Volume 5, 1985	
1. Extracorporeal Shock Wave Lithotripsy (ESWL) Procedures for the Treatment of Kidney Stones	Covered
2. Percutaneous Ultrasound Procedures for the Treatment of Kidney Stones	Covered
3. Transurethral Ureteroscopic Lithotripsy Procedures for the Treatment of Kidney Stones	Not covered
4. Debridement and Other Treatment of Mycotic Toenails	Covered with guidelines
5. 24-Hour Ambulatory Esophageal pH Monitoring	Covered with guidelines
6. Thermography for Indications Other than Breast Lesions	[a]
7. Allogeneic Bone Marrow Transplantation for Indications Other than Aplastic Anemia and Leukemia	Covered with guidelines
8. Autologous Bone Marrow Transplantation (ABMT)	Not covered
9. Stereotactic Cingulotomy as a Means of Psychosurgery	Not covered
10. Reassessment of Cardiokymography	Not covered
11. Patient Selection Criteria for Percutaneous Coronary Angioplasty of a Stenotic Lesion in a Single Coronary Artery	Covered with guidelines
12. Bilateral Carotid Body Resection	[a]
13. Portable Hand-Held X-Ray Instrument (Lixiscope)	[a]
14. Magnetic Resonance Imaging (MRI)	[a]
15. Apheresis in the Treatment of Guillain-Barré Syndrome	[a]
16. Dual Photon Absorptiometry for Measuring Bone Mineral Density	[a]

NOTE: In this table are titles of OHTA assessment reports and the respective coverage recommendations made to HCFA. OHTA assessment reports are available in annual bound volumes (*NCHSR Health Technology Assessment Series: Health Technology Assessment Reports*) from the National Technical Information Service, and individual reports and recommendations are available from the NCHSRHCTA. See the reports for the full wording of the assessment topics and complete report narratives. The recommendations cited here do not reflect fully the discussion presented in the assessment reports.
[a]No instructions issued as of July 1985.
SOURCE: OHTA, 1985.

technologies involving drugs and/or medical devices, HCFA considers whether FDA has found the product safe and effective. HCFA generally does not approve coverage of such a technology unless FDA has already approved it. HCFA considers it to be necessary but not sufficient that a technology be safe and effective in order for it to be reasonable and necessary. HCFA will not necessarily approve coverage for all technologies that FDA has approved, largely because the two agencies differ in their respective definitions of effectiveness. FDA deems a technology effective if it does what the manufacturer claims it will do, whereas HCFA considers the effectiveness of the technology with respect to health outcome.

If a new technology in question is a medical product and has received FDA approval for commercial distribution, the thrust of the OHTA assessment is toward the use of that product in a nonidealized setting, i.e., the setting in which providers in conventional practice circumstances have demonstrated the safety and clinical effectiveness of the procedure. However, if the technology in question is a health care service, not product dependent, the thrust of the OHTA assessment encompasses safety and clinical effectiveness data as determined by clinical and scientific information published in peer review journals, as well as input from NIH and medical specialty societies.

Requests

Questions on the coverage of a particular technology under the Medicare program are forwarded to OHTA from HCFA. These requests may originate in an organization in the public or private sector or be initiated by an individual or group having an interest in the safety and effectiveness of health care technologies. Sources have included the regional offices of HCFA, Congress, commercial insurers and other fiscal intermediaries, clinical centers, medical societies, private physicians, and medical device manufacturers.

Selection

Before HCFA requests OHTA to assess a health care technology, HCFA's Physicians Panel decides whether the question raised warrants an assessment. The panel considers the importance of the issue, the adequacy of the database, and the status of FDA approval before recommending that an assessment be conducted by OHTA.

Process

The OHTA assessment process has four stages, as follows.

1. *Initiation*. Prior to conducting a full assessment, OHTA in conjunction with HCFA reviews the questions to be addressed by the assessment to determine the information need that initiated the original inquiry. OHTA staff work with the HCFA Bureau of Eligibility, Reimbursement and Coverage (BERC) and Physicians Panel to ensure that the questions posed are appropriate and clearly defined. Then OHTA conducts a preliminary analysis of the issues and reports back to BERC and the HCFA Physicians Panel if further clarification is required.

2. *Collection of Information*. OHTA announces the impending assessment in the *Federal Register*, generally providing 90 days for public response. The agency also conducts a literature search with MEDLARS II computer retrieval service and *Index Medicus*. OHTA routinely contacts medical societies such as the Council on Medical Specialty Societies, the American Medical Association, and the American College of Physicians and manufacturers' associations for information on the technology under consideration. OHTA also seeks advice and assistance from appropriate federal agencies. These agencies may supply scientific information, clinical trial data, bibliographic material, or other pertinent information. Agencies that OHTA contacts frequently, including NIH, FDA, HRSA, ADAMHA, CDC, and VA, have developed formal procedures for responding to OHTA's requests.

3. *Synthesis of Information*. The third stage in the assessment is the synthesis of the available information by OHTA staff in order to develop the PHS recommendations. The synthesis involves three steps:

a. All pertinent information, including expert opinions, is summarized.
b. Logical, or at least defensible, conclusions are formulated about the technology's safety and effectiveness.
c. OHTA's policy recommendations to HCFA regarding Medicare coverage of the technology are developed. OHTA coverage recommendations are not included in the assessment reports, but are submitted separately.

4. *Distribution of Results*. The final stage in the process is the dissemination of OHTA's synthesis and findings after HCFA has made

its coverage decision. Assessment reports are made available to the public.

The OHTA assessment process is continually subject to review and adoption of improved assessment techniques.

Assessors

OHTA assessments are conducted by OHTA staff in cooperation with outside experts and other federal agencies, as described above. Coverage recommendations made by the director of OHTA are approved by the Office of the Assistant Secretary for Health before being forwarded to HCFA. The OHTA staff has seven professionals (five of whom perform assessments, including four physicians) and three support staff members.

Turnaround

The time between receipt of a request from HCFA to the time of transmittal of an evaluation and recommendation from OHTA is approximately 6 to 12 months. This normally includes time for advance notice of assessment, sending out requests for and receiving information, and drafting and review of the assessment report.

Reporting

Under the working agreement between HCFA and PHS, OHTA may publish and disseminate results of its assessments. However, the OHTA report is usually not released prior to the time HCFA issues instructions regarding coverage of the technology in question. Once the actual decision concerning Medicare coverage is made, HCFA notifies its contractors and fiscal intermediaries of its decision through formal instruction. State Medicaid agencies are also notified because they often base their determination for coverage on the OHTA assessment. The assessments are disseminated to physicians, hospital administrators, health insurers, manufacturers, and others in the health field. From 1981 through early 1985, PHS has provided over 100 assessment reports, with recommendations, to HCFA. These reports are available in annual bound volumes (*NCHSR Health Technology Assessment Series: Health Technology Assessment Reports*) from the National Technical Information Service, and are published in the *American Hospital Association Hospital Technology Series Guideline Reports*, which are provided to over 1,200 hospitals. Table A-10 shows the general outline of OHTA assessment reports.

Impact

HCFA has always accepted the medical and scientific aspects of OHTA recommendations, although it implements coverage recommendations in keeping with legal and administrative requirements (Young, 1983). Of the 103 OHTA assessments listed in Table A-9, OHTA recommended coverage for 52 and noncoverage for 51. After receiving PHS recommendations, HCFA generally requests PHS to review the new Medicare Manual Statement, which reflects those recommendations, prior to the issuance of a coverage policy. Then HCFA independently makes the actual coverage decision and notifies Medicare intermediaries and the state Medicare agencies.

Reassessment

HCFA or other agencies or persons may request OHTA to reassess a technology in light of new information. This process is similar to the original assessment initiation process except that OHTA requests other PHS agencies to review additional information. OHTA synthesizes the findings and develops a position on the need for reassessment. The resulting recommendations are forwarded to HCFA for consideration by its Physicians Panel. If the Physicians Panel determines that a reassessment is necessary, OHTA initiates the assessment described above.

An example of a reassessment is that of the treatment of senile macular degeneration by argon laser photocoagulation. The September 1980 PHS recommendation to HCFA was that this therapeutic procedure not be covered. During the following year, the National Eye Institute (NEI) supported a randomized clinical trial of safety and clinical effectiveness of the procedure, and concluded that it is safe and clinically effective. In light of these findings, OHTA recom-

TABLE A-10 General Outline of OHTA Technology Assessments

Technology name (generic terminology, if appropriate)
Description of the technology
1. What is it?
2. Who does it?
3. On whom?
4. Why is it done (objective)?
   Is the intervention intended to be *therapeutic*?
   Is the intervention intended to *palliate* or *prevent further regression* or deterioration?
   If the intervention is *diagnostic*, is the information obtained unique when compared with conventional procedures?
   Will this diagnostic information affect therapy when compared with conventional practice?
5. Are there conventional procedures used to achieve the same objective?
6. Where is it done?
7. How is it done?
8. How often is it done?
9. Is there a national demand/need for this technology?
10. Is the technology permanent, temporary, or replaceable in terms of its application and/or patient contact?

Rationale
A statement outlining the theoretical basis for the use of this technology for this indication.

Review of published peer-reviewed medical and scientific literature to include a summary of the:
1. Issues to be addressed in the published literature
2. Study design (double blind, multicentered cooperative, comparative, serial clinical experience, etc.)
3. Size of patient population
4. Characterization of patient population
5. Length of follow-up
6. Recurrence rate, if any
7. Statistical analysis of data
8. Animal or cadaver studies, if appropriate
9. Analyses of matrix data table (reliability, significance of data to determine if the evidence supports the conclusions)
10. Other information

Discussion
1. Have the issues been addressed in the literature?
2. Problems, if any, with the published clinical studies:
   a. Design of clinical studies (controlled, serial experience, multicentered cooperative, etc.)
   b. Size of patient population (large, small, representative, homogeneous, heterogeneous, etc.)
   c. Follow-up: consistency, duration, epidemiologic disciplines used
   d. Recurrence rate, if any
   e. Statistical analysis of data, if any
   f. Animal studies, cadaver studies, etc., if appropriate
3. Safety considerations:
   a. Known risks—probable/predictable risks
   b. Criteria, if any, for use (provider) performance (experienced hands. . .)
   c. Secondary, harmful effects of the intervention, if any
4. Citations of review articles that draw comparisons between the new technology and conventional practices
5. Regulatory status, if a product is under review
6. Other nonmedical, nonscientific controversies, if any

Summary
Statement should contain:
1. Description of differences, if any
2. A statement regarding the supportability of the rationale
3. A description of evidence
4. Level of acceptance of the technology by both the research and clinical practice communities
5. The appropriateness of the new technology as an adjunct or alternative to conventional practice or standard accepted practice
6. Degree of difficulty/sophistication as it affects the needs for special resources and skills
7. Specific characteristics of institution, medical team, etc., involved in use of technology

References—All published studies/reports reviewed in this submittal, attach cited literature

SOURCE: OHTA, 1983.

mended in June 1982 that the procedure be covered under Medicare. Other technologies that have been reassessed include liver transplants, hyperthermia for the treatment of cancer, and implantable chemotherapy infusion pumps.

Funding/Budget

OHTA budgeted approximately $0.7 million in 1985 for technology assessments for HCFA and related activities.

Example

On the following pages is the full text of the 1984 OHTA assessment of percutaneous transluminal angioplasty for obstructive lesions of arteriovenous dialysis fistulas.

Sources

Brandt, E. N. 1984. Technology assessment, a private-public partnership. Public Health Reports 99:329–330.

Carter, E., Director, Office of Health Technology Assessment. 1985. Personal communications.

Department of Health and Human Services, Office of the Assistant Secretary for Planning and Evaluation. 1984. Technology Assessment and Coverage Decisionmaking in the Department of Health and Human Services. Prepared by Macro Systems, Inc.

Erlichman, M., Evaluation Staff, Office of Health Technology Assessment. 1985. Personal communications.

Federal Register. January 19, 1983; Vol. 48, No. 13, p. 2444.

Margulies, H., Director (former), Office of Health Technology Assessment. 1983. Personal communications.

National Center for Health Services Research. 1984. Health Technology Assessment Series: Health Technology Assessment Reports, 1981, nos. 1-25. DHHS Publication No. (PHS) 84-3370. Springfield, Va.: National Technical Information Service.

National Center for Health Services Research. 1984. Health Technology Assessment Series: Health Technology Assessment Reports, 1982, nos. 1-26. DHHS Publication No. (PHS) 84-3371. Springfield, Va.: National Technical Information Service.

National Center for Health Services Research. 1984. Health Technology Assessment Series: Health Technology Assessment Reports, 1983, nos. 1-22. DHHS Publication No. (PHS) 84-3372. Springfield, Va.: National Technical Information Service.

Office of Health Technology Assessment, National Center for Health Services Research and Health Care Technology Assessment, Department of Health and Human Services. 1984. Public Health Service Assessment of Percutaneous Transluminal Angioplasty for Obstructive Lesions of Arteriovenous Dialysis Fistulas. Rockville, Md.

OHTA. 1982. Memorandum regarding coverage of treatment of senile macular degeneration by argon laser photocoagulation, June 9. Rockville, Md.

OHTA. Listing of requests returned from PHS, October 1979 through April 1983. Rockville, Md.

OHTA. 1983. Public Health Service Procedures for Evaluating Health Care Technologies for Purposes of Medicare Coverage. Rockville, Md.

Young, D., Deputy Director, Bureau of Eligibility, Reimbursement and Coverage, Health Care Financing Administration. 1983. Personal communication.

PUBLIC HEALTH SERVICE ASSESSMENT OF PERCUTANEOUS TRANSLUMINAL ANGIOPLASTY FOR OBSTRUCTIVE LESIONS OF ARTERIOVENOUS DIALYSIS FISTULAS

1984

INTRODUCTION

Percutaneous transluminal angioplasty (PTA) is an angiographic treatment for vascular occlusive disease. The technique consists of vascular dilation and recanalization that is associated with the restoration of blood flow through segmentally diseased arteries (1). PTA involves passage of a balloon-tipped catheter to the site of arterial narrowing and inflation of the balloon to reduce the obstruction (2). The first clinical dilation of blood vessels was described by Dotter and Judkins in 1964 (3). They used a "stiff," coaxial catheter system to develop the technique of PTA. Initially, the catheter system was applied to short segment obstructions of the femoro-popliteal region and later to iliac arteries (4). In the early 1970's Gruntzig's development of a "flexible," double lumen, balloon-dilating catheter permitted extension of the technique from the iliofemoral vessels to previously inaccessible sites such as coronary and renal arteries (5,6). In recent years, PTA has been used to treat stenoses of aortic arch vessels and stenotic segments of failing arteriovenous (AV) fistulas.

The creation of an AV fistula in the forearm is used to facilitate access to the vessels in patients with end-stage renal failure treated by hemodialysis. Presently, the surgically created subcutaneous AV fistula is the primary mode of vascular access for chronic hemodialysis. Complications associated with vascular access include stenosis, thrombosis, infection, and cardiac failure associated with high fistula flow. Access malfunction may be manifested by graft and fistula thrombosis, elevated venous pressure resulting in excessive ultrafiltration, and decreased blood flow resulting in inefficient dialysis. The most common etiology of vascular access thrombosis is the occurrence of stenosis at sites of arterial or venous anastomosis, or the development of fibrosis at sites of repeated needle punctures (7).

The conventional surgical management of patients with obstructive lesions of failing AV dialysis fistulas has been revision or replacement of the fistula. Revision includes excision or bypass of the stenotic area and reanastomosis (8). As complications occur, increasingly proximal revisions are performed using any suitable vessels. When the fistula is not amenable to revision, placement of a new fistula is required. Often the patient will receive an AV forearm fistula in the other arm (8). When an autogenous fistula is no longer feasible, extended procedures with prosthetic grafts are used. Forearm brachioantecubital loop grafts, radioantecubital straight grafts, as well as upper arm brachiobasilic loops have been employed routinely (9). The demand for AV access fistulas in chronic renal failure is clearly defined by a yearly incidence of about 24,000 patients treated by chronic dialysis with a prevalence of about 72,000 patients (personal communication, HCFA). Studies of the surgical mangement of fistula complications have indicated that fistulas require revision or replacement at an average of 0.6 times per year per patient. (9). PTA has been offered as an alternative method for restoration of flow in the arteriovenous dialysis fistulas obviating the need for conventional surgery. The purpose of this report is to assess the safety, clinical effectiveness and use of PTA in the treatment of obstructive lesions of AV dialysis fistulas.

BACKGROUND

Chronic hemodialysis became an accepted method of treatment for end-stage renal disease with the development of the Quinton-Scribner external shunt in 1960 (8). With this technique, Teflon Silastic cannulas are inserted into the radial artery and into an adjacent forearm vein. The two ends of the cannulas that exit from the skin are then connected by a U-shaped external shunt that can be disconnected for dialysis (10). Despite improvements in the use of the external shunt, serious complications such as frequent clotting, local and systemic infection, and erosion of the skin overlying the shunt, precluded long-term patency (11). Mennes and coworkers (8) reviewed numerous reports where the duration of function of such shunts was from 3 to 12 months. They found that infection, clotting, or bleeding, necessitated removal and replacement of the cannula in the majority of cases. However, as a result of the external shunt more and more patients were maintained on chronic dialysis for longer periods. This necessitated repeated shunt revisions and reinsertions and made the problem of chronic access to the circulation an even more important consideration in their care.

In 1966, the internal fistula and the use of repeated venipuncture, for dialysis appeared as an alternative. Brescia and coworkers surgically created a subcutaneous AV fistula by anastomosis of the radial artery to an adjacent branch of the cephalic vein in the forearm (12). The internal fistula provides a sufficient blood flow for dialysis through the arterialized vein. Hemodialysis is accomplished by two separate punctures of the enlarged arterialized vein with a No. 15 or 16 gauge needle. The arterial needle is placed distally toward the wrist and is used for withdrawal of blood from the patient, while the venous needle, placed proximally toward the elbow, returns the blood from the dialyzer to the patient. Satisfactory hemodialysis requires three 6-hour sessions per week at a minimal flow rate of 200-300 ml per minute and an ideal fistula flow of 400-500 ml per minute (13).

The distal forearm is the most practical site for fistula creation. Though fistulas mature in about 10 days, it takes three to six weeks for the vein to become "arterialized (i.e., large and thick enough to permit repeated dialysis). During maturation, the overlying skin heals, a thrill develops in the veins continuous with the shunt, and these veins enlarge and become readily palpable (13). In most patients the fistula can be constructed without difficulty. Arteries of the upper extremities are preferred since they tend to be less atherosclerotic. The usual surgery is a side-to-side fistula between the radial artery and the cephalic vein near the wrist. The radial artery is the artery of choice, since it is larger in most patients and can be easily anastomosed to the adjacent cephalic vein. The cephalic vein is also of adequate size in most patients and has an anatomic pattern in the forearm most suitable for arterialization. If the radial artery is not available because of previous cannulations, the ulnar artery can be used. Also, the basilic vein can be used if the cephalic vein is not available and anastomosed to the ulnar artery or mobilized and anastomosed to the radial artery (14). Though a radial-cephalic side-to-side anastomosis was originally described by Brescia and coworkers (12) other authors prefer the end vein-to-side artery anastomosis while some recommend the use of an end-to-end anastomosis (14). Glanz and associates reported that because of blood flow characteristics, these techniques have not proved as durable as the side-to-side anastomosis (15). Additionally, when an internal AV fistula is not feasible, a graft fistula may be inserted between an appropriate artery and vein. Various materials such as bovine carotid artery heterograft and Gore-tex expanded polytetrafluoroethylene have been used.

Despite the type of anastomosis used in the formation of the subcutaneous AV fistula, complications associated with vascular access still represent one of the most frequent and significant problems encountered in a chronic hemodialysis center. Thrombosis, stenosis, venous aneurysms, infections, and cardiac failure associated with high fistula flow all contribute to the morbidity and mortality of the hemodialysis patient. Initial failure rates for most AV fistulas range from about 8 to 16 percent; however, once the fistula is established and successfully used for dialysis, the incidence of late failures drops to less than 5 percent after six months on dialysis (14,16). Kinnaert and associates have reported a 72 percent survival rate for 314 internal AV fistulas at three years (16). These surgically created AV fistulas fail in the late postoperative period because of intimal hyperplasia at the site of anastomosis or at the site of repeated fistula punctures (17). Occlusions or stenoses may involve the connecting artery, the anastomosis, and the main or collateral veins singly or in combination. The most common cause of fistula failure has been found to be stenosis of the venous anastomosis. Fistula failure frequently is manifested by a high venous resistance if the venous end is stenotic or a reduction in flow rate if the stenosis is in the proximal artery, at or near the anastomosis (18). In a study by Mennes and associates 40 percent of the 75 cases evaluated for vascular access difficulties demonstrated significant stenosis (8). Stenosis was the most frequent complication associated with repeated use of the AV fistula. The study, using venous angiography of the fistula, also demonstrated total occlusion by thrombus in 9 percent of the cases (8). Similar findings of vascular stenoses and occlusions were also reported by Anderson and coworkers (19) and Glanz and associates (15). However, the most serious complication of internal AV fistulas is thrombosis, which can result in the complete loss of the fistula (18,20). Poor venous runoff due to a narrow anastomosis or an unsuspected proximal venous obstruction is the most frequent cause of early thrombosis. Late thrombosis is usually caused by thickening of the central venous limb from repeated cannulations (15). Kinnaert and coworkers reported that thromboses were responsible for about 87 percent of the 109 late fistulas losses in a series of 274 AV fistulas. Thrombosis is also the most frequent cause of graft failure. Early graft thrombosis has been reported to occur in 10-20 percent of bovine carotid heterograft cases. Causes include surgical twisting or kinking during implantation, a narrow venous anastomosis, or an unsuspected proximal venous obstruction (15).

The objective of PTA is to improve flow through the diseased segment of the vessel so that vessel patency is increased. The main principle of PTA is the same whether the procedure is used in the lower extremities, renal, coronary, or AV fistulas. A double lumen dilation catheter, with a strong, non-elastic balloon made of polyethylene annealed to the tip, is introduced into a vessel near the anastomotic site (21). The double-lumen dilating catheter consists of a main and a side lumen. The main lumen serves several purposes, such as the passage of a guide wire, pressure recording, or contrast material injection necessary to monitor the position of the guide wire and catheter with fluoroscopy. At the tip of the catheter is the sausage-shaped balloon segment. When deflated it surrounds the catheter like an umbrella and is guided to the site of the lesion and positioned so that the balloon segment lies within the area of the vascular stenosis. By means of the side channel, the balloon is filled with a dilute contrast medium solution and inflated within the stenotic segment up to a pressure of 10 atmospheres (3). Though the mechanism of balloon angioplasty is not fully understood, its result is an increase in lumen size with an increased blood flow through the previously stenotic vascular segment. Successful PTA results in a reduction of the vascular stenosis and decrease in the trans-stenotic pressure gradient (22).

The precise role and importance of anticoagulant therapy before, during, and after PTA is undetermined. Some angiographers believe that the success or failure of PTA depends not only on the nature of the lesion and the skill and experience of the angiographer, but also on the use of appropriate adjunctive medical therapy to prevent complications and to keep the new lumen open (23). Athanasoulis reported that most European authors with extensive PTA experience advocate 3-6 months of anticoagulant therapy after the procedure because this regimen appears to improve long-term patency rates (24). Recent clinical and experimental observations on the pathophysiology of recurrent stenoses have shown that the exposed subendothelial elements of the vessel wall promote local platelet aggregation and stimulate thrombus formation (25). Based on these findings some angiographers performing balloon angioplasty advocate systemic heparinzation during the procedure and low dose aspirin as a platelet inhibitor one or two days before and 3-6 months after dilatation. Some routinely add heparin for several days after dilatation and others institute warfarin anticoagulation for several months (1). Some clinicians who perform PTA on dialysis patients do not favor the use of anticoagulants after PTA due to coagulation abnormalities that exist in some uremic patients (8). To date, no controlled trials of the efficacy of the various post-PTA anticoagulation regimens have been reported.

PTA has become a widely used technique for dilating lesions of the ileofemoral, popliteal, renal and coronary arteries. The Office of Health Technology Assessment has previously assessed the use of PTA in the treatment of stenotic lesions of these vessels and found the technique safe and clinically effective (4,5,6,). Until recently there has been a hesitancy to dilate obstructive lesions in veins and grafts. However, recent studies have reported the outcome of PTA treatment for stenotic lesions of AV dialysis fistulas. Since the use of PTA in AV fistulas has been used for a limited period of time in the United States only a few American studies have been reported in the recent literature. This report examines these and other studies in the published literature as well as other available evidence that pertains to the safety and clinical effectiveness of this technique.

RATIONALE

Proponents of PTA believe that this technique offers a safe and effective alternative to the surgical revision or replacement of AV fistulas with stenotic or occlusive lesions. Additionally, they propose that intervention with PTA at the stenotic stage of access malfunction could prevent access occlusion and/or thrombosis. They cite several advantages of this approach including its use in ambulatory patients, the prolongation of fistula survival and its effectiveness with multiple stenoses. Proponents of PTA argue that it is a less invasive procedure that can be repeated in the event of restenosis and it neither precludes nor prejudices the outcome of subsequent surgery. Moreover, the cost of conventional surgery and hospitalization are certainly more than would be anticipated with PTA (26).

REVIEW OF AVAILABLE INFORMATION

In 1981, Lawrence and associates reported treating six hemodialysis patients with stenotic segments of failing AV fistulas by balloon catheter dilatation (17). These patients were considered candidates for PTA because they developed hemodynamic problems while on dialysis. Three of the six patients had successful dilatation of the AV fistulas. They included one patient with a stenosis of the midportion of a Brescia-Cimino forearm fistula, one patient with a tight stenosis 4 cm from the anastomotic site of a Brescia-Cimino AV fistula and one patient with a stenosis just distal to the venous anastomosis of a straight forearm bovine graft. Two of these fistulas were still functioning at 8 and 10 months followup and the third fistula functioned up to the patient's death (two months). Dilatation was unsuccessful in two patients because the stenosis located adjacent to the AV anastomosis could not be approached with the balloon. The third failure was due to the inability to pass a catheter through a very tortuous vein leading from the anastomotic site. The authors reported no complications secondary to the technique and found that the dilatation attempt did not preclude surgical revision when it failed (17).

In a related report, Spinowitz and associates attemped PTA in 12 hemodialysis patients with vascular access stenoses (7). Though successful dilatation was achieved in six patients, vascular access patency lasted from only 3 weeks to 11 months postangioplasty; at which time surgical correction was performed in the surviving patients. The authors stated that there were no episodes of distal embolization, significant hematoma formation, or rupture of the dilated vascular access. Spinowitz and associates concluded that stenoses of short segments in the venous limb of polytetrafluoroethylene grafts, as well as Brescia-Cimino fistulas are amenable to PTA with a high degree of success and no morbidity.

Recently, Glanz and colleagues reported on their 4-year experience of 56 balloon dilatations in 51 patients with failing dialysis access fistulas (27). Internal fistulas and grafts were evaluated and then dilated in patients presenting increased venous pressure during dialysis, arm edema, venous or graft aneurysms and pseudoaneurysms, and arterial sucking during dialysis. Forty-five lesions in graft fistulas were dilated. Of these, 38 stenoses were located at or near the venous anastomosis, three at the arterial anastomoses and four in a far proximal vein. Eleven lesions were dilated in internal AV fistulas. Of these, six venous stenoses were located within 8cm of the anastomosis and five were in a far proximal vein. The majority of procedures were performed on an outpatient basis. Glanz and colleagues found that 39 of 56 dilatations (70 percent) were initially successful, as shown by morphologic improvement of the lesion and reduction in pressure gradient (27). Of the initial successes, 28/35 (80 percent) were patent at 3 months, 19/27 (70 percent) at 6 months, 12/22 (55 percent) at 1 year, 7/14 (50 percent) at 2 years, and 3/9 (33 percent) at 3 years. The authors reported three complications (5 percent); one internal fistula thrombosis, and one graft thrombosis within 24 hours of the procedure and one pseudoaneurysm at the dilatation site 1 year postprocedure. Because the authors did not have any successful dilatations of lesions longer than 4 cm they recommended that patients with these lesions receive surgical revision (27). Although the long-term patency rates of fistula dilatations using PTA were not high, Glanz and colleagues believe that the nonsurgical prolongation of the life of a fistula by one or more years is still of benefit to dialysis patients who have already undergone and are still likely to undergo numerous surgical procedures during their lifetimes. Especially since repeat dilatation can be performed on recurrent lesions and patients with failed angioplasty can still undergo the surgical revision that would have been done prior to PTA (27).

Satisfactory results with PTA for stenotic segments of failing AV fistulas was also reported by Hunter and coworkers (28). A total of 31 patients with 45 episodes of failing AV dialysis fistulas were evaluated and treated by PTA and occasionally streptokinase infusion. Fistula failure was usually due to venous and/or anastomotic stenosis, often in conjunction with thrombosis. There were 28 occlusions and 17 stenoses treated. Success, defined as having remained patent for at least 6 months of continuous use, being currently patent (less than 6 months) at the time of the review, or remaining patent until the patient's death or successful transplantation, was achieved in 10 of the 28 occluded episodes and in 14 of the 17 stenotic episodes (28).

The authors found occlusions associated with AV fistulas extremely resistant to dilation and the treatment of occlusions with associated thrombus even more difficult to treat. About forty-three percent (6/14) of the occlusions without thrombus were successfully dilated while only twenty-nine percent (4/14) of the occlusions with thrombus were successfully dilated. Streptokinase and/or heparin played a critical role in three of the four "occlusions with thrombus" that were successfully dilated.

The authors found stenoses associated with AV fistulas also resistant to dilation. These abnormalities were much more amenable to PTA treatment. The average patency for the 14 successfully dilated stenoses was almost 10 months. Only three stenoses could not be dilated by PTA and two of these involved multiple stenoses. Hunter and coworkers determined that most complications and failures occurred either in patients with recently created fistulas or in those with multiple or long segment stenosis associated with thrombosis. They recommend PTA as the treatment of choice in patients with a single nonobstructing stenotic AV fistula (28).

DISCUSSION

Recently, PTA has been used to dilate stenotic lesions of failing dialysis access fistulas and shunts. While recent experience suggests that there may be a wider spectrum of applications for PTA than dilating lesions of the ileofemoral, popliteal, renal and coronary arteries, there exists a paucity of published literature describing the use and safety of PTA in AV fistulas in a significant number of patients. AV fistulas are the favored vascular access for chronic hemodialysis and when an internal fistula is no longer feasible a graft may be inserted. Stenotic lesions are a common problem, however, in patients with internal and graft fistulas and many of these patients have had numerous fistulas inserted and multiple revisions in an attempt to maintain adequate access for dialysis. Presently, several authors have reported the successful use of PTA to maintain adequate access for dialysis. All stress the advantages of PTA to surgery and the importance of proper selection of patients. Their experience so far, with small numbers of patients, suggests a promising technique with a low complication rate when a careful selection of patients is made and the angioplasty is performed by an experienced individual. Although recent developments, such as high-pressure balloons and long inflation time procedural refinements, of PTA have permitted clinicians to apply this technology to the problem of access stenosis, many stenoses and occlusions associated with AV fistulas have proved resistant to dilation (27-28). Dense perivenous and endovenous fibrosis make venous anastomotic lesions quite resistant to dilatation. Far proximal venous stenoses with endovenous fibrosis only, are easier and more successfully dilated. Glanz and coworkers suggest that the turbulence and shear stresses of arterial blood flowing into a low-resistance vein may act as the initiating event in the deposition of platelets and fibrin, resulting in mural thrombus and eventual fibrosis (15). They reported needing as many as 8-10 balloon inflations for up to 30 seconds before a successful result was effected (27). In order to generate the higher pressures needed to dilate fibrotic lesions, Glanz and coworkers used polyethylene, rather than polyvinyl chloride balloons. In some cases, they have also had to increase balloon inflation time from 30 seconds to 5 minutes in order to dilate several resistant venous stenoses (27). Hunter and associates found that even strenuous balloon dilation can be unsuccessful with fibrotic stenotic lesions. Seven of their 10 successful dilations of occlusions and four of their five successful dilations of anastomotic stenoses required the followup use of semirigid dilators (coaxial dilation) after unsuccessful attempts with balloon dilation. Presently, rates of late patency of the dilated internal and graft fistulas are not high, and substantially more experience with PTA in AV dialysis fistulas is needed in controlled studies to better define the safety and clinical effectiveness of the procedure. The treatment of patients with obstructive AV fistulas with PTA is a relatively new procedure that lacks adequate experience.

Advice concerning the safety and efficacy of PTA for stenotic lesions of AV dialysis fistulas has been sought from groups and organizations, both within and outside of the Federal Government. However, due to the newness of this application of PTA, and the lack of adequate data and experience in its use, those organizations contacted have been unable to establish positions at this time.

The Food and Drug Administration (FDA) states that percutaneous transluminal balloon dilatation catheter type devices were marketed in the U.S. before May 28, 1976, but have not been classified. Several devices of this type are currently being marketed under the terms of section 510(k) of the Medical Device Amendments of May 28, 1976, to the Food, Drug, and Cosmetic Act. According to the FDA, the indicated use of this type of device is to percutaneously dilate certain stenotic peripheral arteries, including the iliac, femoral, popliteal, tibial, and renal arteries. The FDA has not received any 510(k) premarket notification submissions for use of this type of device in dilating AV fistulas.

SUMMARY

PTA is the percutaneous, fluoroscopically guided use of balloon-tipped catheters to remove or relieve stenotic or occlusive lesions of the vascular system. Since its introduction in 1964, PTA has been widely used to treat atherosclerotic occlusive disease of the coronary, renal, iliac, and femoral arteries. However, dilation of failing AV access fistulas has been only rarely performed due to the newness of this application of PTA. Maintenance of a patent vascular access is one of the most vexing and frequent problems facing the physician who cares for patients on maintenance hemodialysis. While several authors have reported the successful use of PTA in these vessels, their experience, so far, with series of small numbers of patients, suggests a promising application of PTA with a low complication rate when careful selection of patients is made and the angioplasty is performed by an experienced individual. The treatment of patients with obstructive lesions of AV dialysis access fistulas with PTA is a relatively new procedure that lacks adequate experience. Substantially more experience with PTA in failing AV dialysis fistulas and shunts is needed in controlled studies to better define the safety and clinical effectiveness of the procedure.

Prepared by: Martin Erlichman, M.S.

References

1. Moore, T.S., et al. Percutaneous transluminal angioplasty in subclavian steal syndrome: Recurrent stenosis and retreatment in two patients. Neurosurgery. 11 (4): 512-17 (1982).

2. American College of Physicians: Health and Public Policy Committee. Percutaneous transluminal angioplasty. Annals of Internal Medicine. 99 (6): 864-68 (1983).

3. Gruntzig, A. Recanalization of Arterial Stenosis with a Dilatation Catheter. D. Dobbelstein (ed). CEPID, Munich, 1980.

4. National Center for Health Care Technology. Percutaneous transluminal angioplasty in treatment of the lower extremities. Assessment Report Series. 1 (14):1-12 (1981).

5. National Center for Health Care Technology. Percutaneous transluminal angioplasty for treatment of stenotic lesions of a single coronary artery. Assessment Report Series. 2 (24):1-21 (1981).

6. National Center for Health Care Technology. Percutaneous transluminal angioplasty in treatment of stenotic lesions of the renal arteries. Assessment Report Series. 2 (24):1-13 (1984).

7. Spinowitz, BS., Carsen, G., Meisell, R. et al. Percutaneous transluminal dilatation for vascular access. Nephron. 35:201-204(1983.

8. Mennes, PA., Gilula, LA., Anderson, CB., et al. Complications associated with arteriovenous fistulas in patients undergoing chronic hemodialysis. Arch Intern Med. 138:117-21(July 1978).

9. Giacchimo, JL, Geis, P., Buckingham, JM., et al. Vascular access: Long-term results, new techniques. Arch Surg. 114:403-408(1979).

10. Lewis, SM. (1983) Acute and chronic renal failure in: Lewis, SM., Collier, IC., (eds) Medical Surgical Nursing. McGraw-Hill, New York, p.1128-30.

11. Bailey, GL., Morgan, AP. (1972) Circulatory access for hemodialysis in: Bailey, GL., (ed) Hemodialysis. Academic Press., New York and London, p. 211-31.

12. Brescia, MJ., et al. Chronic hemodialysis using venipuncture and surgically created arteriovenous fistula. New England J Med. 275:1089-92(1966).

13. Gilula, LA., Staple, TW., Anderson, CB., et al. Venous angiography of hemodialysis fistulas. Radiology 115:555-62(June 1975).

14. Ilaimov, M. Vascular access for hemodialysis. Surgery Gynec. Obstet. 141:619-629(1975).

15. Glanz, S., Bashist, B., Gordon, DH., et al. Angiography of upper extremity access fistulas for dialysis. Radiology. 143:45-52(April 1982).

16. Kinnaert, P., Vereerstraeten, P., Toussaint, C., et al. Nine years experience with internal arteriovenous fistulas for haemodialysis: a study of some factors influencing the results. Br. J. Surg. 64:242-46(1977).

17. Lawrence, PF., Miller, FJ., Minneau, DC. Balloon catheter dilatation in patients with failing arteriovenous fistulas. Surgery. 89:439-442(1981).

18. Hunter, DW., So, SKS., Cataneda-Zuniga, WR., et al. Failing or thrombosed Brescia-Cimino arteriovenous dialysis fistulas. Radiology. 149:105-109(1983).

19. Anderson, CB., Gilula, LA., Harter, H., et al. Venous angiography and the surgical management of subcutaneous hemodialysis fistulas. Ann Surg. 187(2):194-204(1978).

20. Gothlin, J., Lindstedt, E. Angiographic features of Cimino-Brescia fistulas. AJR. 125(3):582-90(1975).

21. American Medical Association. Percutaneous transluminal angioplasty. Report H of the Council on Scientific Affairs. 269-71 (1982).

22. Abele, J.E. Balloon catheters and transluminal dilatation: Technical considerations. AJR. 135:901-06 (1980).

23. Sos, T.A., Sniderman, K.W. Percutaneous transluminal angioplasty. Seminars in Roentgenology. XVI (1):26-41 (1981).

24. Athanasoulis, CA. Percutaneous transluminal angioplasty: General principles. AJR. 135:893-900(1980).

25. Block, PC. et al. Morphology after transluminal angioplasty in human beings. N ENGL J Med. 305382-85(1981).

26. Damuth, HD. et al. Angioplasty of subclavian artery stenosis proximal to the vertebral origin. AJNR. 41239-42(1983).

27. Glanz, S., Gordon, D., Butt, KMH., et al. Dialysis access fistulas: Treatment of stenoses by transluminal angioplasty. Radiology. 152:637-42(1984).

28. Hunter, DW., Castaneda-Zuniga, WR., Coleman, CC., et al. Failing arteriovenous dialysis fistulas: Evaluation and treatment. Radiology. 152:631-35(1984).

National Heart, Lung, and Blood Institute
Office of Program Planning and Evaluation
Bldg. 31 Room 5A-03
National Institutes of Health
Bethesda, MD 20205
(301) 496-6331

Major Emphases of Technology Assessment Activities

Technology	Concerns: Safety	Efficacy/ Effectiveness	Cost/Cost-Effect/ Cost-Benefit	Ethical/Legal/ Social
Drugs	X	X		
Medical Devices/Equipment/Supplies	X	X		X
Medical/Surgical Procedures	X	X		X
Support Systems	X	X		
Organizational/Administrative				

Stage of Technologies Assessed
_X_ Emerging/new
_X_ Accepted use
_X_ Possibly obsolete, outmoded

Application of Technologies
_X_ Prevention
_X_ Diagnosis/screening
_X_ Treatment
____ Rehabilitation

Assessment Methods
_X_ Laboratory testing
_X_ Clinical trials
_X_ Epidemiological and other observational methods
____ Cost analyses
____ Simulation/modeling
_X_ Group judgment
_X_ Expert opinion
_X_ Literature syntheses

Approximate 1985 budget for technology assessment: $26,000,000*

* This estimate covers NHLBI clinical trials expenditures and expenditures for consensus development and related assessment activities. The total fiscal year (FY) 1984 NHLBI budget was over $700 million.

NATIONAL HEART, LUNG, AND BLOOD INSTITUTE NATIONAL INSTITUTES OF HEALTH

Introduction

The National Institutes of Health (NIH) is the principal biomedical research agency of the federal government. NIH accounts for 69 percent of all federal expenditures for health R&D and 36 percent of total national support for health R&D. NIH is composed of 12 bureaus and institutes (hereafter all referred to as institutes), and six research and support divisions. The National Heart, Lung, and Blood Institute (NHLBI) is the second largest in terms of funding, after the National Cancer Institute (NCI).

NHLBI was established in 1948 under authority of the National Heart Act as the National Heart Institute. With a growing awareness of national health problems, it was redesignated as the National Heart and Lung Institute in 1969. The activities of the institute were expanded in 1972 by the National Heart, Blood Vessel, Lung, and Blood Act (P.L. 92-423) to advance the national effort against diseases of the heart, blood vessels, lungs, and blood. With the passage of the Health Research and Health Services Amendment in 1976 (P.L. 94-278), and its redesignation as the National Heart, Lung, and Blood Institute, the authority was further enlarged to include research on the use of blood and blood products and on the management of blood resources.

The mission of the National Heart, Lung, and Blood Institute is to advance the nation's capabilities to prevent, diagnose, and treat heart, lung, and blood diseases. NHLBI plans, fosters, and supports an integrated and coordinated program of research, investigations, clinical trials, and demonstrations relating to the causes, prevention, methods of diagnosis, and treatment of heart, lung, blood vessel, and blood diseases, including the uses and management of blood and blood products.

Other federal agencies support cardiovascular, lung, and blood research as well. The Interagency Technical Committee (IATC), chaired by the director of NHLBI, coordinates federal health programs and activities in these areas.

The 1972 act mandated that the NHLBI director, with the advice of the National Heart, Lung, and Blood Advisory Council, develop a national plan for attacking heart, blood vessel, lung, and blood diseases. The 1972 act also requires the director and Advisory Council of NHLBI to submit an annual report to the President, for transmittal to Congress, on the accomplishments of the national program during the preceding year and on plans for the next 5 years. NHLBI assessment activities described in this profile are determined largely through the institute's ongoing program cycle of planning, implementation, and evaluation.

The major components of NHLBI are the Office of the Director, Division of Heart and Vascular Diseases, Division of Lung Diseases, Division of Blood Diseases and Resources, Division of Epidemiology and Clinical Applications, Division of Extramural Affairs, Division of Intramural Research, Office of Program Planning and Evaluation, Office of Administrative Management, Office of Prevention and Control, and Office of Special Concerns. The Office of Program Planning and Evaluation (OPPE) coordinates technology assessment and technology transfer activities, and its director represents NHLBI on the NIH Coordinating Committee on Assessment and Transfer of Technology.

Major program areas of NHLBI are as follows.

Heart and Blood Vessel Diseases

arteriosclerosis*
hypertension
cerebrovascular disease
coronary heart disease
peripheral vascular diseases
arrhythmias
heart failure and shock
congenital and rheumatic heart diseases
cardiomyopathies and infections of the heart
circulatory assistance

Lung Diseases

structure and function of the lung
chronic obstructive pulmonary diseases
pediatric pulmonary diseases
occupational and immunologic lung diseases
respiratory failure
pulmonary vascular diseases

Blood Diseases and Resources

bleeding and clotting disorders
red blood cell disorders
sickle cell disease
blood resources

NHLBI supports extramural research and conducts intramural research in the three categorical disease areas. The Division of Epidemiology and Clinical Applications plans and directs a program of epidemiological studies, clinical trials, basic and applied behavioral research, demonstration and education research, and projects for disease prevention and health promotion in all three areas.

* Although NHLBI does not have direct programmatic responsibility for diabetes mellitus, it supports investigations on the metabolic effects and cardiovascular consequences of diabetes.

Like other institutes, NHLBI has several advisory bodies, the foremost of which is the National Heart, Lung, and Blood Advisory Council. The council has 5 ex officio members, including the directors of NHLBI and NIH, and 18 appointed members from outside the federal government, including scientists and lay community members with a demonstrated interest in relevant health areas. Among its major activities, the council makes recommendations regarding areas and relative emphasis of institute research support, reviews grant applications, and submits an annual report to the President and Congress on the progress of the national program.

The Board of Scientific Counselors advises NHLBI regarding the intramural research program. The NHLBI Clinical Trials Review Committee, Research Review Committees A and B, and Research Manpower Review Committee advise the institute by providing initial scientific merit review for studies seeking grant or contract support. Other program advisory committees composed of nonfederal experts review and evaluate ongoing extramural and intramural programs, identify future research needs and opportunities, and conduct other advisory tasks.

Purpose

This profile deals primarily with NHLBI clinical trials and other assessment activities such as consensus development conferences and workshops. The purpose of NHLBI technology assessment activity is to serve the overriding strategy of the institute's national program. This strategy is represented by the biomedical research and clinical applications spectrum illustrated below (Figure A-1). Although the institute recognizes that the development and use of many medical technologies have not evolved through this sequence, NHLBI efforts to guide technological evolution through this spectrum are intended to maximize the beneficial effects of research findings on clinical practice and on the health-related behavior of the population. Evaluation is integral throughout this model spectrum because some aspect of evaluation is built into it in all stages. Formalized evaluation and validation in the form of clinical trials or other validation research often occur before a technology is disseminated for general use. Existing technology is continually evaluated and reevaluated by practitioners, by patients and, in some cases, by regulatory and research agencies. Consensus development conferences, task force reports, workshops, review articles, and related reports evaluate the available scientific evidence on medical technologies, and identify problems needing further research.

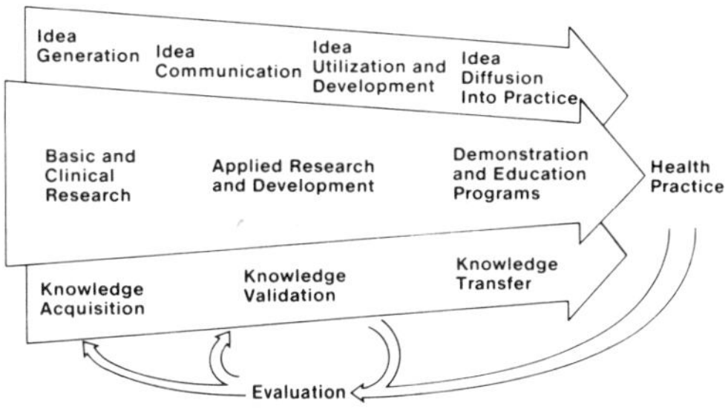

FIGURE A-1 NHLBI conception of the biomedical research spectrum. SOURCE: Moskowitz et al. (1981).

Subjects of Assessment

The principal types of technology assessed by NHLBI are drugs, medical devices, medical and surgical procedures, and support systems used in prevention, diagnosis, screening, and treatment. NHLBI also devotes considerable attention to the roles of smoking, diet, and other aspects of life-style and the environment in heart and vascular diseases, lung diseases, and blood diseases. One of the major NHLBI efforts addressing support systems is that of the Division of Blood Diseases and Resources, which plans and directs programs to improve national systems of blood procurement, management, and distribution. The institute does some work in evaluating the organization of health care, e.g., assessing alternative hypertension management programs, various educational programs, and delivery of care by state health departments. Furthermore, it administers and evaluates the National Heart, Blood Vessel, Lung, and Blood Program.

Topics of ongoing and completed NHLBI clinical trials are shown in Table A-7, with

TABLE A-7 NHLBI Clinical Trials Since 1965

Trial	Initiation/ Duration (years)[a]	Actual/Projected Total Cost (in millions of $)
Heart and Vascular Diseases Program		
Coronary Drug Project	1965/18	41.6
Coronary Drug Project Mortality Surveillance	1981/3.5	0.2
Lipid Research Clinics Coronary Primary Prevention Trial	1973/15	172.0
Multiple Risk Factor Intervention Trial for the Prevention of Coronary Heart Disease	1972/13	115.3
Hypertension Detection and Follow-Up Program	1971/14	71.6
Unstable Angina Pectoris Trial	1972/10	0.6
Coronary Artery Surgery Study	1973/14	26.9
Program on Surgical Control of Hyperlipidemias	1973/12	51.1
Aspirin-Myocardial Infarction Study	1974/6	16.9
Beta-Blocker Heart Attack Trial	1977/7	18.4
Multicenter Investigation of Limitation of Infarct Size	1977/8	19.0
Treatment of Hypertension	1966/12	3.1
Management of Patent Ductus in Premature Infants	1978/4	4.3
Systolic Hypertension in the Elderly Program (Pilot Study)	1980/5	3.7
Randomized Trial of Aspirin and Mortality in Physicians	1981/9	8.0
Hypertension Prevention Trial	1981/5	10.6
Cardiac Arrhythmia Pilot Study	1982/5	7.9
Randomized Clinical Trial of Non-Surgical Reperfusion of the Coronary Arteries	1982/5	4.2
Thrombolysis in Myocardial Infarction	1983/4	10.2
Dietary Intervention Study for Hypertension	1980/3	10.2
Control of Hypertension by Non-Pharmacologic Means	1980/5	2.3
Risk Factor Intervention in Coronary Disease	1983/5	2.9
Intravenous Streptokinase in Acute Myocardial Infarction	1983/4	1.3
Platelet Drug Trial in Coronary Disease Progression	1979/8	1.9
Platelet-Inhibitor Drug Trial in Coronary Angioplasty	1983/5	1.6
Evaluation of SC-V Versus Conventional CPR	1981/3	0.9
Systolic Hypertension in the Elderly Program	1984/9	48.0
Studies of Left Ventricular Dysfunction	1985/5	30.1
Lung Diseases Program		
Prevention of Neonatal Respiratory Distress Syndrome with Antenatal Steroid Administration	1976/7	5.5
Clinical Study of Intermittent Positive Pressure Breathing	1976/7	8.9
Nocturnal Oxygen Therapy	1976/4	4.0
Extracorporeal Support for Respiratory Insufficiency	1974/3	5.6
Prospective Investigation of Pulmonary Embolism Diagnosis	1983/5	7.6
Prevention of Chronic Obstructive Pulmonary Disease	1984/7.5	20.9
High Frequency Ventilation in Premature Infants	1984/3	7.0
Blood Diseases and Resources Program		
Granulocyte Transfusion Study	1976/4	1.6
Interruption of Maternal-to-Infant Transmission of Hepatitis B by Means of Hepatitis B Immune Globulin	1975/3	0.1
Cooperative Study of Factor VIII Inhibitors	1978/2	0.8
Hepatitis B Vaccine Clinical Trial	1978/3	0.2
Transfusion-Transmitted Cytomegalovirus Prevention in Neonates	1983/3	0.7
Division of Intramural Research		
NHLBI Type II Coronary Intervention Study	1971/10	0.5
Diffuse Fibrotic Lung Disease	1978/5	69.1 man-years
Evaluation of Subcutaneous Desferrioxamine as Treatment for Transfusional Hemochromatosis and a Controlled Trial to Determine the Value of Supplemental Ascorbic Acid	1978/5	13.5 man-years

[a] Total duration, including patient recruitment, intervention, analysis, follow-up.

the initiation year, duration, and actual or projected total cost of each. Other assessment topics are addressed in group efforts such as consensus development conferences, special task forces and other working groups, and in state-of-the-art review articles. Many of the group efforts are cosponsored by other federal agencies and by professional and voluntary organizations. NHLBI has cosponsored with the NIH Office of Medical Applications of Research (OMAR) the following eight NIH consensus development conferences:

- Tranfusion Therapy in Pregnant Sickle Cell Disease Patients (1979)
- Improving Clinical and Consumer Blood Pressure Measuring Devices (1979)
- Thrombolytic Therapy in Thrombosis (1980)
- Coronary Bypass Surgery (1980) (A second conference was cosponsored with the National Center for Health Care Technology)
- Treatment of Hypertriglyceridemias (1983)
- Fresh Frozen Plasma: Indications and Risks (1984)
- Lowering Blood Cholesterol to Prevent Heart Disease (1984)
- Health Implications of Obesity (1985).

The following are examples of publications covering other recent group efforts conducted or cosponsored by NHLBI on subjects related to technology assessment.

- Fourteenth Bethesda Conference: Noninvasive Diagnostic Instrumentation for Assessment of Cardiovascular Diseases in the Young
- Third Report of the Joint National Committee on the Detection, Evaluation, and Treatment of High Blood Pressure
- Proceedings of a Workshop on Apolipoprotein Qualification
- Report of the Working Group to Define Critical Behaviors in the Dietary Management of High Blood Pressure
- Working Papers, NHLBI Conference on the Implications of the Hypertension Detection and Followup Program
- Workshop on Arachidonic Acid Metabolism and the Pulmonary Circulation
- Report of the Working Group on Arteriosclerosis of the National Heart, Lung, and Blood Institute
- Artificial Heart and Assist Devices: Directions, Needs, Costs, Societal and Ethical Issues. Report of the Working Group on Mechanical Circulatory Support of the National Heart, Lung, and Blood Institute
- Legal and Ethical Issues Surrounding Organ Transplantation

Through OMAR, NHLBI participates in the technology coverage decision process for the Health Care Financing Administration (HCFA). In FY 1983 and 1984, OMAR referred 22 HCFA coverage issues to NHLBI for review and analysis. Examples of technologies that were subjects of these inquiries are outpatient cardiac catheterization, cardiac pacemakers, fully automated blood pressure monitoring, and streptokinase infusion for acute myocardial infarction.

(The profile of OMAR describes the NIH Consensus Development Program in detail and OMAR's role in coordinating NIH responses to HCFA inquiries. See the Office of Health Technology Assessment [OHTA] profile for discussion of its role in coordinating Public Health Service responses to HCFA coverage inquiries.)

Stage of Diffusion

NHLBI's technology assessment activities address emerging and new technologies and established technologies in transition. According to the institute, emerging technologies are those under development that appear likely to be used in the practice of medicine within 5 years. New technologies are those that may have passed the stage of clinical trials but are not yet widely disseminated, or those that are moving into general use without benefit of clinical trials. The last group are those established technologies that are currently undergoing or likely to undergo major changes in use or costs as a result of new research findings, or for which serious concerns have been raised concerning safety and effectiveness. Examples of clinical trials involving established technologies in transition are the Coronary Artery Surgery Study and the Clinical Study of Intermittent Positive Pressure Breathing.

Concerns

The principal concerns of NHLBI assessment activities are safety and efficacy. The institute also continues to address certain ethical, social, and legal implications of technologies such as the artificial heart and ventricular assist devices, coronary artery bypass surgery, and organ transplantation. (Examples are the efforts of the NHLBI Working Group on Mechanical Circulatory Support, and the 1985 conference cosponsored by the institute on the legal and ethical issues surrounding organ transplantation.) Of course, the planning and conduct of research supported by NHLBI—particularly clinical trials—are subject to detailed review of ethical considerations. The institute does conduct some cost studies, such as in-house studies to demonstrate the cost-effectiveness of its clinical trials. It must also evaluate the cost-effectiveness of the federal investment in the National Heart, Blood Vessel, Lung, and Blood Program, and make recommendations regarding future resource allocations.

Requests

(The descriptions under Requests, Selection, and Process address NHLBI clinical trials. Other assessment activities conducted by NHLBI, i.e., consensus development conferences and the technology coverage decision process for HCFA, are described in the profiles of OMAR and OHTA.) The process of initiating a clinical trial begins with discussions among institute staff, institute advisory groups, and other biomedical scientists and health care researchers. Suggestions may also originate from workshops, conferences, and various professional organizations. In most cases, a clinical trial is part of the progression of an idea as it emerges from basic science through clinical research to the point at which large-scale testing is required to determine the safety and efficacy of a technology. Activities leading up to a clinical trial frequently include feasibility studies and pilot studies of intervention.

Of the 43 NHLBI clinical trials initiated since 1965, 17 have been funded by grants, 22 by contract, 2 were intramural studies, and the others were combinations of these. Clinical trials account for a minority of all NIH grants and contracts, which are also provided for laboratory research and other R&D activities. (The definition and use of the term *clinical trial* varies among NIH bureaus, institutes, and divisions. NIH is considering the implementation of a standardized inventory of clinical trials that will use common definitions of this and related terms.)

Most grants are not solicited by the institute. In general, the investigator (through an eligible institution) who applies for a grant is formally responsible for developing the ideas, concepts, methods, and approach for a research project. In contrast, for projects that would be supported by contracts, the institute is responsible for establishing the plans, parameters, and detailed requirements. Contracts are generally solicited through requests for proposals (RFPs). In certain circumstances, grant applications are invited to support areas of special interest to the institute, in which case requests for applications (RFAs) and program announcements are issued.

For solicited contracts, institute advisory groups generally recommend types of projects that should be undertaken by the respective institutes. In NHLBI, these groups include the Arteriosclerosis, Hypertension and Lipid Metabolism Advisory Committee; Blood Diseases and Resources Advisory Committee; Cardiology Advisory Committee; Clinical Applications and Prevention Advisory Committee; Pulmonary Diseases Advisory Committee; and Sickle Cell Disease Advisory Committee. The institute advisory groups review the contract concept to recommend whether the anticipated results will be beneficial to NIH and whether the necessary technology and resources are available. If the contract concept is approved by the institute, an RFP is prepared and advertised. The RFP defines the program requirements and describes the criteria by which the proposals will be evaluated.

Selection

Proposed clinical trials generally go through a peer review process twice—the first time for approval to plan the trial and develop a detailed trial protocol; the second time for review of the detailed proposals for conducting the trial.

Review of a proposal to plan a trial entails consideration of the state of the science, feasibility, required resources, potential impact, and ethical considerations. Approval commits resources to plan the trial and develop its protocol. This approval does not commit NHLBI to conduct the trial itself, although its fiscal planning is made with the assumption that the planning phase will develop a scientifically appropriate and feasible protocol. Once a proposal to plan a trial is approved, a planning committee composed of principal investigators and other key project staff and institute staff oversees a detailed trial planning process generally involving subcommittees on trial design, patient eligibility, pharmacology, end points, recruitment, and others as appropriate.

The major factors considered in review of a proposal to conduct a trial are the feasibility of the trial based on the detailed planning, the state of the science, and the projected cost of the trial. Although these have been reviewed earlier in the decision to approve planning of the trial, they are considered in great detail here. Approval to conduct the trial commits defined resources for an extended period—several years in the case of major long-term trials. (For an example of a detailed clinical trial protocol, see NHLBI [1978].)

The peer review system for grant applications used by the NIH is based on two sequential levels of review, referred to as the *dual review system*. The dual review system is intended to separate the scientific assessment of proposed projects from policy decisions about scientific areas to be supported and the level of resources to be allocated. Grant applications submitted to NIH are received and processed centrally by the Division of Research Grants, which is one of the research and support divisions of NIH.

For most institutes, the first level of review is undertaken by panels of experts—referred to as *study sections*—established by the Division of Research Grants according to scientific disciplines or current research areas for the primary purpose of evaluating the scientific and technical merit of grant applications. There are approximately 95 study sections in the Division of Research Grants. In the case of NHLBI, the Division of Research Grants also may forward grant applications to the NHLBI Division of Extramural Affairs, which establishes ad hoc study sections to carry out the first level of review. (This is usually the case for program project grants and institute-solicited programs, including clinical trials.) These study sections usually consist of 12 to 20 members each and are composed primarily of nonfederal scientists selected for their competence in the particular scientific areas for which that study section has review responsibilities. An NIH health scientist administrator serves as executive secretary of each study section. The study sections provide initial scientific and technical merit review of grant applications, but they make no funding decisions and do not set program priorities. The study sections may recommend that a grant application be approved, disapproved, or deferred for further information. For approved applications, they assign a technical merit priority rating and make specific budget recommendations.

The second level of review is conducted by the institute and includes review by appropriate division staff, the institute director, and a national advisory board or council of the institute. For NHLBI, this is the National Heart, Lung, and Blood Advisory Council. Council recommendations are based not only on considerations of scientific merit, as judged by the study sections, but also on the relevance of the proposed study, as outlined in a grant application, to the institute's programs and priorities. The council assesses the quality of study section review of grant applications, makes recommendations to institute staff on funding, and evaluates program priorities and relevance. It also advises on policy and matters of significance to the mission and goals of the institute.

Variations on this process are required for review of solicited and unsolicited contract proposals and for proposals responding to solicitations for R&D support. All of these review, approval, and award processes are conducted in accordance with requirements of federal and DHHS procurement regulations.

Process

If the institute makes a commitment to conduct a trial, subject recruitment and clinical intervention begin. In general, subjects are not recruited simultaneously, and thus the recruitment and intervention activities proceed together.

Once the trial is under way, it is managed by a complex of committees composed of the investigators, advisors, and institute staff. Often, the central organizational element of the trial is a steering committee that provides overall scientific direction for the study at the operational level. Various subcommittees appointed by the steering committee are responsible for reviewing such matters as patient adherence, quality control, nonfatal events, natural history, mortality classification, bibliography, and editorial review. An assembly of investigators representing all of the clinical and logistical coordinating centers reports to the steering committee. A policy data-monitoring board which does not include any of the trial investigators acts in a senior advisory capacity to NHLBI on policy matters throughout the duration of the trial. It periodically reviews study results and evaluates the study treatments for beneficial and adverse effects, and consults on such major policy decisions as trial safety and termination, changes in protocol, measurement procedures, and publication.

Analysis continues during the trial. By the time the trial is ended, much of the analysis concerning the major question may already have been completed. However, only in rare cases—such as those in which a trial is not double-blind and the trends are extraordinary—might the findings of a trial be published during its course.

Assessors

NHLBI technology assessment activities entail the participation of the full complement of biomedical research and health care delivery personnel. Various advisory groups also include representatives of other professions. As noted above, members of the National Heart, Lung, and Blood Advisory Council include scientists and others who are lay community members with a demonstrated interest in health areas relevant to the program area of the institute. The study sections that review proposals are composed of nonfederal scientists selected for their competence in the particular scientific areas for which a study section has review responsibilities.

Turnaround

The duration of clinical trials supported by NHLBI has ranged from 2 to 18 years (including patient follow-up), averaging about 6.6 years, although interim assessments and other reports are made during the longer trials. Consensus conferences, state-of-the-art conferences, and workshops generally take about 1 year to plan.

Reporting

Reports of NHLBI clinical trials and other assessment activities appear in many medical and other scientific journals; books; technical reports; conference proceedings; annual reports of the National Heart, Lung, and Blood Advisory Council; and reports from the directors of NIH and NHLBI, and OMAR. For example, reports of the 13-year Multiple Risk Factor Intervention Trial for the Prevention of Coronary Heart Disease (MRFIT) have appeared in the *American Journal of Epidemiology*, *American Journal of Medicine*, *American Journal of Public Health*, *Annals of the New York Academy of Sciences*, *Circulation*, *International Journal of Mental Health*, *Journal of the American Dietetic Association*, *Journal of the American Medical Association*, *Journal of Chronic Diseases*, *Preventive Medicine*, and various NIH reports and conference proceedings.

Among the other journals in which NHLBI assessment activities are often reported are the *American Heart Journal*, *American Journal of Cardiology*, *Annals of Internal Medi-*

cine, Chest, Circulation Research, Hypertension, Controlled Clinical Trials, Journal of the American College of Cardiology, Journal of Community Health, Journal of Medical Virology, Medical Care, New England Journal of Medicine, and *Symposia Reporter*.

NHLBI promotes and disseminates assessment findings through workshops; information centers; and prevention, education, and control programs. The institute also disseminates information through professional societies, educational programs such as the National High Blood Pressure Education Program, clearinghouses such as the High Blood Pressure Information Center, interactions with industry representatives, and activities of the institute's Office of Prevention, Education, and Control.

NHLBI's Specialized Centers of Research (SCORs) and National Research and Demonstration Centers Program are important means of technology transfer. SCORs were initiated to provide a program of basic and clinical research in institutions that are fully equipped and staffed to support sophisticated investigations of specific diseases.

Impact

NHLBI is the leading research organization addressing cardiovascular, pulmonary, and hematologic diseases. There has been a concurrent expansion of NHLBI's functions and funding, and the sharp decline in adult cardiovascular mortality in the United States. Over the 20-year period 1963 to 1983, the death rates for coronary heart disease and cerebrovascular disease dropped 40 and 55 percent, respectively. The death rate for all cardiovascular diseases combined declined much more rapidly over that period than did the rate for all other causes of death combined. The decline in the death rate from coronary heart disease has resulted in the prevention of an estimated 114,000 deaths annually. Improvements in rates of mortality and morbidity are not only desirable for human well-being, but there are also sizeable economic benefits. The decrease in mortality from cardiovascular disease has been attributed to advances in diagnosis and treatment (e.g., early noninvasive diagnostic techniques and coronary care units), preventive measures, and changes in life-style. Among 26 industrialized countries, the United States has shown the steepest decline in cardiovascular mortality in middle-aged men, and the steepest decline in mortality from coronary heart disease in men and women ages 35–74 years.

Over the last generation, no advance in the prevention, diagnosis, or treatment of diseases of the heart and blood vessels, the lungs, and the blood has been unaffected in some measure by NHLBI, and most major technological advances in these areas have come as a direct result of NHLBI support. These have certainly resulted in improvement in the health of the American people and others throughout the world. However, it is not possible to quantify causal connections between the wide spectrum of NHLBI activities and improvements in the health of the American people.

According to the institute, a number of NHLBI clinical trials have had major implications for practice, including the following.

- The Beta-Blocker Heart Attack Trial to determine whether the regular administration of propranolol would prevent sudden death in patients with myocardial infarction. In this trial, mortality in patients on propranolol was reduced 26 percent (from 9.8 to 7.2 percent) when compared to the control group. This would amount to a savings of at least 6,000 lives annually if put into widespread practice.
- The Coronary Primary Prevention Trial showed that lowering blood cholesterol reduces risk of coronary heart disease. The results of this trial have immediate applicability to the estimated one to two million hypercholesterolemic men in the country, and the results could be extended to women with elevated cholesterol levels.
- The implications of the Coronary Artery Surgery Study, which compared surgical and medical treatment of patients with mild to moderate heart pain or in those who survived a heart attack and were free of angina, are that mildly affected patients can be managed with medical rather than surgical treatment

unless or until the condition becomes worse and surgery is clearly indicated. Results of this trial should make it possible to select patients for bypass surgery more appropriately.

- The Type II Coronary Intervention Study of the effects of diet and drug therapy on the rate of progression of coronary heart disease showed that the greater the reduction in cholesterol obtained through treatment, the less the progression of coronary artery disease.
- The Intermittent Positive Pressure Breathing (IPPB) Study provided scientific evidence to the medical community that IPPB provides no benefit as a therapy for ambulatory patients with chronic obstructive pulmonary disease.

NHLBI also evaluates its technology transfer and information dissemination processes, e.g., the Evaluation of Health Hazard Appraisal Strategies in Industrial Cardiovascular Risk Reduction Programs, and the Evaluation of Sickle Cell Education. OMAR has conducted and sponsored evaluations of the NIH Consensus Development Program, which has included consensus conferences cosponsored by NHLBI.

Reassessment

NHLBI reassesses technologies in light of new scientific evidence of efficacy or of long-term adverse effects not apparent in short-term studies, and given suggested new uses for established technologies. Two examples of such reassessment are the reappraisals of arteriosclerosis and the institute's artificial heart program.

NHLBI sponsored expert panel reports in 1971, 1978, and 1981 on arteriosclerosis. The first task group on arteriosclerosis was formed in response to the magnitude of the national and personal toll exacted by the disease, and issued its report in 1971. This report was instrumental in the passage of the National Heart, Blood Vessel, Lung, and Blood Act of 1972. The 1981 report of this group summarized the current understanding of basic processes of the disease; its prevention, diagnosis, and treatment; and rehabilitation of persons suffering from it. It also identified opportunities for research, with particular attention to preventive measures, therapies, and technologies ready for clinical trials or application in practice.

The institute's artificial heart program, formally established in 1964, has evolved during a period characterized by marked changes in technology; cost considerations; and ethical, legal, and social concerns relevant to the program. The institute has sponsored periodic reviews of the artificial heart program, reports of which were published in 1969, 1973, 1977, 1980, 1981, and most recently in 1985 by the NHLBI Working Group on Mechanical Circulatory Support.

Funding/Budget

NIH is funded by congressional appropriation. In terms of appropriations, NHLBI is the second largest institute after the National Cancer Institute (NCI). In FY 1984, NHLBI appropriations were $703.2 million, or nearly 16 percent of the total NIH appropriations. In constant dollars, NHLBI funding rose during the 1970s, but was reduced by 1982 to 85 percent of its 1979 level. By FY 1984, it had risen again to nearly the 1979 level.

NHLBI funding is broken down by program areas roughly as follows: heart and vascular diseases (67 percent), lung diseases (17 percent), and blood diseases and resources (16 percent). By type of activity, funding consists of extramural research (86 percent), intramural research (8 percent), direct operations (5 percent), and program management (1 percent).

Clinical trials expenditures by NHLBI were $22.9 million in FY 1984 and an estimated $25.2 million in FY 1985, accounting for about 9 percent of total NIH clinical trials expenditures. (Total NIH clinical trials expenditures are an estimated $275.7 million for FY 1985, of which NCI accounts for 59 percent.) Due to uncertainties in funding and competing priorities, NHLBI has postponed initiating new large-scale clinical trials since 1978; its support of clinical trials overall dropped from the $40 million–$60 million range of the mid- to late 1970s to $25.2 million in FY 1985 (current dollars not corrected for inflation). Whereas clinical trials expenditures accounted for 11 percent of NHLBI expenditures in 1979, they accounted for only 3.2 percent of 1984 NHLBI expenditures.

Example

On the following pages is a brief description of the Coronary Artery Surgery Study, a major long-term trial supported by NHLBI comparing surgical and medical treatment of coronary heart disease. This description is given in the May 1984 NHLBI Clinical Trials Reference Document, as updated in June 1985.

Sources

DeMets, D. L., R. Hardy, L. M. Friedman, and K. K. Gordon. 1984. Statistical aspects of early termination in the beta-blocker heart attack trial. Controlled Clinical Trials 5:362–372.

Levy, R. I., and J. Moskowitz. 1982. Cardiovascular research: Decades of progress, a decade of promise. Science 217:121–129.

Levy, R. I., and E. J. Sondik. 1978. Decision-making in planning large-scale comparative studies. Annals of the New York Academy of Sciences 304:441–457.

Moskowitz, J., Director, Office of Program Planning and Evaluation, National Heart, Lung, and Blood Institute. 1985. Personal communication. Assistance was also provided by W. T. Friedewald, Director of the Division of Epidemiology and Clinical Applications, NHLBI; L. M. Friedman, Chief, Clinical Trials Branch, Division of Epidemiology and Clinical Applications, NHLBI; P. L. Frommer, Deputy Director, NHLBI; and J. G. Green, Director of Extramural Affairs, NHLBI.

Moskowitz, J., S. N. Finkelstein, R.I. Levy, et al. 1981. Biomedical innovation: The challenge and the process. In E. B. Roberts, R. I. Levy, S. N. Finkelstein, et al. (eds). Biomedical Innovation. Cambridge, Mass.: MIT Press.

National Heart, Lung, and Blood Institute. 1978. Beta-Blocker Heart Attack Trial Study Protocol (with July 1980 update). Bethesda, Md.

National Heart, Lung, and Blood Institute. 1982. Tenth Report of the Director, National Heart, Lung, Blood Institute. Volume 1: Progress and Promise. Bethesda, Md.

National Heart, Lung, and Blood Institute. 1983. Guidelines for Demonstration and Education Research Grants. Bethesda, Md.

National Heart, Lung, and Blood Institute. 1983. Eleventh Report of the National Heart, Lung, and Blood Advisory Council. Bethesda, Md.

National Heart, Lung, and Blood Institute. 1984. Clinical Trials Reference Document. Bethesda, Md.

National Heart, Lung, and Blood Institute. 1984. Fiscal Year 1984 Fact Book. Bethesda, Md.

National Heart, Lung, and Blood Institute Working Group on Arteriosclerosis. 1981. Arteriosclerosis 1981. Volume 1: Summary, Conclusions, and Recommendations. Bethesda, Md.

National Heart, Lung, and Blood Institute Working Group on Mechanical Circulatory Support. 1985. Artificial Heart and Assist Devices: Directions, Needs, Costs, Societal and Ethical Issues. Bethesda, Md.

National Institutes of Health. 1982. Orientation Handbook for Members of Scientific Review Groups. Bethesda, Md.

National Institutes of Health. 1983. NIH Public Advisory Groups: Authority, Structure, Functions, Members. Bethesda, Md.

National Institutes of Health. 1983. National Institutes of Health Organization Handbook. Bethesda, Md.

National Institutes of Health. 1984. NIH Data Book. Bethesda, Md.

National Institutes of Health. 1985. Report on the Patterns of Funding Clinical Research. Bethesda, Md.

Office of Medical Applications of Research, National Institutes of Health. 1984. Technology Assessment and Technology Transfer in DHHS: A Report Submitted to the Department of Commerce in Compliance with the Stevenson-Wydler Technology Innovation Act of 1980 (P.L. 96-480). Bethesda, Md.

Office of Technology Assessment. 1982. Technology Transfer at the National Institutes of Health. Washington, D.C.: U.S. Government Printing Office.

CORONARY ARTERY SURGERY STUDY (CASS)

Objective

To compare coronary artery surgery with medical management in patients with coronary artery disease and to maintain a registry on all patients undergoing coronary arteriography, whether operatively or medically managed.

Summary Data

Mechanism:	Contract	
Initiation:	June 1973	
Total Duration:	14 years	
Funding:		
Total funding prior to FY 1984		$23,958,615
FY 1984 support		2,924,971
Support projected beyond FY 1984		0
Total support		$26,883,586

Subjects

Randomized: males and females, under 66 years of age with ischemic heart disease and specific history, symptoms, and angiographic findings.

Registry: All patients undergoing coronary angiography for ischemic heart disease.

Experimental Design

Randomized: non-blind, sequential. Some 780 patients meeting the criteria of specific subsets based on history, physical exam, laboratory tests, catheterization, and angiography were randomized to either surgical or medical therapy. Primary endpoints included death and myocardial infarction.

Registry: Essentially identical data, but no randomization.

Current Phase

(As of June 1985): Analysis and dissemination.

Background

Although it is generally agreed that many patients with severe angina pectoris improve symptomatically after coronary artery surgery, there is less consensus concerning, for example, other effects of the procedure, such as its long-term benefit and the criteria for patient selection. In addition, there are fewer data and less agreement on the effects and proper role of this procedure in other clinical circumstances. Both the surgical procedure and the prior diagnostic procedures represent substantial costs in both monetary and manpower terms; moreover, they entail morbidity and mortality risks.

There exists an urgent need for reliable and quantitative information regarding the effects of coronary artery surgery in patients with coronary ischemic heart disease. To be meaningful, these data must be set into the perspective of the clinical course of such patients under medical treatment. This assessment presupposes a meaningful classification of these patients and of the therapeutic interventions as well as evaluations of the effects of surgical and medical regimens in terms of mortality, the quality of life, and objective hemodynamic and other physiological measurements. Only such information can provide sufficient background for determining the suitability of coronary artery surgery for a particular patient.

In 1972, the National Heart and Lung Advisory Council identified these questions as topics of high priority, and the National Heart and Lung Institute established an Ad Hoc Policy Advisory Board on Coronary Artery Surgery to assist it in developing a program of research activities. In its report, the board noted a "critical need for objective data on the long- and short-term effects of coronary artery surgery." Requests for proposals were issued to carry out the recommendations of the board.

Planning of the trial was conducted between June 1973 and April 1975 and included protocol design, the development of a manual of operations, and a pilot study of the registry. In August 1975, registry patients' entry and randomization began at the 11 clinical centers and coordinating center. Initial projections of patient population numbers were underestimated; therefore, five clinical centers were added to the trial in 1976.

The five clinical subgroups of patients in the randomized studies included stable angina with normal resting left ventricular function; stable angina with impaired left ventricular function; postmyocardial infarction without angina; congestive heart failure due primarily to ischemic heart disease; and patients previously asymptomatic who were discovered to have serious coronary artery disease. All of the above subgroups must have met specifically outlined clinical and angiographic criteria to be placed in the randomized subset. The other two subsets (as distinguished from subgroups) of the study included those patients who were unsuitable for randomization because surgery was the treatment of choice in the judgment of many physicians and those patients for whom medical management was the treatment of choice. The patients enrolled in both the registry and randomized trial were followed for a 10-year period. This allowed evaluation of the primary endpoints, death and myocardial infarctions, and the secondary endpoints, angina, status, and quality of life.

A total of 24,959 patients were entered into the registry; 780 patients were entered into the trial. Recruitment ended in 1979. Intervention ended in June 1983. Follow-up has been extended for an additional four years to 1988.

Trial Results

The randomized collaborative Coronary Artery Surgery Study showed that coronary artery bypass graft surgery improves the quality-of-life as manifested by relief of chest pain, by improvement in both subjective and objective measurements of functional status, and by a diminished requirement for pharmacological therapy. However, no significant effect on employment or recreational status was observed. The excellent survival observed in both medically and surgically assigned CASS patients and the similarity of survival rates in groups of patients assigned to either treatment strategy in this randomized trial leads to the conclusion that patients similar to those enrolled in this trial can safely defer bypass surgery until worsening symptoms require surgical palliation.

From August 1975 to May 1979, 780 patients with stable moderate or milder ischemic heart disease were randomly assigned to surgical (390) or nonsurgical (390) management and followed through April 15, 1983. At five years, the average annual mortality rate in patients assigned to surgery was 1.1%. The annual mortality rate in those randomized to medicine was 1.6%. The annual mortality rates in surgically assigned patients with single, double, and triple vessel disease were 0.7%, 1.0%, and 1.5%; the corresponding rates in medically assigned patients were 1.4%, 1.2%, and 2.1%. None of the differences were statistically significant. The annual rate of bypass surgery in all medically assigned patients was 4.7%.

In order to evaluate the comparative effects of medical and surgical therapy on "quality-of-life" in patients with stable manifestations of ischemic heart disease, the 780 randomized patients were systematically followed for a mean of 5.5 years. Analysis was performed according to original treatment assignment. Surgically assigned patients had significantly less chest pain, fewer activity limitations, and less utilization of nitrates and beta-blockers. Treadmill exercise tests documented significantly longer treadmill time, less exercise-induced angina, and less ST-segment depression among surgical patients. However, employment status and recreational status did not differ significantly between medical and surgical groups, although employment status related significantly to chest pain severity. Total hospitalizations following randomization were greater in the surgical group owing primarily to rehospitalization during the first year of follow-up for the coronary artery bypass graft surgical procedure.

Consensus Development Program
Office of Medical Applications of Research
National Institutes of Health
Building 1, Room 216
Bethesda, MD 20205
(301) 496-1143

Major Emphases of Technology Assessment Activities

Technology	Concerns: Safety	Efficacy/ Effectiveness	Cost/Cost-Effect/ Cost-Benefit	Ethical/Legal/ Social
Drugs	X	X		
Medical Devices/Equipment/Supplies	X	X		
Medical/Surgical Procedures	X	X		
Support Systems	X	X		
Organizational/Administrative				

Stage of Technologies Assessed
_X_ Emerging/new
_X_ Accepted use
____ Possibly obsolete, outmoded

Application of Technologies
_X_ Prevention
_X_ Diagnosis/screening
_X_ Treatment
____ Rehabilitation

Assessment Methods
____ Laboratory testing
____ Clinical trials
____ Epidemiological and other observational methods
____ Cost analyses
____ Simulation/modeling
_X_ Group judgment
_X_ Expert opinion
_X_ Literature syntheses

Approximate 1985 budget for technology assessment: $1,789,000*

* This is the approximate total OMAR budget for 1985. The average total cost of a consensus conference is approximately $145,000.

OFFICE OF MEDICAL APPLICATIONS OF RESEARCH NATIONAL INSTITUTES OF HEALTH

Introduction

The Office of Medical Applications of Research (OMAR) was informally established in 1977 with the initiation of the Consensus Development Program, and was formally established in the Office of the Director of NIH in 1978. OMAR is the focal point for activities aimed at improving the assessment and translation of results from NIH-supported biomedical research into knowledge that can be applied safely and effectively in the practice of medicine and public health. OMAR's functions, as published in the *Federal Register* of October 13, 1978, may be summarized as follows (OMAR, 1983a).

- Advise the NIH director and his senior staff, and provide guidance to the NIH Bureaus, Institutes, and Divisions (BIDs) on medical applications of research.
- Coordinate, review, and facilitate the

systematic identification and evaluation of clinically relevant NIH program information.

• Promote the effective transfer of such information to the health care community and to other agencies requiring such information.

• Provide a link between technology assessment activities for the BIDs and the Office of Health Technology Assessment (OHTA) of the National Center for Health Services Research (NCHSR).

• Monitor the effectiveness and progress of NIH assessment and transfer activities.

A primary vehicle for OMAR's efforts in systematic assessment of biomedical technologies is the Consensus Development Program (CDP). Each CDP conference is a cooperative effort of OMAR and one or more BID cosponsors. Other OMAR technology assessment and transfer activities include the following.

Administration of the NIH/DHHS Patent Program The NIH/DHHS patent program fosters commercialization of federally funded inventions. The director of NIH designated OMAR to act as the central clearinghouse for all NIH patent-related activities. The director of OMAR also serves as chairperson of the NIH Patent Board.

Review and Analysis of HCFA Medicare Coverage Questions OMAR coordinates NIH medical and scientific review of the Health Care Financing Administration (HCFA) Medicare coverage issues referred to NIH by the Office of Health Technology Assessment of the National Center for Health Services Research and Health Care Technology Assessment (NCHSRHCTA). During FY 1981 and 1982, OMAR coordinated the assessment of nearly 100 HCFA Medicare coverage issues raised by Medicare contractors, practitioners, private industry, and others. Depending upon the nature of the specific technology in question, the coverage issue is forwarded by OMAR to one or more appropriate BIDs. OMAR reviews and integrates the BID responses and forwards them to OHTA.

Research and Evaluation Activities OMAR undertakes and awards contracts for special studies to evaluate and improve assessment and transfer efforts. Studies in FY 1981 and 1982 have included evaluations of

• the impact of discoveries in biomedical research that have been adopted by industry for commercial application outside the health-care sector;

• the NIH/DHHS Patent Program;

• physician awareness of the Consensus Development Program; and

• the process and the impact on health practice behavior of the Consensus Development Program and possible alternative approaches for biomedical technology assessment and transfer.

NIH Coordinating Committee on Assessment and Transfer of Technology The director of OMAR serves as chairperson of the NIH Coordinating Committee on Assessment and Transfer of Technology, established by the director of NIH to provide a mechanism for the coordination of NIH policy and activities related to health technology assessment and transfer. The committee is composed of one representative from each of the BIDs. Liaison representatives from ADAMHA, FDA, CDC, OHTA, NCHSRHCTA, NCHS, and the DHHS Office of the Assistant Secretary for Health also participate.

The remainder of this profile addresses the NIH Consensus Development Program, which is coordinated by OMAR.

Purpose

The purpose of the CDP is to evaluate publicly scientific information concerning biomedical technologies and arrive at consensus statements that will be useful to health care providers and the public at large and that will serve as contributions to scientific thinking about the technologies under consideration (OMAR, Participants' Guide).

The CDP has three primary objectives:

1. to provide a setting for the evaluation and review of the scientific soundness of a health or health-related technology, with emphasis on safety and efficacy;

2. to aid in the diffusion of knowledge of advances in biomedical technology, through dissemination of the findings from the consensus development process to physicians and consumers; and

3. to facilitate the diffusion, adoption, and appropriate use of technologies found to be sound.

It is intended that

> as a result of the Consensus Development evaluations . . . the use of those technologies found to be scientifically sound will increase and those that receive no such endorsement will diminish, thus adding something to the quality of health care (NIH, 1980).

The CDP is not meant to dictate the practice of medicine. Rather than being guidelines or regulations, consensus statements are intended to aid the physician and the public, and to be influential by weight of the prestige of the consensus process and the members of the panel (Jacoby, 1983). The consensus statement is an independent report and is not a policy statement of NIH or the federal government.

Subjects of Assessment

A broad variety of technologies have been topics of consensus conferences, including medical and dental drugs, devices, procedures, facilities, and support systems used in prevention, diagnosis, and treatment. Table A-11 lists the CDP conferences held since the program's inception in 1977.

Stage of Diffusion

Although the CDP originally was to have focused on emerging technologies, most of the conferences have addressed technologies already in clinical use, especially new or widely used technologies. This is largely because evaluative information regarding many emerging technologies is insufficient for the level of validity sought for CDP conferences, and because many technologies already in widespread use have not been carefully scrutinized for safety and efficacy (Jacoby, 1984; Perry and Kalberer, 1980).

Concerns

The CDP is primarily concerned with the safety, efficacy, and clinical application of technologies. It does not normally address social, ethical, legal, economic, or political issues surrounding technologies.

At the time of the establishment of OMAR, NIH identified two types of consensus development: technical consensus development, the assessment of the scientific and medical aspects of the technology in question, and interface consensus development, the assessment of the economic, social, legal, and ethical implications as well as the scientific and medical issues (NIH, 1977). In these terms, the CDP involves technical consensus development.

The focus of each consensus conference is established by a set of predetermined questions. The questions identify the relevant issues and define the scope of the conference. These questions, the answers as determined by the consensus panel, and a conclusion comprise the final consensus statement. As discussed below under Process, program planning committees composed of NIH staff and outside experts cooperate with OMAR in posing and editing conference questions. Examples of CDP conference questions are shown in Table A-12.

Requests

Suggestions for consensus conferences come from many sources, including the staff or director of a sponsoring NIH BID, OMAR staff, the director of NIH, consumer groups, government agencies such as HCFA, or Congress. Requests may coincide with the planning or completion of a major clinical trial.

Selection

Although the criteria for selecting topics for consensus development conferences have varied somewhat since the program's inception, current criteria are as follows.

1. The subject under consideration should be medically important.

2. There should be a scientific controversy

TABLE A-11 NIH Consensus Development Conferences, 1977–1986

Date	Conference Title	Cosponsor[a]
1977		
Sep. 14–16	Breast Cancer Screening	NCI
1978		
May 22	Educational Needs of Physicians and Public Regarding Asbestos Exposure	NCI
June 13–14	Dental Implants Benefit and Risk	NIDR
June 26–28	Mass Screening for Colo-Rectal Cancer	NCI
July 10–11	Treatable Brain Diseases in the Elderly	NIA
July 20	Indications for Tonsillectomy and Adenoidectomy: Phase I	NINCDS
Sep. 14	Availability of Insect Sting Kits to Non-Physicians	NIAID
Sep. 18–20	Mass Screening for Lung Cancer	NCI
Nov. 10–11	Supportive Therapy in Burn Care	NIGMS
Dec. 4–5	Surgical Treatment of Morbid Obesity	NIADDK
1979		
Feb. 15–16	Pain, Discomfort, and Humanitarian Care	(HHS)
Mar. 5–7	Antenatal Diagnosis	NICHD
Apr. 23–24	Transfusion Therapy in Pregnant Sickle Cell Disease Patients	NHLBI
Apr. 26–27	Improving Clinical and Consumer Blood Pressure Measuring Devices	NHLBI
June 5	Primary Breast Cancer: Management of Local Diseases	NCI
June 27–29	Steroid Receptors in Breast Cancer	NCI
Sep. 10–11	Intraocular Lens Implantation	NEI
Sep. 13–14	Estrogen Use and Postmenopausal Women	NIA
Oct. 15	Amantadine in the Prevention and Treatment of Influenza	NIAID
Oct. 17–19	The Use of Microprocessor-Based "Intelligent" Machines in Patient Care	DRS
Nov. 28–30	Removal of Third Molars	NIDR
1980		
Apr. 10–12	Thrombolytic Therapy in Thrombosis	NHLBI
May 19–20	Febrile Seizures	NINCDS
July 14–16	Adjuvant Chemotherapy of Breast Cancer	NCI
July 23–25	Cervical Cancer Screening: The Pap Smear	NCI/NIA/NICHD
Aug. 20–22	Endoscopy in Upper GI Bleeding	NIADDK
Sep. 22–24	Childbirth by Cesarean Delivery	NICHD
Sep. 29–Oct. 1	CEA: Its Role as a Marker in the Management of Cancer	NCI
Dec. 3–5	Coronary Bypass Surgery	NHLBI
1981		
Mar. 2–4	Reye's Syndrome	NINCDS/NIAID NICHD/NIEHS/DRS
Nov. 4–6	CT Scan of the Brain	NINCDS/NCI
1982		
Jan. 13–15	Defined Diets and Childhood Hyperactivity	NIADDK/NICHD
Mar. 1–3	Total Hip Joint Replacement	NIADDK
Nov. 1–3	Clinical Applications of Biomaterials	DRS
1983		
Mar. 7–9	Critical Care Medicine	NIH Clinical Center
June 20–23	Liver Transplantation	NIADDK
Sep. 27–29	Treatment of Hypertriglyceridemias	NHLBI
Oct. 24–26	Precursors to Malignant Melanoma	NCI

TABLE A-11 *Continued*

Nov. 15–17	Drugs and Insomnia: The Use of Medications to Promote Sleep	(NIMH)
Dec. 5–7	Dental Sealants in the Prevention of Tooth Decay	NIDR
1984		
Feb. 6–8	Diagnostic Ultrasound Imaging in Pregnancy	NICHD/(FDA)
Feb. 27–29	Analgesic-Associated Kidney Disease	NIADDK
Apr. 2–4	Treatment and Prevention of Osteoporosis	NIADDK
Apr. 24–26	Drug Therapy for Depression	(NIMH)
Sep. 24–26	Fresh Frozen Plasma: Indications and Risks	NHLBI/(FDA)
Dec. 3–5	Limb-Sparing Treatment: Adult Soft-Tissue and Osteogenic Sarcomas	NCI
Dec. 10–12	Lowering Blood Cholesterol to Prevent Heart Disease	NHLBI
1985		
Jan. 28–30	Travelers' Diarrhea	NIAID
Feb. 11–13	Health Implications of Obesity	NIADDK/NHLBI
Apr. 22–25	Anesthesia and Sedation in the Dentist's Office	NIDR
June 10–12	Electroconvulsive Therapy	(NIMH)
Sep. 9–11	Adjuvant Chemotherapy for Breast Cancer	NCI
1986		
Feb.[b]	Smokeless Tobacco	NCI/NIDR
Apr. 21–23	Neurological Applications of Positron Emission Tomography (PET)	NIH Clinical Center/ NINCDS/NIA/(NIMH)
Apr.[b]	Role of Nursing in the Management of Chronic Pain	NIH Clinical Center
Apr.[b]	Health Maintenance Needs of the Elderly	NIA
July[b]	Impact of HTLV-III Antibody Screening on Blood Banks	NHLBI
Aug.[b]	Preventing the Spread of Infectious Disease in Dental Practice	NIDR
Sep.[b]	Infantile Apnea and Home Monitoring	NICHD
Sep.[b]	Magnetic Resonance Imaging	NIH Clinical Center
[b]	The Utility of Plasmapheresis in Neurological Disorder	NINCDS

[a]Each conference is normally sponsored by OMAR and one or more Bureau, Institute, or Division of NIH:

NCI: National Cancer Institute
NHLBI: National Heart, Lung and Blood Institute
NLM: National Library of Medicine
NIADDK: National Institute of Arthritis, Diabetes, and Digestive and Kidney Diseases
NIAID: National Institute of Allergy and Infectious Diseases
NICHD: National Institute of Child Health and Human Development
NIDR: National Institute of Dental Research
NIEHS: National Institute of Environmental Health Sciences
NIGMS: National Institute of General Medical Sciences
NINCDS: National Institute of Neurological and Communicative Disorders and Stroke
NEI: National Eye Institute
NIA: National Institute on Aging
DRS: Division of Research Services

Sponsors from organizations outside NIH are shown in parentheses:

HHS: Department of Health and Human Services
NIMH: National Institute of Mental Health
FDA: Food and Drug Administration

[b]Date not set as of July 1985.
SOURCE: OMAR.

TABLE A-12 Examples of NIH Consensus Conference Questions

Total Hip Joint Replacement, March 1–3, 1982.
What are the indications and contraindications for total hip joint replacement?
What are the current scientific principles guiding selection of materials, devices, and procedures for total hip joint replacement?
What is the short-term and long-term prognosis for medical status and functional activity after total hip joint replacement?
What are the medical and surgical complications of total hip joint replacement?
What are the problems related to revision surgery for total hip joint replacement?
In what directions should the science base and techniques of total hip joint replacement be advanced?

Lowering Blood Cholesterol to Prevent Heart Disease, December 10–12, 1984.
Is the relationship between blood cholesterol levels and coronary heart disease causal?
Will reduction of cholesterol levels prevent coronary heart disease?
Under what circumstances and at what level of blood cholesterol should dietary or drug treatment be started?
Should an attempt be made to reduce the blood cholesterol levels of the general population?
What are the directions for future research?

Health Implications of Obesity, February 11–13, 1985
What is obesity?
What is the evidence that obesity has adverse effects on health?
What is the evidence that obesity affects longevity?
What are the appropriate uses and limitations of existing height-weight tables?
For what medical conditions can weight reduction be recommended?
What should be the future directions of future research in this area?

that would be clarified by the consensus approach or a gap between current knowledge and practice that a conference might help to narrow.

3. The topic must have an adequately defined and available base of scientific information to answer the previously posed questions.

4. The topic should be amenable to clarification on technical grounds and the outcome should not depend mainly on the impressions or value judgments of panelists.

5. The timing of the conference should be such that it is likely to have a meaningful impact; i.e., it should neither be so early in the developmental course of a new technology that data are insufficient nor so late that the conference merely reiterates a consensus already arrived at by the profession.

The following additional elements are desirable for positive consideration of a consensus topic:

1. Public health importance. The topic should affect a significant number of people.
2. Health care cost impact. The topic may have implications for reimbursement by agencies such as the Health Care Financing Administration.
3. Preventive impact.
4. Public interest.

Before a conference topic is finally selected, it is agreed to by the directors of the BID and OMAR, and approved by the director of NIH. Forthcoming or pending conferences are discussed by the NIH Coordinating Committee on Assessment and Transfer of Technology to elicit suggestions and interest from other BIDs.

Process

Once a conference topic has been selected, a planning committee composed of OMAR, BID staff, the conference chairperson, and outside experts is formed to delineate key conference issues and specific questions relating to the technology being assessed. These questions identify the most important issues concerning safety and efficacy and define the dimensions of the conference. The questions have normally been confined to those issues on which there is enough factual evidence to serve as a basis for consensus. The planning committees also recommend panelists, program format, and speakers. Background reports may also be prepared, and individual experts may be commissioned to compile summaries of the state of the science. The consensus process is designed to produce a published document, called a consensus statement, which will be useful to clinicians, researchers, and the public.

Consensus conferences are open meetings to which members of the public and the medical community are invited, and usually last 2½ days. The first 1½ days are normally devoted to a plenary session in which experts or representatives of task forces present information on the state of the science and the safety and efficacy of the technology. These presentations are followed by an open discussion involving speakers, panelists, and questions from the audience.

Following the plenary session, the panel convenes to draft consensus answers to the predetermined questions, considering the expert opinions of the conference speakers and other views expressed at the meeting. The consensus view of the panel is not necessarily that of all panelists. If a panel cannot achieve full agreement on a particular point, the consensus statement may identify opposing or alternative opinions and/or majority-minority viewpoints.

This document is read to the audience on the morning of the third day for further comment and discussion among the panel and audience. The panel may choose to incorporate comments received during this session for inclusion in the final consensus statement. The conference concludes with a press conference.

Assessors

Conference program planning committees cooperate with the BID and OMAR in choosing panelists. Chairpersons are selected for their stature as distinguished physicians and scientists and for their personal skills in chairing the open symposium portion of the conference and in leading the consensus panel. Chairpersons usually participate on the planning committee and participate in framing the questions and selection of panelists and speakers. The size of panels has varied from 8 to 16 members; most have had 10 to 12 members. OMAR seeks balanced representation from various sectors from professional and community life, including at least two individuals from each of the following four categories:

1. Research investigators in the field, i.e., academic clinicians and scientists who are active in the area of consideration but who are not professionally identified with advocacy or promotional positions with respect to the consensus topic.
2. Health professionals who are users of the technology, including practicing internists, surgeons, pediatricians, family practitioners, nurses, and other members of the health care team.
3. Methodologists or evaluators such as epidemiologists and biostatisticians.
4. Public representatives such as ethicists, lawyers, theologians, economists, public interest group representatives, and patients.

Although both adversary panels—composed of persons having espoused opposing viewpoints—and neutral panels—composed of persons not having publicly established positions—were used early on, the program now seeks neutral panels. Each CDP conference involves participation of approximately three staff members from the NIH institute concerned, three staff members from OMAR, and logistical support provided by an outside contractor.

Turnaround

The current NIH pattern is to devote about 1 year to conference preparation and another 3 to 6 months to dissemination of conference results. A final consensus statement is normally submitted for publication approximately 1 to 3 weeks following the conference.

Reporting

By the end of 1985, the CDP will have conducted more than 50 conferences. Table A-11 lists the conferences held since the time of the program's inception in late 1977.

At the conclusion of each conference, the panel presents its findings to the news media in a public briefing. After a final consensus statement is approved by the panel, the document is published by OMAR and widely disseminated to health care providers and administrators, the biomedical research and education community, and the public. Conference reports and summaries are published in medical and science journals pertaining to the conference topic. Most consensus statements are published in the *Journal of the American Medical Association* (*JAMA*).

Within 3 months after each conference, printed copies of consensus statements are mailed to over 20,000 individuals and organizations with interests relevant to the particular conference topic. Copies of the consensus statement are also available from OMAR on request. Copies of background papers and task force reports may also be made available, and the sponsoring bureaus may distribute more detailed reports of the proceedings. An example of pre- and postconference reporting activity is shown in Table A-13.

Impact

The CDP is one of few medical technology assessment programs which has undergone formal evaluation. In addition to formal evaluation, the CDP has been subject to considerable discussion in various publications (e.g., Perry and Kalberer, 1980; Rennie, 1981; Blue Sheet, 1983; Kolata, 1983, 1985) and government reports (e.g., OTA, 1982).

Through experience and in response to program evaluations, the CDP has undergone various modifications. The procedures for conference planning, formulation of questions, and report dissemination have become more standardized, as have the formats for conducting the conferences and the final consensus statements. Greater attention is given to including on the panels the various types of expertise needed for technology assessment.

One indication of the program's impact is that it has served as a model for similar efforts in Britain, Sweden, Denmark, and The Netherlands (see, e.g., Smith, 1984). NIH and Swedish representatives agreed to conduct in 1982 consensus development conferences following similar formats on hip joint replacement. The Swedish conference was the first such conference held outside the United States (Rogers et al., 1982). Britain's first consensus development conference, on coronary artery bypass grafting, was held in November 1984 (British Medical Journal, 1984).

Certain consensus statements have fallen short of addressing directly certain prominent issues. Consistent with CDP policy, conferences usually examine only the safety and efficacy of medical technology, and conference questions are limited to issues for which sufficient data exist for reaching scientifically valid findings. Because the conferences do not address such matters as cost and availability of other resources, some consensus statements may be of limited use in setting guidelines for clinical use of medical technology, e.g., frequency of Pap smears or the use of mammography. In the consensus statement issued on the diagnosis and treatment of Reye's Syndrome, none of the 15 conference questions was addressed to the controversial role of salicylates (aspirin), although limitations of studies indicating its association with Reye's Syndrome were cited (OTA, 1982). Although the panel on liver transplantation

TABLE A-13 Information Dissemination Activities for November 1981 NIH Consensus Conference on Computed Tomographic Scanning of the Brain

Preconference	
Journals receiving announcements	112
Flyers mailed	4,750
Special invitation letters to professional society presidents	36
Media press releases	125
Telephone calls to local media	60
Miscellaneous announcements (including *Federal Register*, NIH publications, posters, etc.)	Yes
Ads in *JAMA* and *NEJM*[a]	Yes
Postconference	
Consensus statements mailed	19,000
Full statement published in *JAMA*	Yes
Journals receiving availability announcements	43
Statements mailed in response to personal requests	1,100

[a]*JAMA, Journal of the American Medical Association; NEJM, New England Journal of Medicine.*

SOURCE: Jacoby, 1983.

concluded that the procedure has merit, especially because many transplant patients would otherwise die, the panel did not address the prominent issues of payment for liver transplants or the number needed should the procedure become generally available (Kolata, 1983).

The conference on liver transplantation was held despite the preferences of OMAR to avoid conference topics for which limited data are available. Panel members noted the lack of data regarding frequency of liver disease and success of liver transplants (Kolata, 1983).

Because published final consensus statements generally do not reflect the debate which is likely to have been present among panel members, expert speakers, and audiences, concern has been raised that consensus statements are prone to consist of generalities representing the lowest common denominator of discussion, i.e, the only points on which panel members can fully agree. An Office of Technology Assessment report (1982) noted that the CDP conference format is not designed to limit problems associated with face-to-face interaction (e.g., relative dominance of viewpoints due to social or hierarchical factors) in group settings, as are Delphi, nominal group, and other group processes. Rennie (1981) has suggested that consensus statements make fuller recommendations about further research, and that panels be kept intact to obtain their opinion on funding research projects in their areas.

Group judgment efforts such as the NIH program often seek to bridge gaps in and otherwise make sense of available research, to provide guidance for clinical practice. In so doing, expert panels may render recommendations relying to some extent on suggestive but not rigorously founded clinical evidence, e.g., derived from weaker epidemiological studies as opposed to randomized clinical trials. One recommendation of the NIH consensus panel on lowering blood cholesterol—to lower dietary cholesterol for all Americans age two onward—may have been such an instance. (See Kolata [1985], Lenfant et al. [1985], and Steinberg [1985] for discussion.) This is a methodological concern of any group judgment effort, and is best addressed with documentation of group judgment methodology and the characteristics of the research considered and assumptions made by the panelists.

A number of concerns about the CDP which were voiced at its inception have not materialized. The program has been successful in clarifying its role as one of provider of information, rather than as government regulator dictating methods of clinical practice. The issuance of consensus statements has not precipitated a flurry of malpractice action based upon consensus panel findings. There is no evidence that the program has stifled innovation. Consensus statements now routinely identify areas in which further development is needed. For example, the statement on total hip joint replacement highlighted several materials innovations and areas for further study of implant failure mechanisms, and the statement on clinical applications of biomaterials identified specific areas in great clinical need of new biomaterials.

Below are overviews of several formal studies of the process and impact of the program.

Consensus Development Process The Center for Research on Utilization of Scientific Knowledge (CRUSK), University of Michigan, conducted a detailed study (Wortman and Vinokur, 1982) of the CDP process to develop suggestions for strengthening the activity. The study employed measures of consensus conference outcome (e.g., quality of consensus statements), process (e.g., establishment and adherence to procedural arrangements that facilitate panels' deliberations), and technology (e.g., controversy) in examining eight conferences held between July 1980 and March 1982. Data for the study were collected through direct observations of conferences, personal interviews, analysis of consensus statements, and questionnaires. Although CRUSK found that the process "operates well in meeting its major objectives . . . and is evaluated quite positively," it did cite certain problems in the conduct of several of the conferences which may "disrupt [the process] and result in an unsatisfactory product." CRUSK made recommendations regarding selection of panelists, speakers and questions, conference format, and drafting of consensus statements. Many of the CRUSK recommendations have been adopted by the CDP.

Impact of OMAR Information Dissemination OMAR conducted a survey to measure the effectiveness of NIH consensus conference studies as evidenced by the extent to which physicians were aware of the conferences and the conclusions reached at each (Jacoby, 1983). The survey probed whether physicians in related specialties knew (1) that the conference was to be held, (2) that it was held, and (3) if they knew of the principal findings. More than 2,700 randomly sampled physicians in selected specialties were interviewed in two separate two-part telephone surveys (pre- and postconference) to test their awareness of NIH consensus development activities, especially the scheduling and conclusions of two consensus conferences. The conferences involved were the computed tomography (CT) scan of the brain (November 1981) and hip joint replacement (March 1982).

These surveys determined that awareness of the conference varied greatly among different physician specialties. Among the 10 physician specialties targeted for special dissemination efforts, between 3 and 37 percent of the specialists contacted had heard of either conference, and between 1 and 15 percent were aware of the conclusions of either conference. Across specialties, respondents' main sources of information were the *Journal of the American Medical Association*, other professional publications, and statements mailed by OMAR. The highest awareness of the CT scan conference was among neurologists: 37 percent of the neurologists surveyed were aware that the conference took place, and 15 percent were aware of the conclusions. The highest awareness of the hip joint conference was among orthopedic surgeons: 21 percent were aware of the conference, and 10 percent were aware of the conclusions. The study concluded that there is much room for improvement in information dissemination and that it would be fruitful to examine physicians' information-seeking habits, such as examining the role of opinion leaders, so as to better design strategies that more effectively disseminate conference results.

Impact of Conference on Burn Therapy An impact study of the November 1978 NIH Consensus Conference on Supportive Therapy in Burn Care was conducted by Burke et al. (1981) using a survey of the 25 burn centers at 6 burn care demonstration project sites of the National Burn Demonstration Project.

The survey found, among the 25 center directors, an overall average of 95 percent awareness for the conference's recommendations regarding 12 specific treatment approaches. Although the use level at the time of the conference was already relatively high for many of the recommended approaches, the survey found that an average of 68 percent of facility directors who were not already using specific recommended approaches reported an actual or potential practice change based on information received from the conference proceedings. All responding facility directors thought that the conference was important to their clinical practice, and most of those who indicated that they conduct ongoing research considered the conference important to their research.

The study findings indicated that the publication of the proceedings of the conference in a supplement to the November 1979 *Journal of Trauma* was a major factor contributing to the observed impact of the conference.

Program-Wide Impact The Rand Corporation is conducting a study, to be completed by 1985, of how consensus conferences have affected the knowledge, attitudes, and practices of health care professionals. The study has the following four major components:

1. a content analysis of the published consensus statements to identify message characteristics that may affect outcomes;
2. analyses of the professional literature for selected conference topics, covering periods both before and after publication of conference findings;
3. design and analysis of a study of changes in hospital-based procedures that

have been the subject of consensus conference recommendations;

4. design and analysis of a survey of physicians, which will cover their knowledge, attitudes, and self-reported practices with respect to one or more relevant technologies, while also eliciting information about their background, type of practice, and usual information sources.

Reassessment

As of 1985, no technology has been reassessed in a consensus conference. However, the program is prepared to undertake the reassessment of any technology in which such reassessment is merited by new developments.

Funding/Budget

The 1985 OMAR budget is approximately $1.8 million. The average cost of a conference is approximately $145,000, including contractor costs, NIH staff time, and printing and other information dissemination costs.

Example

On the following pages is the full text of the questions, answers, and conclusion of the CDP conference on Liver Transplantation, held June 20–23, 1983.

Sources

Blue Sheet. June 29, 1983. Liver transplantation: randomized clinical trials "Much in Doubt."

British Medical Journal. 1984. Consensus Development Conference: Coronary Artery Bypass Grafting. 289:1527–1529.

Clark, S., Office of Medical Applications of Research, National Institutes of Health. 1985. Personal communication.

Jacoby, I. 1983. Biomedical technology information dissemination and the NIH consensus development process. Knowledge: Creation, Diffusion, Utilization 5(2):245–261.

Jacoby, I., Acting Director, Office of Medical Applications of Research, National Institutes of Health. 1984. Personal communication.

Kolata, G. 1985. Heart Panel's conclusions questioned. Science 227:40–41.

Kolata, G. 1983. Liver transplants endorsed. Science 221:139.

Lenfant, C., B. Rifkind, and I. Jacoby. 1985. Heart Panel's conclusions (letter). Science 227:582–583.

National Institutes of Health. 1977. The Responsibilities of NIH at the Health Research/Health Care Interface. Bethesda, Md.

National Institutes of Health. 1980. Consensus Development Conference Summaries: Volume 3. Washington, D.C.: U.S. Government Printing Office.

National Institute of General Medical Sciences, National Institutes of Health. 1981. An Impact Study of the 1978 Consensus Development Conference on Supportive Therapy in Burn Care. Bethesda, Md.

National Institutes of Health Consensus Development Panel. 1978. Statement of recommendations on breast cancer screening. Clinical Research 26:118–120.

OMAR. Undated. Participants' Guide to Consensus Development Conferences. Bethesda, Md.

OMAR. 1978. Criteria for Identification of Candidate Technologies for Consensus Development. Bethesda, Md.

OMAR. 1983a. Technology Assessment and Technology Transfer in DHHS: A Report Submitted to the Department of Commerce in Compliance with the Stevenson-Wydler Technology Innovation Act of 1980. Bethesda, Md.

OMAR. 1983b. Liver Transplantation: National Institutes of Health Consensus Development Conference Summary. Volume 4, Number 7. Bethesda, Md.

OMAR. 1983c. Guidelines for the Selection and Management of Consensus Development Conferences. Bethesda, Md.

Office of Technology Assessment, U.S. Congress. 1982. Strategies for Medical Technology Assessment. Washington, D.C.: U.S. Government Printing Office.

Perry, S., and J. T. Kalberer, Jr. 1980. The NIH consensus-development program and the assessment of health-care technologies: The first two years. New England Journal of Medicine 303:169–172.

Rand Corporation. 1983. Submission to the Office of Management and Budget of Supporting Statement and Data Collection Instruments for Assessing the Effectiveness of the NIH Consensus Development Program. Volume I: Supporting Statement. Bethesda, Md.

Rennie, D. 1981. Consensus statements. New England Journal of Medicine 34:665–666.

Rogers, E. M., J. K. Larsen, and C. U. Lowe. 1982. The consensus development process for medical technologies: A cross-cultural comparison of Sweden and the United States. Journal of the American Medical Association 248:1880–1882.

Shires, G. T., and E. A. Black, eds. 1981. Second

Conference on Supportive Therapy in Burn Care. Journal of Trauma 21:665–752 (supplement).

Smith, T. 1984. Consensus on cabbage. British Medical Journal 289:1477–1478.

Steinberg, D. 1985. Heart Panel's conclusions (letter). Science 227:582.

Their, S. O. 1977. Breast-cancer screening: A view from outside the controversy. New England Journal of Medicine 297:1063–1065.

Wortman, P. M., and A. Vinokur. 1982. Evaluation of NIH Consensus Development Process. Phase I: Final Report. Ann Arbor, Mich.: Center for Research on Utilization of Scientific Knowledge, University of Michigan.

Liver Transplantation

National Institutes of Health
Consensus Development
Conference Summary
Volume 4 Number 7

Introduction

Since performance of the first human orthotopic liver transplantation in 1963, over 540 such operations have been carried out in four medical centers in the United States and Western Europe. Additional liver tranplantation procedures have been performed in other parts of the world, and more recently in several other American medical centers. Although extremely demanding and expensive, the operation has been shown to be technically feasible, and interpretable results have been reported from all four primary transplant centers. These clearly demonstrate that liver transplantation offers an alternative therapeutic approach which may prolong life in some patients suffering from severe liver disease that has progressed beyond the reach of currently available treatment and consequently carries a predictably poor prognosis. However, substantial questions remain regarding selection of patients who may benefit from liver transplantation; the stage of their liver disease at which transplantation should be performed; survival and clinical condition of patients beyond the initial year after transplantation; and overall long-range benefits and risks of transplantation in the management of specific liver diseases.

In order to resolve some of these questions, the National Institutes of Health on June 20-23, 1983, convened a Consensus Development Conference on Liver Transplantation. After 2 days of expert presentation of the available data, a Consensus Panel consisting of hepatologists, surgeons, internists, pediatricians, immunologists, biostatisticians, ethicists, and public representatives considered the offered evidence to arrive at answers to the following key questions:

1. Are there groups of patients for whom transplantation of the liver should be considered appropriate therapy?
2. What is the outcome (current survival rates, complications) in different groups?

3. In a potential candidate for transplantation, what are the principles guiding selection of the appropriate time for surgery?
4. What are the skills, resources, and institutional support needed for liver transplantation?
5. What are the directions for future research?

1.
Are there groups of patients for whom transplantation of the liver should be considered appropriate therapy?

Liver transplantation is a promising alternative to current therapy in the management of the late phase of several forms of serious liver disease. Candidates include children and adults suffering from irreversible liver injury who have exhausted alternative medical and surgical treatments and are approaching the terminal phase of their illness. In many forms of liver disease the precise indications and timing of liver transplantation remain uncertain or controversial.

Prolongation of life of good quality for patients who would otherwise have died has been reported in the following conditions:

- *Extrahepatic biliary atresia* is the most common cause of bile duct obstruction in the young infant. Patients who fail to respond to hepatoportoenterostomy (Kasai procedure) often benefit from liver transplantation. Recent data suggest that as many as two-thirds of these patients survive for 1 year or more after transplantation.
- *Chronic active hepatitis* is caused by viral infections or drug reactions, but many cases remain unexplained. Some patients with progressive liver failure are candidates for transplantation. Currently, exceptions seem to include drug-induced chronic active hepatitis, which usually responds to removal of the chemical agent, and hepatitis B-induced disease in which viremia persists. In the latter instance, rapid reappearance of infection with progressive liver failure has been reported following transplantation.
- *Primary biliary cirrhosis* is a slowly progressive cholestatic liver disease. Results of transplantation appear favorable for patients with end-stage liver injury. The procedure may improve the quality of life.
- *Inborn errors of metabolism* may cause end-stage liver damage or irreversible extrahepatic complications. Transplantation may be appropriate for such patients.
- *Hepatic vein thrombosis* (Budd-Chiari syndrome) often results in progressive liver failure, ascites, and death. Patients who have not responded to anticoagulation or appropriate surgery for portal decompression may be candidates for transplantation.
- *Sclerosing cholangitis,* a chronic nonsuppurative inflammatory process of the bile ducts, may cause liver failure. Less favorable results following transplantation in this group may be due to prior multiple surgical procedures, a diseased extrahepatic bile duct, the presence of biliary infection, or other factors.
- *Primary hepatic malignancy* confined to the liver but not amenable to resection may be an indication for transplantation. Results to date indicate a strong likelihood of recurrence of the malignancy. Nonetheless, the procedure may achieve significant palliation.
- *Alcohol-related liver cirrhosis and alcoholic hepatitis* are the most common forms of fatal liver disease in America. Patients who are judged likely to abstain from alcohol and who have established clinical indicators of fatal outcome may be candidates for transplantation. Only a small proportion of alcoholic patients

with liver disease would be expected to meet these rigorous criteria.

Although *fulminant hepatic failure* with massive hepatocellular necrosis induced by hepatitis viruses, hepatotoxins, or certain drugs may warrant liver transplantation, rapid progression of the disease and multi-organ system failure frequently preclude this option.

2.
What is the outcome (current survival rates, complications) in different groups?

The survival and complication rates of patients who have undergone liver transplantation are the major criteria for judging efficacy. Data are available from four locations (Pittsburgh; Cambridge, England; Hanover, Germany; and Groningen, The Netherlands). The interpretation of the existing data on survival is extremely difficult because no control data are given for comparison, surgical techniques and drug therapies varied over time, and patient selection criteria and management differed across centers.

While sufficient data for thorough assessment of liver transplantation are not available to date, today certain trends appear to emerge:

- Patients currently being accepted for transplantation have a high probability of imminent death and a low quality of life in the absence of transplantation.
- Patients undergoing transplantation have an operative mortality (within 1 month) of 20 to 40 percent.
- One-year survival among transplant recipients since 1980 is favorable when compared with their expected course in the absence of transplantation.
- Since 1980, 1-year survival appears improved over the earlier transplant experience.
- Individual patients have survived for many years with good quality of life after transplantation.
- Data are insufficient to evaluate survival rates beyond 1 year following transplantation with current technologies.
- Short-term quality of life is probably enhanced in many transplant survivors. We lack systematically gathered information on quality of life among long-term survivors.

Severe non-lethal complications of transplantation frequently occur and must be taken into account in judging efficacy of this procedure. Massive hemorrhage is the most serious intraoperative and early postoperative problem. Other postoperative complications include renal dysfunction, rejection, biliary tract complications, graft vascular obstruction, and infection. With accumulating expertise in medical and surgical management and with new developments in technology (e.g., intraoperative veno-venous bypass and cyclosporine), these complications can be expected to diminish.

3.
In a potential candidate for transplantation, what are the principles guiding selection of the appropriate time for surgery?

Selecting an appropriate stage for a given illness for liver transplantation is a complex issue: transplantation just prior to death may significantly diminish the life-saving potential of the procedure since hepatic decompensation in its latest stages poses a formidable surgical risk. Transplantation early in the course of hepatic decompensation may deprive a patient of an additional period of useful life.

An ideally timed liver transplantation procedure would be in a late enough phase of disease to offer the patient all opportunity for spontaneous stabilization or recovery, but in an early enough phase to give the surgical procedure a fair chance of success. For most patients, these phases are difficult to define prospectively. While no single best time for surgery can be specified, transplantation should be reserved for patients in any of the following phases of disease:

- When death is imminent.
- When irreversible damage to the central nervous system is inevitable.
- When quality of life has deteriorated to unacceptable levels.

The exact choice of the time for liver transplantation in an individual requires the judgment of a qualified medical team and a well-informed patient. The following are offered as guidelines for individual liver diseases.

- *Extrahepatic Biliary Atresia*

Biliary enteric anastomosis (hepatoportoenterostomy of Kasai) performed in the first 2 months of life provides significant improvement for at least 5 years in one-third of the patients, although cirrhosis and disappearance of the intrahepatic bile ducts occur with increasing age. While success of this procedure cannot be predicted for the individual patient, it should be used as initial therapy for extrahepatic biliary atresia. In the absence of severe hepatic decompensation in these children, liver transplantation should be delayed as long as possible to permit the child to achieve maximum growth. In children with successful hepatoportoenterostomy, liver transplantation should be deferred until progressive cholestasis, hepatocellular decompensation, or severe portal hypertension supervene.

Multiple attempts at hepatoportoenterostomy or surgical porto-systemic shunting render eventual transplant surgery technically more difficult and operationally more dangerous and therefore should be avoided in favor of liver transplantation.

- *Chronic Active Hepatitis*

The potential for spontaneous remission and the complex course of chronic active hepatitis make valid predictions of the subsequent course difficult except in the latest stages of the disease. Using strict criteria, patients can be identified who have almost no chance of survival beyond 6 months. Such patients may be suitable candidates for transplantation.

- *Primary Biliary Cirrhosis*

The indolent course of primary biliary cirrhosis and the potential for spontaneous improvement even in patients with advanced disease make transplantation potentially suitable only in the final stages of liver failure or when the quality of life has deteriorated to an unacceptable level.

- *Alpha-1-Antitrypsin Deficiency*

Of the some 20 phenotypes in this genetic disorder, only Pi ZZ is associated with significant hepatic disease in children. Of infants with this phenotype, neonatal cholestasis occurs in 5.5 percent. Jaundice usually is transient, clearing before 6 months of age although biochemical evidence of activity may persist. Liver transplantation is indicated in children with Pi ZZ phenotype only when cirrhosis has developed and when evidence of hepatic failure is present.

Adults with alpha-1-antitrypsin deficiency may have liver disease associated with phenotype Pi ZZ, MZ, or SZ. If hepatic failure occurs, liver transplantation may be indicated.

- *Wilson's Disease*

Patients with Wilson's disease usually are responsive to chelation therapy with penicillamine. However, some patients present with fulminant hepatic failure and/or progressive disease unresponsive to adequate chelation therapy. Liver transplantation may be indicated in these instances.

- *Crigler-Najjar Syndrome*

Of the two types of this genetic disorder associated with severe unconjugated hyperbilirubinemia, patients with Type I invariably develop bilirubin encephalopathy usually before 15 months of age. Because of the inevitability of central nervous system damage and the limitations of phototherapy, liver transplantation is indicated in such patients at an early age.

- *Miscellaneous Metabolic Diseases*

A number of rare genetic diseases may involve the liver and cause cirrhosis and eventual hepatic failure.

Patients with tyrosinemia, Byler's disease, Wolman's disease, and glycogen storage diseases Types O and IV may be candidates for hepatic transplantation.

Liver transplantation may also be indicated for patients with certain genetic diseases associated with severe neurological complications, such as hereditary deficiency of urea cycle enzymes and disorders of lactate/pyruvate or amino acid metabolism.

- *Hepatic Vein Thrombosis*

The course of hepatic vein thrombosis is variable, and therefore transplantation should be reserved for patients with severe hepatic decompensation. The possibility of later transplant surgery should not discourage the use of portal venous decompression when otherwise indicated.

- *Primary Sclerosing Cholangitis*

No clinical, biochemical, serologic, or histologic factors have proved to be of value in predicting outcome. When appropriate attempts at biliary tract diversion and dilatation have failed, and death from liver failure is imminent, liver transplantation should be considered.

- *Alcoholic Liver Disease*

At least 50 percent of the cases of cirrhosis in the United States are attributable to the abuse of alcohol, and alcohol abuse is the leading cause of hepatic morbidity and mortality.

Alcoholic liver disease is most favorably affected by abstinence. The natural history of untreated alcoholic hepatitis and/or cirrhosis is extremely variable, and there are few precise prognostic indicators in any but the terminal phase of the disease.

Liver transplantation may be considered for the patients who develop evidence of progressive liver failure despite medical treatment and abstinence from alcohol.

4.
What are the skills, resources, and institutional support needed for liver transplantation?

The requirements for conducting a liver transplantation program by a sponsoring institution are formidable. Accordingly, any institution embarking on this program must make a major commitment to its support. In addition to the full array of services required of a tertiary care facility and a program in graduate medical education, an active organ transplantation program should exist. Few hospitals are likely to meet these prerequisites.

Liver transplant recipients are seriously ill before surgery. The transplant effort is prodigious, and the postoperative intensive care interval, averaging 2 weeks, is punctuated by complications and frequent need for reoperation.

In this context, experts in hepatology, pediatrics, infectious disease, nephrology with dialysis capability, pulmonary medicine with respiratory therapy support, pathology, immunology, and anesthesiology are needed to complement a qualified transplantation team. Extensive blood bank support to provide the needed copious quantities of blood components is mandatory. Similarly, sophisticated microbiology, clinical chemistry, and radiology assistance are required. Emotional support for patient and family warrants psychiatric participation. Availability of effective social services to assist patients and families is indispensable.

The transplantation surgeon must be trained specifically for liver grafting and must assemble and train a team to function whenever a donor organ is available. Institutional commitment to the program mandates that operating room, recovery room, laboratory, and blood bank support exist at all times. Allocation of intensive care and general surgical beds is important. Recruitment of a cohort of specialized nurses and technicians to staff these areas is necessary. Access to tissue typing capability; ongoing research programs in liver disease, organ preservation, and transplantation immunology; and available hemoperfusion and microsurgical techniques are desirable attributes of a transplantation effort.

Participation in a donor procurement program and network is essential, and an interdisciplinary deliberative body should exist to determine on an equitable basis the suitability of candidates for transplantation.

Institutions conducting liver transplantation are obligated to prospectively collect and share data in a coordinated, systematic, and comprehensive manner in all patients selected as transplantation candidates, so that the role of liver transplantation in the management of patients with liver disease can be assessed properly. Additional information permitting cost-benefit analysis should be secured.

Finally, the panel feels that adherence to these guidelines detailing the essentials to conduct a transplantation program offers the best assurance of high quality in performing this very difficult operation.

5.
What are the directions for future research?

The Consensus Panel identified several broad areas related to liver transplantation in which critically important information is either unavailable or so incomplete as to defy meaningful interpretation. It is recommended that a registry or clearinghouse be established for collection and evaluation of all available data on liver transplantation. Such a center would develop unified criteria for selection of patients for transplantation and for reporting and evaluating all data related to the outcome of the operation and the patients' postoperative and long-term condition. As methods of immunosuppression improve and the logistic obstacles are resolved, the feasibility and desirability of randomized clinical trials of liver transplantation should be explored for suitable subgroups of patients with specific liver diseases.

High priority also should be given to research projects related to several aspects of the transplant procedure itself. Means should be developed to improve preservation of human liver *ex vivo* and criteria should be established to evaluate its viability. Improved control of organ rejection requires urgent attention; this includes thorough evaluation of the benefits and risks of cyclosporine as an immunosuppressive agent in liver transplantation. The design of the hemodynamic support system during transplantation needs evaluation and potential improvement. Research should be encouraged for developing better supportive measures for patients in liver failure, including maintenance of proper renal and cerebral function.

In the broad areas of the cause, pathogenesis, and natural course of chronic liver disease, present knowledge is fragmentary and incomplete, and research in these areas should be fostered and supported by all available means. Particular attempts should be made to determine the possible role of liver transplantation in the management of hepatocellular carcinoma at a stage when metastatic spread appears remote. Similarly, approaches should be sought to limit infection of the transplanted liver by hepatotropic viruses. Finally, liver transplantation should be explored as a modality of replacement therapy in genetically determined multi-organ enzyme deficiencies.

Conclusion

After extensive review and consideration of all available data, this panel concludes that liver transplantation is a therapeutic modality for end-stage liver disease that deserves broader application. However, in order for liver transplantation to gain its full therapeutic potential, the indications for and results of the procedure must be the object of comprehensive, coordinated, and ongoing evaluation in the years ahead. This can best be achieved by expansion of this technology to a limited number of centers where performance of liver transplantation can be carried out under optimal conditions.

Members of the Consensus Development Panel were:

Rudi Schmid, M.D. (Panel Chairman)
Professor of Medicine and Dean
University of California, San Francisco
School of Medicine
San Francisco Medical Center
San Francisco, California

Donald M. Berwick, M.D.
Assistant Professor of Pediatrics
Harvard Medical School
Acting Director of Research
Harvard Community Health Plan
Boston, Massachusetts

Burton Combes, M.D.
Professor of Internal Medicine
University of Texas Health Science
Center at Dallas
Dallas, Texas

Ralph B. D'Agostino, Ph.D.
Professor of Mathematics and Statistics
Boston University
Boston, Massachusetts

Stuart H. Danovitch, M.D.
Private Practice of Gastroenterology
Washington, D.C.

Harold J. Fallon, M.D.
Professor and Chairman
Department of Medicine
Medical College of Virginia
Richmond, Virginia

Olga Jonasson, M.D.
Professor of Surgery
University of Illinois
Chief of Surgery
Cook County Hospital
Chicago, Illinois

Charles E. Millard, M.D., A.B.F.P.
Family Practitioner
Medical Associates of Bristol County
Vice Chairman
Biomedical Ethics Commission
Roman Catholic Diocese of Providence
Bristol, Rhode Island

Linda Miller, M.S.
Executive Director
Volunteer Trustees of Not for Profit
Hospitals
Washington, D.C.

Frank G. Moody, M.D.
Professor and Chairman
Department of Surgery
University of Texas Medical
School at Houston
Surgeon-in-Chief
Hermann Hospital
Houston, Texas

William K. Schubert, M.D.
Professor and Chairman
Department of Pediatrics
University of Cincinnati College
of Medicine
Physician Executive Director
Children's Hospital Medical Center
Cincinnati, Ohio

Laurence Shandler, M.D.
Private Practice of Pediatrics
Santa Fe, New Mexico

Henry J. Winn, Ph.D.
Senior Associate in Surgery
Harvard Medical School
Immunologist
General Surgical Services
Massachusetts General Hospital
Boston, Massachusetts

Members of the Planning Committee were:

Steven Schenker, M.D. (Chairman)
Professor of Medicine and Pharmacology
Chief, Division of Gastroenterology and Nutrition
Department of Medicine
University of Texas Health Science Center
San Antonio, Texas

Itzhak Jacoby, Ph.D.
Deputy Director
Office of Medical Applications of Research
National Institutes of Health
Bethesda, Maryland

Sarah C. Kalser, Ph.D.
Program Director for Liver and Biliary Diseases
National Institute of Arthritis, Diabetes, and Digestive and Kidney Diseases
National Institutes of Health
Bethesda, Maryland

Curtis Meinert, Ph.D.
Professor of Epidemiology and Biostatistics
School of Hygiene and Public Health
Johns Hopkins University
Baltimore, Maryland

Harold P. Roth, M.D.
Director
Division of Digestive Diseases and Nutrition
National Institute of Arthritis, Diabetes, and Digestive and Kidney Diseases
National Institutes of Health
Bethesda, Maryland

Paul S. Russell, M.D.
John Homans Professor of Surgery
Harvard Medical School
Boston, Massachusetts

The conference was sponsored by:

National Institute of Arthritis, Diabetes, and Digestive and Kidney Diseases
Lester B. Salans, M.D.
Director

Office of Medical Applications of Research
J. Richard Crout, M.D.
Director

National Library of Medicine
National Institutes of Health
8600 Rockville Pike
Bethesda, MD 20209
(301) 496-4725

Major Emphases of Technology Assessment Activities

Technology	Concerns: Safety	Efficacy/ Effectiveness	Cost/Cost-Effect/ Cost-Benefit	Ethical/Legal/ Social
Drugs				
Medical Devices/Equipment/Supplies				
Medical/Surgical Procedures				
Support Systems		X	X	
Organizational/Administrative				

Stage of Technologies Assessed
- X Emerging/new
- X Accepted use
- X Possibly obsolete, outmoded

Application of Technologies
- X Prevention
- X Diagnosis/screening
- X Treatment
- X Rehabilitation

Assessment Methods
- X Laboratory testing
- ___ Clinical trials
- X Epidemiological and other observational methods
- X Cost analyses
- X Simulation/modeling
- X Group judgment
- X Expert opinion
- X Literature syntheses

Approximate 1985 budget for technology assessment: $300,000*

* This amount covers intramural technology assessment activities only. A significant but undocumented fraction of the $7.5 million spent extramurally in 1984, via the grants mechanism, includes functions that may be classified as technology assessment.

NATIONAL LIBRARY OF MEDICINE NATIONAL INSTITUTES OF HEALTH

Introduction

The National Library of Medicine (NLM) is the world's largest research library in a single scientific and professional field. The library collects materials exhaustively in all major areas of health sciences and to a lesser degree in such areas as chemistry, physics, botany, and zoology. The collection stands at 3.3 million items, including books, journals, technical reports, manuscripts, microfilms, and pictorial materials. The library was established in 1836 as the Library of the Army Surgeon General's Office, and it remained in the military until 1956, when it was transferred to the Public Health Service and upgraded to the National Library of Medicine.

NLM serves as a national resource for all U.S. health science libraries. Lending and other services are provided through the Regional Medical Library Network consisting of more than 2,000 basic unit libraries (mostly at hospitals), 125 resource libraries (at medical schools), 7 regional medical libraries, and the NLM as a national resource for the entire network. The library also provides a variety of educational, audiovisual, and publication services; support for medical library development; training for health information specialists; and technical consultation and research assistance.

NLM's computer-based Medical Literature Analysis and Retrieval System (MEDLARS) was established to achieve rapid bibliographic access to the library's store of biomedical information. The establishment of this system was a pioneering effort in the emerging computer technology of the early 1960s for the production of bibliographic publications and for conducting individualized searches of the literature.

The best known of the MEDLARS family of 20 databases is MEDLINE. *Index Medicus* is the monthly subject/author guide to articles in nearly 3,000 journals prepared from MEDLINE. Other MEDLARS databases are TOXLINE (Toxicology Information Online), HEALTH PLANNING AND ADMIN, CANCERLIT, and BIOETHICSLINE. More than four million references to current and historical journal articles, books, and audiovisual materials are stored in MEDLARS databases. Some MEDLARS databases are available through commercial database vendors such as DIALOG and BRS. Today, MEDLARS search services are available online to researchers at 2,500 MEDLARS centers at biomedical libraries and other institutions in the United States and are available to individuals via personal computers and dial-in lines. In addition, there are 14 overseas national or regional MEDLARS centers. The U.S. institutions performed 2.8 million searches in 1984. The design and initial implementation of MEDLARS III is being coordinated by the NLM Office of Computer and Communications Systems.

The major components of NLM are the Office of the Director, Office of Administration, Office of Computer and Communications Systems, Division of Library Operations, Division of Extramural Programs, Division of Specialized Information Services, and the Lister Hill National Center for Biomedical Communications. The Extramural Programs Division supports research at universities and not-for-profit organizations in the areas of generation, organization, and utilization of health information.

The Lister Hill National Center for Biomedical Communications is the research and development arm of NLM. The Center was established in 1968 and reorganized in 1983 to include the functions of NLM's National Medical Audiovisual Center. Through the Lister Hill Center, NLM conducts and supports research in techniques and methods for recording, storing, retrieving, and communicating health information. The Lister Hill Center has six branches: Communications Engineering, Computer Science, Information Technology, Audiovisual Program Development, Health Professions Applications, and Training and Consultation. Other Lister Hill Center resources are the new National Learning Center for Educational Technology, which provides an environment for demonstrating new technologies in computer-based education for the health sciences.

Purpose

The purpose of NLM assessment activities is to evaluate new and existing biomedical information technologies for the enhancement of information dissemination and utilization among health professionals and other users. It is intended that assessments be carried out as an integral part of the research and development process, and of efforts to improve ongoing operations of the library. The NLM Board of Regents intends that the American public receive rapid and easy access to biomedical information disseminated by NLM and other sources. To this end, NLM seeks to work cooperatively with database producers and vendors in the private sector to create linkages, reduce production costs, and to otherwise facilitate access to all relevant health information.

Subjects of Assessment

NLM assesses a major subgroup of support systems related to biomedical information including but not limited to systems for information storage, retrieval, and dissemination; teaching/learning systems; and artificial intelligence or expert systems. A number of new and emerging technologies that are being applied in other fields are also being assessed by NLM for use in biomedical information systems. Examples are laser discs, microprocessors, microcomputers, microwave and cable television, satellite communication systems, computer-assisted instruction, and speech recognition systems. Table A-8 briefly describes intramural NLM projects in related areas.

The Lister Hill Center is also investigating the potential of optical videodisc technology for document preservation, storage, and retrieval, and has under way several projects that combine videodisc technology with microcomputers to develop new health-science teaching materials.

NLM has made a number of extramural grants and contracts for assessing the management of health information. At Mount Sinai School of Medicine in New York City, reports of controlled clinical trials are analyzed to determine how valid the trial procedures are. At Case Western Reserve University in

TABLE A-8 Descriptions of Selected Research and Development Projects Coordinated by the Lister Hill Center, NLM

• The Technological Innovations in Medical Education (TIME) Project involves several Lister Hill branches and addresses the potential application of the new technologies of microprocessor, interactive laser disc, and speech recognition to the education of medical practitioners and students. The project is exploring educational capabilities by developing a series of problem-based, patient-related clinical simulations.

• The Electronic Document Storage and Retrieval (EDSR) Program is an effort to design, develop, and evaluate a laboratory facility that will serve as an engineering prototype to electronically store, retrieve, and display documents acquired by the library. The development of this experimental system involves integrating various components such as a document capture subsystem, high density storage media, document display subsystem, and system controller. The resulting engineering prototype enables both technical and operational evaluation. The prototype will be used to evaluate and correct problems encountered in capturing images, transferring images on output devices, and evaluating factors such as display image quality, system reliability, maintainability, the man-machine interface, and the utility of such a system for NLM information processing needs.

• The Automated Classification and Retrieval Program investigates, develops, and evaluates information science, computational linguistics, and artificial intelligence techniques supporting the automated classification and retrieval of biomedical literature. The program includes projects in the areas of natural language understanding, knowledge representation, and information retrieval. The goal of these projects is to explore their application to the development of automated systems for identifying relevant concepts and main ideas from printed documents.

• The Distributed Information System (DIS) Program encompasses several projects related to the effective distribution of advanced information systems technology. The Interactive Information Management System (IIMS) project is designed to produce a working model for testing and demonstrating advanced information management and retrieval techniques that can be applied to full-text databases. The Network Access Information Workstation Project is to develop a user-friendly microcomputer workstation that can facilitate access to different on-line information sources. The Information Retrieval Testbed System, which evolved from earlier work in the area of natural-language queries and statistical retrieval techniques, is intended to create a system that will enable evaluation of the performance of statistically based information retrieval systems.

• The NLM Audiovisual Program Development Branch applies current and emerging video communication technologies and audiovisual techniques to Lister Hill projects. Among its projects, videodisc slides of skin disorders are being tested in medical education settings to evaluate their utility as a teaching/learning tool and as an aid in diagnostic decision making. Experiments are under way to ascertain if optical videodisc recording provides sufficient resolution for cataloging and analyzing brain sections, and to determine whether photographic copies can be used in the videodisc production process, rather than actual brain sections.

Cleveland, the usage of medical libraries has been surveyed in a study that combines usage statistics with data on information service costs.

In the area of medical informatics, Stanford University research in computerized representation of medical knowledge has yielded a computer program that represents and assesses treatment planning for cancer patients. At Latter Day Saints Hospital in Salt Lake City, computer-based logic is being studied for diagnosis and treatment of coronary artery disease and other diseases. The vast amount of biomedical information now available and the increasing sophistication of computer and communications technology have prompted the use of artificial intelligence techniques in the development of *expert systems*, or systems that will aid clinicians in making patient-related decisions. A full cycle of national field testing to validate the automated consultative systems has yet to be completed.

NLM is committed to developing prototypes of the Integrated Academic Information Management System in the coming years. This far-reaching effort would integrate the myriad sources of health-related information within the modern academic health center. The system would pull together a variety of information sources—patient records, laboratory results, clinical decision-making systems, and the vast professional literature of biomedicine—for instant access by health professionals, faculty, and students.

The lack of a standardized language continues to be a fundamental impediment to the widespread adoption of computer-based information systems in medicine. NLM is embarking on a long-term coordinative effort to develop, implement, and evaluate a unified medical language system that integrates terminology in biomedical research, patient care, and hospital management.

The Lister Hill Center holds monthly seminars in which outside experts in areas of increasing interest to biomedical communications researchers discuss their recent efforts. Among the 1984 topics were:

- human factors design of computer dialogues
- physician's judgments about estrogen replacement therapy
- a study of clinical decision making
- feedback systems for improving clinical judgment
- information compression techniques
- artificial intelligence: problems in knowledge representation
- optical disk technology and library information
- computer simulation of the patient-physician encounter
- designing interactive computer systems

Stage of Diffusion

NLM assesses biomedical information technologies that are new and emerging, in accepted use, and possibly obsolete or outmoded.

Concerns

NLM assessment activities are concerned with effectiveness (including technical performance), cost, and cost-effectiveness.

Requests

Requests for assessment may originate with intramural R&D staff, NLM management, and officials of NIH, DHHS, and Congress. Extramural requests follow the procedures governing the grants process; these are typically investigator-initiated projects submitted by universities and not-for-profit organizations.

Selection

Priorities for selecting candidate assessment projects are influenced by the source of the request, current and anticipated information needs of the biomedical community, potential impact on the performance of NLM's statutory mission, and availability of funds.

Process

NLM assessment processes vary according to subject. Assessments may involve field testing and evaluation, simulation, experiments with prototypes, cost analyses, consensus development, and literature syntheses. For instance, the NLM Hepatitis Knowledge Base Project (active from 1977 to 1983) was a computer-based synthesis of information on viral hepatitis formulated by consensus of geographically dispersed experts who were linked to each other and to project staff via a computer conferencing network. A full-scale field test and evaluation of the prototype Hepatitis Knowledge Base addressed its technical performance, degree of user acceptance, and cost-effectiveness in light of other sources of viral hepatitis information. Information in the Toxicology Data Bank is being similarly assessed using computer conferencing technology. NLM is planning a consensus development conference for late 1986 on computer-based clinical consultation systems, to be cosponsored by the NIH Office of Medical Applications of Research. The recent NLM assessment of on-line catalog systems, as reported under Example below, involved testing of prototype systems and user surveys. The educational capabilities of the Technological Innovations in Medical Education (TIME) project are being tested using problem-based patient-related clinical simulations.

Some technologies supported by the Extramural Programs Division have been assessed in clinical settings. These include the expert systems HELP, which has been installed at the Latter Day Saints Hospital in Salt Lake City, and CADUCEUS, which is undergoing testing at the University of Pittsburgh Medical Center.

Assessors

Assessment activities are performed intramurally by in-house R&D and operations staff and extramurally within the framework of NLM's grants process. Projects involving multiple library divisions are carried out by a specially constituted Operations Research Group (ORG) located in the NLM's Office of Planning and Evaluation. ORG also serves to coordinate all planned and ongoing evaluations within NLM. Whenever feasible, evaluations are designed to allow for the participation of the community ultimately affected by the product or service in question, including health professionals, researchers, educators, practitioners, and students.

NLM has three public advisory groups that participate with staff in the assessment process. The Board of Regents of NLM advises the Office of the Director on all important matters of library policy, among which are final review of proposals for support of research in biomedical information systems and special scientific projects. The Biomedical Library Review Committee advises NLM and reviews applications and makes recommendations to the Board of Regents regarding research and other proposals submitted to NLM. The Board of Scientific Counselors reviews the library's intramural research and development programs. Ad hoc advisory or oversight committees, which may include non-NLM staff such as library professionals, computer scientists, and other researchers, are often an important adjunct to NLM-sponsored evaluations.

Turnaround

Assessments are generally carried out within a period of 6–18 months. Evaluations lasting up to 3 years may be appropriate in certain instances wherein the study design incorporates both formative and summarative features.

Reporting

Reports of NLM technical assessment activities are routinely transmitted to the source of the request. Study reports may also be filed with National Technical Information Service (NTIS), Educational Resources Information Center (ERIC), and similar document distribution centers. NLM staff are also encouraged to report study findings at professional meetings and conferences, and in the open scientific and technical literature.

Impact

Evaluation studies performed by NLM have affected R&D activities as well as the scope and availability of the library's products and services. Examples are the following.

- The field test and evaluation of the Hepatitis Knowledge Base system demonstrated the utility and cost-effectiveness of computer conferencing technology as a means for validating and updating the contents of a database by expert consensus. The technology has since been adopted as an important feature of other fact-based information systems developed and operated by NLM.
- A survey of users of NLM's Videocassette Loan Program resulted in a management decision to expand the program to videocassettes in NLM's collection, thereby partially achieving the goal of providing access to materials in this medium comparable to the access for print media.
- A study of NLM's coverage of the medical behavioral services compared the performance of MEDLARS with that of alternative health-related databases. The finding served to document the impact of the library's present coverage and indexing policies, and has led to a reconsideration of these policies and the use of the research technologies with other subject literatures.

Reassessment

Products and services for the nation's biomedical community are reassessed as part of the R&D process, and technologies involved in NLM's own internal operations are evaluated and improved periodically. Reassessment is especially important given the rapidly evolving nature of computer technology and other innovations applicable to biomedical information systems. The MEDLARS system, which governs both inhouse technical processing and the on-line availability of the derivative bibliographic databases is now undergoing its third major reassessment and updating. The controlled indexing vocabulary, MeSH, is itself continuously reassessed as is the list of journals selected for inclusion in *Index Medicus* and MEDLINE.

Funding/Budget

The FY 1984 budget for NLM was approximately $50.2 million. Although NLM's budget has increased in most years since 1972, in constant dollars its budget has dropped 22 percent since 1974. The R&D budget for FY 1984 was approximately $14.1 million, including $8.2 million for the Lister Hill National Center for Biomedical Communication. In FY 1984, NLM obligated $7.5 million for grants and made 103 new and renewal grant awards. These included grants for library resources and publications, as well as research in biomedical communications.

There are no budget line items for technology assessment as such; however, it is estimated that NLM devoted $0.3 million to intramural technology assessment activities in FY 1984. A significant but unknown amount of the $7.5 million FY 1984 extramural grant program was devoted to technology assessment. Of course, the bulk of the library's operating budget can be said to be devoted to biomedical information transfer.

Example

On the following pages is a report of an NLM intramural assessment of two prototype public-access on-line catalog systems designed to replace conventional card catalogs. This report was published in *Information Technology and Libraries* in 1984 and is reproduced here with permission.

Sources

Bernstein, L. M., E. R. Siegel, and C. M. Goldstein. 1980. The hepatitis knowledge base: A prototype information transfer system. Annals of Internal Medicine 93:169–181.

National Institutes of Health. 1983. National Institutes of Health Organization Handbook. Bethesda, Md.

National Institutes of Health. 1983. NIH Public Advisory Groups: Authority, Structure, Functions, Members. Bethesda, Md.

National Institutes of Health. 1984. NIH Data Book. Bethesda, Md.

National Library of Medicine. 1985. National Library of Medicine Programs and Services Fiscal Year 1984. Bethesda, Md.

National Library of Medicine. 1985. Fact Sheet. Bethesda, Md.

Office of Medical Applications of Research, National Institutes of Health. 1984. Technology Assessment and Technology Transfer in DHHS: A Report Submitted to the Department of Commerce in Compliance with the Stevenson-Wydler Technology Innovation Act of 1980 (P.L. 96-480). Bethesda, Md.

Siegel, E. R., Special Assistant for Operations Research, National Library of Medicine. 1985. Personal communication.

Siegel, E. R., K. Kameen, S. K. Sinn, and F. O. Weise. 1984. A comparative technical performance and user acceptance of two prototype online catalog systems. Information Technology and Libraries 3(1):35–46.

Smith, K. A., Deputy Director, National Library of Medicine. 1985. Personal communication.

A Comparative Evaluation of the Technical Performance and User Acceptance of Two Prototype Online Catalog Systems*

Elliot R. Siegel, Karen Kameen, Sally K. Sinn, and Frieda O. Weise

The National Library of Medicine (NLM) conducted a comparative evaluation of two prototype patron accessible online catalog systems within the same operational environment. The study design provided for the assessment of both systems on the basis of technical performance and user acceptance by NLM's patrons and staff. This article describes the study's research strategy and methods, some aspects of which are unique to the evaluation of online information systems. Included is a description of verification and limits testing that were used to determine and document the extent to which both systems met the technical performance requirements specified a priori for an NLM-based online catalog. User acceptance was addressed in three ways, each complementary in scope and methodology: a Sample Search Experiment designed to provide control over potentially confounding variables; a Comparison Search Experiment intended to maximize the authenticity of study conditions; and a User Survey characterizing users' catalog information needs and searching behavior. The results of technical performance testing were separately corroborated by a strong and consistent pattern of findings from the three studies of user acceptance. Overall, users of the online catalog at NLM are relatively infrequent library visitors and represent a broad cross section of professional roles and occupations. Most users of the online catalog come with subject-related information, are looking for books on a subject, and search by subject. The decision to adopt one of the two prototypes tested was largely based on that system's relatively superior performance in conducting subject-related searches that, as has also been reported recently in other studies of online public access catalogs, is the most important determinant of user satisfaction and acceptance of this new technology.

*Portions of this paper were presented at the Fourth National Online Meeting, New York, New York, April 12–14, 1983; and the Eighty-third Annual Meeting of the Medical Library Association, Houston, Texas, May 27–June 2, 1983.

BACKGROUND

Movement toward the design and development of patron accessible online information systems is receiving substantial im-

Elliot R. Siegel is special assistant for Operations Research, Office of the Director; Karen Kameen is librarian, Bibliographic Services Division; and Sally K. Sinn is assistant head, Catalog Section, Technical Services Division; all at the National Library of Medicine, Bethesda, Maryland. Frieda O. Weise was formerly assistant head, Reference Section, Reference Services Division at NLM and is now assistant director for Public Services, Health Sciences Library, University of Maryland, Baltimore.

petus from the nation's library community. An important aspect of this trend is the increasing availability of computer-based public access catalog systems, developed either as part of an integrated effort at library automation or as a separate patron service. The economic incentive is frequently significant given the increasingly prohibitive costs of maintaining, updating, and revising the conventional card catalog.

To the credit of the library community, the proliferation of "homegrown" and commercially available public access catalog systems has also seen the advent of several noteworthy attempts at conducting formalized assessments of these systems. See, for example, the Council on Library Resources' nationwide survey of user responses to public online catalogs,[1] Hildreth's detailed analysis of user interface features,[2] and Markey's study using the focus group interview technique with library patrons and staff.[3] However, as with other studies of online information systems, these frequently suffer from a methodological weakness in which the confounding influence of a "novelty effect" can make even a relatively poor system appear better than whatever it is replacing. This is especially true for single system studies, but it also applies to studies purporting to assess multiple systems, but which for a variety of political, logistical, or economic reasons are unable to examine the technical performance and/or user acceptance of more than one system within a single operational environment.

Recently, the National Library of Medicine (NLM) was fortunate to be in a position in which it was feasible to mount a comparative evaluation of two prototype patron accessible online catalog systems within the same operational environment. This study was intended to provide an objective, comparative assessment of the candidate systems, using the same physical space, library staff, computer terminals, database, and user populations. This paper describes the study's research strategy and methodology, some aspects of which are unique to the evaluation of online information systems. The major study findings that led to the adoption of one of the two prototype online catalogs are summarized.

APPROACH

Initial study plans specified that the study would be performed in-house over the course of nine months. While this placed a heavy burden on already busy library staff, we were in a position to draw upon the unique technical skills and capacities of persons from nearly all divisions of the library who were familiar with one another and their respective job functions. The learning curve for those involved was probably shorter than if the study had been delegated to an outside group.

In January 1982, the study group undertook as its first task the specification of requirements and capabilities of an NLM-based online catalog system intended for use by NLM patrons and nontechnical staff. Existing publications and NLM staff members were consulted. What resulted was a detailed list of specifications that addressed the key areas of database content, composition of records, search/access features, user cordiality, and display features. Each area was further categorized as to whether a feature or attribute was to be "required" for the prototype test version; "necessary" for a fully implemented system, but not required for the initial test version; or "optional," its need not yet having been determined for an NLM-based system. These specifications were organized as a "technical requirements" or criteria document, against which the candidate online catalog systems would be evaluated.[4]

Two experimental in-house systems were selected for test and evaluation based upon their potential for meeting the technical requirements as specified. They are CITE (*C*urrent *I*nformation *T*ransfer in *E*nglish), incorporating a user-friendly front end to the CATLINE* system operating on the library's IBM 3033 multiprocessor; and the public access catalog module of the ILS (*I*ntegrated *L*ibrary *S*ystem), which, for this study, uses the current contents of the

*Designed for staff access, CATLINE is used by the library's reference and technical staff for information retrieval and file maintenance. At the time of the study, the database contained some 225,000 current and an additional 245,000 retrospective machine-readable records for the library's collection of printed materials.

CATLINE database and operates on a dedicated Data General S230 minicomputer. CITE and ILS are going research-and-development efforts in NLM's Specialized Information Services division and the Lister Hill National Center for Biomedical Communications, respectively.[5] In March, the designers of both systems were requested further to develop and equip their prototypes to conform to the technical requirements for an NLM-based online catalog. In the case of CITE—hereafter referred to as System A—this involved continuing with the production and refinement of new software. For ILS—hereafter referred to as System B—the principal hurdle was to create a functionally acceptable database suitable for operational use by library patrons during the test period. This involved the conversion of nearly one-quarter of a million current (post-1966) CATLINE records to MARC format, and their loading and indexing on the host minicomputer. The time allotted for these activities was very short given the planned duration of the study. System A was successfully established and made ready for testing in April, and System B in June.

Concurrently with the above, another working group proceeded with the development of context-specific online HELP facilities for both systems, printed instruction materials, signs informing patrons of the impending experiment, and modification of terminals to highlight certain function keys (e.g., RETURN), and disable others (e.g., BREAK). A battery of six Hewlett-Packard 2626A CRT terminals, with internal printers, was assembled immediately adjacent to the main entrance of the public catalog area. A separate working group focused on refinement of the preliminary study design and construction of the several data collection instruments that would be used during the various phases of the study.

The study design provides for the independent and comparative assessment of System A and System B as to both technical performance and user acceptance (i.e., effectiveness from the users' standpoint). The assessment of technical performance deals primarily with the systematic determination and documentation of the extent to which the candidate systems meet the technical specifications for an NLM-based online catalog system, as defined by the study group in its "requirements" document. This approach has the virtue of making known to the systems designers, in advance, the criteria against which their systems would be evaluated; ensuring that both systems would be evaluated against the same performance criteria; and ensuring that if shortcomings were discovered, documentation would be sufficient to identify clearly the weakness or malfunction and, whenever possible, suggest a strategy for improvement. In addition, "stress" or "limits" testing would seek to elicit additional data on the outer ranges of system search capabilities, should the above methods prove insufficiently sensitive to discriminate between the two systems.

The concept of "user acceptance," while more difficult to operationally define and measure, is addressed in three ways—each complementary in scope and methodology: (1) a questionnaire User Survey characterizing the nature of users' catalog searching requirements, relevant demographic factors, and satisfaction with search outcomes on Systems A and B, judged separately and independently; (2) a partially controlled but authentic Comparison Search Experiment in which members of a smaller sample of library patrons conduct a search of their own choosing—sequentially—on both Systems A and B and briefly record comparative system preferences in several key areas relating to search outcome; and (3) a controlled field experiment, the Sample Search Experiment, utilizing a panel of NLM staff conducting equivalent—but different—searches on both systems, simulating representative uses of an online catalog. The Sample Search Experiment controls for important variables that the Comparison Search Experiment does not; namely, the searcher's professional role/occupation, type of search performed, database size, and a potentially confounding "transfer effect" stemming from the conduct of identical searches on both systems.

The research strategy underlying this approach to user acceptance seeks to produce a comprehensive data set pertaining to online catalog use at the NLM; distribute equitably and realistically the response

Table 1. User Acceptance of System A and System B: Key Variables Measured in the Three Study Methods

Study Variables	Sample Search Experiment (n = 20)	Comparison Search Experiment (n = 60)	User Survey (n = 600)
Dependent Variables			
Amount of information retrieved	x	x	x
Proportion of retrieved items judged relevant	x		
Number of known relevant items retrieved	x		
Time to complete search	x		
Ease of system use	x	x	x
Satisfaction with search results	x	x	x
Satisfaction with terminal display	x		x
Satisfaction with online instructions, prompts, HELP messages	x		x
Satisfaction with system response time	x		x
Overall satisfaction with system	x	x	x
Independent or "Predictor" Variables			
Type of search performed	x*	x	x
Professional role/occupation	x	x	x
Primary use for information			x
Frequency of library and catalog use			x
Prior experience with other computer systems			x
Age, sex, education			x

*Variable manipulated by experimenter.

burden among participating patrons and staff; and weave across the three study methods a common thread of similarly worded questions relating to a core set of dependent and independent variables (i.e., measures defining the nature and extent of user acceptance of Systems A and B, and definable user attributes or behaviors thought to be potentially related to, or predicting, user acceptance and system preference). Assigning these variables in an overlapping fashion across the three study methods would, it was hoped, yield a high degree of confidence in the strength and reliability of study findings obtained under different experimental conditions with different user populations. Table 1 lists the study's dependent variables and selected independent or predictor variables, and their respective usage in each of the three study methods. The approach taken is not unlike that advocated by Shneiderman, who makes a strong case for the use of controlled field experimentation in the study of human-computer interaction.[6]

METHODS AND PROCEDURES

Data collection activities relating to the user acceptance dimension took five months, beginning with administration of the System A User Survey of patrons and staff in late April and May; administration of the System B User Survey in early June through August; conduct of the Sample Search Experiment with staff in August; and conduct of the Comparison Search Experiment with patrons in September.* Technical performance testing was carried out by a separate data collection team during the period July through September.

Assessing User Acceptance

Sample Search Experiment

The Sample Search Experiment provided the most effective control over potentially confounding variables. In this experiment, a panel of twenty NLM professional staff, comprising librarians and nonlibrarians uninvolved in the development of either candidate system, was randomly se-

*It should be noted that hardware downtime, both planned and unplanned, was the source of several interruptions to the data collection schedule. Prudent investigators will make allowances accordingly, especially when attempting to evaluate prototype systems within an operational environment containing a heavy service obligation. On the other hand, we were fortunate to experience a minimum of disruptions due to software malfunctions.

lected, assigned to one of two experimental conditions (odd/even), and scheduled for individual search sessions. Fourteen specially selected paired search queries, simulating representative uses of an online catalog across six common search types, were presented to each respondent for execution. Each sample search pair was selected from a larger group that had undergone thorough pretesting on both candidate systems using uninstructed searchers. Those assigned to the "odd" condition performed the first half of the paired searches on System A and the second on System B ("even" condition respondents used the two systems in reverse order), thus respondents did not repeat the same search query on both systems. While the order of system use varied according to experimental condition, the order of search query pairs remained constant. Search query pairs were matched by type (i.e., personal and corporate author, conference, series, title, and subject), by level of search difficulty, and by size of the expected retrieval. Respondents were instructed to base their judgments of retrieval relevance to post-1974 records to control for the unequal size of the two systems' database. Conduct of the Sample Search Experiment took place in the NLM's public catalog area where two adjacent terminals, separately hard-wired to the System A and System B hosts, were reserved for the experiment. Following execution of each search pair on Systems A and B, which was stopwatch-timed by the experimenter, the respondent was instructed to check relevant records on the hard-copy printouts retrieved and to answer a series of structured questions dealing specifically with system preference when conducting that particular type of search. Upon completion of all fourteen searches, global attitude measures of user satisfaction and comparative system preference were obtained. Individual, open-ended interviews, probing specific user interface features liked and disliked, were also conducted by the experimenter.[7] The time burden for this in-depth system comparison was high, averaging $1^1/_4$ hours per respondent.

Comparison Search Experiment

In contrast to the more controlled but less realistic Sample Search Experiment, the Comparison Search Experiment served to maximize the authenticity of study conditions. In this experiment, sixty library patrons conducted a self-initiated search of their own choosing on both System A and System B, sequentially. The procedure was that patrons entering the public catalog area during randomly selected periods were asked to participate in the experiment; approximately 75 percent agreed to participate. Each was assigned to one of two odd/even experimental conditions; "odd" numbered respondents began their search on a terminal connected to System A and "even" numbered respondents started with System B. The experimenters, the same two-person team conducting the Sample Search Experiment, closely monitored the respondents' searches and recorded them on hard-copy printouts for subsequent analysis. The experimenters determined when it was appropriate for respondents to switch systems and repeat their searches. They also conducted brief postsearch interviews with each respondent, using a subset of the same structured questions used in the Sample Search Experiment (see table 1). Total completion time for each respondent, including a short orientation to both systems, was under thirty minutes.

User Survey

The User Survey was intended to provide a detailed characterization of the information needs and behaviors of the NLM's computer catalog users and to indicate their acceptance of each candidate system. A self-administered sixty-item survey questionnaire, requiring fifteen minutes to complete, was given to all patrons and staff who conducted a computer catalog search during the test periods in which System A, and later System B, were available for use in the public catalog area. Initial plans to counterbalance the availability of Systems A and B (an ABBA design) and, thus, to help ensure equality of the two user samples, were abandoned due to scheduling difficulties and the need to adhere to a tight study timetable. Also, the relatively limited number of visitors to the public catalog area precluded a sampling protocol—for example, every tenth person—if the quota of three hundred respondents per system was to be achieved. (A compliance rate in excess of 80 percent was a plus in this regard.) In all other respects, data collection procedures mirrored those established for the Council on Library Resources' (CLR) noncomparative study of fifteen online catalog systems.[8] Use of the CLR instrument, slightly modified to provide more precise demographic data concerning NLM's user population, permits comparisons with the findings of that study. The companion CLR nonuser questionnaire was also administered to a sample of three hundred patrons who had not used either online catalog. However, its principal value for the NLM study proved to be that of a control instrument, indicating that despite the nonrandom selection of catalog users surveyed, they did not differ appreciably from nonusers on such important demographic variables as professional role/occupation and frequency of library use.

Assessing Technical Performance

The assessment of system performance was intended to be a comprehensive and in-depth comparative examination covering all categories of system features and attributes:

- database contents (e.g., number and type of records, currency)
- composition of records (e.g., author, title, call number)
- search/access (e.g., searchable data elements, indexes, truncation)
- user cordiality (e.g., prompts, menus, HELP messages, leniency of punctuation and spacing)
- display (e.g., full and abbreviated records, paging forward and backward).

Performance testing was carried out by a two-person team highly skilled in and knowledgeable about the technical aspects of cataloging and online searching and who were uninvolved in the design and development of System A and System B. Because these testing activities were time-consuming and physically fatiguing, they were carried out over an extended period. Results were periodically reviewed to resolve discrepancies in findings and to ensure consistent interpretation of the recommended procedures.

Verification Testing

Using specially constructed verification protocols and checklists, each tester—independently of the other—systematically exercised both systems so as to verify the presence or availability of all "required" and (selected) "necessary" system features and attributes, as specified by the study group. They also documented, with detailed annotation, the strengths and weaknesses of each system with respect to the listed features and attributes. For example, in the course of obtaining information on the availability of prompts, the testers noted all junctures at which a system automatically generates prompts or HELP messages and those which must be user-generated. Verification of user cordiality also included testers' comments on the appropriateness and clarity of all HELP messages.

Limits Testing

Deliberately complex and ambiguous test queries were conducted for the purpose of "stressing" the limits of both systems in an effort to determine the systems' abilities to handle a variety of potential search problems. These included common and compound surnames, incomplete titles, and long titles beginning with generic words.

FINDINGS

The results of technical performance testing were separately corroborated by a strong and consistent pattern of findings from the three studies of user acceptance. The major evaluation findings are summarized below:[9]

- *Users of the Computer Catalog.* Users of the online catalog at NLM (survey data merged for System A and System B users) represent a broad cross section of professional roles and occupations: one-third students, one-quarter researchers, and one-tenth health care practitioners, with the remaining third distributed across several categories of "other." Most users of the online catalog are infrequent visitors to the library: 80 percent report visiting monthly or less often, and one-quarter are first-time visitors. This latter finding underscores the need for effective instructions, prompts,

Table 2. Amount of Information Retreived when Using System A and System B

Corresponding Questionnaire Items	% Respondents System A	System B	No Difference
Sample Search Experiment (n = 20)			
"Considering only current items published since 1974, in general do you think you found more of the information you were looking for using . . ."	75	5	20
Comparison Search Experiment (n = 35)*			
"Do you think you found more of the information you were looking for using . . ."	71	18	11
User Survey (n = 600)			
"In this computer search I found:			
More than/all that I was looking for . . .	50	36	N/A
Some of what I was looking for . . .	44	49	N/A
Nothing of what I was looking for . . ."	6	15	N/A

*A total of sixty patrons participated in the Comparison Search Experiment; of these, thirty-five conducted subject searches and were asked this question.

and HELP messages, inasmuch as most catalog users will be novices. Such users are also unlikely to benefit from quick search techniques (i.e., use of a command language rather than menus) that are better suited to more practiced users.

• *Characteristics of Catalog Searches.* Most online catalog users (53 percent) come with subject-related information, are looking for books on a topic (68 percent), and search by subject or topic (57 percent). This finding obtained in the User Survey and confirmed in the Comparison Search Experiment is consistent with other studies of computer catalog systems; it is inconsistent with studies of the conventional card catalog that generally report a proportionately greater incidence of known-item searching.[10] This may well represent an instance in which the availability of a technology conducive to subject searching has brought about a behavior change in the user.

• *Online Catalog versus Card Catalog and COMCAT.* The online catalog is clearly preferred to the library's card catalog and computer output microform catalog (COMCAT). System A users preferred the computer catalog to the card catalog in higher numbers, with 91 percent of the System A users surveyed rating it "better," as compared to 76 percent of the System B users.* Among patrons who have used COMCAT (50 percent of those surveyed), preference for the computer catalog is equivalent for System A and System B users, with 83 percent and 75 percent rating it as "better."

• *User Satisfaction with System A and System B.* A consistent pattern of findings indicates that more information was generally found by users of System A. As shown in table 2, 75 percent of staff users in the Sample Search Experiment and 71 percent of patrons in the Comparison Search Experiment selected the searches performed on System A as yielding more information. Similarly, 50 percent of the System A users as compared to only 36 percent of the System B respondents in the User Survey indicated that they found "more than" or "all the information" that they were looking for.

Satisfaction with search results was also higher among users of System A. Fifty-two percent of the patrons in the Comparison Search Experiment thought their search results were most satisfactory on System A, while 23 percent preferred System B and 25 percent indicated no difference. In the user survey, 62 percent of the System A users rated their search results as "very satisfactory" compared to 39 percent of the System B users; in the other extreme, only 4 percent of the System A users rated their search as "very unsatisfactory" compared to 10 percent of the System B users.

Overall satisfaction was higher among System A users. As may be seen in table 3,

*All User Survey findings in which System A and System B are reported to differ have a statistically significant chi-square value of at least $p > .001$.

Table 3. Overall Satisfaction with System A and System B

Corresponding Questionnaire Items	% Respondents System A	System B	No Preference
Sample Search Experiment (n = *20)*			
"Overall, do you have a preference for . . ."	60	15	25
Comparison Search Experiment (n = *60)*			
"The next time you need to conduct a catalog search, will you want to use . . ."	55	20	25
User Survey (n = *600)*			
"My overall or general attitude toward the computer catalog is:			
Very Favorable . . .	84	65	N/A
Somewhat Favorable . . .	13	22	N/A
Somewhat Unfavorable . . .	2	8	N/A
Very Unfavorable . . ."	1	5	N/A

60 percent of Sample Search Experiment respondents expressed a moderate to strong preference for System A; only one-quarter of the staff persons queried expressed a preference for System B. Fifty-five percent of the patrons participating in the Comparison Search Experiment indicated that they "would use System A again," whereas 20 percent selected System B and 25 percent had no preference. In the User Survey, 84 percent of those who had used System A responded that they had a "very favorable" attitude toward the computer catalog; in contrast only 65 percent of the System B users did so. Whereas 13 percent of the System B users surveyed indicated an unfavorable overall attitude, less than 3 percent of the System A users expressed this view.

What accounts for this observed preference for System A? The professional role or occupation of the user appears to be unrelated to satisfaction with System A and System B. In the Sample Search Experiment, preference for System A was equivalent for librarian and nonlibrarian staff persons. In the Comparison Search Experiment and in the User Survey, researchers, educators, practitioners, and students did not differ appreciably from one another in their preference for System A over System B. Other demographic variables thought to be potentially related to, or predicting, user acceptance, and that were not found to be related to satisfaction with one system as compared to the other, included such variables as the intended use of the information, frequency of library use, frequency of card catalog use, previous computer experience, age, gender, and education.

• *Preference for System A/System B and Search Type.* Preference for System A among patron and staff users is clearly related to the type of search performed. Table 4 shows that two out of three respondents in the Sample Search Experiment thought that they "found the largest proportion of relevant information," and four out of five reported that their "search was easier" and "most satisfactory" using System A to conduct subject searches. Significantly, only one of forty sample subject searches failed on System A; nearly half failed on System B. A sample search was termed a "failure" under one of two conditions: the searcher gave up, deciding to discontinue searching for relevant records; or the search was terminated by the experimenter, elapsed time having exceeded ten minutes. Among patrons conducting subject searches in the Comparison Search Experiment (see table 5), nearly three out of four favored System A, stating that they "found more information," that their search was "most satisfactory using [this system]," and that they "would use that system again." Postsearch interview comments made by both patrons and staff indicated that system users were aware of the presence or absence of specific system interface features that are supportive of subject searching and that they perceived them to be related to the conduct of a successful search. System A, for example, supports common treatment of controlled vocabulary and text word searching, an ability to search on multiple terms simultaneously, and provides for an automatic weighting and ranked display of closest matching

Table 4. Acceptance of System A and System B among Staff Conducting Subject Searches in the Sample Search Experiment (n = 20)

Dependent Variables and Corresponding Questionnaire Items	% Respondents System A	System B	No Difference
Proportion of Retrieved Items Judged Relevant "Considering only current items published since 1974, of the information retrieved, would you say that the largest proportion of relevant information was found using . . ."	65	10	25
Ease of System Use "In terms of user friendliness, did you find it easier to conduct this type of search [subject] using . . ."	80	10	10
Satisfaction with Search Results "In relation to what you were looking for, would you say that this type of search [subject] was most satisfactory using . . ."	80	5	15

Table 5. Acceptance of System A and System B among Patrons Conducting Subject Searches in the Comparison Search Experiment (n = 35)*

Dependent Variables and Corresponding Questionnaire Items	% Respondents System A	System B	No Difference
Amount of Information Retrieved "Do you think you found more of the information you were looking for using . . ."	71	18	11
Ease of System Use "In general, did you find it easier to use . . ."	46	11	43
Satisfaction with Search Results "In relation to what you were looking for, would you say your search was most satisfactory using . . ."	71	20	9
Overall Satisfaction with System "The next time you need to conduct a catalog search, will you want to use . . ."	66	14	20

*A total of sixty patrons participated in the Comparison Search Experiment; of these, fifteen persons limited their searching to known items only and are not included in this analysis.

items by frequency of the search terms' occurrence within the records. All are features demonstrated to be consistent with and supportive of user preferences and actual searching behavior. Comparable findings favoring System A in performing subject-related searches were also obtained in the User Survey (see table 6). In the present study, and as was reported in the CLR study,[11] the most important determinant of user satisfaction with the online catalog is effective subject searching.

In contrast to the clear preference for System A in performing subject searches, both systems were generally preferred equally well in performing known-item searches. A possible exception is the title search, due largely to the requirement that the System B user know the first word of the title sought. This restriction does not apply to System A in which a user may execute a multiword title search without regard to word order. Table 7 displays the verification testers' findings vis-à-vis system leniency with regard to inconsistencies in syntax, including "order of words." The importance of this difference, observed and documented in verification testing, was subsequently corroborated by the finding that no title search failures occurred in the Sample Search Experiment using System A, whereas thirteen of twenty such searches failed on System B.

• *System A and System B Displays.* Although substantially different in appearance, with System B emulating the conven-

Table 6. Acceptance of the Online Catalog among User Survey Respondents Using System A (n = 222) and System B (n = 182) to Conduct Subject Searches

Dependent Variables and Corresponding Questionnaire Items*	% Respondents System A	System B
Amount of Information Retrieved		
"In this computer search I found:		
More than/all that I was looking for . . .	44	27
Nothing I was looking for . . ."	5	13
Satisfaction with Search Results		
"In relation to what I was looking for, this computer search was:		
Very Satisfactory . . .	55	30
Very Unsatisfactory . . ."	4	10
Overall Satisfaction with System		
"My overall or general attitude toward the computer catalog is:		
Very Favorable . . .	84	61
Very Unfavorable . . ."	<1	6
Ease of System Use		
"A computer search by subject is difficult:		
Strongly Agree . . .	6	12
Strongly Disagree . . .	36	21

*Only "extreme" ratings are shown; total responses on these 4- and 5-point scales equal 100%.

*Table 7. Technical Performance Testing: Excerpt From Verification Testers' Report**

Feature/Attribute	Status	System A	System B	Comment
System is lenient with regard to inconsistencies in syntax				System A: Will tolerate some inconsistencies in spacing and punctuation only in subject search. It is rigorous in requiring exact input for series, names, call numbers, etc. System B: Intolerant of inconsistencies in spacing and punctuation for all searches except term (which must be single word).
Spacing	Required	No	No	
Punctuation	Required	No	No	
Order of words	Required	Yes—for subject and title searches.	No	
Completeness of name	Required	Yes	Yes—to a degree.	(See truncation) Neither system will tolerate incomplete terms imbedded in a name or series search, e.g., Natl. Lib. of Med.
Variant spelling	Required	Yes—to a degree, only under subject search. Terms not found in the index are displayed to user for response—they may be retyped in case of typo or misspelling, or omitted from the search at the user's discretion.		

*The interested reader is referred to the study's technical report (*Siegel, Online Catalog Study Final Report*) for a detailed presentation of all available study data, including the results of technical performance testing as it relates to the "required" and necessary system features and attributes specified in the Study Group.

tional card catalog image and System A utilizing a continuous "wraparound" array of record elements, both displays were found to be equally acceptable (or unacceptable) to patron and staff users. That is, just as many respondents in the Sample Search Experiment and the User Survey preferred one display format as the other.

- *Other Measures of User Acceptance.* Although System A operates on a large mainframe computer and System B on a minicomputer, users were equally satisfied with computer response time on both systems. User ratings and comments concerning the adequacy of online instructions, prompts, and "help" messages, however, suggest the need for additional work in this area, with System A's user aids being perceived as somewhat more effective. Finally, Sample Search Experiment data pertaining to "number of known relevant items retrieved" and "time to complete search" were collected but only partially analyzed, inasmuch as preliminary examination indicated their consistency with other dependent measures of user acceptance favoring System A.

CONCLUSIONS

1. From a methodological standpoint, the present study has demonstrated the feasibility of conducting an objective, comparative evaluation of two prototype online catalog systems within the same library. The research strategy and methods developed and used here should prove useful elsewhere in evaluating other patron accessible online information systems.

2. The study findings resulted in a decision to adopt CITE (System A) for in-house use by the NLM's patrons and nontechnical staff. This decision was based on the determination that CITE has no critical shortcomings and is essentially acceptable as is to the large majority of online catalog users at the NLM. ILS (System B) was also found to possess most system features and attributes required for an NLM-based online catalog. However, its performance on subject-related searches, an especially important requirement for online catalog users, was not equal to that of CITE. Specific suggestions for enhancing the user interface in this area (some of which had already been planned by the system designers) have been identified and documented.

3. While this evaluation study was designed primarily to provide an objective basis for choosing among the candidate online catalog systems, it has also yielded important insight into catalog users' information needs and searching strategies. In this instance, it has provided an empirical basis for pursuing continued development of both systems. In the larger sense, it illustrates the value of conducting formal evaluations—with actual user groups—as a logical step within the overall system development process.

ACKNOWLEDGMENTS

This study involved the participation and close collaboration of many persons throughout the NLM, in particular, system designers Tamas Doszkocs and Charles Goldstein. Their contributions are gratefully acknowledged. Special thanks is due Pauline Cochrane, Syracuse University, for her many helpful suggestions. Members of the Online Catalog Study Group were John Anderson, Clifford Bachrach, Lois Ann Colaianni, Karen Kameen, Henry Riecken, Warren Seibert, Manfred Waserman, and Elliot R. Siegel (chair).

REFERENCES

1. Douglas Ferguson and others, "The CLR Public Online Catalog Study: An Overview," *Information Technology and Libraries* 1: 84–97 (June 1982); University of California, Division of Library Automation and Library Research and Analysis Group, *Results of a National Survey of Users and Non-Users of Online Public Access Catalogs* (final report to the Council on Library Resources, Berkeley: Univ. of California, Office of the Assistant Vice President for Library Plans and Policies, Nov. 1982).
2. Charles Hildreth, *Online Public Access Catalogs: The User Interface* (Dublin, Ohio:

OCLC, Inc., 1982).

3. Karen Markey, *Online Catalog Use: Results of Surveys and Focus Group Interviews in Several Libraries* (final report to the Council on Library Resources, V.2, Dublin, Ohio: OCLC, Inc., Mar. 1983), OCLC/OPR/RR-83/3.
4. NLM Online Catalog Study Group, "Requirements and Capabilities of an NLM-Based Online Catalog System" (unpublished report, Bethesda, Md.: National Library of Medicine, Feb. 1982).
5. Tamas E. Doszkocs, "CITE NLM: Natural Language Searching in an Online Catalog," *Information Technology and Libraries* 2:364–80 (Dec. 1983); Charles M. Goldstein, Elizabeth A. Payne, and Richard S. Dick, *The Integrated Library System (ILS): System Overview* (TR 81-05) (Bethesda, Md.: Lister Hill National Center for Biomedical Communications, National Library of Medicine, July 1981), NTIS PB 81-188039.
6. Ben Shneiderman, "Fighting for the User: How to Test and Evaluate Human Performance with Information Systems," *ASIS Bulletin* 9: 27–29 (Dec. 1982).
7. Copies of all data collection instruments can be found in Elliot R. Siegel, *Online Catalog Study Final Report* (Bethesda, Md.: National Library of Medicine, Dec. 1982), ERIC/IR ED 229 051.
8. Ferguson, "The CLR Online Catalog Study," *Results of a National Survey of Users and Non-Users of Online Public Access Catalogs.*
9. The interested reader is referred to the study's technical report for a detailed presentation of all available study data: Siegel, *Online Catalog Study Final Report.*
10. Pauline Atherton Cochrane, "Guest Editorial: A Paradigm Shift in Library Science," *Information Technology and Libraries* 2:3–4 (Mar. 1983).
11. *Results of a National Survey of Users and Non-Users of Online Public Access Catalogs.* ■■

Office of Technology Assessment Health Program
Congress of the United States
Washington, DC 20510
(202) 226-2070

Major Emphases of Technology Assessment Activities

Technology	Concerns: Safety	Efficacy/ Effectiveness	Cost/Cost-Effect/ Cost-Benefit	Ethical/Legal/ Social
Drugs	X	X	X	X
Medical Devices/Equipment/Supplies	X	X	X	X
Medical/Surgical Procedures	X	X	X	X
Support Systems	X	X	X	X
Organizational/Administrative		X	X	X

Stage of Technologies Assessed
X Emerging/new
X Accepted use
X Possibly obsolete, outmoded

Application of Technologies
X Prevention
X Diagnosis/screening
X Treatment
X Rehabilitation

Assessment Methods
___ Laboratory testing
___ Clinical trials
___ Epidemiological and other observational methods
X Cost analyses
___ Simulation/modeling
___ Group judgment
X Expert opinion
X Literature syntheses

Approximate 1985 budget for technology assessment: $1,600,000

OFFICE OF TECHNOLOGY ASSESSMENT HEALTH PROGRAM

Introduction

The Office of Technology Assessment (OTA) is a nonpartisan analytical support agency which serves the U.S. Congress. OTA works directly with and for committees of Congress. It was authorized in 1972, funded in late 1973, and began full operations in 1974.

OTA has three operating divisions: The Energy, Materials, and International Security Division; the Science, Information and Natural Resources Division; and the Health and Life Sciences Division. Within the Health and Life Sciences Division are three programs: the Food and Renewable Resources Program; the Biological Applications Program; and the Health Program. This profile deals primarily with assessment activities of the Health Program.

OTA is governed by a 12-member bipartisan congressional board of six senators and six representatives. The board is advised by an Advisory Council of 10 public members eminent in science, technology, and education, appointed by the board. The Comptroller General of the United States and the director of the Congressional Research Service of the Library of Congress are also members. The OTA director is appointed by the board and serves as a nonvoting member. The director has full authority and responsibility for organizing and managing OTA's resources according to board policies. OTA is currently funded at about $15.8 million per year, with a staff ceiling of 143.

Assessments of health-related technologies have been conducted by OTA since its inception. Established in 1975, the Health Program has issued reports on a wide variety of topics such as postmarketing surveillance of drugs, medical information systems, carcinogenesis testing technologies, technology for handicapped people, vaccine policies, the computed tomography (CT) scanner, the medical devices industry, tropical diseases, diagnosis-related groups (DRGs), and blood policy. Studies on generic issues related to social impacts, efficacy and safety, and cost-effectiveness have also been conducted. Current topics of assessment include Indian health, physician payment,and techniques for measuring human mutations.

OTA has several other important health-related activities. OTA was mandated by Congress to select and appoint the 15 members of the Prospective Payment Assessment Commission (ProPAC), which advises the secretary of DHHS regarding the hospital prospective payment system used for Medicare. The appointments were first made in late 1983. OTA acts as an observer and evaluator of ProPAC, is to report annually to Congress on the functioning of the Commission, and is responsible for appointment of replacement commissioners each year. OTA is mandated to approve the study protocol and monitor the conduct of the Veterans Administration (VA) study of agent orange being carried out by the Centers for Disease Control. OTA was also mandated to judge the feasibility of and study the protocol for the VA study of the health effects of exposure of servicemen to radiation from atomic bomb testing.

Purpose

The purpose of OTA is to help Congress anticipate and plan for the consequences of technological applications, and to examine the ways, expected and unexpected, in which technology affects people's lives. OTA clarifies for Congress both the range of policy options and the potential impacts of adopting each option, but it makes no formal recommendations. OTA also provides advice to congressional committee members and staff, presents testimony at hearings, and conducts workshops with committees. Although OTA is responsible to the needs of the Congress and its products are designed for use by the Congress, they clearly have a much wider applicability.

Subjects of Assessment

OTA Health Program evaluations have encompassed a broad variety of technologies, including drugs, devices, procedures, and organizational and support technologies used in diagnosis, prevention, and treatment and rehabilitation. OTA focuses its evaluation efforts on either generic technological issues (such as evaluation) or on case studies from which further research questions or generalizable lessons can be gained.

Stage of Diffusion

OTA Health Program evaluations have addressed new, emerging, and widely accepted technologies.

Concerns

Compared to most medical technology assessment programs, the scope of OTA Health Program efforts is quite broad, reflecting the extent to which legislative policy issues are influenced by developments in technology. Assessments are primarily concerned with economic implications, cost, and cost-effectiveness of technologies, and are usually concerned with safety, effectiveness, and efficacy. Assessments also address cost-benefit, social, ethical, and legal aspects of technologies where they are relevant.

Requests

Under OTA statute, studies may be initiated by a request from a chairman of a congressional committee, the OTA Congressional Board, or the director of OTA. The congressional board approves all studies before they are undertaken. The director of

OTA does have the authority to initiate small studies (under $30,000). In addition, OTA will respond formally to requests for information from any member of Congress or any congressional committee. In practice, OTA staff are very much involved in discussions with congressional staff, and study topics emerge from a continual iterative process.

Selection

The OTA Board decides whether or not OTA will undertake a requested assessment. First, the OTA staff screens the proposed study to determine what resources and time it might require and what modifications it might need to suit OTA's resources and congressional needs. The staff then presents a formal study proposal to the board, which makes the final decision.

Process

OTA generally does not support original research, but synthesizes existing knowledge from the medical and health policy literature with the help of expert advisers. OTA multidisciplinary staff teams plan, direct, and draft all assessments. The teams rely extensively on the broad technical and professional resources of the private sector, including the universities, research organizations, industry, and public interest groups. The staff identifies and works with an expert advisory panel and consultants and contractors as appropriate, analyzes and integrates their work, and drafts the final report.

The staff develops an initial draft with advice from an expert advisory panel appointed for each main report, and then the draft is circulated for review and comment to groups and experts both in the government and in the private sector. Advisory panel assistance includes review and comment, although its consensus is not sought for report content or findings and reports are not formally approved by the panels. Case studies of specific technologies have been used often in conjunction with reports dealing with broad issues such as in studies of cost-effectiveness and cost-benefit analyses of technologies. Such case studies usually are prepared by experts under commissions from the OTA and occasionally by OTA staff.

Assessors

The OTA Health Program has 13 permanent, multidisciplinary full-time staff, and approximately 12–14 other in-house staff on temporary appointments at any time. Outside contract work is usually for special material to be included in OTA reports, such as appendixes to main reports, case studies, etc.

OTA uses the expert advisory panels as a way of ensuring that reports are objective, fair, and authoritative. The Health Program is advised regarding overall planning by a standing 15-member Health Program Advisory Committee composed of experts in a variety of fields relevant to health care technology assessment. This committee generally is not involved directly in specific studies.

The private sector is heavily involved in OTA studies as a source of expertise and perspectives while an assessment is in progress. Contractors and consultants are drawn from industry, universities, private research organizations, and public interest groups.

OTA works to ensure that the views of the public are fairly reflected in its assessments. OTA involves the public in many ways—through advisory panels, workshops, surveys, and formal and informal public meetings.

Turnaround

The bulk of OTA's work involves comprehensive, in-depth assessments that may take 18 months or more to complete. It also provides shorter responses to meet congressional needs, largely based on information in past and current assessments. OTA can structure longer-range assessments so that the results, in various stages, can be sent to Congress in the form of interim reports.

Reporting

After a completed assessment has been approved by the director of OTA, copies are sent to the Technology Assessment Board. If a majority of the board does not object, the report is forwarded to the requesting congressional committee(s), and summaries are sent to all members of Congress. The report and summary are then released to the public.

OTA's reports are all published by the U.S. Government Printing Office, and are frequently reprinted by commercial publishers. Several hundred copies are ordinarily sent to people and organizations which OTA expects have interests in particular topics. Summaries of all OTA reports are available free from OTA. Reports are released to the press with an accompanying press release. OTA studies are also available through the National Technical Information Service. Table A-14 lists titles of OTA Health Program main reports, technical memoranda, background papers, and health technology case studies.

TABLE A-14 OTA Health Program Reports

Main Reports

Drug Bioequivalence. July 1974.

Development of Medical Technology: Opportunities for Assessment. August 1976.

Cancer Testing Technology and Saccharin. October 1977.

Policy Implications of Medical Information Systems. November 1977.

Policy Implications of the Computed Tomography Scanner. August 1978.

Assessing the Efficacy and Safety of Medical Technologies. September 1978.

Selected Topics in Federal Health Statistics. June 1979.

A Review of Selected Vaccine and Immunization Policies Based on Case Studies of Pneumococcal Vaccine. September 1979.

Forecasts of Physician Supply and Requirements. April 1980.

The Implications of Cost-Effectiveness Analysis of Medical Technology. August 1980.

Assessment of Technologies for Determining Cancer Risks from the Environment. June 1981.

Cost-Effectiveness Analysis of Inactivated Influenza Vaccine. December 1981.

Technology and Handicapped People. May 1982.

Strategies for Medical Technology Assessment. September 1982.

Medical Technology Under Proposals to Increase Competition in Health Care. October 1982.

Postmarketing Surveillance of Prescription Drugs. November 1982.

Medical Technology and Costs of the Medicare Program. July 1984.

Federal Policies and the Medical Devices Industry. October 1984.

Blood Policy and Technology. February 1985.

Medical Devices and the Veterans Administration. February 1985.

Preventing Illness and Injury in the Workplace. April 1985.

Biomedical Research and Related Technology for Tropical Diseases. August 1985.

Technical Memoranda

Compensation for Vaccine-Related Injuries. November 1980.

Technology Transfer at the National Institutes of Health. March 1982.

MEDLARS and Heath Information Policy. September 1982.

Diagnosis Related Groups (DRGs) and the Medicare Program: Implications for Medical Technology. July 1983.

Quality and Relevance of Research and Related Activities at the Gorgas Memorial Laboratory. August 1983.

Scientific Validity of Polygraph Testing: A Research Review and Evaluation. November 1983.

Update of Federal Policies Regarding the Use of Pneumococcal Vaccine. May 1984.

Review of the Public Health Service's Response to AIDS. February 1985.

Background Papers

Computer Technology in Medical Education and Assessment. September 1979.

Methodological Issues and Literature Review. September 1980.

The Management of Health Care Technology in Ten Countries. October 1980.

Policy Implications of Computed Tomography (CT) Scanner: An Update. January 1981.

The Information Context of Premanufacture Notices. April 1983.

The Impact of Randomized Clinical Trials on Health Policy and Medical Practice. August 1983.

Case Study Series

Case Study No.

1. Formal Analysis, Policy Formulation, and End-Stage Renal Disease. April 1981.
2. The Feasibility of Economic Evaluation of Diagnostic Procedures: The Case of CT Scanning. April 1981.
3. Screening for Colon Cancer. April 1981.
4. Cost Effectiveness of Automated Multichannel Chemistry Analyzers. April 1981.

TABLE A-14 *Continued*

5. Periodontal Disease: Assessing the Effectiveness and Costs of the Keyes Technique. May 1981.
6. The Cost Effectiveness of Bone Marrow Transplant Therapy and Its Policy Implications. May 1981.
7. Allocating Costs and Benefits in Disease Prevention. May 1981.
8. The Cost Effectiveness of Upper Gastrointestinal Endoscopy. May 1981.
9. The Artificial Heart: Cost, Risks, and Benefits. May 1982.
10. The Costs and Effectiveness of Neonatal Intensive Care. August 1981.
11. Benefit and Cost Analysis of Medical Interventions: The Case of Cimetidine and Peptic Ulcer Disease. September 1981.
12. Assessing Selected Respiratory Therapy Modalities: Trends and Relative Costs in the Washington, D.C. Area. July 1981.
13. Cardiac Radionuclide Imaging and Cost Effectiveness. May 1982.
14. Cost Benefit/Cost Effectiveness of Medical Technologies: A Case Study of Orthopedic Joint Implants. September 1981.
15. Elective Hysterectomy: Costs, Risks, and Benefits. October 1981.
16. The Costs and Effectiveness of Nurse Practitioners. July 1981.
17. Surgery for Breast Cancer. October 1981.
18. The Efficacy and Cost Effectiveness of Psychotherapy. October 1980.
19. Assessment of Four Common X-Ray Procedures. April 1982.
20. Mandatory Passive Restraint Systems in Automobiles. September 1982.
21. Selected Telecommunications Devices for Hearing-Impaired Persons. December 1982.
22. The Effectiveness and Costs of Alcoholism Treatment. March 1983.
23. The Safety, Efficacy, and Cost Effectiveness of Therapeutic Apheresis. July 1983.
24. Variations in Hospital Length of Stay: Their Relationships to Health Outcomes. August 1983.
25. Technology and Learning Disabilities. December 1983.
26. Assistive Devices for Severe Speech Impairments. December 1983.
27. Nuclear Magnetic Resonance Imaging Technology: A Clinical Industrial, and Policy Analysis. September 1984.
28. Intensive Care Units: Clinical Outcomes, Costs, and Decisionmaking. November 1984.
29. The Boston Elbow. November 1984.
30. Market for Wheelchairs: Innovation and Federal Policy. November 1984.
31. The Contact Lens Industry: Structure, Competition, and Public Policy. December 1984.
32. The Hemodialysis Equipment and Disposables Industry. December 1984.
33. Technologies for Managing Urinary Incontinence. July 1985.
34. Cost-Effectiveness of Digital Subtraction Angiography in the Diagnosis of Cerebrovascular Disease. May 1985.

NOTE: Also available is the booklet "Abstracts of Case Studies in the Health Technology Case Study Series," updated annually.

Impact

OTA reports have generally been well-received by Congress and the various sectors of the health care industry. Because of the nature of congressional decisions, it is difficult to attribute legislative change or other congressional actions to any one factor. However, there are some specific examples, such as the following:

- Based in substantial part on data and analysis in OTA's cost-effectiveness analysis of pneumococcal vaccine, Congress amended the Social Security Act to pay for the vaccine under Medicare (the first such preventive measure covered).
- In 1983, the administration requested no money for the Gorgas Memorial Institute (a private, but federally supported, tropical disease research laboratory in Panama). The Senate Appropriations Committee asked OTA to examine whether the zeroing out was justified on the basis of quality and relevance of Gorgas's research. (The General Accounting Office [GAO] pursued a separate set of questions regarding the institute.) The OTA report indicated that Gorgas was a good value for the amount of federal support in terms of quality and relevance. Congress restored the funding for Gorgas and directed Gorgas to report back to it with its plan for addressing the shortcomings noted in the OTA and GAO reports.
- OTA analysis was one of the elements used in developing the legislation for the National Center for Health Care Technology. A

final draft of the OTA report *Assessing the Efficacy and Safety of Medical Technologies* was available during the course of the staff work and legislative deliberations.

- The OTA study on the scientific status of polygraph validity has been used as a basis for strong oversight of the administration's directives concerning increased use of the polygraph for national security.

Reassessment

Reassessments would be made upon congressional request, especially for any significant level of resources to be devoted to such study. Substantial congressional staff interest led to the 1981 updating of the 1978 CT report. Similarly, a 1979 analysis of pneumococcal vaccine was updated by congressional request in May 1984, and the earlier OTA study on nurse practitioners is being updated and expanded at the request of the Senate Appropriations Committee. Other than those instances, there has not been significant interest in reassessment.

Funding/Budget

OTA is funded by direct congressional appropriation each year and does not accept funding from other sources. Program budgets at OTA change as new projects are approved and initiated. The FY 1985 budget for the Health Program is approximately $1.6 million.

Examples

Due to their length, full OTA assessment reports are not included here. The following pages include summaries from the OTA case studies of assistive devices for severe speech impairments (1983), nuclear magnetic resonance (1984), intensive care units (1984), the Boston Elbow (1984), and the market for wheelchairs (1984).

Sources

Behney, C. J., Health Program Manager, Congressional Office of Technology Assessment. 1985. Personal communications.

Gibbons, J. H. 1984. Technology Assessment for the Congress. The Bridge. Summer:2–8.

Office of the Federal Register. 1982. The United States Government Manual 1982/83. Washington, D.C.: General Services Administration.

OTA. 1982. What OTA Is, What OTA Does, How OTA Works. Washington, D.C.

OTA. 1983. Health Technology Case Study 23: The Safety, Efficacy, and Cost Effectiveness of Therapeutic Apheresis. Washington D.C.: U.S. Government Printing Office.

OTA. 1983. Assessment Activities: Current Projects, Publications in Press, Recent Publications, Selected Publications of Interest. Washington, D.C.

OTA. 1984. List of Publications. Washington, D.C.

CASE STUDY #26

Assistive Devices for Severe Speech Impairments

Lack of speech is a serious disability. When combined with other disabilities that render a person functionally unable to write or type, it is more serious still. Whatever their age and whether or not they are of normal intelligence, people with such disabilities are very likely to be placed in institutional care. And if they are people who—because of a genetic defect, an accident during gestation or an injury at birth—have never talked, chances are they will be assumed to be profoundly mentally retarded and so will also have been deprived of that education without which no one in this society can aspire to enter the work force or to live as an independent adult.

As recently as the mid-1970's, there was little or no remedy for either the congenital or the acquired inability to speak when accompanied by severe physical disability. Affected individuals could often communicate with those in their immediate circles by resorting to eye signals, other forms of private language, or the use of primitive language boards. But the emotional and intellectual content of such interactions was limited, consigning these people to social isolation, passivity, and custodial care.

This case study is about the revolution in communication aids that has since changed the outlook for this population, its accomplishments to date, its promise for the future, and its problems. It also discusses related public policy and the barriers to fully utilizing the technology now available for the benefit of the individuals in question, their friends and families, and society as a whole.

Prepared by: Judith Randal. Published in December 1983 as Case Study #26 (50 pp., 52 refs.). Associated main report was Office of Technology Assessment, U.S. Congress, *Technology and Handicapped People* (Washington, D.C.: U.S. Government Printing Office, May 1982).
Available from: U.S. Government Printing Office, stock #052-003-00940-4, $2.50.

CASE STUDY #27

Nuclear Magnetic Resonance Imaging Technology: A Clinical, Industrial, and Policy Analysis

The case study entitled "Nuclear Magnetic Resonance Imaging Technology: A Clinical, Industrial, and Policy Analysis" provides a "snapshot" view of the scientific and clinical status of nuclear magnetic resonance (NMR) imaging, as well as an overview and analysis of the impact of various Federal and non-Federal policies and practices on the development and diffusion of NMR imagers as of August 1984. The policies examined include the Food and Drug Administration (FDA) premarket approval (PMA) process; Health Care Financing Administration (HCFA), Blue Cross/Blue Shield (BC/BS), and commercial insurance company reimbursement decisions; State certificate-of-need (CON) policies, and Federal financial support for research and development.

NMR imaging is an exciting new diagnostic imaging modality that has captured the interest of the medical and scientific communities and the general public. NMR imagers employ radiowaves and magnetic fields rather than ionizing radiation, thus eliminating the risk of X-irradiation associated with use of devices such as X-ray computed tomography (CT) scanners. NMR imagers not only produce images with excellent spatial and contrast resolution without the need for injection of potentially toxic contrast agents, but also enable physicians to visualize areas such as the posterior fossa, brain stem, and spinal cord that until now have not been well seen with other noninvasive imaging techniques. In addition, because NMR imagers are sensitive to fundamental physical and chemical characteristics of cells, the technique offers the *possibility* of detecting diseases at earlier stages than is currently possible and of permitting accurate diagnoses to be made noninvasively.

NMR imagers are diffusing very rapidly. In January 1983, 14 units were installed in the United States. By October 1983, 34 units were in place in the United States, and by August 1984, at least 145 units had been installed worldwide, of which 93 were in the United States.

NMR imagers are the first imaging devices for which FDA premarket approval has been required under the 1976 Medical Device Amendments. In the case of NMR, the PMA process appears to be playing primarily a quality assurance role. PMA does not appear to have constrained NMR technological development or the number of NMR imagers that could be installed in the United States on an experimental basis. The PMA process may prove capable of conferring an important competitive advantage upon those manufacturers who are first to receive PMA, a possibility which could affect the speed with which manufacturers pursue development of new technologies in the future.

Third-party payers are now in a position of major influence over the rate at which NMR imagers are acquired. Although some local BC/BS plans and some commercial insurers have begun to pay for NMR scans, neither HCFA nor national BC/BS have completed the assessments that will determine their payment policies and recommendations. Delays in reimbursement coverage will slow diffusion of NMR imagers. Future HCFA decisions regarding recalibration of diagnosis related groups (DRG) payment rates as part of Medicare's prospective hospital payment system will also affect hospital decisions regarding acquisition of NMR scanners in the future.

State CON policies appear to be having several effects on the diffusion of NMR imagers. They are delaying the acquisition of NMR devices by some hospitals, speeding acquisition by others, and promoting the placement of NMR imagers in outpatient diagnostic centers, which are not subject to the same CON controls as hospitals. The status of State CON policies and decisions is reviewed in the case study.

Prepared by: Earl P. Steinberg and Alan B. Cohen. Published in September 1984 as Case Study #27 (156 pp., 207 refs.). Associated main report was Office of Technology Assessment, U.S. Congress, *Federal Policies and the Medical Devices Industry* (Washington, D.C.: U.S. Government Printing Office, October 1984).

Available from: U.S. Government Printing Office, stock #052-003-00961-7, $5.50.

CASE STUDY #28

Intensive Care Units: Costs, Outcome, and Decisionmaking

This case study was prepared as part of OTA's project on "Medical Technology and Costs of the Medicare Program." This case study provides an overview of the development of intensive care units (ICU) and their rapid diffusion into medical practice. It presents information on their utilization costs and reimbursement. It also describes various measures of outcomes of intensive care and reviews the outcome literature. Finally, the intricacies of decisionmaking in the ICU are discussed, and policy implications are presented.

Almost 80 percent of short-term general hospitals have at least one intensive care unit. Overall, in 1982, 5.9 percent of total hospital beds in non-Federal, short-term community hospitals were beds in intensive and coronary care units. Over the 6 years to 1982, the number of ICU beds rose about 5 percent a year, compared to a rise in general hospital beds of only 1 percent a year.

For a number of reasons, an accurate estimate of the national cost of ICU care is difficult to make. The national average per diem charge in 1982 was $408 compared to a regular bed per diem charge of $167, a ratio of about 2.5:1. However, it is likely that the true cost ratio is closer to 3.5:1. In addition, ICU patients consume a greater proportion of ancillary services than patients on regular floors. Based on these and other considerations, it is estimated that the costs of adult intensive care—the cost to the hospital of patients while they are in the intensive care unit—represents about 14 to 17 percent of total inpatient, community hospital costs, or $13 billion to $15 billion in 1982. Inclusion of the other types of specialized, intensive care units, such as burn units and neonatal intensive care units, would bring the percentage of total inpatient hospital costs attributable to intensive care to about 20 percent.

Unfortunately, it is difficult to separate the intensity of care from the setting in which it is provided, and therefore, to know whether intensive care would be as effective if provided on the general medical floor as on the physically and administratively separate ICU. A recent consensus panel sponsored by the National Institutes of Health found that it is impossible to generalize about whether ICU care improves outcome for the varied ICU patient population. Nevertheless, for most severely ill and injured patients, care in an ICU has become the accepted and standard mode of treatment in the United States.

The representation of the elderly in ICUs seems to be the same or slightly more than in the hospital as a whole. Poor chronic health status, rather than age, appears to be a predominant factor that limits the use of ICUs in individual cases in the United States.

Recent data have emphasized the inverse relationship between the cost of care and survival. At this time, there are no accepted methods for determining ahead of time which patients will benefit from additional ICU care. From a number of studies it is clear that the sickest ICU patients, many of whom do not survive consume a highly disproportionate share of ICU costs.

Under the new Medicare prospective pricing payment system, based on diagnosis-related groups (DRGs), the sicker ICU patients will become financial "losers" to the hospital. Yet, the new incentives of the DRG payment system are being imposed on a decisionmaking environment in which the cost of ICU care has been of relatively minor concern. Indeed, the traditional decisionmaking process related to ICU patients has often led physicians to provide ongoing intensive care after the initial rationale for doing so no longer exists. The relatively recent concern about health care costs as well as the increasing desire by patients and families to forego life-sustaining treatment in some situations may alter prevailing provider attitudes regarding provision of intensive care. ICU decisionmaking will become even more difficult than it has in the past due to potential financial, moral, and ethical conflicts between patients, physicians and hospitals.

Prepared by: Robert Berenson. Published in November 1984 as Case Study #28. Associated main report was Office of Technology Asessment, U.S. Congress, *Medical Technology and Costs of the Medicare Program* (Washington, D.C.: U.S. Government Printing Office, July 1984).

Available from: U.S. Government Printing Office, contact OTA Publishing Office for price information (202/224-8996).

CASE STUDY #29

The Boston Elbow

The Boston Elbow is an artificial arm, battery-powered and myoelectrically controlled—i.e., controlled by signals from an amputee's stump muscles. It reproduces one active movement of the human arm, elbow flexion and extension. The Boston Elbow is technologically distinctive, but it is only one way to compensate for the loss of an arm. Nonprosthetic measures as well as competing prostheses are available to most amputees.

Distribution of the Boston Elbow and other compensatory options is at least in part a function of public policy, especially the design and implementation of disability benefits programs. For policy purposes, people (excluding children) with disabilities seem to fall into three groups—veterans, workers, and citizens—each with eligibility criteria set by law. The amputee-veteran has many alternatives to the Boston Elbow, including an elbow prosthesis that originated at the Veterans Administration. The amputee-worker faces three sets of circumstances:

- If injured in the workplace, he or she is eligible for workers' compensation benefits, including monetary compensation and prosthetic devices.
- Amputees are most likely to be fitted with a Boston Elbow if their employer's insurer is the Liberty Mutual Insurance Co.; Liberty Mutual financed design of the device and continues to develop and manufacture it.
- Workers with long-term disabilities who have paid into the Social Security system receive Disability Insurance benefits in the form of cash payments and Medicare program coverage.

The latter may provide a Boston Elbow, but program coverage becomes a benefit only 24 months after the onset of disability.

Disabled individuals judged to be potential workers are entitled to enter the Federal/State Vocational Rehabilitation Program and receive the services required for their rehabilitation. Potential workers are thus entitled to a Boston Elbow, but they must compete for limited Vocational Rehabilitation moneys. The amputee-citizen is unlikely to be provided with a Boston Elbow, but Federal policies do create relevant research by the National Institute of Handicapped Research, regulation by the Food and Drug Administration, and legislated restatements of disability issues, such as the Rehabilitation Act of 1973. The Boston Elbow fares differently in different programs, and although this can be difficult for the amputee, it is the result of explicit mandates, institutional histories, and ongoing allocation of public resources.

Prepared by: Sandra J. Tanenbaum. Published in November 1984 as Case Study #29. Associated main report was Office of Technology Assessment, U.S. Congress, *Federal Policies and the Medical Devices Industry* (Washington D.C.: U.S. Government Printing Office, October 1984)

Available from: U.S. Government Printing Office, contact OTA Publishing Office for price information (202/224-8996).

CASE STUDY #30

The Market for Wheelchairs: Innovations and Federal Policy

Wheelchairs, for many disabled persons, are essential medical devices for work, mobility, and recreation. The characteristics, prices, and durability of these chairs are critical both to the quality of life of their users and to the costs incurred by the users, insurers, and government agencies. This case study focuses on how Federal policies affect innovations in wheelchair characteristics.

The case study examines the wheelchair market and notes that one American in 200 (approximately 1.2 million total in 1977) is a wheelchair user. In 1982, an estimated 338,000 wheelchairs of all types were sold in the United States, for total retail sales of $126 million. The market is dominated by a few large firms, which suggests that the wheelchair market is oligopolistic.

Purchase costs of a wheelchair vary from $200 to $3,000, depending on the type of wheelchair (manual, power, sports, or power alternative), the number of accessories and custom features, the quality of the construction and materials, and the manufacturer. Maintenance and repair costs of wheelchairs are substantial. Over an average 3- to 4-year wheelchair lifetime, cumulative repair costs are sometimes more than initial purchase costs. The study compares the costs of different wheelchair models using total annualized costs.

The wheelchair market is dominated by third-party reimbursement. About half of all wheelchair purchases are at least partially funded by government and another 40 to 45 percent by private insurers. Only 5 to 10 percent are paid for totally by the user. The extensive amount of third-party reimbursement steers innovation to devices that can expect to receive such funds. Although all insurers will pay for a wheelchair that is "medically necessary," the meaning of this term and insurers' policies vary. The emphasis on price over performance in the reimbursement procedures for general manual wheelchairs has probably discouraged innovation.

The case study also discusses Federal policies relating to wheelchairs. Government research and development efforts on wheelchairs appear modest in relation to the number of users. However, the Federal Government is a major purchaser of wheelchairs through the Veterans Administration, Medicaid, and Medicare.

Wheelchairs themselves are covered under legislation concerning medical devices. The Food and Drug Administration classifies and regulates the marketing of medical devices, including wheelchairs.

Eleven wheelchair manufacturers were surveyed by telephone interview regarding their innovations in the last decade, their research and development efforts, their marketing methods, and the effect of government policies upon their operations. The results indicated that most innovations have been refinements of existing products, with an emphasis on usefulness to active users.

The case study also presents two examples of innovations in wheelchair design, the Power Rolls© IV, made by Invacare Corp., and a curb-climbing wheelchair available in parts of Europe, but not the United States. Finally, public policy issues related to the wheelchair industry are discussed.

Prepared by: Donald S. Shepard and Sarita L. Karon. Published in November 1984 as Case Study #30. Associated main report was: Office of Technology Assessment, U.S. Congress, *Federal Policies and the Medical Devices Industry* (Washington, DC: U.S. Government Printing Office, October 1984).

Available from: U.S. Government Printing Office, contact OTA Publishing Office for price information (202/224-8996).

Prospective Payment Assessment Commission

300 7th Street, S.W., Suite 301B
Washington, DC 20024
(202) 453-3986

Major Emphases of Technology Assessment Activities

Technology	Concerns: Safety	Efficacy/ Effectiveness	Cost/Cost-Effect/ Cost-Benefit	Ethical/Legal/ Social
Drugs	X	X	X	X
Medical Devices/Equipment/Supplies	X	X	X	X
Medical/Surgical Procedures	X	X	X	X
Support Systems	X	X	X	X
Organizational/Administrative		X	X	X

Stage of Technologies Assessed
X Emerging/new
X Accepted use
X Possibly obsolete, outmoded

Application of Technologies
___ Prevention
X Diagnosis/screening
X Treatment
X Rehabilitation

Assessment Methods
___ Laboratory testing
* Clinical trials
* Epidemiological and other observational methods
X Cost analyses
___ Simulation/modeling
X Group judgment
X Expert opinion
X Literature syntheses

Approximate 1985 budget for technology assessment: $3,100,000†

* ProPAC has the authority to collect original data using these methods, but has not done so thus far.

† This amount constitutes the full ProPAC budget for FY 1985, including funds for technology assessment and other ProPAC functions. It includes $2.4 million in the FY 1985 budget, plus $0.7 million carried over from the FY 1984 budget.

PROSPECTIVE PAYMENT ASSESSMENT COMMISSION

Introduction

The Prospective Payment Assessment Commission (ProPAC) was established by Congress under the Social Security Act Amendments of 1983 (P.L. 98-21), when the new Medicare prospective payment system was enacted. ProPAC was established as a permanent, independent commission of the legislative branch of government‡ to advise and assist the Congress and the secretary of the Department of Health and Human Services (DHHS) in maintaining and updating

‡ The intent of the original statutory language regarding the placement of ProPAC in the Legislative Branch of government rather than the Executive Branch has been subject to some controversy between the Congressional Office of Technology Assessment

the Medicare prospective payment system (PPS).

Under PPS, Medicare pays a predetermined, fixed amount per hospital inpatient discharge. This amount is determined in advance (i.e., prospectively) for each type of case based on the classification system in which patient diagnoses are categorized into 468 diagnosis-related groups (DRGs). (Two additional DRGs are used for administrative purposes.) If a hospital's costs are less than the payment, it may keep the profit; if costs exceed payments, the hospital must absorb the loss. PPS replaces a retrospective, cost-based payment method in which hospitals essentially were reimbursed for most costs incurred in providing hospital inpatient care to Medicare beneficiaries.

Implementation of PPS began in October 1983 with individual hospitals' accounting years, to be phased in over 3 years, during which a hospital's payments are based on a combination of its own experience, the average of hospitals in its census division, and the average of hospitals nationwide. During the first year, a hospital's payment reflected its own cost experience most strongly with some contribution of the experience of other hospitals in its region. In the next 2 years, the payments are based on a decreasing percentage of a hospital's experience with increasing contributions of regional and national averages. For hospitals' fiscal years starting on or after October 1, 1986, payments are to be based only on the national standardized amount.

The PPS payment rates will be updated each year by the Department of Health and Human Services. For the FY 1984 and 1985 DRG rates, the law stipulated that DHHS increase the rates by the "hospital market-basket," i.e., a measure of price changes for the goods and services hospitals use to produce care, plus a 1 percent "discretionary adjustment factor" that was subsequently lowered to 0.25 percent by the Deficit Reduction Act of 1984. Starting in FY 1986, DHHS is to have the discretion to modify the payment rates annually by any amount. The discretionary adjustment factor will take into account such elements as hospital productivity, changes in the hospital product, and technological advances.

DHHS is to adjust the DRG classifications and weighting factors for FY 1986 and at least every 4 years thereafter to reflect changes in treatment patterns, technology, and other factors that may change the relative use of hospital resources. The reclassification of DRGs may include the establishment of new DRGs. The weighting factor for each DRG is to reflect the relative hospital resources required for the diagnoses included in that DRG, compared to those classified in other DRGs.

Given the far-reaching effects of PPS on the health care system and Medicare beneficiaries, Congress thought that an independent body—ProPAC—was needed for assisting in updating and maintaining the new payment system. ProPAC also was designed to assist in addressing questions that were previously of lesser priority, such as what reasons are behind variation of medical practice across the country and which new technologies should be included in the system.

Purpose

The formal responsibilities of ProPAC are mandated by law.* The primary responsibilities of ProPAC are (1) recommending annually to the secretary of DHHS the appropriate percentage change in the payments made under Medicare for inpatient hospital care, and (2) consulting with and recommending to

and congressional staffers, and the Office of Management and Budget in the Executive Branch. At present, the opinion of the ProPAC and OTA general counsels that Congress intended ProPAC to be placed in the Legislative Branch prevails. Language in the Deficit Reduction Act of 1984 and letters from Senator Dole and Congressman Rostenkowski further clarify the matter. See OTA (1985) for discussion of this matter.

* ProPAC's responsibilities are set forth in Section 1886 of the Social Security Act as amended by P.L. 98-21, and by P.L. 98-369, the Deficit Reduction Act of 1984. Further responsibilities are set forth in the report of the House Appropriations Committee, House Report No. 911, 98th Congress., 2d Sess. (1984) 139,140, accompanying the appropriations legislation for ProPAC for FY 1985, P.L. 98-619.

DHHS and reporting to Congress necessary changes in the DRGs including reclassifying DRGs and changing their relative weights. ProPAC is also required to evaluate adjustments in the DRG system made by DHHS and to report its findings to Congress.

The Deficit Reduction Act of 1984 (P.L. 98-369) gave ProPAC two additional specific tasks: (1) to study cardiac pacemakers and the relative weights assigned to those DRGs in which pacemakers are used, and (2) to make a recommendation regarding the overall annual rate of increase for non-PPS hospitals.

Finally, in 1984 the House Appropriations Committee set forth ProPAC's role as evaluator of the impact of P.L. 98-21 on the American health care system. ProPAC was therefore directed to submit an annual report to Congress expressing its views on this broader matter. Other responsibilities will be pursued to the limit of available staff and resources.

ProPAC is not an appeals body and has no regulatory functions. ProPAC does not make coverage decisions.

Subjects of Assessment

A critical area of ProPAC responsibility is to evaluate and make recommendations regarding an administrative technology, i.e., prospective payment using diagnosis-related groups for inpatient hospital services. In order to advise DHHS regarding PPS payment rates and DRG classification and weighting, ProPAC may evaluate drugs, medical devices, medical and surgical procedures, support systems, and various organizational and administrative aspects of health care.

Technologies that may have important effects on hospital inpatient reimbursement will be selected for consideration by ProPAC. The technologies and diagnoses considered thus far by ProPAC (in particular by its Subcommittee on Diagnostic and Therapeutic Practices) are the following.

In-depth analyses for April 1985 report to DHHS:

- intraocular lens implants
- percutaneous transluminal coronary angioplasty
- cardiac pacemaker implantation

In-depth analyses in 1985 (no recommendation in April 1985 report):

- cyclosporine use in renal transplantation
- magnetic resonance imaging
- dual joint procedures in one hospitalization
- treatment for alcohol dependence
- cochlear implants
- extracorporeal shock wave lithotripsy
- dermatologic disorders

Considered, but no in-depth analyses planned at present (a decision for no recommendation was made):

- bone marrow transplantation
- treatment for infective endocarditis
- treatment for cystic fibrosis

Stage of Diffusion

ProPAC may examine technologies that are new, emerging, in accepted use, and those that may be obsolete.

Concerns

ProPAC is required to collect and assess information on the safety, efficacy, and cost-effectiveness of technologies in order to carry out its responsibility to identify medically appropriate patterns of health resources use. It is also to take into account the hospital market basket of goods and services that hospitals purchase, hospital productivity, length of hospitalization, technological and scientific advances, quality of care provided in hospitals, site of service delivery (e.g., outpatient versus inpatient), and regional variation in medical practice patterns and resource utilization.

ProPAC's information needs and work focus on changes—both general and specific—in the delivery of hospital services to Medicare patients. The changes occurring in medical and hospital service delivery must be identified and reflected in ProPAC's recommendations regarding the appropriate percentage change in Medicare payments and the DRG classification and weighting system. Adjustments may be needed due to new technologies that may be costly but quality enhancing, or because a technology is becoming obsolete and its cost may exceed its value.

ProPAC will consider the issue of appropriate reimbursement levels for technologies as they diffuse into wider use. (The initial costs for emerging technologies are often high, reflecting the investment in research and development. However, contrary to what might be expected under market forces, the price tags on these technologies, once established, generally have not gone down, even though the technologies become more widely applied by providers who did not make the initial investments in research and development.)

To the extent that DHHS and Congress accept ProPAC's recommendations regarding the PPS, ProPAC's decisions may have significant ethical, legal, and social implications. Because of the magnitude of the Medicare program, and because most other third-party payers—Medicaid, commercial insurers, and others—closely observe Medicare when making their own coverage decisions, Medicare policies regarding coverage for medical technologies may have sweeping effects on particular groups of people. As in the exemplary case of the federal end-stage renal disease program begun in 1972, major third-party payer coverage of new technologies may make these widely available where they had not been before. Eligibility for coverage by various third-party payers varies according to such factors as age, income, and employment status, so coverage decisions may affect groups of people along these lines. Thus, when considering the role of certain technologies in the configuration of the PPS—and the future of the system itself—ProPAC may take into account certain ethical, legal, and social consequences.

Requests

Issues for ProPAC consideration may be suggested by outside parties such as medical specialty societies, the hospital industry, the medical products industry, Congress, and staff and commission members. Notices in the *Federal Register* solicit various types of input from the public. The commission encourages consumers, hospitals, physicians, business firms, and other individuals and groups to submit information in writing concerning medical and surgical procedures, services, practices, and technologies, or other information relevant to its responsibilities.

Selection

ProPAC usually operates within a structure in which issues and information are brought by staff to the attention of appropriate ProPAC subcommittees, and then brought to the attention of the full commission. Candidate assessment topics are first screened by ProPAC staff before being addressed by the commission, as described below.

Process

The flow of work at ProPAC generally proceeds from staff to subcommittee to full commission for final approval. Methods used thus far have been literature syntheses, consultation of experts, various cost and other data analyses, and informal group judgments.

ProPAC is to use existing information and its staff for analysis to the fullest extent possible. Where information is inadequate and where the desired scope of analysis exceeds staff capabilities, ProPAC has the authority to carry out, or award grants or contracts for, original research and experimentation, including clinical research, in order to meet specific needs for making well-informed recommendations. However, the commission has neither plans nor the budget for any clinical research at this time.

To date, three subcommittees have been appointed. The Diagnostic and Therapeutic Practices Subcommittee is responsible for assessing individual technologies and making the recommendations regarding DRG classification and weights. In the conduct of its work, it will assess the safety, efficacy, and relative cost-effectiveness of technologies. Special attention will be given to revising the DRG system to reflect appropriate differences in hospital resource consumption that result from changing health care practices. This subcommittee uses a two-step process for evaluating diagnostic and therapeutic technologies and their relationship to the DRG system. The first step is a screening analysis in which ProPAC staff summarizes available information regarding a specific technology for safety, efficacy, practice patterns, affected populations, costs, quality, availability of data, and current DRG classification and weighting. The second step is an in-depth analysis by the subcommittee and staff of options that could be used to decide whether changes should be recommended in the DRGs.

The Hospital Productivity and Cost-Effectiveness Subcommittee is responsible for making the annual update factor recommendations. This subcommittee has concentrated its work in two areas: the hospital market basket of goods and services and the discretionary adjustment factor. It will determine indicators of change and measures of productivity to be considered in determining the overall rate of change for inpatient payments. It is to identify and examine changes in staffing arrangements, type and patterns of service delivery, lengths of hospitalization, and other issues related to productivity and cost of care.

The Data Development and Research Subcommittee has assumed responsibility for organizing the outside research agenda. It will identify data needs and availability of data sources relevant to the commission's responsibilities. Data sources will be evaluated according to such standards as reliability and validity of information and generalizability of results. It is also responsible for developing an analytic plan for areas in which data are needed but unavailable. The subcommittee has developed a candidate list of extramural research topics. The subcommittee will seek to ensure that research projects are timely enough to assist the commission on DRG recalibrating and reweighting, on the overall system update factor, and on its report on the effects of PPS on the health care system.

Assessors

The commission has 15 members appointed to staggered 3-year terms by the Director of the Congressional Office of Technology Assessment (OTA). ProPAC commissioners were first appointed in November 1983. The membership is to have expertise and experience in the provision and financing of health care, including physicians and nurses, employers, third-party payers, researchers in health services and health economics, and research and development of health care technologies. Nominations are accepted from national organizations of physicians and other health care providers, hospitals, health care product manufacturers, business, health benefits programs, labor, the elderly, and other sources.

By statute, the commission is to be assisted in its work by a staff of not more than 25, which is the current size of the ProPAC staff. The staff has two physicians (including the director) and members with backgrounds in nursing, statistics, hospital financial management, health services research, public health, economics, public policy, law, biomedical engineering, and medical records. Staff members have held previous positions with the Health Care Financing Administration, Food and Drug Administration, National Center for Health Care Technology, National Center for Health Services Research, Office of the DHHS Secretary, Office of the Assistant Secretary for Health, the Veterans Administration, various congressional offices and other federal agencies, institutional provider organizations, the medical product industry, and private third-party payers.

Turnaround

The turnaround time for ProPAC reports may vary from several months to more than a year. The commission's reports of recommendations for adjusting PPS are due annually, in accordance with the statute. The cardiac pacemaker report was delivered on time on March 1, 1985, as specified in the Deficit Reduction Act passed less than 8 months earlier.

The period between statutorily mandated DRG recalibrations has raised an important consideration for ProPAC regarding the diffusion of new technologies. By law, recalibrations are to occur at least every 4 years, and they may be more frequent. *DRG lag* refers to the period of time between the availability of a new technology in the marketplace and the reflection in DRG payment rates of its effect on the cost of delivering health care. DRG recalibrations are necessarily based on historical data. If DRG payment rates are recalibrated no more frequently than every 4 years, hospitals may face having to wait several years before the acquisition of new technology may be rewarded by a concomitant increase in the appropriate DRG payment rate. The prospect of such lags may affect the diffusion of new, cost-raising technologies (see, e.g., Anderson and Steinberg, 1984). ProPAC will consider a number of strategies for addressing DRG lag. These might include a fund that would allow the technology a temporary payment for a period of time, or a transitional DRG that evaporates within a specified period of time.

Reporting

The first full report of ProPAC, with recommendations to the secretary of DHHS regarding the percentage change in the payments made under Medicare for inpatient hospital care and changes in the DRGs, was submitted April 1, 1985. It included a recommendation regarding the overall annual rate of increase for non-PPS hospitals. The cardiac pacemaker study was submitted on March 1, 1985. By late 1985, ProPAC will evaluate and report to Congress regarding the adjustments actually made by DHHS in the PPS. A third major report on the impact of PPS on the American health care system, requested by the House Committee on Appropriations, is scheduled to be completed by February 1986 and every year thereafter. These reports are to be made available to the public.

ProPAC maintains a mailing list in order to keep the interested public informed of its meeting and other activities. Meetings of the commission are held every 2 to 3 months and are open to the public.

Impact

The director of OTA reports at least annually to Congress on the activities of ProPAC. The first such report was made available in March 1985. In it, OTA concluded that in its first year of operation, ProPAC's overall performance was of a high order, and in some respects exceptionally high. OTA found that ProPAC's resources are adequate and necessary for its current functions. The report noted several areas for future consideration, including the intended breadth of ProPAC's responsibility and the emphasis to be placed on assessing specific drugs, medical devices, and medical and surgical procedures. See OTA (1985) for full findings.

A discussion of the substance and content of the April 1985 ProPAC report and the responses stemming from it is to be addressed in an OTA report to be delivered to Congress in late 1985. That report also is to cover ProPAC's comments on the DHHS secretary's FY 1986 PPS regulations. ProPAC is subject to periodic audit by the General Accounting Office.

Much has been speculated regarding the impact of the Medicare prospective payment system. Its major effect will be to shift a variety of hospital incentives. Implementation of PPS will certainly affect overall health expenditures, perhaps in the tens of billions of dollars, and will probably mean significant shifting of health care resources via changing case-mix and utilization of technologies. The extent to which ProPAC, an advisory but not a policy-setting group, affects the system remains to be seen.

The impact of ProPAC will depend on the extent to which the secretary of DHHS and Congress accept the commission's recommendations and use in policymaking the data and information generated by the commission. Recent actions of Congress and the administration—to alter the 1983 Social Security Act's provisions for hospital market basket increases and the lowering of the discretionary adjustment factor from 1 to 0.25 percent—suggest that the net effect of ProPAC recommendations regarding DRG adjustments will be subject to congressional and administration moves. ProPAC's evaluation of the prospective payment system may be considered carefully by Congress, or it may be superfluous to other congressional action on the program.

As noted earlier, DRG lag may affect diffusion of expensive technologies, and Pro-

PAC decisions regarding the assimilation of technologies into DRGs may affect their diffusion and pricing. Such developments would likely depend on many factors, including the time between DRG reclassifications.

Reassessment

ProPAC would reassess a technology based on new developments regarding its relative importance in hospital inpatient reimbursement.

Funding/Budget

ProPAC is funded through congressional appropriations. A total of 85 percent of the commission's appropriations comes from the Federal Hospital Insurance Trust Fund, and 15 percent comes from the Federal Supplementary Medical Insurance Trust Fund. Congress appropriated $1.5 million for ProPAC in FY 1984, but less than one-third of that amount was spent because the commission was in operation for less than the full year. Thus, about $1.05 million was carried over and added to a FY 1985 $2.4 million appropriation, for an estimated FY 1985 budget of $3.1 million, plus a FY 1986 carry-over of $0.35 million. A budget of approximately $3.2 million was requested for FY 1986.

Example

The following pages include the executive summary only of the ProPAC Report and Recommendations to the Secretary, U.S. Department of Health and Human Services, April 1, 1985. The full report and accompanying technical appendixes are available from ProPAC and the U.S. Government Printing Office.

Sources

Anderson, G., and E. Steinberg. 1984. To buy or not to buy: Technology acquisition under prospective payment. New England Journal of Medicine 311:182–185.

Congressional Record. 1983. Social Security Act Amendments of 1983: Title VI—Prospective Payments for Medicare Inpatient Hospital Services. H.R. 1900:H1749–H1756.

Hospitals. 1984. 'An honest broker' for fine-tuning Medicare. 58(19):102–105.

Moore, J., Prospective Payment Assessment Commission. 1985. Personal communications.

Omenn, G. S., and D. A. Conrad. 1984. Implications of DRGs for clinicians. New England Journal of Medicine 311:1314–1317.

Office of Technology Assessment. 1985. First Report on the Prospective Payment Assessment Commission (ProPAC). Washington, D.C.

Prospective Payment Assessment Commission. Undated. Fact Sheet. Washington, D.C.

Prospective Payment Assessment Commission. 1985. Report and Recommendations to the Secretary, U.S. Department of Health and Human Services, April 1, 1985. Washington, D.C.: U.S. Government Printing Office.

Prospective Payment Assessment Commission. 1985. Technical Appendixes to the Report and Recommendations to the Secretary, U.S. Department of Health and Human Services, April 1, 1985. Washington, D.C.: U.S. Government Printing Office.

Prospective Payment Assessment Commission. 1985. A Report on the Appropriateness of Medicare Hospital Payments for Pacemaker Implantation. Presented to the Committee on Finance, U.S. Senate, and the Committee on Ways and Means, U.S. House of Representatives. March 1.

Washington Report on Medicine & Health. March 28, 1983. Congress Begins Prospective Payment Experiment. Washington, D.C.

Washington Report on Medicine & Health. January 7, 1985. DRGs and Quality of Care. Washington, D.C.

Young, D. A. 1984. Prospective Payment Assessment Commission: Mandate, structure, and relationships. Nursing Economics 2:309–311.

Young, D. A. 1984. Testimony before the Senate Committee on Labor & Human Services. June 6.

PROSPECTIVE PAYMENT
ASSESSMENT COMMISSION

REPORT AND RECOMMENDATIONS TO THE SECRETARY, U.S. DEPARTMENT OF HEALTH AND HUMAN SERVICES

APRIL 1, 1985

—ProPAC—

Executive Summary

In 1983 Congress enacted the most far reaching changes in the Medicare program since its establishment in 1965. Left behind was a cost reimbursement system that by general agreement had produced unacceptable hospital cost inflation. Congress mandated that the inpatient hospital care rendered Medicare beneficiaries would henceforth be paid on the basis of a prospective payment per case, using diagnosis-related groups (DRGs) to classify and label the hospital product being purchased.

This report is the product of the congressionally-established Prospective Payment Assessment Commission, fifteen individuals knowledgeable about the health industry who were vested with the responsibility of analyzing the new prospective payment system (PPS) and advising the Secretary of the Department of Health and Human Services and the Congress on ways of improving it. The recommendations emanate from a profound concern that the fundamental changes introduced October 1, 1983 be implemented in as fair, cost-effective, and quality-enhancing a manner as possible.

The Commission, which began meeting in December 1983, has focused its attention on two major questions:

1. By what percentage should Medicare's payments for hospital discharges in fiscal year 1986 increase or decrease (the "Update Factor")?
2. What changes, if any, should be made concerning payments to hospitals for specific treatments or procedures by the Medicare program (adjustments of DRG classifications and weights)?

The body of this report and accompanying technical appendixes explain the Commission's actions and decisions in substantial and technical detail. For purposes of this summary, six major points should be emphasized:

- The Commission's unanimous recommendations reflect five major priorities: maintaining access to high-quality health care; encouraging hospital productivity and long-term cost-effectiveness; facilitating innovation and appropriate technological change; maintaining stability for providers, consumers, and other payers; and basing decisions upon reliable and timely data and information.

- The Commission recommends that next year's Medicare hospital payments incorporate inflation in hospital input prices and higher costs due to treating sicker patients, minus one percentage point. This recommendation would result in payment increases significantly less than those of recent years. The inflation minus one percentage point represents the Commission's best judgment as to the net change in payments needed to provide scientific and technological advances in the hospital industry, balanced by changes in hospital productivity and in the hospital product. In particular, the Commission's calculations reflect a judgment and belief that appropriate, sustained, and necessary technological growth in the health care industry can be achieved in part by savings generated through improvements in hospital productivity.

- The Commission recommends action on two problems arising from PPS implementation. Specifically, the Commission urges the Secretary of the Department of Health and Human Services to move quickly to improve the current definition of hospital labor market areas, in order to better adjust PPS rates for area wage differences. The Commission also urges the Secretary to institute adjustments for hospitals that incur higher Medicare costs per case associated with treating a greater proportion of low income patients ("disproportionate share hospitals").

- For fiscal year 1986, the Commission recommends adjusting all of the DRG weights using newer, more complete, and more accurate data. Such adjustment or "recalibration" is intended to enable PPS to reflect changes in hospital practice during recent years. As part of the recalibration process, the weights should also be adjusted to avoid building changes in coding practice into future PPS payments. The Commission's recommendations incorporate its review of a number of specific medical practices and technologies. Additional data collection and analysis regarding other such practices and technologies are required in order to reach well-informed conclusions.

- While making no recommendation at this time on the pace of transition to national payment rates, the Commission is aware of concerns that have arisen regarding the impact of that transition on different hospitals and regions. The transition issue involves weighing the desirability of continued implementation of a system already clearly yielding positive results, against the possible harms of delaying that transition to correct PPS inequities and shortcomings. The Commission will continue to analyze this important issue.
- The Commission offers its analysis and recommendations in an environment of debate concerning future directions in health care delivery and financing. The recommendations themselves are predicated on continued implementation of the current PPS system. They seek to address as sensibly as possible the tension among several compelling and competing considerations: Federal budgetary constraints; maintenance of Medicare beneficiaries' access to high-quality care; and changes in the hospital industry. Should any health policy proposals affecting PPS be adopted, the Commission will respond with appropriate analytical work.

The report that follows is by design and necessity a technical document. The Commission issuing it, however, remains mindful of the fact that the report's analysis, discussion, and recommendations will directly affect millions of Medicare beneficiaries—individuals for whom the pluses and minuses of the "Update Factor" will translate into a significant impact on the kind of life-giving treatment they receive.

OVERVIEW OF THE COMMISSION'S RECOMMENDATIONS

The Commission's 21 recommendations fall into two major categories: recommendations regarding the update factor and recommendations regarding adjustments of DRG classifications and weights.

The first 16 recommendations address the update factor. In recommendation 1, the Commission proposes updating the standardized amount by the projected increase in the hospital market basket, minus one percentage point, plus an allowance for the estimated increase in real case-mix complexity during fiscal year 1985. Several of the first 16 recommendations involve specific market basket issues, including the desirable number of such market baskets, wage components, and correction of forecast errors.

Recommendations 13 through 15 address distributional concerns. The Commission selected the definition of hospital labor market areas and disproportionate share hospitals as two problem areas of PPS deserving immediate attention in the establishment of the fiscal year 1986 payment rates. This does not imply that other problem areas are not also of great importance, but the Commission believes that the distributional consequences of these two problems are sufficiently severe, and the potential for finding workable solutions is sufficiently high, that immediate attention is warranted.

Recommendation 17 recommends recalibration of the DRG weights with a data base that is newer, more complete, and more accurate than the 1981 data used to create the current DRG weights. The Commission's recommendation reflects its belief that, because of potential inaccuracies in the data originally used to establish the DRG weights and changes in hospital practice patterns since 1981, a full recalibration for the 1986 rates is advisable.

Recommendations 18 through 20 pertain to specific DRG weight, classification, and assignment issues concerning three procedures: pacemaker implantation; cataract extraction and intraocular lens implantation; and percutaneous transluminal coronary angioplasty. Recommendation 21 concludes that two additional procedures, bone marrow transplantation and treatment of infective endocarditis, do not require in-depth analysis at this time.

The Commission will make future recommendations concerning these and many other DRG weight, classification, and assignment issues, as new information becomes available.

THE COMMISSION'S FUTURE AGENDA

While much has been accomplished during the Commission's first year, many important PPS-related issues require further evaluation. The Commission looks forward to analyzing a variety of complex matters including:

- The measurement of case mix used for PPS and evaluation of alternative case-mix systems.
- Improvement in the methods used to account for resources consumed during specific types of hospital stays. Special emphasis will be placed on analyzing the allocation of nursing costs to DRGs.
- PPS payment policies, with emphasis on adjustments for differing costs of hospitals serving large numbers of low income patients, definitions of hospital market areas, and effects of the transition to national payment rates.
- System responsiveness to changes in practice patterns, focusing on payment mechanisms for new or changing technologies. In addition, a number of specific diagnostic and therapeutic practices are currently being examined:

  —Cyclosporine used in renal transplantation
  —Magnetic resonance imaging
  —Dual joint procedures in one hospitalization
  —Treatment for alcohol dependence
  —Cochlear implants
  —Extracorporeal shock wave lithotripsy
  —Dermatologic disorders

- The effects of PPS on health care delivery, such as changes in quality of care and health outcomes, changes in types of patients treated in hospitals, changes in the hospital product, and regional practice pattern variations.

STRUCTURE OF THE REPORT AND APPENDIXES

The Commission's report consists of two volumes. In this volume, the Commission's first chapter presents background information concerning establishment of the prospective payment system. Chapter 2 identifies the major priorities and approaches underlying the Commission's recommendations. The recommendations themselves, along with explanatory material, appear in Chapter 3. The fourth and final chapter of the first volume explores areas and issues requiring substantial Commission attention in the year and years to come.

In developing its recommendations the Commission considered staff analyses and the views of numerous technical experts. The purpose of volume 2—the Technical Appendixes—is to present much of this background material to afford greater insight into the Commission's decisions.

The appendixes consist of both descriptive and analytical pieces covering the origins of the prospective payment system, the determination of prospective payments, the update factor, and DRG recalibration. They underscore many of the dilemmas and issues confronting the Commission during its deliberations.

LIST OF RECOMMENDATIONS

The Update Factor

Recommendation 1: Amount of the Update Factor

For fiscal year 1986, the standardized amounts should be updated by the projected increase in the hospital market basket, minus one percentage point, plus an allowance for the estimated increase in real case-mix complexity during fiscal year 1985. The negative one percentage point is a combined adjustment of a positive allowance for scientific and technological advancement and a negative allowance for productivity improvement and hospital product change.

This recommendation reflects the Commission's collective judgment of the appropriate increase in the level of payment per Medicare discharge under PPS, assuming that the Commission's other concerns regarding the market basket component of the update factor, the DRG weighting factors, and the distribution of payments across PPS hospitals are also addressed in the fiscal year 1986 payment rates. Further, this recommendation is based on the premise that no net reductions or increases in average per case payments to hospitals will be effected through measures other than the update factor, such as reducing the indirect teaching adjustment, incorporating capital payment under PPS at a budget-saving level, adjusting for coding changes occurring before fiscal year 1985, or any other changes in total payments per discharge under PPS.

The Hospital Market Basket

Recommendation 2: The Number of Market Baskets

For fiscal year 1986, a single market basket should be continued for those hospitals under PPS. The Commission will undertake a study to determine the appropriateness of developing market basket measures that reflect variation in economic factors across hospitals. The use of multiple market baskets by region and classes of hospitals within regions will be examined. If the analysis indicates that multiple market baskets are appropriate, the study will also include an assessment of the data required for implementation.

Recommendation 3: Market Basket for Psychiatric, Rehabilitation, and Long-Term Care Hospitals

Separate market basket weights should be used for the group of psychiatric, rehabilitation, and long-term care hospitals and related distinct-part units that are exempt from PPS, but subject to the TEFRA rate of increase limitation. Separate market basket weights need not be developed for children's hospitals.

Recommendation 4: Market Basket Wage Component—Occupational Groups

The wage component of the market basket should be split into three categories, each with separate weights: Managers and Administrators, Professionals and Technicians, and Other Hospital Workers. Changes in wages for these categories should be measured as follows:

- Managers and Administrators: the Employment Cost Index (ECI) for Managers and Administrators.
- Professionals and Technicians: a 50-50 blend of the Average Hourly Earnings (AHE) for the hospital industry and the ECI for Professionals and Technicians.
- Other Hospital Workers: a 50-50 blend of the AHE for the hospital industry and the ECI for all private industry.

Recommendation 5: Employment Cost Index Feasibility Study

For the long run, the Secretary should work with the Bureau of Labor Statistics to study the advantages and feasibility of developing an Employment Cost Index for the hospital industry that includes both public and private hospitals and covers increases in both wages and fringe benefits.

Recommendation 6: Study Effects of Changes in the Minimum Wage Law on Hospital Workers

The Commission plans to study the extent to which hospital workers would be affected by changes in the Federal minimum wage law. The intent of the study is to detect whether, under PPS, workers who earn more than the minimum wage are differentially affected by statutory increases in the minimum wage compared with workers in other industries. If a differential effect is found to exist, the Commission will consider requesting the Secretary to take appropriate action.

Recommendation 7: Correction of Market Basket Forecast Errors

The update factor should include a correction for substantial errors made in the previous year's forecast of changes in the external price measures used in the hospital market basket. In the judgment of the Commission, substantial errors are those that equal or exceed 0.25 percentage points (or, when rounded in the published forecasts, 0.3 percentage points). The Commission will undertake a study to determine the extent to which differences between forecasted and actual increases in the internal price change measures are due to factors beyond the hospitals' control. Substantial errors determined after study to be due to factors beyond the hospitals' control should be corrected in the update factor.

Recommendation 8: Statutory Change for Forecast Error Correction

The Secretary has determined that she does not have the statutory authority to correct for market basket forecast errors. Therefore, the Secretary should seek statutory change to provide explicitly that the update factor include a correction for errors in forecasting the market basket beginning in fiscal year 1986.

Recommendation 9: Rebasing of Market Basket Weights

Market basket weights should be rebased at least every five years. Rebasing should be performed more frequently if significant changes in the weights occur. In addition, the market basket weights will need to be rebased if payment for capital or direct medical education is included in the PPS rates.

Discretionary Adjustment Factor

Recommendation 10: Allowance for Productivity and Scientific and Technological Advancement Goals

For the fiscal year 1986 payment rates, the allowance in the discretionary adjustment factor for scientific and technological advancement, productivity improvement, and hospital product change should be set at minus one percentage point.

Recommendation 11: Adjustment for Case-Mix Change

Prospective payments to individual hospitals and in the aggregate should reflect real changes in case mix. Changes in reported case mix that are unrelated to actual differences in the types of patients treated should not be built into future PPS payments.

Recommendation 12: Update Factor for Exempt Hospitals

In addition to the projected increase in the market basket, hospitals and hospital distinct-part units exempt from PPS should receive a minus one percentage point adjustment in their fiscal year 1986 update factor for productivity improvement and scientific and technological advancement.

Hospital Labor Market Areas—Area Wage Index

Recommendation 13: Improvement of Labor Market Area Definitions

In order to better reflect hospital labor markets, the Secretary should improve, as soon as possible, the current definition of a hospital labor market area used to adjust PPS rates for area wage differences, taking into account variations in wages paid in the inner city compared with suburban areas within a metropolitan area, and variations paid in different rural locations within a state. Implementation of this recommendation should not result in any change in aggregate payments.

Disproportionate Share Hospitals

Recommendation 14: Disproportionate Share Adjustment for Fiscal Year 1986

The Secretary should develop a methodology for adjusting PPS rates for disproportionate share hospitals and implement the adjustment in fiscal year 1986. The adjustment should be implemented so that it does not change aggregate payments.

Recommendation 15: Definition of Disproportionate Share Hospitals

The Secretary should complete the development of a definition of disproportionate share hospitals in ample time to include adjustments for these hospitals in the fiscal year 1986 PPS payment rates. The Secretary should consider broader definitions of low income than simply the percentage of patients who are Medicaid recipients and should determine whether the share of Medicare Part A patients should be excluded from the definition.

Rebasing the Standardized Amounts

Recommendation 16: Rebasing the Standardized Amounts

The standardized amounts used to determine hospital payments under PPS should be recalculated using cost data that reflect hospital behavior under PPS. The results of such a recalculation, with appropriate modifications, could be used to rebase the standardized amounts. Although recent cost data are not available to recalculate the standardized amounts for the fiscal year 1986 payment rates, the Secretary should implement a process for timely collection of the cost data necessary for future recalculation. The Commission will later consider more specific recommendations regarding the timing, data sources, and process for rebasing the standardized amounts.

DRG Classifications and Relative Weighting Factors

Recommendation 17: Recalibrating the DRG Weights

For fiscal year 1986, all DRG weights should be recalibrated using the 1984 PATBILL data set. The newly recalibrated weights should be:

(1) Normalized so that the average case weight is the same as it was at the beginning of fiscal year 1985, thereby incorporating DRG weight adjustments made before the start of fiscal year 1985

(2) Adjusted for any demonstrable changes in reported case mix occurring during fiscal year 1985

Recommendation 18: Cardiac Pacemaker Implantation

The DRGs involving cardiac pacemakers, DRGs 115, 116, 117, and 118, should be recalibrated in the same manner as other DRGs to reflect changes in practice since 1981. The Commission will continue to analyze diagnosis and procedure coding and DRG classification related to pacemaker implantation and replacement; the distribution of costs and payments across discharges, hospitals, and DRGs; and the impact of PPS on the quality of patient care.

Recommendation 19: Cataract Extraction and Intraocular Lens Implantation

DRG 39, Lens Procedures, should be recalibrated in the same manner as other DRGs to reflect changes in practice since 1981, including the more frequent implantation of an intraocular lens following cataract removal. The Commission will continue to monitor resource use in this DRG to determine whether the types of patients treated as hospital inpatients change with increased outpatient surgery for cataract removal.

Recommendation 20: Percutaneous Transluminal Coronary Angioplasty

Cases in which Percutaneous Transluminal Coronary Angioplasty (PTCA) is the principal procedure should be removed from DRG 108 and temporarily assigned to DRG 112 before recalibration. The Secretary should immediately implement a mechanism to identify bills for cases in which PTCA is performed in order to provide data for analysis and additional adjustments as appropriate.

Recommendation 21: No Change Recommended for Bone Marrow Transplantation and Infective Endocarditis

The Commission has examined Bone Marrow Transplantation and Treatment for Infective Endocarditis and is recommending no changes in DRG classification or weights at this time, other than those that would occur with recalibration. Information will continue to be gathered and the subjects reconsidered at an appropriate time.

Cost-Benefit Studies Program

Smith Kline & French Laboratories
1900 Market Street
P.O. Box 7929, Suite #410
Philadelphia, PA 19101
(215) 751-4000

Major Emphases of Technology Assessment Activities

	Concerns			
Technology	Safety	Efficacy/ Effectiveness	Cost/Cost-Effect/ Cost-Benefit	Ethical/Legal/ Social
Drugs			X	
Medical Devices/Equipment/Supplies				
Medical/Surgical Procedures				
Support Systems				
Organizational/Administrative				

Stage of Technologies Assessed
X Emerging/new
X Accepted use
___ Possibly obsolete, outmoded

Application of Technologies
___ Prevention
___ Diagnosis/screening
X Treatment
___ Rehabilitation

Assessment Methods
___ Laboratory testing
X* Clinical trials
X* Epidemiological and other observational methods
X Cost analyses
___ Simulation/modeling
___ Group judgment
___ Expert opinion
___ Literature syntheses

Approximate 1985 budget for technology assessment: $550,000†

* SK&F-CBS may "piggyback" cost studies on clinical trials and epidemiological studies conducted by SK&F for establishing safety and efficacy of drugs.

† This amount is the estimated budget of the SK&F-CBS Program only. The SmithKline Beckman Corporation spent nearly $300 million on research and development in 1984, or over 9 percent of total sales.

SMITH KLINE & FRENCH COST-BENEFIT STUDIES

Introduction

In order to place the Smith Kline & French Cost-Benefit Studies (SK&F-CBS) program in proper context of the company's drug assessment activities, this introduction begins with an overview of Smith Kline & French Laboratories.

Smith Kline & French Laboratories (SK&F) is the pharmaceutical division of SmithKline Beckman Corporation. Its main business is the research, development, and marketing of prescription pharmaceutical products. SmithKline Beckman's total assets as of December 31, 1984, were $3.2 billion. Its major product areas are ethical pharmaceuticals (52 percent contribution to 1984 revenues), instruments and chemistries (20 percent), clinical laboratory (8 percent), eye and skin care (8 percent), consumer health care (5 percent), and animal health care (7 percent).

SK&F markets its products worldwide. A major share of SK&F sales, particularly of SK&F's leading product, the antiulcer drug Tagamet (active ingredient, cimetidine), comes from overseas markets.

SK&F markets 24 brand-name prescription pharmaceutical products in the United States. Worldwide sales in 1984 were approximately $1.5 billion. Tagamet is the world's largest-selling drug, with worldwide sales in 1984 of approximately $900 million and U.S. sales of about $450 million. Tagamet accounted for 30 percent of all sales for the SmithKline Beckman Corporation, and 60 percent of its prescription pharmaceutical sales (SmithKline Beckman, 1984). SK&F's second leading product is the diuretic Dyazide (active ingredients, hydrochlorothiazide and triamterene) introduced in 1965. Dyazide is the major product of SK&F's cardiovascular products group, which had $304 million in 1984 sales. In the 1984 U.S. retail sales market, Tagamet ranked first and Dyazide third among all prescription drugs.

SK&F's third major product area is antibiotics, with three cephalosporin products. Other major products are the tranquilizer Thorazine (active ingredient chlorpromazine) developed in the mid-1950s, and cough-cold products. As of the end of 1984, SK&F was awaiting approval from the Food and Drug Administration (FDA) to market an oral gold antiarthritic compound, Ridaura (active ingredient, auranofin).

SK&F's assessment activities involve the full range of research and development and testing required for prescription drugs. This includes synthesis of new chemical entities, testing in animals, and establishing evidence of safety and efficacy in humans. The company has a pharmaceutical research staff of 1,800. Evidence of safety and efficacy (the characteristics or the effect of the drug when used under ideal conditions) in humans is normally developed through randomized, double-blind clinical trials. The findings of such trials usually cite the effects that the drug has, compared to placebos and/or standard treatments, on various biological end points for appropriate levels of statistical significance and confidence intervals. For example, measured end points of efficacy for cimetidine include healing of the ulcer, concomitant use of antacids, side effects, and relief of other symptoms. For the rheumatoid arthritis drug auranofin, measured end points include the number of swollen or tender joints, the time to onset of fatigue in the morning, the number of seconds taken to walk 50 feet, and various chemical determinations.

In addition to the clinical trials used for establishing evidence for safety and efficacy, other data are gathered in nonrandomized studies using surveillance and other epidemiological methods before and after introduction of the drug into the market. These so-called phase IV studies provide longer-range, experiential information about drug safety and efficacy which may not be evident from premarketing, double-blind clinical trials alone. Typically, a thousand or more patients may be studied in one form or another before marketing, and several thousand may be studied after the drug is on the market. See Chapter 4 for further discussion of technology assessment in the drug industry.

The *SK&F Cost-Benefit Studies* effort (SK&F-CBS) was initiated in 1977 as a result of the developing marketing experience with cimetidine, which had been introduced in overseas markets in 1976 and in the United States in 1977. Immediately following its introduction, the worldwide sales of cimetidine increased much faster than had been forecast. Although cimetidine was in great demand by physicians and patients, its price at the time (about $1.20 per day to the patient) was considerably higher than that of older drugs used in the treatment of duodenal ulcer, such as anticholinergic agents (about $0.38 per day) and antacids (about $0.50 per day). The price of cimetidine was set to be comparable with that of recent drug innovations in other disease areas and to reflect the

10 years of gastrointestinal and related R&D preceding the introduction of the drug. Since its introduction, other duodenal ulcer products have been marketed at prices comparable or exceeding the current price of cimetidine (e.g., ranitidine at $1.45 per day).

SK&F-CBS was introduced to document, in addition to its medical advantages, the cost advantages of cimetidine to physicians, third-party payers, and health services programs (e.g., national health services, state Medicaid programs, commercial insurance companies, health maintenance organizations [HMOs]) in an environment of increasing cost-containment and price justification pressures. The decisions of these parties to prescribe, purchase, and pay for cimetidine affect the demand for the drug for large groups of patients. (In certain countries, introductory prices and rates of reimbursement and price increases must be negotiated.) In a broader sense, cimetidine appeared to offer an excellent opportunity for demonstrating the economic contributions to society of major new pharmaceutical products.

Purpose

The purpose of SK&F-CBS is to document the cost-benefit and cost-effectiveness of SK&F's major prescription pharmaceutical products. This is done in addition to the biological/medical evaluations which are conducted at SK&F. SK&F-CBS principally addresses the implications of cost considerations on potential limitations of use of and reimbursement for SK&F prescription pharmaceuticals. It is also intended that the program document the value of pharmaceuticals in general, and SK&F products in particular.

Subjects of Assessment

The subjects of assessment are chemical entities anticipated to be marketed as prescription drugs. In 1984, the antiarthritic drug auranofin and the antibiotics cefonicid and ceftizoxime were the primary subjects of SK&F-CBS studies. Other SmithKline Beckman companies conduct assessments of diagnostic and bioanalytic instruments and services, and animal, eye care, and consumer (over-the-counter) drug and health care products.

Stage of Diffusion

The drugs assessed are those being brought onto the market, including those awaiting approval by the FDA. The program does not routinely study products put on the market prior to 1977–1978, when the program was initiated.

Concerns

The particular concerns of SK&F-CBS include market price, cost-benefit, cost-effectiveness, and quality-of-life, in addition to SK&F's traditional assessment concerns of safety and efficacy.

Requests

Candidates for assessment are the new chemical entities developed by SK&F. As is typical for a firm in the prescription drug industry, only one or two major products may be introduced in any one year.

Selection

If a product in research and development meets expectations in clinical trials for safety and efficacy and promises to be marketed, it becomes a subject for SK&F-CBS evaluation.

Process

SK&F-CBS cost-benefit and cost-effectiveness evaluations for any one product may involve several types of analyses. SK&F contracts with academic research institutes and other agencies to conduct studies and data analyses; data are used from published sources (e.g., medical/epidemiological literature, National Center for Health Statistics, and other national data); data may be purchased by SK&F from other sources; and SK&F-CBS conducts its own analyses.

The SK&F-CBS managers and the SK&F product management staff jointly develop an evaluation plan. Consultation is sought from SK&F and outside clinical personnel as appropriate, such as cases in which cost-benefit evaluations involving clinical trials are to be conducted.

Types of studies that are conducted for the cost-benefit and/or cost-effectiveness evaluation of a drug may include the following:

- cost of disease determinations using surveys and other data sources;
- economic/cost inquiries in premarketing randomized clinical trials;
- expert estimates of treatment costs with and without a drug;
- postmarketing epidemiological studies (e.g., time-series studies of populations before and after using a drug, and cross-sectional comparisons of patients undergoing treatment with and without the drug);
- quality-of-life studies using patient questionnaires; and
- decision-tree analyses of alternative treatments.

Results of randomized clinical trials conducted and sponsored by SK&F for investigating drug safety and efficacy are also used as appropriate.

Assessors

Although these studies are usually sponsored by SK&F, they are generally conducted by persons outside the organization. As is evident from the various study types, the assessors include a diverse range of personnel, both from within SK&F and from outside organizations, often research institutes with academic ties. These include research design personnel, epidemiologists, economists, and physicians and other health care personnel.

Turnaround

Turnaround varies according to study type. It may vary from 2 months for decision-tree analyses using existing cost data, to 2 or 3 years for studies involving clinical trials, to 5 years or more for longitudinal studies. It has been the experience of SK&F that 10 to 12 years on average are required from synthesis and testing of new chemical entities through FDA approval of a prescription drug.

Reporting

The outside, independent investigators who conduct SK&F-sponsored studies are free to publish their findings. These are usually published in the appropriate medical and other literature. Prepublication drafts of SK&F-sponsored research are sometimes circulated to appropriate SK&F personnel. Since 1977–1978, when the SK&F-CBS program began with cimetidine, approximately 20 papers and reports have been published on cimetidine studies conducted and/or sponsored by SK&F. Publication sources have included such journals as *Lancet*, the *Journal of Clinical Gastroenterology*, and *Social Science and Medicine*; publications of the Congressional Office of Technology Assessment (OTA), the Stanford Research Institute, and Robinson Associates (Bryn Mawr, Pa.); and a number of foreign publications and international conference proceedings.

Study results may be distributed to physicians and others with special interests in the particular area of research. Quality-of-life study findings may be provided to physicians to assist them in weighing efficacy and side effects of drugs in prescribing decisions. The SK&F corporate affairs and marketing departments send reports to leaders in the private and public sectors, such as professional health economists and Medicaid program administrators, to provide economic perspectives regarding the reimbursement of SK&F prescription drugs.

Impact

SK&F-CBS findings are intended to have an impact particularly on commercial and government third-party payers, and on domestic and foreign government agencies charged with the regulatory approval of drugs, introductory pricing of drugs (e.g., in Japan), reimbursement of drugs at particular rates (e.g., in France), and allowing price increases. Specific impacts are hard to determine; however, SK&F attributes the addition and retention of cimetidine on the formularies of several Medicaid jurisdictions to evidence of the effectiveness of cimetidine in reducing ulcer surgery and patient treatment costs. It is likely that the original pricing and/or reimbursement status of cimetidine in various countries overseas was at least partly dependent on studies of its cost-effectiveness, according to SK&F.

Reassessment

SK&F-CBS has not yet conducted reassessments. However, the introduction of competitive drugs may prompt reassessment in which SK&F-CBS would seek to supply new comparative cost-benefit and cost-effectiveness evidence. SK&F has traditionally conducted clinical reassessments for newly reported side effects or indications of a drug.

Funding/Budget

Though varying within a wide range, the annual budget for SK&F-CBS has averaged about $700,000. The estimated 1985 budget for the program is $550,000. Funds have been allotted from SmithKline Beckman and from various SK&F departments such as state government affairs, product management, and medical affairs. Studies range in cost from $5,000 for small desk-top analyses to over $1 million for certain clinical and time-series studies.

Example

On the following pages is an article describing approaches used in SK&F-CBS and an overview of such studies of cimetidine. The article was published in *Managerial and Decision Economics*, 4(1):50–62, 1983, and is reproduced here with permission.

Sources

Kleinfield, N. R. May 29, 1984. SmithKline: One-drug image. New York Times. D1.

Koenig, R. December 23, 1983. SmithKline's Beckman unit off to slow start. Wall Street Journal.

Neuhauser, D. 1982. New drug evaluation: Cimetidine. Medical Care 20:755–757.

Office of Technology Assessment. 1981. The Implications of Cost-Effectiveness Analysis of Medical Technology. Washington, D.C.: U.S. Government Printing Office.

Paterson, M. L. 1983a. Cost-Benefit Evaluation of a New Technology for Treatment of Peptic Ulcer Disease. Managerial and Decision Economics 4:50–62.

Paterson, M. L. 1983b. Measuring the socio-economic benefits of auranofin. In G. T. Smith (ed.), Measuring the Social Benefits of Medicine. London: Office of Health Economics.

Paterson, M. L., Manager, Cost-Benefit Studies, Smith Kline & French Laboratories. 1985. Personal communication.

SmithKline Beckman. 1984. Annual Report 1983. Philadelphia.

Standard & Poor's Corporation. 1983. Industry Surveys, Health Care: Basic Analysis 151:H13-H35.

Cost-Benefit Evaluation of a New Technology for Treatment of Peptic Ulcer Disease

MORTON L. PATERSON
Smith Kline & French Laboratories, Philadelphia, USA

Psychosocial benefit resists monetary expression. However, reduction in costs, with no loss of benefits assumed, improves a cost-benefit ratio. The effect of cimetidine on the costs of ulcer has been widely studied. Randomized clinical trials show reductions in surgery and work loss among cimetidine-treated patients versus placebo controls. In the community, time series studies have documented drops in ulcer surgery, averaging about 25% below the expected trend line, following marketing introduction of the drug. These, plus a cross-sectional study of Medicaid patients with and without use of cimetidine, indicate that the drug has reduced the net direct costs of ulcer disease.

INTRODUCTION

Smith Kline & French's new drug product for ulcer disease, cimetidine, was forecast in 1977 to achieve a substantial sales volume. The forecast was made just as pressures were increasing to contain the fast-rising costs of health care. Since then the drug has become conspicuous as both an unusually efficacious new technology and as a leading, if not *the* leading, item on many pharmaceutical reimbursement budgets around the world. Cost-benefit matters regarding cimetidine have become important indeed. Do the benefits of cimetidine in the community exceed its costs? This is an economic question, testing whether the cimetidine undertaking – its research and development, widespread adoption and effect on society – has in the broadest sense been worthwhile.

COST–BENEFIT ANALYSIS

There are objectors to cost–benefit questions of this kind. Some might like to let a free marketplace answer the question: consumers will pay for a drug what it is worth to them. Imperfectly informed consumers and the physician's role as product prescriber are not typical of a free market; nor is patent protection, and certainly not reimbursement of costs by third parties so, the free market objector is probably a straw man. However, he makes the point that cost-benefit analysis is a substitute for market forces. In fact, it began with evaluation of public works: Should a dam be built, an airport? More recently, the cost-effectiveness of different national defense systems has been evaluated: Which gives more 'bang for the buck'? Put crudely, a national concern today is more 'health for the buck'.

This leads to a different objector to cost-benefit analysis in health. Hippocratic in spirit, he or she must be taken quite seriously. In fact, it is this person most of us want for our physician. He says, in effect, let us do everything medically possible for the patient. The economist will tell him that is not possible; society has other goals; resources are not infinite. Yet the physician feels it unethical, if not impossible, to deny a particular patient a treatment or test on the basis of predicted other patients who may need it instead. Usually, in the end, someone other than the physician sets the dollar limit and probably the rationing rules. Economic, not just medical, evaluation becomes necessary.

When examining the benefits and costs of cimetidine the following equation was used as a model:

Present value of an investment over time:

$$V = \sum_{t=1}^{T} \frac{(B_t - C_t)}{(1+r)^t}$$

where:

V = value

$\sum_{t}^{T}$ = sum of years $t_1 + t_2 + \cdots$ etc.

B = benefits

C = costs

r = rate of discount

CCC-0143-6570/83/0004-0050$06.50

The symbols indicate that the value of an investment over time is the benefits in a given year, t, minus the cost in that year, with the difference discounted at a rate, r, reflecting the value of money over time. That means that all the years over the lifetime of the investment must be considered. Since most of what follows concerns only one year at a time, we can simplify the equation in the following manner:

Value when all benefits and costs occur in same year:

$$V = B - C$$

where:

V = value

B = benefits

C = costs

Value equals benefits minus costs during one year.

The important point this brings out is that we cannot fill in B in the equation! We know that cimetidine inhibits the secretion of gastric acid, heals ulcers, relieves gastrointestinal pain and distress, reduces the need for concomitant antacids and forestalls ulcer surgery. This has been proven in clinical trials. We have heard of and talked to people who could eat normally, sleep all night, work more regularly and enjoy family life again because of cimetidine. But we have not quantified these changes in quality of life – not most of them – and certainly have no single number for B to put in the equation. Moreover, if we did have a number, it would need to be translated into dollars, so that C, the dollar costs, could be subtracted from it. What is the dollar value to patients of pain-free nights, of a pleasant disposition, of not having to swallow antacids, of not getting anesthetized and cut in an operating room? Economists would dearly love to be able to find out. (You can ask patients questions about their willingness to pay to avoid these things. We might have tried that with cimetidine, but it is obviously a very tricky and controversial matter.) Are we thus stymied by the lack of numbers before we start?

Not necessarily. What we want is a net gain in benefits from the investment which the payers for health care make in cimetidine. This is shown thus:

Gain from an investment comes from raising benefits:

$$V = B - C$$

$$10 = 15 - 5$$

$$\text{Invest: } 12 = 17 - 5 \text{ gain} = 2$$

Raising benefits and reducing costs:

$$V = B - C$$

$$10 = 15 - 5$$

$$\text{Invest: } 14 = 17 - 3 \text{ gain} = 4$$

Reducing costs:

$$V = B - C$$

$$10 = 15 - 5$$

$$\text{Invest: } 12 = 15 - 3 \text{ gain} = 2$$

This shows at least three ways of producing a gain. The most obvious is to increase the benefit, in the sense of health-related quality of life. Let us use the number 15 to represent the benefit of therapy before or without cimetidine and 5 to represent the cost needed to produce that benefit – the drugs, doctor visits, tests, operations, bed days and so on. The value, V, then equals 10, benefit minus cost. If with cimetidine the benefit is increased to 17, the investment has produced a gain of 2. If with cimetidine the benefit is 17 and the cost drops to 3, the gain is 4. Now, let us assume that cimetidine has no effect on quality of life – that is, produces no new health benefit, even though we know it does – but that cost declines to 3. We still have a net gain of 2. Therein lies the hope of doing a cost-benefit study of cimetidine; because cost reduction is always cost-beneficial, as long as the benefit – the health status – at least holds constant. If cimetidine can pass this cost-reduction test, it is 'home free'. If it does not pass, it may perfectly well still be cost-beneficial because it increases benefits *more* than costs. Cost reduction is an unfair test, to be undergone by only the hardiest of new technologies – or by the hardiest of cost-benefit analysts.

CIMETIDINE AND EPIDEMIOLOGY

Our question has now become: What is the effect of cimetidine on the costs of ulcer disease? The first country studied was the Netherlands (Bulthuis *et al.*, 1977). It can be seen from Table 1 that there are two kinds of cost: medical or treatment costs, called direct; and productivity-related costs, called indirect. These are traditional groupings. The major direct cost in 1975 was hospitalization, at

Table 1. The Netherlands: Peptic Ulcer Costs (in million dollars)

	1975
Hospitalization	20.8
Surgeon fees	1.7
Polyclinics	1.3
Consultations	1.4
Diagnoses	1.9
Drugs	0.9
Total direct	27.8
Absenteeism	82.9
Disability	—
Mortality	—
Total indirect	82.9
Total	110.7
Population	13 650 000

Table 2. United States: Duodenal Ulcer Costs (in million dollars)

	1977
Hospitalization	732
Surgeon fees	74
Consultations	46
Diagnoses	66
Drugs	85
Nursing home	11
Other	2
Total direct	1016
Absenteeism	455
Disability	476
Mortality	245
Total indirect	1176
Total	2192
Population	215 000 000

Table 3. United States: Duodenal Ulcer Costs if Cimetidine Used in 50% of Patients (in million dollars)

	1977	Cimetidine Effect
Hospitalization	571	−22%
Surgeon fees	55	−25%
Consultations	41	−11%
Diagnoses	60	−9%
Drugs	106	+25%
Nursing home	11	0
Other	2	0
Total direct	846	−17%
Absenteeism	362	−20%
Disability	363	−24%
Mortality	218	−11%
Total indirect	943	−20%
Total	1789	−18%

$20.8 million. Drugs were a very small share in the Netherlands. Total direct costs were $27.8 million. Indirect costs were much larger, even with only absenteeism considered. Total costs of ulcer disease to the Dutch economy were $110.7 million.

Table 2 refers to the United States, and only duodenal ulcer costs, in 1977 (adapted from Chandler and von Haunalter, 1977). About 80% of ulcers in the United States are in the duodenum; the other 20% are in the stomach. In the United States direct costs almost equal indirect costs. Hospitalization is again the major medical cost and a tempting area in which to look for savings. A 12% reduction in hospital costs, for example, would more than offset a 100% increase in drug costs.

Similar studies were done in several European countries. As one ranges into the Latin countries of Europe, hospital costs still constitute the largest direct cost, but less so than in the north; and drugs are a larger share than in the north. One value of a cost-of-disease study is that it shows the cost categories which the new technology may increase or decrease. Of course, it is the net cost effect we want to know.

In the United States a survey was done in 1977 among the early clinical investigators of cimetidine in duodenal ulcer (Olitsky *et al.*, 1978). They were asked to judge from their experience what the specific treatment and response patterns of duodenal ulcer patients would be over a year both with and without cimetidine. Their answers were costed out and the results projected to the national level. Table 3 shows that cimetidine was estimated to reduce hospitalization costs by 22%, raise drug costs by 25%, reduce indirect costs by 20% and produce a total net saving of 18% – assuming that the drug had been used in 50% of duodenal ulcer patients in 1977. A similar exercise in the Netherlands produced similar results. These are estimations only, needing verification by hard data, but they are useful to show what we mean by a net effect of cimetidine on the cost of ulcer disease.

What hard economic data do we have? One kind is from clinical trials of cimetidine in ulcer disease, those done to prove efficacy and safety to regulatory authorities. Economists are intrigued by such trials, because economists almost never get to do controlled experiments, particularly the randomized double-blind kind in which nobody knows until the trial is over which group got the experimental treatment and which got the placebo. We put a simple one-line item in the U.S.A. patients' case report forms: number of days of work missed last week because of ulcer disease. That is about all gastroenterologists would take time to ask.

Figure 1 shows the results from a subset of work-missing patients in the clinical trial. The horizontal axis shows the pretreatment through six-week-treatment points. The vertical axis shows the average number of work days missed per patient per week. The cimetidine and placebo groups start off about equal, missing about three and a half to four days per week for each patient. By the end of the second week, the cimetidine group was averaging about one day of missed work and the placebo group about two. The difference holds through the end of the trial. When the results were published by Drs Ricardo-Campbell and Wardell (1980), they expressed the effect of

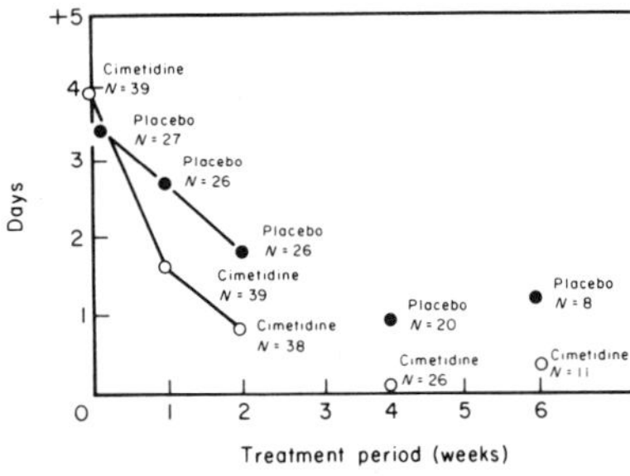

Figure 1. Average time lost from work per patient per week.

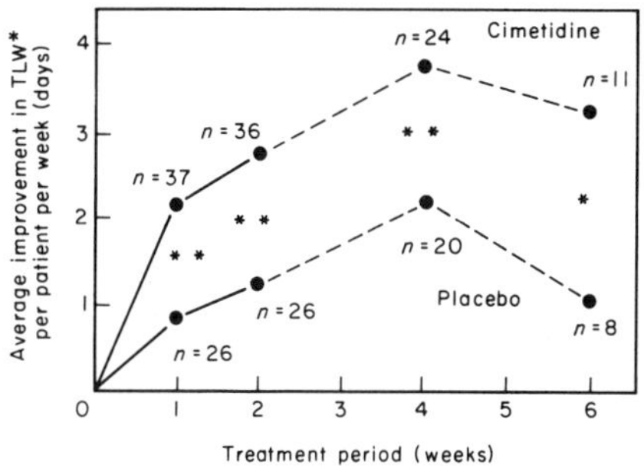

Figure 2. The solid line connecting data points at pre-, 1 and 2 weeks indicates that data from these weeks were common to all three studies (i.e. 2-, 4- and 6-week). In contrast, data from weeks 4 and 6 were not common to all three studies. Hence a broken line connects the data points at weeks 4 and 6* (TLW = Time Lost from Work.)

cimetidine in terms of improvement in worktime and inverted the data accordingly, as shown in Fig. 2.

At the same time, in Sweden Drs Bodemar and Walan asked the same question of ulcer patients during a year-long double-blind trial of cimetidine maintenance therapy. Sixty-eight patients took part, 32 on cimetidine and 36 on placebo.

	Cimetidine 400 mg twice daily (32 patients)	Placebo twice daily (36 patients)
Number missing work	1	23
Work-days lost	79	1405
Average workdays lost per patient	2.8	49.3

As reported in the *Lancet* (Bodemar and Walan, 1978), these figures tell us that one of the 32 cimetidine patients was off work for 79 days, giving a mean of 2.8 days per patient; while 23 of the 36 patients on placebo were off work for a total of 1405 days, giving a mean 49.3 workdays missed per patient during the year. This is an outstanding difference. Drs Bodemar and Walan went further and noted how many in each group went to surgery.

	Cimetidine 400 mg twice daily (32 patients)	Placebo twice daily (36 patients)
With recurrences	6 (19%)	30 (83%)
With two recurrences	1 (3%)	12 (33%)
With complications	0	4 (11%)
Receiving surgery	1 (3%)	15 (42%)

We see that recurrences were much less frequent in the cimetidine group – 19% versus 83% – leading to only one case of surgery versus 15 in the placebo group. This has obvious economic implications for the health care system.

Is our cost-reduction question answered by such findings? Unfortunately not. While randomized clinical trials have internal validity and therewith clearly isolate cause and effect, they are not necessarily valid externally in the community. At least three artificialities of the controlled conditions in most randomized trials limit projection to average conditions in the 'real world'. First, although patients are assigned at random to treatment or placebo, those patients are not obtained initially in a random manner: they must meet certain disease characteristics, often tending toward more severe status. Second, the patients are regularly observed and examined medically and are required to take their medication according to a strict protocol. Third, placebo is not a common alternative in medical practice; most doctors will give an active drug regimen of some sort.

Is it not possible, then, to do a randomized experiment in the community itself? We can with consumer products, in test marketing for example, or with technologies like insulin infusion pumps or water fluoridation; but with prescription drugs it is probably impossible. Once the drug is approved legally as safe and effective, based on the double-blind clinical trials, it is known and demanded. We cannot dictate use in a randomized design, allowing it in Liverpool and denying it in Manchester, for instance. Thus, we are hampered in the pre-approval stage by artificial conditions and in the post-approval stage by the impossibility of randomization. It is ironic, in a way, that drugs, because look-alike placebos can be easily supplied, must be proven efficacious in controlled trials, whereas vastly more expensive and drastic intervention like heart-bypass surgery, where treating with a placebo is much more difficult, have no approval requirements at all.

What, then, do we turn to for hard data on the economic effect of cimetidine in the community? The answer is to epidemiology, meaning the study of disease events in a natural population. As Prof. A. J. Culyer, the eminent health economist, has said: 'The first essential for a cost-effectiveness study is good epidemiology.'

Ulcer disease seems to have been declining for ten to twenty years. At least, deaths, hospitalization and surgery due to ulcer have been declining in various populations. No one knows why, although this writer's personal guess is that improved treatment, including tranquilizers, and exclusion of non-ulcers through more specific diagnosis have contributed. In any case, if cimetidine has affected any of these events, they must be found to have fallen, or fallen faster, after its introduction. Its adoption in most countries, it should be pointed out, was rapid and extensive. Typically, use occurred in over 50% of ulcer patient visits within six to nine months after market introduction. The opportunity for an effect was indeed present.

Figure 3 shows the first of several time-series suggesting that an effect has occurred. We see here the number of operations for duodenal ulcer performed over the last several years by a group of six hospitals in the UK. The data, from Dr Wyllie *et al.*, appear in the *Lancet* (1981). Cimetidine was

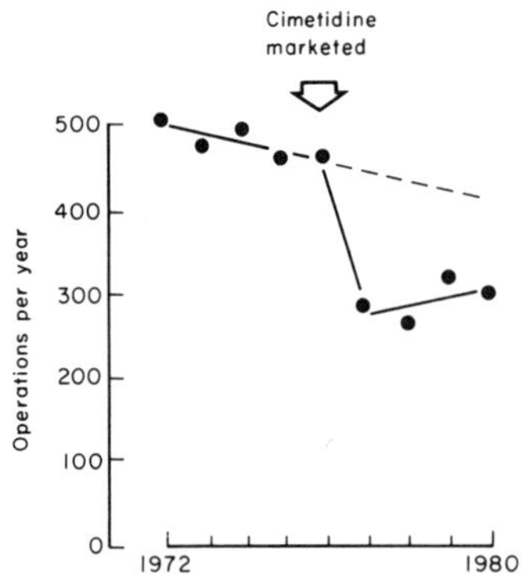

Figure 3. Operations for duodenal ulcer by a group of six medical centers in the UK from 1972 to 1980.

introduced at the end of 1976. We see a sharp drop in operations in the following year. The trend line would have predicted a much higher number than that observed. By the ruler and eyeball method, the average difference between the expected and observed points is roughly 32% during the four-year cimetidine period.

Figure 4 shows surgery data through 1979 from another area of the UK, the Northern Health Authority, collected by Venables (1981), a surgeon at Newcastle-on-Tyne. Though not as striking as in the previous data, the steeper drop after cimetidine is apparent. Moreover, no sign of a rebound in ulcer surgery is seen. Mr. Venables has presented data through 1978 for all of England and Wales, and these are displayed in Fig. 5.

Note the drop in surgery in 1975, before cimetidine was introduced. Such are the anomalies to be reckoned with in time-series analysis. The explanation, according to Venables and others, is a labor dispute, a kind of strike, among younger physicians in 1975. We can see that general surgery for all conditions, not just ulcer, declined in that year

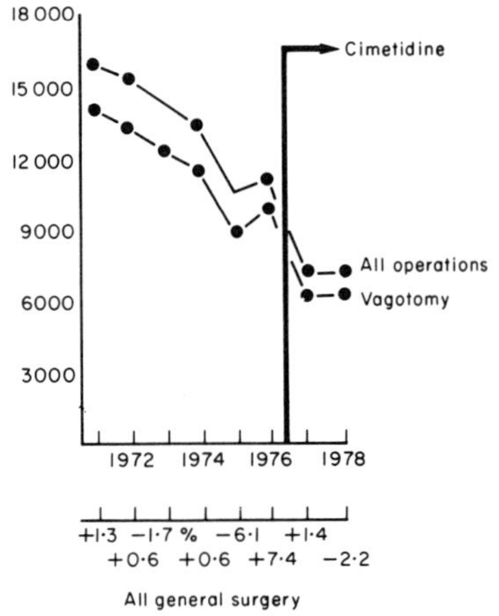

Figure 5. Operations for duodenal ulcer in England and Wales (HIPE) from 1971 to 1978.

(−6.1%) and then rebounded in 1976, along with the ulcer surgery (Hospital In-Patient Enquiry, OPCS, UK). In many cases it can be postponed. Again, with ruler and eyeball, the drop below trend following cimetidine can be calculated at 21%, averaged during 1977 and 1978.

It is time to raise the *post hoc ergo propter hoc* fallacy to remind us that because the sharp drop in surgery followed cimetidine it was not necessarily caused by cimetidine. No one has observed other sudden changes in therapy or the health care system that might explain the drop, but theoretically they may exist. The following data from the United States may elucidate causality.

Figure 6 illustrates the number of partial gastrectomies and vagotomies performed in the United States over the last several years. The data were obtained from the National Center for Health Statistics by Dr Fineberg of Harvard and appear (through 1979) in the *Lancet* (1981). Vagotomy and partial gastrectomy are the leading operations for ulcer and a clear indication of the trend in ulcer

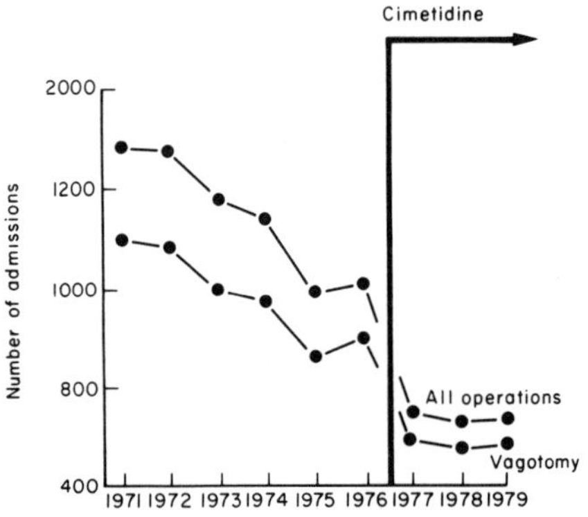

Figure 4. All operations for duodenal ulcer in the Northern Health Region of the UK from 1971 to 1979 (excludes perforations).

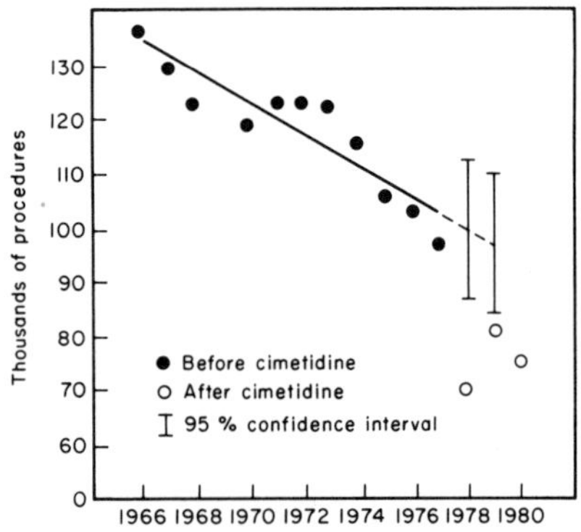

Figure 6. Partial gastrectomy and vagotomy surgery in the United States from 1966 to 1980.

Table 4. Selected Abdominal Surgical Procedures in the United States: Rate per 10 000 Population

Procedure	1970	1975	1976	1978
All abdominal surgery	122	138	133	132
Partial gastrectomy and vagotomy	6	5	5	3
Appendicectomy	16	15	14	14
Cholecystectomy	18	21	21	20
Herniorrhaphy	25	26	24	24

Source: National Center for Health Statistics, National Hospital Discharge Survey.

surgery. Had the trend continued as expected, the dashed line with its confidence bracket would represent the number of operations in 1978. Cimetidine was introduced in the fall of 1977. The actual number of operations in 1978 was much lower than expected, as shown. There was a rebound in 1979 but not up to the prior trend line. The 1980 point (added after a personal communication from Dr Fineberg) is down again, strongly suggesting that the level of procedures has established itself below the prior trend line. Note that cimetidine was introduced a year later than in the UK but that the drop in surgery again followed. This temporal relationship greatly strengthens the probability that cimetidine caused the drop.

The data provided in Table 4 from Dr Fineberg's article further reinforce that probability. We see the number of appendectomies, cholecystectomies, and herniorrhaphies over the same period and find no decline in the rate per 10 000 population, and none in all abdominal surgery. Only ulcer surgery dropped. This appears to rule out general changes in health care procedures as the cause of the drop. Again, it should be pointed out that during 1978 in the United States cimetidine usage grew rapidly, with prescriptions occurring in over 50% of that year's office visits for ulcer.

Dr Fineberg's data on vagotomy and partial gastrectomy show surgery for both duodenal and gastric ulcer. However, in the United States cimetidine had not yet been cleared by the FDA for gastric ulcer. Thus more precise data on duodenal ulcer only are desirable. They are provided by Dr Murray Wylie of the University of Michigan and appear in the *Journal of Clinical Gastroenterology* (Wylie, 1981).

Dr Wylie's trend data include all operations for ulcer, not just vagotomy and partial gastrectomy; and only operations performed on patients hospitalized with an ulcer diagnosis are counted. The data come from a nearly constant cohort of 790 hospitals across the United States. Figure 7 shows the trend in hospitalizations for duodenal and for gastric ulcer.

We see that for duodenal ulcer the trend has again been downward and that in 1978, the year after the introduction of cimetidine, it did not drop faster than before. Gastric ulcer hospitalizations appear essentially level.

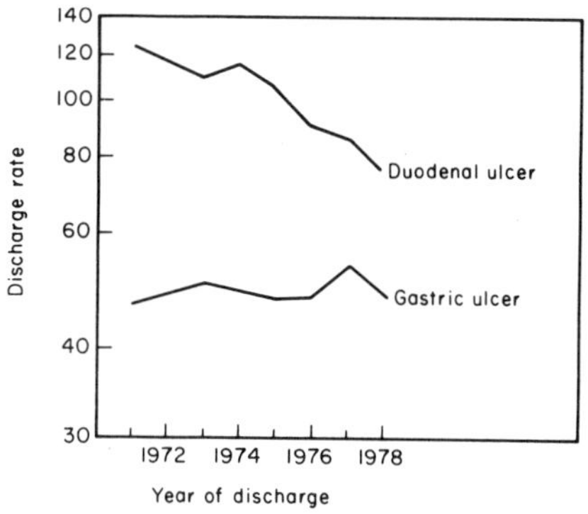

Figure 7. Time trends in the United States in hospital discharge rates for duodenal and gastric ulcer per 100 000 population, by diagnosis and year, short-term hospitals, from 1971 to 1978. (Source: National Center for Health Statistics, Hospital Discharge Survey.)

As shown in Table 5, Dr Wylie finds, starting in 1977, a growth in the share of admissions with complications, meaning bleeding or a perforation of the intestinal wall. He then notes (Fig. 8) the percentage of ulcer admissions receiving gastrointestinal surgery.

Again a sharp drop in the rate of surgery following cimetidine's introduction is seen, reversing a slightly rising trend in the rate. As Dr Wylie points out, the greater share of complicated cases would normally be expected to produce more surgery, not the lesser amount observed. The drop did not occur in gastric ulcer, neither complicated nor uncomplicated, for which cimetidine was not approved. However, in duodenal ulcer the drop occurred in both the complicated and uncomplicated kinds. Also, the drop started quite promptly after the introduction of cimetidine.

Dr Wylie also noted the case fatality rate among hospital admissions (Fig. 9). He observes that at a time when the mix of cases changed to increase the risk of dying – that is, from the greater share of hemorrhages and perforations – the death rate clearly dropped, particularly so in 1978 for duodenal ulcer. The decline in ulcer surgery is suggested as the cause of this drop. Dr Wylie also finds that the

Table 5. Percentage of patients with complications of Duodenal and Gastric Ulcer Admissions to 790 PAS Participating Hospitals in the United States

Year of admission	Duodenal ulcer	Gastric ulcer
1974	33.0	32.5
1975	32.9	32.8
1976	33.1	32.6
1977	35.4	34.5
1978	37.7	37.1
1979	39.6	37.4

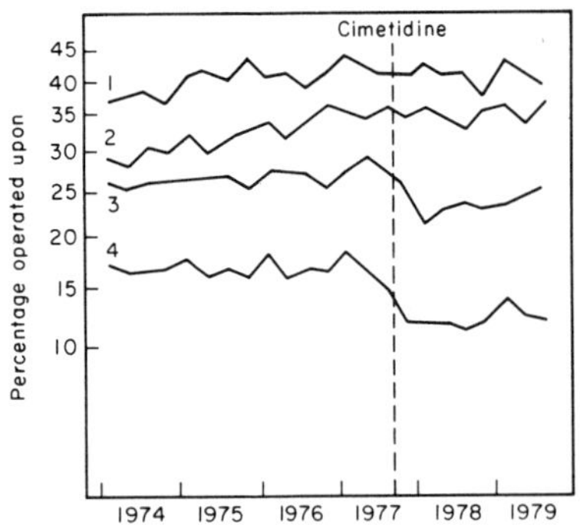

Figure 8. Percentage operated upon duodenal and gastric ulcer admissions to 790 PAS participating hospitals in the United States by year and quarter of admission, 1974–1979. (1) Gastric ulcer with complications; (2) uncomplicated gastric ulcer; (3) duodenal ulcer with complications; (4) uncomplicated duodenal ulcer.

average length of hospital stay fell more rapidly after 1977. In all, Dr Wylie concludes, 'the use of cimetidine, plus the high expectations before its impending release, probably caused the change in trends documented in this study'.

Finally, Fig. 10 provides one other time series in the United States, useful because it shows the frequency of ulcer surgery as a rate per population. The small state of Rhode Island collects such data and thus controls for demographic shifts which theoretically may confound results. The data are from a study by Rhode Island Health Services Research (Norton *et al.*., 1980) and have been submitted for publication. We see the same drop after cimetidine's introduction. The number of vagotomies and partial gastrectomies for duodenal ulcer per 100 000 population was projected along the trend line but actually fell well below it, saving about 10 operations per 100 000 residents of the

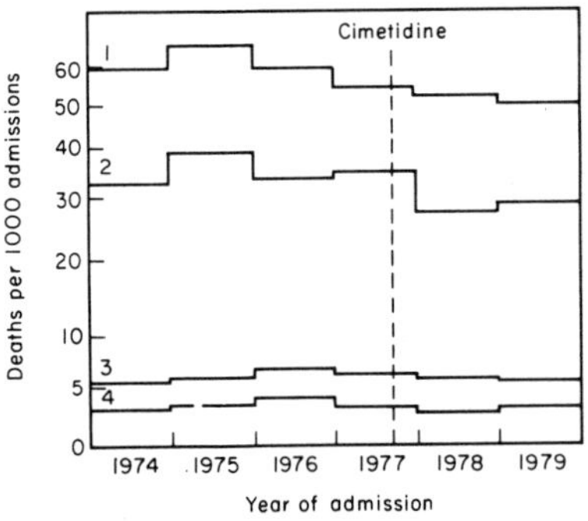

Figure 9. Deaths per thousand admissions in the United States of duodenal and gastric ulcer by presence or absence of complications, by year of admission, 1974–1979. (1) Complicated gastric ulcers; (2) complicated duodenal ulcer; (3) uncomplicated duodenal ulcer; (4) uncomplicated gastric ulcer.

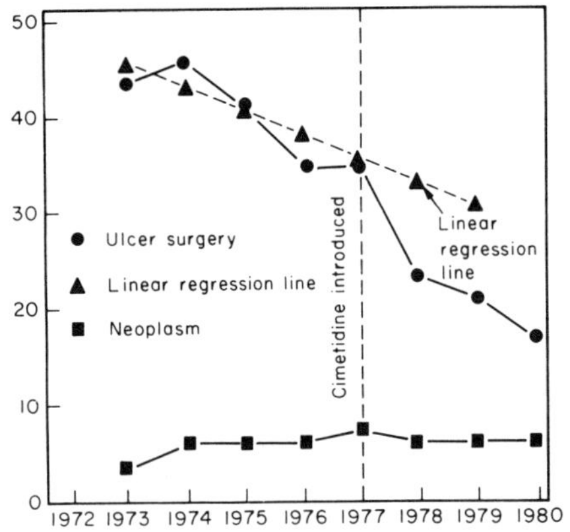

Figure 10. Rates per 100 000 persons of partial gastrectomy and/or vagotomy for Rhode Island residents for the twelve months ending 31 August 1973 through 1980.

state in 1978 and 1979, and somewhat more in 1980. No sign of a rebound is seen. Since partial gastrectomies are sometimes done for cancer, all cancer cases have been separated and appear along the bottom of the graph. This serves as a kind of control in the data, and we see no drop after cimetidine.

So much for the epidemiologic data in the United States. In this writer's view, simply by reproducing the UK data one year later – given that cimetidine was introduced in the United States one year later than in the UK – evidence clearly is established for cimetidine as the cause of the sudden drop observed.

The same decline can be found in the two other countries where time-series data have been collected so far. First, in France data were collected by Lambert–Yves Conseil (1980), research consultants, in a special survey of 25 university and regional hospital centers (CHU and CHR). The results have not yet appeared in the medical literature:

	1976	1977	1978	1979
Number of ulcer operations	1456	1376	988	1026
1976 base = 100	100	95	68	70

Although the series is shorter than in the United States, the number of operations for peptic ulcer dropped sharply after the introduction of cimetidine in the fall of 1977. There were two other samples of hospitals supplying such data. Table 6 shows the findings for each. The drop also occurred in medium-size hospitals and in private clinics; although the decline in 1977 in the former is difficult to explain and may be spurious. Appendectomies and cholecystectomies were recorded as a control and national projections made (Table 7). As in the United States' data earlier, we see no fall

Table 6. Number of Operations for Duodenal and Gastric Ulcers in France

	1976	1977	1978	1979
Eight medium-size public hospitals				
Number of operations	202	152	142	124
1976 base = 100	100	75	70	61
Twelve centers for private care				
Number of operations	353	335	229	254
1976 base = 100	100	95	65	72

in these other gastrointestinal interventions, only in surgery for ulcer, down 30%.

Next, and last, the Netherlands has excellent data at the national level on most aspects of medical care. The data on ulcer surgery have been collected by the Netherlands Economic Institute and are presented very briefly in *Economisch Statistische Berichten* (Bulthuis, 1981). A full article will be published based on a presentation by Bulthuis (1981). Hospitalization for ulcer, in terms of both admissions and length of stay, has been declining in the Netherlands, as have total operations for ulcer. Figure 11 details the operations performed for

Table 7. National Projection of Appendectomies and Cholecystectomies in France

	1972	1976	1979
Appendectomies	333 000	340 000	340 000
Cholecystectomies	69 000	85 000	85 000
Ulcers Operated	15 600	15 600	10 700(−30%)

duodenal ulcer patients since 1972, with the total through 1980. Both gastrectomies and vagotomies dropped sharply after cimetidine was introduced in the fall of 1977. The latter operation was becoming more popular but reversed its uptrend.

Figure 12 shows operations for gastric ulcer, for which cimetidine was approved. Again, the same drop is seen, with no sign of a rebound in 1980 (updated NEI report in press). Because the Netherlands have impressively complete data, Dr Bulthuis was able to do a multiple regression analysis of a number of variables possibly causing the drop in

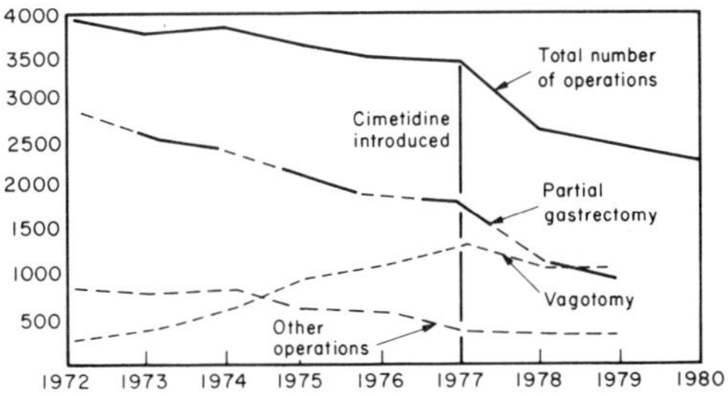

Figure 11. Trend in the number of operated hospitalizations for duodenal ulcer in the Netherlands, by type of operation.

surgery. Those variables include fiber-optic endoscopies (a popular new procedure for looking into the gastrointestinal tract with a tube), drug usage, physician visits and even a change in 1975 in government policies toward hospital reimbursement. While no absolute proof of cause and effect, multiple regression analysis allows the contribution of the different variables to the change in trend to be calculated and tested for statistical significance. Table 8 shows the findings of Dr Bulthuis.

The table shows the only two things accounting for the decline in ulcer operations between 1972 and 1979, the general trend and cimetidine. In admissions for gastric ulcer without surgery, the trend explains all of the reduction, some 300 operations. With surgery, cimetidine and the trend each contributes equally to the reduction. In

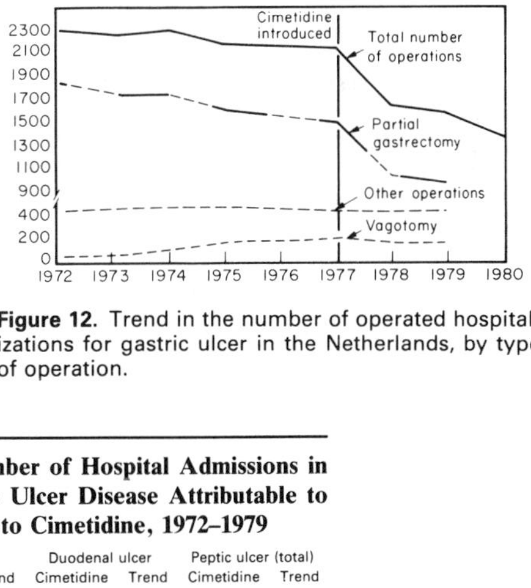

Figure 12. Trend in the number of operated hospitalizations for gastric ulcer in the Netherlands, by type of operation.

Table 8. The Reduction in the Number of Hospital Admissions in the Netherlands for Peptic Ulcer Disease Attributable to the Established Trend and to Cimetidine, 1972–1979

	Gastric ulcer		Duodenal ulcer		Peptic ulcer (total)	
	Cimetidine	Trend	Cimetidine	Trend	Cimetidine	Trend
Hospital admissions without surgery	n.a.	300	n.a.	1700	n.a.	2000
Hospital admissions with partial gastrectomy or vagotomy	400	400	1000	n.a.	1400	400
Hospital admissions with other operations	n.a.	n.a.	n.a.	500	n.a.	500
Total	400	700	1000	2200	1400	2900

duodenal ulcer without surgery, the trend accounts for the entire reduction; whereas with surgery, cimetidine accounts for all the 1000 operations avoided.

To summarize the international data so far. (1) Hospitalization and surgery are major components of the direct cost of ulcer disease. (2) Randomized double-blind clinical trials have proven that cimetidine not only heals ulcers and prevents their recurrence but also can keep ulcer patients working and away from surgery. (3) Cimetidine was rapidly and widely adopted in the treatment of ulcer disease. (4) The reduction in surgery suggested by Bodemar and Walan's clinical trial of cimetidine has now been clearly observed in a number of different data series covering four countries and two different years of introduction. (5) Factors such as abdominal surgery generally and other specific variables examined do not explain the sudden reduction seen. Surely, until some other explanation is provided, we should accept cimetidine as the cause of the recent sharp drop in ulcer surgery.

CIMETIDINE AND TREATMENT COST REDUCTION

Now, what about costs? As mentioned above, a conservative approach is forced on us. Psychosocial benefit to patients from changes in treatment methods, the gain in wellbeing, is too intangible to measure in money terms. We could quantify the gain in terms of total years of wellness, or as Dr Weinstein puts it, 'quality-adjusted life years' or more simply in terms of operations and absenteeism avoided. If a dollar spent on a new technology produces more of these indications of health than a dollar spent on another technology, then the newer one is more cost-effective. Thus, one technology may increase costs but nevertheless be more cost-effective than another. It may offer more health for the money. While that sounds reasonable, budget administrators today simply have less money to spend and want technologies to help them to cut expenses. So, we come back to the cost-reduction criterion, which perhaps only the luckiest of cost-benefit analysts should grapple with. Does cimetidine reduce the treatment costs of ulcer disease?

Most epidemiological studies do not go into costs, but three of the above do: the French, the Rhode Island and the Dutch. The French study (Lambert–Yves Conseil, 1980) relates its trend data in the sample of hospitals to national counts of ulcer surgery to project a national figure in 1979 of 4900 ulcer operations avoided. Using national cost schedules for operations and for a hospital day as well as the average length of stay of ulcer surgery patients, the study calculates a national saving in hospital costs in 1978 of about 43 million francs.

Table 9. Charges for Hospitalization of Blue Cross and Blue Shield Patients in Rhode Island, January–June 1976 (in dollars)

	Routine charges	Blue Cross Ancillary charges	Blue Shield Surgery physicians' fees	Total
Partial gastrectomy	1775	1519	700	3994
Vagotomy	1824	1210	535	3569
Ulcer and ulcer-related without ulcer surgery	1189	465		1654

Source: Blue Cross and Blue Shield of Rhode Island and *CPHA Abstracts.*

The above is based on the straightforward assumption that none of the patients avoiding surgery go into the hospital at all. The data on trends in total admissions for ulcer, surgical or not, do not as yet show statistically significant sharper drops after the introduction of cimetidine; however, the relatively few ulcer surgery candidates – perhaps 15% or 20% of ulcer admissions in the United States – could indeed all stay out of the hospital without affecting total admissions to a statistically significant degree, given the natural yearly variability of the trend line. Of course, it is also possible that most of the patients saved from surgery nevertheless enter and stay for some time in the hospital for diagnosis, bed rest, other treatment or observation.

With that in mind, we return to the Rhode Island study (Norton *et al.*, 1980). Table 9 shows the cost of surgical and non-surgical stays in Rhode Island in 1976. These costs are averaged from the records of reimbursement payments to hospitals and surgeons and anesthetists in Rhode Island for individuals hospitalized under Blue Cross and Blue Shield, the dominant private health insurance programs in the United States. A surgical stay, which is longer, of course, generates over twice the reimbursement costs of a non-surgical stay for ulcer. A weighted average of the vagotomy and partial gastrectomy costs and the non-surgical costs were adjusted upward for inflation through 1978, giving the figures of Table 10.

This shows that if the surgical candidate does not enter the hospital at all, $4874 is saved. If he enters but avoids surgery, $2799 is saved. Recall from Table 9 that in Rhode Island about ten operations per 100 000 population were avoided in 1978 after the introduction of cimetidine. If this rate is directly applied to the United States population of about 215 million people the figures in Table 11 emerge.

We calculate a saving of about $104 million if hospitalization for surgery candidates is avoided altogether and about $60 million if they are hospitalized with only medical treatment. The Rhode Island research group was able to make some refinements in the projection by adjusting for Rhode Island's higher per capita share of health expenditures versus the United States average. The more accurate national projections of cost savings

Table 10. Charges per Hospital Stay in Rhode Island (in dollars)

		Routine plus ancillary charges	Surgery physicians' fees	Total
With partial gastrectomy or vagotomy (weighted average)	1976	3252	674	3926
	1978[a]	4081	793	4874
Ulcer and ulcer-related without ulcer surgery	1976	1654	—	1654
	1978[a]	2075	—	2075
Savings of admission avoiding ulcer surgery	1978	2006	793	2799

[a] Inflation from 1976 to 1978: routine plus ancillary charges = +25.5% (R.I. Blue Cross average daily hospitalization costs); surgery physician's fee = +17.7% (physician services, consumer price index)

are shown as about \$97 million and \$59 million. The lower figure might be termed a worst case for 1978. For 1980, the range is \$82 million to \$135 million.

Finally, we turn again to data from the Netherlands. Table 12 shows the reductions in days and guilders resulting from the reduced operations in that country. The reductions are separated into those explained by trend and by cimetidine. Using cost and fee schedules in the Netherlands, Dr Bulthuis has translated the days into the costs shown (Bulthius, 1981). We see that the cost reduction contributed by cimetidine comes to 10 million guilders in 1978 and 1979 together. Drug costs for treating ulcer were increased by 5.5 million, leaving a net reduction in ulcer treatment costs contributed by cimetidine of 4.5 million guilders. Dr Bulthuis' conclusion is that new technologies in health do not necessarily increase treatment costs. More importantly, perhaps, his analysis shows what can be learned from multiple regression analysis when sufficient data are available. In a sense, he shows what must be learned if we are to put the obvious purchase or reimbursement costs of a technological innovation into the

Table 11. Projection of Rhode Island Savings to National United States Population

	US population	= 215 000 000
	÷ 100 000	= 2150
	× ten operations avoided per 100 000	= 21 500
	× \$4874 saved if no admission	= \$104 791 000
or	× \$2799 saved if admission but no surgery	= \$60 178 500

Adjusted for Rhode Island versus US per capita expenditures on hospital and physician services:

\$104 791 000 → \$97 175 500

\$60 178 500 → \$59 162 500

Table 12. Contribution of Factors in the Netherlands Responsible for the Decreasing Importance of Hospitalization Costs among the Total Costs of Peptic Ulcer (million guilders)

(1) Decrease in number of hospitalizations since 1972:

(a) Due to trend, *non-operated*: 85 500 days = 22.0

(b) Due to trend, *Operated*: 37 500 days = 10.8

Due to cimetidine, *Operated*: 30 000 days = 8.7

Total operated 19.5

Subtotal 41.5

(2) Decrease of operation costs (not included under (a) and (b) above)

Due to trend 0.8

Due to cimetidine 1.2

2.0

Total 43.5

Overall due to trend	33.5
Due to cimetidine	10.0
Drug costs	−5.5
	4.5 million guilders

perspective of the much less obvious cost reductions it may cause.

The final data presented are unique. They come from the computerized reimbursement records of Michigan Medicaid, the state's health care program for the poor and disabled, and were analysed by the eminent American health economist, Dr Burton Weisbrod of the University of Wisconsin, along with his colleague, Dr John Geweke. They have been submitted for publication (Geweke and Weisbrod, 1981). The Medicaid records are invaluable, since they show all treatment events and costs as they occur for each patient in the program. Drs Weisbrod and Geweke constructed an experiment retrospectively after the marketing of cimetidine. They compared all ulcer-related costs of cimetidine-treated patients with those of ulcer patients not treated with cimetidine, that is, treated traditionally.

The costs were counted starting with a duodenal ulcer episode and continuing for the remaining months of the patient year. Now, comparing two such groups after they have manifested themselves naturally in the community can be faulty and very misleading, because the cimetidine and the traditional treatment were obviously not assigned at random. Unlike the case of most clinical trials, selectivity bias will almost certainly arise. In fact, the researchers found that cimetidine was given to the more severe patients, that is, those who had histories of much higher reimbursement costs prior to the initiation of cimetidine. Obviously, a meaningful comparison must be based on equally severe or costly cases in each treatment group. Therefore, Weisbrod and Geweke controlled for severity by regression analysis, meaning in this instance adjusting treatment cost averages for the two groups to start out equal. Their findings may be displayed as in Fig. 13. The horizontal axis shows

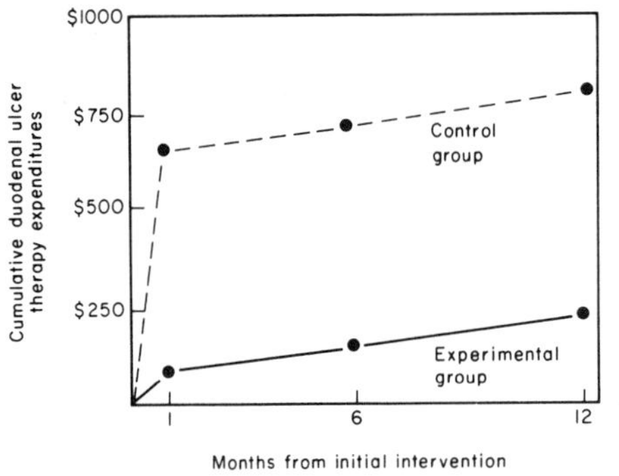

Figure 13. Average annual Michigan Medicaid expenditures per patient with duodenal ulcer, by month of expenditure.

Table 13

Estimated reductions in rate of surgical/ physician intervention (%)	Savings per capita (cimetidine and non-cimetidine) (patients) in duodenal ulcer related care	
	$	%
Pessimistic (19.5)	68	9.4
Best guess (39.0)	187	26.0
Optimistic (69.5)	375	51.9

the twelve months following onset of the duodenal ulcer episode, and the vertical axis shows cumulative treatment costs for the average patient over the twelve months. The broken line shows the traditionally treated patients, the solid line the cimetidine patients. The difference at the end of the year is $500. This is due mainly to reduced hospitalization costs among the cimetidine patients, as Fig. 14 illustrates.

As all the data seen so far would have predicted, hospital charges are much lower among the cimetidine patients. The researchers have not yet focused on reduced admissions, surgery and lengths of stay so as to present just where the hospital savings are generated; but fewer hospital days per average patient were observed for the cimetidine group. Also, the first month of the patient's episode is critical, since it is then that many cimetidine-treated patients avoided hospitalization altogether.

Note also that physician costs are lower for the average cimetidine patient, and that drug costs are higher. One *caveat*, however, is that Michigan Medicaid does not reimburse antacids, the only widely used alternative to cimetidine in the United States. If antacids were included at recommended doses, the $10 drug costs for the non-cimetidine patient would be at least $50 higher, and somewhat higher for the cimetidine patient, who may well take some antacids in the early days of the episode. Finally, in a sensitivity analysis (Table 13), the researchers calculate what the total net savings per duodenal ulcer patient would be if various reductions in the frequency of surgical and physician intervention were achieved.

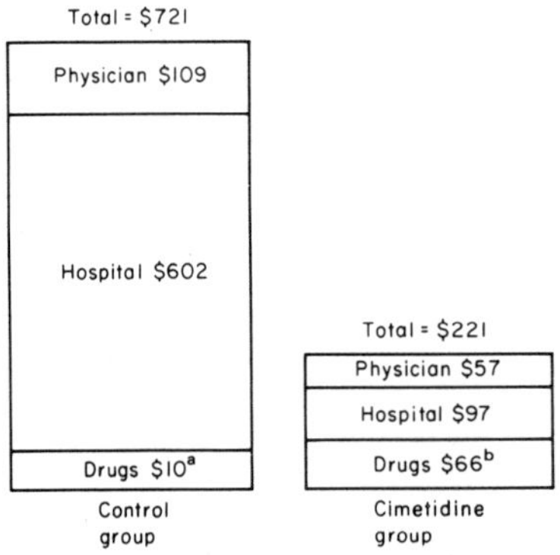

Figure 14. Average annual Michigan Medicaid expenditures per patient with duodenal ulcer. [a]Does not include antacids which are excluded from Michigan Medicaid; [b] includes cost of cimetidine therapy.

We see that in the pessimistic case $68 in treatment costs are saved for every duodenal ulcer patient in the Medicaid program. This is net, with the cimetidine costs included. Actually, a reduction in frequency of surgical intervention among the cimetidine-treated patients would seem to fall between 39% and 69.5%. This is because we have observed in the trend-analysis data shown earlier an overall average reduction in ulcer surgery of about 25% below the expected trend line. This, of course, represents entire populations, including both cimetidine and non-cimetidine patients. If a 25% reduction is seen for both groups together, then the reduction for the cimetidine group alone must be higher than 25%. If cimetidine over the trend periods studied was used in half the duodenal ulcer patients, then a 50% reduction in surgery among the cimetidine patients would produce the 25% reduction below trend that we have seen in the time-series data. Therefore, perhaps a $250 savings per patient has been realized in the entire duodenal ulcer population – representing the present writer's extrapolation from the Weisbrod–Geweke findings. In any case, let us conclude with a quote from the researchers:

> The empirical results show that treatment with cimetidine is an expenditure reducing alternative compared to previously existing therapeutic intervention . . . The approach used . . . shows the new technology to reduce expenditures by some 70 percent . . . even our more conservative approach predicts expenditure savings attributable to cimetidine.

CONCLUSION

To summarize, the reduction in surgery-related hospitalization costs due to cimetidine use in ulcer disease has ranged from about 10 million guilders over two years to 43 million francs in one year to $135 million per year. From these some increase in drug costs needs to be subtracted; however, from the Dutch and the Weisbrod–Geweke data, the final result shows a net reduction, or savings, in total treatment costs.

Though a businessman and market researcher, not an academic economist, the writer cannot resist speculating on some implications for society of the data we have seen. First, it is not only sick people and their families who have benefited from the innovation under analysis. Everyone else, insofar as they pay taxes or medical insurance premiums, ultimately benefits through lowered, or less increased, total treatment costs. Second, net benefits from a new drug are not unprecedented. To quote von Grebmer (1981) citing Stahl: 'Within the available factors of production for health (e.g., hospital care, physicians' services, medical therapy) the highest productivity increases have originated and will originate from technological advances in drug therapy.' Third, how will this continue so that society obtains for itself the benefits in such areas as cardiovascular disease, cancer and arthritis that cimetidine provided in ulcer disease? The author believes that the most efficient way is through continued investment by industry in the research and development of new chemical entities against disease. We have seen how that worked with cimetidine. Fourth, most Western economists would probably find it elementary that the inducement to intensive drug R & D is the expectation of profit.

What is not widely understood is that the profit on some individual products must be high to offset those new chemical entities which after marketing never repay their R & D investment. Recent data (Joglekar *et al.*, to be published) show that of the new chemical entities introduced in the United States since 1963, two out of three have not sold enough worldwide to repay capitalized R & D costs of the average marketable new entity – some $54 million dollars as of 1978 (Hansen, 1979). Thus the only thing that makes new drug R & D an acceptable gamble – for a large firm able to afford it – is the chance of a 'big winner'.

Fifth, and last (and on admittedly treacherous ground), what might the savings in total treatment cost, such as those from cimetidine use in ulcer disease, mean for the price of the drug producing those savings? Just posing the question raises the possibility, at least, that if we seek efficiency in producing health for a population over a long run, we should accept the notion that some of the savings produced by the drug should be channeled back to the innovator. The probability of that happening, in the case of an innovative firm hovering on the brink of more or less drug R & D, could induce a $54 million investment that otherwise would not occur. Let us reverse things. At one early point the H_2 research program which produced cimetidine was almost shut down; there were limits on research expenditure. The large market for the specific product, cimetidine, was not obvious at that stage. Would the research expenditure have continued if the innovating firm had believed that the price of cimetidine would be held down to that of pre-existing products, many of them generic? Apparently, there is no straightforward economic law telling how much, if any, of the savings realized should go to the innovator – so as to incite the maximum amount of future benefit for society at the lowest possible cost – but the expense and risk of drug R & D and the need for 'big winners' to finance it make it reasonable for economic and political leaders to recognize the possibility of the future innovator sharing equitably in any savings he may generate.

REFERENCES

G. Bodemar and A. Walan (1978). Maintenance treatment of recurrent peptic ulcer by cimetidine. *Lancet* (25 February).

R. Bulthuis, *et al.* (1977). *Present Cost of Peptic Ulceration to the Dutch Economy and Possible Impact of Cimetidine on this Cost.* Netherlands Economic Institute, Rotterdam.

R. Bulthuis (1981). Medicines for health care? *Economisch Statistische Berichten* 66e Jargang, No. 3298 (25 March), Rotterdam.

R. Bulthuis (1981). Surgery trends and costs of peptic ulcer disease in the Netherlands before and after the introduction of cimetidine. Proceedings of NEI–SKF Symposium, Amsterdam, March.

V. Chandler and G. von Haunalter (1977). *The Cost of Ulcer Disease in the United States.* Stanford Research Institute, Menlo Park, Cal.

H. Fineberg and L. A. Pearlman (1981). Surgical treatment of peptic ulcer in the United States. *Lancet* (13 June).

R. W. Hansen (1979). The pharmaceutical development process: estimate of current development costs and times and the effects of regulatory changes, in *Issues in Pharmaceutical Economics,* ed. by R. I. Chien, Lexington Books.

P. Joglekar, *et al.* Investment in the research and development of new chemical entities: the risks and returns. Manuscript in preparation.

J. Norton, *et al.* (1980). *The Effect of Cimetidine on Peptic Ulcer Disease in Rhode Island.* Rhode Island Health Services Research, Inc., Providence, R. I. The 1980 data are from an update report of 26 May 1982.

M. Olitsky, *et al.* (1978). *The Impact of Cimetidine on the National Cost of Duodenal Ulcers.* Robinson Associates, Inc., Bryn Mawr, Pa.

R. Ricardo–Campbell and W. Wardell, *et al.* (1980). Preliminary methodology for controlled cost-benefit study of drug impact: the effect of cimetidine on days of work lost in a short-term trial in duodenal ulcer. *J. Clin. Gastroenterol.* **2,** 37–41.

C. W. Venables (1981). Surgery and hospitalization trends in

the United Kingdom before and after cimetidine. Proceedings of NEI–SKF Symposium, Amsterdam, March.
K. von Grebmer (1981). Competition in a structurally changing pharmaceutical market: some health economic considerations. *Soc. Sci. Med.* **15C,** 77–86.
B. Weisbrod and J. Geweke (1981). Assessing technological change: the case of a new drug. To be published. Used with permission of the authors.
M. Wylie (1981). The complex wane of peptic ulcer. I. Recent national trends in deaths and hospital care in the United States. II. Trends in duodenal and gastric ulcer admissions to 790 hospitals, 1974–1979. *J. Clin. Gastroenterol.* **3,** 327–39.
J. Wyllie, *et al.* (1981). Effect of cimetidine on surgery for duodenal ulcer. *Lancet* (13 June).
Y. Lambert (1980). *Trend in Ulcer Surgery, Gastrointestinal Hemorrhages, Appendectomies and Cholecystectomies 1976–1979.* Lambert–Yves Conseil, LaGarenne, France.

Institute for Health Policy Studies
University of California, San Francisco
1326 Third Avenue
San Francisco, CA 94143
(415) 666-4921

Major Emphases of Technology Assessment Activities

Technology	Concerns: Safety	Efficacy/ Effectiveness	Cost/Cost-Effect/ Cost-Benefit	Ethical/Legal/ Social
Drugs		X	X	X
Medical Devices/Equipment/Supplies		X	X	X
Medical/Surgical Procedures		X	X	X
Support Systems		X	X	X
Organizational/Administrative		X	X	X

Stage of Technologies Assessed
_X_ Emerging/new
_X_ Accepted use
____ Possibly obsolete, outmoded

Application of Technologies
_X_ Prevention
_X_ Diagnosis/screening
_X_ Treatment
____ Rehabilitation

Assessment Methods
____ Laboratory testing
____ Clinical trials
_X_ Epidemiological and other observational methods
_X_ Cost analyses
_X_ Simulation/modeling
____ Group judgment
_X_ Expert opinion
_X_ Literature syntheses

Approximate 1985 budget for technology assessment: $700,000*

* The total Institute budget for the period is approximately $2.5 million. Of this, about 40 percent is devoted to training fellowships. Approximately $700,000 is devoted to assessment of medical technologies, and the remainder is devoted to other health-related studies.

INSTITUTE FOR HEALTH POLICY STUDIES UNIVERSITY OF CALIFORNIA, SAN FRANCISCO

Introduction

The Institute for Health Policy Studies (IHPS) is an academic and research unit of the University of California, San Francisco (UCSF). IHPS was formerly known as the Health Policy Program.

IHPS was established in 1972 within the UCSF School of Medicine. The Institute consists of an interdisciplinary group of faculty members representing medicine, government, education, law, sociology, pharmacology, journalism, and philosophy and ethics. When established, IHPS was the only organized health policy group in the nation based within a university health sciences campus, according to UCSF-IHPS.

From 1972 through 1977, IHPS developed its capacity to conduct independent policy analysis and policy research and to provide technical assistance, primarily to federal and state policymakers, with a major emphasis on health manpower policies; prescription drug policies; ethical issues in health care; long-term care issues; and planning, regulation, and financing issues. IHPS also began to engage in health services research, focusing on the cost of illness and health care, the use and cost of medical technologies, and group practice and prepaid health care settings. A program of education and training for faculty and students in the health professions, law, ethics, economics, planning, public policy, and other disciplines also was developed during this period. The major initial sources of support were UCSF and the Robert Wood Johnson Foundation. Additional support was provided by federal contracts and grants from the Veteran's Administration, the National Center for Health Services Research, the Bureau of Health Planning and Resources Development, and the Health Resources Administration, as well as grants from a number of private foundations.

In 1977, IHPS was awarded a 5-year grant (through April 1983) from the National Center for Health Services Research as the first national Health Services Policy Analysis Center. This grant supported the creation of a strong multidisciplinary group of faculty whose focus was on health policy issues. The Institute was formally designated as an Organizational Research Unit within the School of Medicine, UCSF, in 1982, and officially changed its name from the Health Policy Program to IHPS. IHPS has formal linkages with schools and departments on the UCSF campus, the UCSF hospitals and clinics, the University of California, Berkeley, and the University of California, San Diego.

Purpose

The IHPS has a threefold purpose. First, IHPS provides opportunities in education and training for students and practitioners in the health professions; for students and faculty in other disciplines (e.g., law, economics, sociology, bioethics, planning); and for policymakers, program managers, and others in the field of health. To accomplish this purpose, IHPS develops formal courses for students in the UCSF schools of medicine, nursing, pharmacy, and dentistry; offers training opportunities through fellowships and internships; forms collaborative education and training programs with other institutions; and develops seminars and other educational experiences for individuals and special groups in the health field.

Second, health services research and policy analysis projects are undertaken by Institute faculty in a variety of areas, including the costs of health care, long-term care and chronic illness, health policies and the aged, technology assessment, and reproductive health.

Third, IHPS provides informed advice to federal and state governments and other policymaking bodies on ways of improving the effectiveness and efficiency of health care delivery systems. This profile primarily addresses this aspect of IHPS.

Subjects of Assessment

IHPS is primarily interested in topics of health services research. In recent years, IHPS's priority areas in research and policy analysis have been health maintenance organizations (HMOs) and other organized health care delivery systems, cost containment, impact of medical technology on health care, ethical issues in health care, reproductive health policy, health policies and the aged, child health policies, prescription drug policies, health manpower policies, health planning, health promotion, and disease prevention, and health care for disadvantaged persons. Table A-15 lists the more than 60 research and analysis projects, including major research programs, initiated during the period 1977–1983.

Stage of Diffusion

IHPS addresses new, emerging, and widely accepted technologies and modalities of health services delivery.

TABLE A-15 University of California, San Francisco, Institute for Health Policy Studies Project Listing, 1977–1983

Analysis of the Trends in the Number and Distribution of Pediatricians and Family and General Practitioners in the United States between 1976 and 1979
Assessment of Long-Term Social Outcomes of Total Hip Replacement
Changes in Medical Technology Use Over Time
Child Health Policy
Childhood Chronic Illness: Trends and Determinants
Chronic Disease Care Among Different Specialties
Commonweal-Institute Joint Research Project
Competition and Complementarity in Hospital Services
Competitive and Selection Effects of HMOs
Competitive Impact of Prepaid Medical Plans in California
Correlates of Long-Term Care Expenditure and Service Utilization
Cost and Epidemiology of Catastrophic Illness
Costs and Effectiveness of Neonatal Intensive Care
Costs and Effectiveness of Nurse Practitioners
Costs and Effectiveness of Upper Gastrointestinal Endoscopy
Cost-Effectiveness of Perinatal Access and Obstetrical Access Programs
Determinants of Health
A Diagnosis Study of Utilization Patterns
Drugs and the Elderly
East Bay Hospital Perinatal Study
The Effects of Selective Regulation on Competition in the Long-Term Care Industry
Evaluation of New California Health Insurance Laws
Exercise and the Elderly
The Growth and Utilization of Intensive Care Units
Health Factors Affecting Long-Term Care Policy
Health Maintenance Organizations: Dimensions of Performance
Health Policy and the Aged, Including Long-Term Care
Health Promotion/Disease Prevention
HMOs: The California Experience
Hospital Cost Containment
Hospital Reimbursement: Diagnostic-Related Groups
Incidence of Upper Gastrointestinal Endoscopy
Income and Health
An Inpatient Hospice at Moffitt Hospital: A Feasibility Study
Laguna Honda Project
Long-Term Care: Impact of State Discretionary Policies
Long-Term Care: Implications for California's State Discretionary Policies
Low Income and Health
Medical Care Expenditures in the Last 12 Months of Life
Medical Care Use Under Two Prepaid Plans
Medical Cost Changes of Selected Illnesses, 1971–1981
Multiple Risk Factor Intervention Trial
National Service Health Care Study
Nutrition and the Elderly
Planning and Regulation Research
Poverty and Health
Prescription Drug Policy: Drug Coverage Under National Health Insurance
Prescription Drugs in the Third World
Prescription Drugs: Regulation, Pricing, Cost Containment, Promotion, Irrational Prescribing
Program for the Humane Care of the Dying Patient
Program in Reproductive Health Policy
Refugee Health Services/Refugee Health Manpower
Relationship Between Surgical Volumes and Mortality
Research and Analysis of Health Manpower Issues
Retailing of Health Care Services
Role of Out-of-Pocket Costs in Selection of Health Insurance by University of California Employees
Role of Pharmacy in Health Care in Jamaica
Selection and Competitive Effects of Health Maintenance Organizations
Social Isolation as a Predictor of Hip Fractures
State and Local Long-Term Care Policy Project
A Study of Differences in the Care of Arthritis in HMOs and Fee-for-Service
A Study of the Interactions Between Health Planning Agencies and Area Agencies on Aging in Meeting the Health Needs of the Elderly
Synthesis of Research Findings on the Operations and Performance of Health Maintenance Organizations
Systolic Hypertension in the Elderly Project
Third-Party Methods of Paying Physicians
Why Do the Chronically Ill Stop Working?

Concerns

Most of the Institute's technology-related projects are concerned with effectiveness; cost-effectiveness and other cost-related issues; and certain social, ethical, and legal implications of technologies.

Requests

From 1977 through 1983, IHPS faculty and research staff responded to approximately 800 documented requests for technical assistance. Nearly half of the requests were from federal policymakers or their staffs. IHPS receives requests for information and assistance from foundations, professional organizations and societies, health provider groups and associations, hospitals, employers, unions, insurance companies, universities, health service research centers, consumer groups, advocacy organizations, voluntary associations, and the media. Policymakers from countries outside the United States also seek information and technical assistance.

Federal government recipients of technical assistance have included Congress, Executive Office of the President, Department of Health and Human Services, and the Federal Trade Commission. California governmental recipients of technical assistance have included the state legislature, Office of the Governor, and Health and Welfare Agency. Other technical assistance recipients have included California county and municipal governments, other states, and policymakers in countries outside the United States.

Selection

Selection of projects is generally made by individual faculty and staff members. Projects undertaken must be within a faculty/staff members' area of interest, consistent with the purposes of the IHPS, and subject to university policies regarding grants, contracts, and other arrangements with outside parties.

Process

The wide variety of studies conducted by IHPS include literature syntheses, cost-effectiveness and cost-benefit analyses, and epidemiological studies. Through its formal relationships with other university institutions, IHPS has access to clinical data for study. For instance, in a study of changes from 1972 to 1977 in the use of medical technologies for 10 inpatient diagnoses, IHPS used automated billing data from the UCSF hospital, a 560-bed teaching facility (Showstack et al., 1982).

Assessors

IHPS has approximately 30 faculty members and 28 affiliated faculty, over 20 full-time research staff, approximately 40 predoctoral and postdoctoral fellows and visiting scholars, and approximately 20 full-time support staff. This multidisciplinary staff represents the fields of law, pharmacology, philosophy and ethics, medicine, economics, public policy and administration, planning, statistics, sociology, epidemiology, political science, medical anthropology, and medical information sciences. Many IHPS faculty members have educational responsibilities in addition to their research and analysis activities. As an Organizational Research Unit, IHPS offers joint academic appointments, with the primary appointment in an academic department, such as the Department of Medicine.

Turnaround

The turnaround time varies according to the type of study conducted or other assistance provided. For instance, the case studies on various technologies conducted for the Congressional Office of Technology Assessment took approximately 6 months to complete. Responses to requests for technical assistance may take from 1 day to several weeks, and formal health services research projects are often 2 to 3 years long.

Reporting

Reporting of IHPS findings and related health policy issues is directed to three major audiences: federal and state policymakers, the health services research and health policy research communities, and the general public. From 1977 to 1983, UCSF-IHPS faculty and research staff published 14 books, 15 monographs, 61 book chapters, and 129 journal articles. The journals in which reports of IHPS studies have appeared include the *American Journal of Public Health*, *Annals of Internal Medicine*, *Health Care Financing Review*, *Journal of Health Politics, Policy and Law*, *Medical Care*, *Milbank Memorial Fund Quarterly/Health and Society*, and *New England Journal of Medicine*. IHPS staff have prepared case studies for the Congressional Office of Technology Assessment on the cost-effectiveness of upper gastrointestinal endoscopy (OTA, 1981a), neonatal intensive care (OTA, 1981b), and nurse practitioners (OTA, 1981c). IHPS has its own special publications series and periodicals, including the following:

- *Courses by Newspaper* project on "The Nation's Health" included a 15-part series of newspaper articles, a textbook, a study guide, and examination materials. In 1981, the course was presented on a weekly basis in 362 newspapers and 190 colleges and universities in the United States. These materials are to be re-released to newspapers and other institutions which did not carry the project in 1981.
- *IHPS Report* is the IHPS semiannual newsletter, circulated to more than 1,500 individuals and institutions.
- *HMO Dissemination Project* of 1979–1983 synthesized research findings on the operations and performance of HMOs and communicated these in a series of five regional workshops.
- *Research Highlights* is a quarterly newsletter produced by the IHPS Center for Population and Health Policy.
- *Mobius* is a quarterly journal (circulation 1,000) of continuing education for health science professionals published by the University of California Press.

IHPS has sponsored and cosponsored a number of conferences, mostly in California, on a variety of topics including drug regulation reform, health insurance reform, cost-benefit and cost-effectiveness methods, high-cost illnesses, caring for the terminally ill, and bioethics.

Impact

It is difficult to measure directly the impact of IHPS activities, because IHPS acts as an analytic and advisory body, as opposed to a policymaking body. Results of health services research and policy analysis projects have had wide circulation through publication in peer-reviewed journals and are often cited by other investigators. Technical assistance and policy analyses provided by IHPS have been used in augmenting and guiding legislative efforts and various policy changes.

The primary users of IHPS technical assistance (as measured by the volume of requests answered by IHPS) have been Congress and congressional offices, the Executive Office of the President, the Department of Health and Human Services, and the Federal Trade Commission. For these and other federal agencies, IHPS analyses have contributed to research agendas and policy options in such areas as prescription drugs, health manpower, health promotion and disease prevention, and health planning and regulation. For instance, in the area of prescription drugs, IHPS contributed to analyses of provisions of the Drug Regulation Reform Acts of 1978 and 1979, drug approval processes and drug regulation policies in foreign countries, export of drugs unapproved for use in the United States, generic drugs, drug repackaging houses, drug coverage under Medicare and Medicaid, use of drugs by outpatients to minimize hospitalization, physician education in the area of drug prescription, over-the-counter drugs, federal vaccine and immunization policies, drug labeling and drug promotion, development of drugs for rare diseases, and drugs and the elderly.

For the state of California, IHPS provided analyses of MediCal reform options, the impact of prepaid medical care plans, health and social service policy options in long-term care, the cost-effectiveness of perinatal care, and other areas. The health provider community—individual providers, institutions, and service programs—have benefited from IHPS technical assistance, information, and educational programs.

The expansion of IHPS research and analysis activities has augmented its role in education and training. For instance, what began as a small series of weekend workshops in bioethics offered by IHPS has grown into a bioethics teaching program for medical students and others on the UCSF campus. IHPS faculty have developed some 20 courses in health policy and related areas for students on the UCSF and University of California, Berkeley, campuses. The newly required fourth-year medical school course "Responsibilities of Medical Practice," with content in ethical, legal, economic, and social issues, is designed to prompt in medical students a greater awareness of the broad personal and social responsibilities of medical practice and to encourage more responsible and conscientious exercise of medical skills. IHPS has been instrumental in several major developments in academic programs at UCSF, including the establishment of the Division of General Internal Medicine; the Division of Medical Ethics; the Aging Health Policy Center; and postgraduate programs in health policy research, health policy management, and clinical epidemiology. As an Organizational Research Unit of the University of California, IHPS has an advisory board that meets periodically to review IHPS activities and offer advice on future directions.

Reassessment

IHPS has not yet reassessed any technology.

Funding/Budget

The 1985 budget of the IHPS is approximately $2,500,000. Of this amount, about 40 percent is devoted to training fellowships and is funded primarily by foundations. The remaining 60 percent is devoted to health services and other technology assessment efforts and is funded by foundations and federal and state governments.

Example

The following summarizes a recently completed study of changes in the use of medical technologies in hospitals. This work, to be submitted for publication, follows up on a similar study (see J. Showstack et al. [1982]).

CHANGES IN THE USE OF MEDICAL TECHNOLOGIES: 1972, 1977, 1982

To assess the degree to which the use of medical technologies have changed over time, and the impact of these changes on the costs of medical care, IHPS studied patients admitted to the UCSF hospital over the past decade. Patients discharged during 1972, 1977, or 1982 who had one of the following ten diagnoses were studied: acute asthma, acute myocardial infarction, lung cancer, respiratory distress syndrome of the newborn, cataract excision, delivery (both cesarean and vaginal), kidney transplant, stapedectomy, and total hip replacement. Data were collected from medical and billing records. The principal findings of the study were that the use of older technologies (such as x rays) changed little over the first half of the decade, and length of stay tended to decrease, while the use of newer diagnostic technologies increased substantially. Later in the decade, some substitution of newer for older technologies was observed. The most cost-increasing changes were the use of surgery for certain conditions that would have previously been treated medically and increasingly aggressive care for critically ill patients. This project received funding from the Henry J. Kaiser Family Foundation and the National Center for Health Services Research.

Sources

Lee, P. R., Professor of Social Medicine, Institute for Health Policy Studies, University of California, San Francisco. 1984. Personal communication.

Office of Technology Assessment. 1981a. The Cost Effectiveness of Upper Gastrointestinal Endoscopy. Case Study #8. Washington, D.C.: U.S. Government Printing Office.

Office of Technology Assessment. 1981b. The Costs and Effectiveness of Neonatal Intensive Care. Case

Study #10. Washington, D.C.: U.S. Government Printing Office.

Office of Technology Assessment. 1981c. The Costs and Effectiveness of Nurse Practitioners. Case Study #16. Washington, D.C.: U.S. Government Printing Office.

Showstack, J., Coordinator of Research and Policy Analysis, Institute for Health Policy Studies, University of California, San Francisco. 1985. Personal communication.

Showstack, J. A., S. A. Schroeder, and M. F. Matsumoto. 1982. Changes in the use of medical technologies, 1972–1977: A study of 10 inpatient diagnoses. New England Journal of Medicine 306:706–712.

University of California, San Francisco Institute for Health Policy Studies, School of Medicine. 1983. Health Services Policy Analysis Center—Final Report submitted to the National Center for Health Services Research.

Cooperative Studies Program
Veterans Administration (151I)
810 Vermont Ave., N.W.
Washington, DC 20420
(202) 389-2861

Major Emphases of Technology Assessment Activities

Technology	Concerns: Safety	Efficacy/ Effectiveness	Cost/Cost-Effect/ Cost-Benefit	Ethical/Legal/ Social
Drugs	X	X	X	
Medical Devices/Equipment/Supplies	X	X	X	
Medical/Surgical Procedures	X	X	X	
Support Systems				
Organizational/Administrative				

Stage of Technologies Assessed
_X_ Emerging/new
____ Accepted use
____ Possibly obsolete, outmoded

Application of Technologies
____ Prevention
_X_ Diagnosis/screening
_X_ Treatment
____ Rehabilitation

Assessment Methods
____ Laboratory testing
_X_ Clinical trials
____ Epidemiological and other observational methods
____ Cost analyses
____ Simulation/modeling
____ Group judgment
____ Expert opinion
____ Literature syntheses

Approximate 1985 budget for technology assessment: $12,000,000*

* The 1985 budget for the CSP is approximately $12 million. However, this does not reflect the full cost of the cooperative studies. This amount is primarily for support of the CSP coordinating centers and other nonclinical aspects of the cooperative studies. The clinical cost of these trials is met entirely through VA medical benefits, and is not reflected in the CSP budget.

COOPERATIVE STUDIES PROGRAM VETERANS ADMINISTRATION

Introduction

The Veterans Administration (VA) extends to eligible veterans free or highly subsidized health care services, including hospital, ambulatory, and nursing home care. The VA provides most of its care at its 172 hospital centers, where it also operates outpatient clinics and 101 nursing home units. In 1983, total medical care outlays for the VA system were $8.3 billion. The VA annually assists about 3 million veteran patients, including about 1.4 million inpatients.

The VA has three major research and development services and several activities addressing technology assessment. The VA devoted about $164 million in FY 1984 to research and development activities conducted in the Medical Research Service ($148 million), the Rehabilitation Research and

Development Service ($11 million), and the Health Services Research and Development Service ($5 million). The Rehabilitation Research and Development Evaluation Unit evaluates rehabilitative devices arising from VA research and encourages their production and distribution by private industry. The VA Health Services Research and Development Service supports and conducts evaluations of alternative policies and interventions of care. The VA Supply Service evaluates new equipment for safety and effectiveness for procurement by VA facilities. In 1984, the VA instituted a Technology Assessment Committee to make recommendations to the VA medical director regarding priority technologies for assessment, appropriate assessment methods, and purchasing and deployment of technologies, to track assessment activities of other agencies, and to coordinate these and other agency-wide assessment activities. In 1982 the VA initiated a Prosthetics Technology Evaluation Committee to coordinate the evaluation of VA prosthetic products and devices.

The VA Cooperative Studies Program (CSP) was established in 1972 in the VA Medical Research Service to provide coordination and support for multicenter medical studies that fall within the purview of the Medical Research Service, the Rehabilitation Research and Development Service, and the Health Services Research and Development Service. CSP is involved only in trials requiring participation of more than one VA medical center. The VA conducts other clinical trials in single centers, and the VA is involved in trials funded by other sources, such as NIH and pharmaceutical companies. The VA spent approximately $20 million on clinical trials in 1984, including $11.3 million for the Cooperative Studies Program.

Purpose

Cooperative studies enable investigators from two or more VA medical centers to study collectively a selected problem in a uniform manner, using a common protocol with central coordination.

The multicenter approach of the VA cooperative studies facilitates the accumulation of patient samples that are sufficiently large to provide valid significant findings regarding medical technologies. For medical conditions that are relatively rare, cooperative studies may be the only feasible approach; for other more common conditions, these studies enable accumulation of data more rapidly by pooling the observations of several facilities.

The VA is an especially useful environment for multicenter trials because it has a relatively uniform and large patient base under one management. This enables uniformity of research methodology, adherence to common protocols, patient follow-up, and fiscal management of large trials. Of course, the VA is a most appropriate setting for research that addresses medical problems of the veteran population.

Subjects of Assessment

The technologies assessed in the cooperative studies are drugs, medical devices, and medical and surgical procedures. These reflect the medical problems of the veteran population. Of the ongoing and recently completed studies, the greatest number treat cardiovascular diseases. Other important areas are alcohol-related diseases and dental and mental conditions. Other trials treat acute infectious diseases, diabetes, epilepsy, and conditions associated with disabling injuries. The largest number of studies have tested drug therapies, followed by those testing surgical procedures. Most studies have addressed therapeutic technologies, although a few have focused on prevention of cardiovascular disease through control of hypertension. A total of 81 VA cooperative studies have been conducted since the program's inception, including those ongoing in 1985. Table A-16 lists the subjects of VA cooperative studies.

Stage of Diffusion

Cooperative studies are generally conducted for new technologies that have been subject to preliminary trials in humans.

TABLE A-16 Subjects of Veterans Administration Cooperative Studies (listed by status as of January 1985)

Studies Approved by Medical Research "Triage" Review and Currently in Active Planning

Hepatitis B Vaccine in Patients with Chronic Renal Failure
Percutaneous Transluminal Coronary Angioplasty
Reflux Esophagitis Complicated by Barrett's Esophagus: A Prospective Randomized Trial of Medical and Surgical Therapies
Treatment of Lymphatic Neoplasms Directed by *In Vitro* Chemo-Sensitivity Testing
Toluidine Blue Rinse as a Screening Agent for Detection of Asymptomatic Mucosal Carcinoma
A Double Blinded Randomized Comparison of Nitrendipine with a Diuretic or a Beta Blocker in Mild Hypertension
Natural History of Bronchitis & Emphysema: Predictive Value of Small Airway Tests & Effect of Smoking Cessation
Therapy of Primary Amyloidosis

Studies Approved But Not Yet Funded

Early Detection of Hearing Loss Due to Ototoxic Agents by High Frequency Auditory Evaluation
Decapeptyl in Advanced Prostatic Cancer
The Efficacy of Oral Physostigmine in Alzheimer Disease and Senile Dementia of the Alzheimer Type
Treatment of Specific Types of Status Epilepticus
Vasodilators Used in Chronic Heart Failure-II
A Randomized Study of Prostatic Surgery for Benign Prostatic Hyperplasia in Elderly Men
Protein-Calorie Therapy in Combination with Anabolic Steroids in Alcoholic Hepatitis-II
Primary Treatment of Esophageal Carcinoma

Ongoing Cooperative Studies

Clinical Evaluation of Two New Dental Alloy Systems Used in the Fabrication of Fixed Crown and Bridge Restoration (NIDR-VA)
Coronary Artery Surgery I Stable Angina (Vein Bypass)
Coronary Artery Surgery II Unstable Angina (Vein Bypass)
Dental Implants (Removable vs. Permanent Dentures)
Vasodilators Used in Chronic Heart Failure
Evaluation of Specific & Cross-Protective Immunity in High Risk (Renal Insufficiency, Alcoholic Hepatic Insufficiency & Elderly) Patients Following Pneumococcal Capsular Polysaccharide Vaccine
Percutaneous Transluminal Angioplasty in the Lower Extremity
Evaluations of Corticosteroids Therapy in Severe Sepsis
Asymptomatic Carotid Stenosis: Etiological Importance in Development of Stroke
Randomized Clinical Trial of Total Parenteral Nutrition in Malnourished Surgical Patients
Lithium Treatment in Alcohol Dependence
Treatment of Depression Collaborative (NIMH-VA) Research Program
Prognosis & Outcome Following Heart Valve Replacement (Non-Biological vs. Tissue)
Clinical Comparison of Base Metal Alloys vs. a Gold Alloy Used in the Fabrication of Fixed (Crown & Bridge) Restorations
Anticoagulants in the Treatment of Cancer
Spontaneous Pneumothorax
Antiplatelet Therapy After Coronary Bypass Surgery
Effects of Reduction in Drugs or Dosage After Long Term Control of Hypertension
Treatment of Mild Hypertension in the Aged: Anti-Hypertensive Effectiveness and Patients' Toleration of Different Regimens
Vietnam Experience: Twin Find Study
Comparative Efficacy of Vascular Bypass Graft Materials in Lower Extremity Revascularization
Clinical Studies of Biphasic Calcium Phosphate Ceramic in Periodontal Osseous Defects
Prospective Evaluation of the Efficacy & Tolerance of Oral Trimethoprim Sulfamethoxazole Prophylaxis in Granulocytopenic Patients with Acute Non-Lymphocytic Leukemia
Efficacy and Toxicity of Carbamazepine vs. Valproic Acid for Partial Seizures
A New Strategy to Preserve the Larynx in Treatment of Advanced Laryngeal Cancer
Cooperative Clinical Trial of Sclerotherapy for Esophageal Varices in Alcoholic Liver Disease

TABLE A-16 *Continued*

Cooperative Studies in Final Analysis
Hepatitis and Dentistry
Patient Compliance and Its Role in Dental Plaque Control
A Comparison of Hospital & Home Treatment Programs for Aphasic Patients
Evaluation of Anti-Epileptic Drugs (Phenobarb vs. Phenytoin vs. Primidone vs. Carbamazepine)
Drugs & Sleep Phase III—Comparison of Phenobarb & Dalmane in Insomnia EEG
Antabuse in Treatment of Alcoholism
A Randomized Comparison of the Peritoneo-Venous Shunt (LeVeen) & Conventional Medical Treatment Alone for Ascites in Patients with Alcoholic Cirrhosis
The Treatment & Prevention of Infection-Induced Urinary Stones in Spinal Cord Injury
Recently Completed Studies
Renal Failure Self Care Dialysis (Hemo vs. Peritoneal Dialysis)
Nafcillin Therapy of Staphylococcal Bacteremia
Platelet Aggregation in Diabetes (Use of Aspirin & Persantine)
Community vs. VA Nursing Home Care vs. Hospitalization in Psychiatric Patients
Alcoholic Hepatitis (Steroid Therapy)
Aspirin in Unstable Angina
Vasodilators in Acute MI
Characteristics of Psychiatric Programs & Their Relationship to Treatment Effectiveness
Alcoholic Hepatitis (Steroid Therapy)
Bowel Prep for Elective Colon Surgery

SOURCE: Veterans Administration (1984).

Concerns

The primary concerns of cooperative studies are safety, efficacy, and cost-effectiveness. Although cost-effectiveness is not a concern for all studies, it is receiving greater attention, and its appropriateness will be considered for all future studies. Of the 14 studies in active planning (see Table A-16), at least 6 have an explicit cost-effectiveness component, e.g., in studies of hepatitis B vaccine, percutaneous transluminal coronary angioplasty, and continuous peritoneal dialysis. At least three ongoing studies have explicit cost-effectiveness components, including studies of pneumococcal vaccine immunity in high-risk patients, percutaneous transluminal angioplasty in the lower extremities, and parenteral nutrition in malnourished surgical patients.

Requests

The origination, selection, conduct, and reporting of VA cooperative studies follow well-defined guidelines. A cooperative study usually begins with the submission by a VA researcher—physicians and investigators in VA centers around the United States—of a *planning request*, i.e., an initial study proposal, to the chief of the Cooperative Studies Program. Recently, the CSP office has begun to encourage studies in certain areas of special interest to the VA.

Selection

Planning requests are reviewed by VA program specialists who provide written critiques and are then evaluated by a Triage Review Committee. This committee comprises primarily representatives of the Office of the Associate Chief Medical Director for Research and Development, Medical Research Service and Professional Services. They may decide to reject a request, assign a priority rating, or ask for additional information. The requests with a priority rating are put on a waiting list, and those with the highest priority are chosen for planning.

At the time that a study is approved for planning, and again when a study is approved for funding, VA medical centers are invited to participate. Medical centers seeking to participate are considered based on a number of criteria, including level of interest, availability of appropriate staff resources, and availability of eligible study patients. A medical center's participation in a CSP is voluntary, but an agreement to participate means acceptance of the study protocol without change and acceptance of the practices and guidelines of the CSP program.

When a study is funded for planning, the principal investigator is notified by the CSP. Biostatisticians and, where appropriate, clinical research pharmacists are assigned to the study planning process and the production of a detailed final proposal. The principle investigator is also informed as to which of the four CSP coordinating centers the study has been assigned. The four special centers established by the VA to support and coordinate the CSP are located at VA medical centers in Hines, Illinois; Palo Alto, California; Perry Point, Maryland; and West Haven, Connecticut. These provide the biostatistical and data processing support and administrative coordination for the cooperative studies and ensure their compliance with program guidelines. A CSP clinical research pharmacy coordinating center in Albuquerque, New Mexico, provides additional support and coordination for those studies involving drugs and devices, such as dispensing and monitoring drugs, and liaison with the FDA and pharmaceutical companies.

Ethical, scientific, professional, budgetary, and administrative aspects of the final proposal are evaluated by three groups, a human rights committee, a cooperative studies evaluation committee, and a budget review group, and at least three independent reviewers who provide written critiques of these same areas. Based on the judgment of these groups, proposed studies may be completely rejected, rejected with recommendations for resubmission, given conditional approval, or given unconditional approval.

Process

Almost all VA cooperative studies are randomized clinical trials. A few have been nonrandomized trials and observational studies. Five groups share the responsibility for conducting or monitoring a cooperative study: the study group, the executive committee, the operations committee, the CSP coordinating center human rights committee, and the cooperative studies evaluation committee. In general, the current schedule of meetings for the study group, executive committee, and operations committee consists of an initial meeting for organizational, informational, and training purposes prior to patient intake, a meeting 9 months after the initiation of patient intake, and annual meetings thereafter.

If drugs or devices used in a study require FDA approval, an investigational new drug application or investigational device exemption must be filed with the FDA before the study can begin.

The study group, composed of all participating investigators and permanent consultants to the study and chaired by the study chairperson, reviews the progress of the study, discusses problems encountered, and provides suggestions for improving the study. Results of blind data related to study end points are not discussed with this group.

The executive committee is the management group and major decision-making body for the operational aspects of the study. It includes the study chairperson, the study biostatistician, the clinical research pharmacists, the head(s) of any special central support units(s), two or three participating investigators, and selected consultants. This committee decides on all changes in the study and on any subprotocols or other use of the study data and on publications of study results, and takes actions on medical centers whose performance is unsatisfactory. As with the study group, the results of the blind portions of the study are not presented to this group.

The operations committee usually consists of experts in the subject matter of the study, an independent biostatistician, and other technical or scientific consultants. Nonvoting members include the study chairperson and the study biostatistician. This committee considers from meeting to meeting whether the study should continue, based on study performance, patient accrual, treatment efficacy, adverse effects, and other factors; assesses the performance of each participating center and makes recommendations regarding continuation, termination, or change in support; and reviews and provides recommendations regarding protocol changes.

The human rights committee, besides reviewing the protocol for human rights issues prior to initiating the study, is responsible for ensuring that patients' rights are protected during the course of the study. This committee meets at least once a year for the duration of the study with the operations committee. Each year, the human rights committee conducts three site visits to participating medical centers to ensure that the human rights aspects of the studies are being observed.

All cooperative studies undergo an in-depth review by the cooperative studies evaluation committee at 3-year intervals during their active phase.

Assessors

The assessors include physicians and other health care providers, biostatisticians, clinical pharmacists, and others noted above.

Turnaround

The time from submission of a planning request to approval and initiation of formal planning is generally 4 months. Another 12 months are taken between formal planning of a study and its approval and initiation. Once begun, cooperative studies may range from 1 to 8 years.

Reporting

All VA medical centers conducting medical research must report regularly to the VA Medical Research Service. Summaries of cooperative studies are included in the annual report to Congress of medical research in the VA. Where applicable, sponsors of investigational new drugs and investigational devices are required to submit annual reports to the FDA. The primary means of keeping cooperative study participants informed between meetings are study newsletters prepared and issued regularly by the study chairperson and the study biostatistician or by the executive committee.

The presentation or publication of data collected by investigators on patients entered into VA cooperative studies is under the control of the study's executive committee. The results of cooperative studies are published in major refereed journals as the *New England Journal of Medicine*, *Circulation*, *Journal of the American Medical Association*, *Archives of General Psychiatry*, and others.

Impact

Results from VA cooperative studies have made significant impacts on clinical practice in the VA systems, as well as on clinical practice at large. Among the most significant studies have been those on aspirin therapy of unstable angina, drug treatments for moderate and severe hypertension, chemotherapy for schizophrenia, and coronary artery bypass surgery in chronic stable angina.

Reassessment

There have been several instances of reassessment of drugs, such as reserpine for hypertension and the beta-blocker propranolol for hypertension and for angina. These reassessments occur when new drugs and/or regimens are compared to prevailing treatments in clinical trials.

Funding/Budget

Although most VA cooperative studies are supported by the Medical Research Service, occasionally studies are funded by other VA sources or by outside sources such as NIH or the pharmaceutical industry. The funding level for each cooperative study is determined by the Budget Review Group.

The 1985 budget for the Cooperative Studies Program is approximately $12 million. However, this is deceptively small. These funds are primarily for support of the CSP coordinating centers and other nonpatient care aspects of the cooperative studies. The clinical costs of these trials is met entirely through VA medical benefits, and is not reflected in the CSP budget.

Example

On the following pages is a report by the VA Coronary Artery Bypass Surgery Cooperative Study Group, published in the *New England Journal of Medicine*, November 22, 1984, and is reproduced here with permission.

Sources

Blue Sheet. 1984. VA spending $4.3 million in FY 1984 on prosthetic/amputation R&D. May 30:P&R-8.

Hagans, J., Chief, Cooperative Studies Program, Veterans Administration, Washington, D.C. 1984. Personal communication.

Huang, P., Staff Assistant, Cooperative Studies Program, Veterans Administration, Washington, D.C. 1985. Personal communication.

Congressional Budget Office. 1984. Veterans Administration Health Care: Planning for Future Years. Washington, D.C.

Goldschmidt, P., Director, Health Services Research and Development Service, Veterans Administration, Washington, D.C. 1984. Personal communication.

Office of Technology Assessment. 1983. The Impact of Randomized Clinical Trials on Health Policy and Medical Practice. Washington, D.C.: U.S. Government Printing Office.

Veterans Administration. 1983. Administrator of Veterans Affairs Annual Report 1982. Washington, D.C.

Veterans Administration. 1983. Guidelines for the Planning and Conduct of Cooperative Studies in the Veterans Administration. Sixth Edition. Washington, D.C.

Veterans Administration. 1984. Cooperative Studies Program Status Report. Washington, D.C.

ELEVEN-YEAR SURVIVAL IN THE VETERANS ADMINISTRATION RANDOMIZED TRIAL OF CORONARY BYPASS SURGERY FOR STABLE ANGINA

THE VETERANS ADMINISTRATION CORONARY ARTERY BYPASS SURGERY COOPERATIVE STUDY GROUP

Abstract We evaluated long-term survival after coronary-artery bypass grafting in 686 patients with stable angina who were randomly assigned to medical or surgical treatment at 13 hospitals and followed for an average of 11.2 years. For all patients and for the 595 without left main coronary-artery disease, cumulative survival did not differ significantly at 11 years according to treatment. The 7-year survival rates for all patients were 70 per cent with medical treatment and 77 per cent with surgery (P = 0.043), and the 11-year rates were 57 and 58 per cent, respectively. For patients without left main coronary-artery disease, the 7-year rates were 72 and 77 per cent in medically and surgically treated patients, respectively (P = 0.267), and the 11-year rates were 58 per cent in both groups.

A statistically significant difference in survival suggesting a benefit from surgical treatment was found in patients without left main coronary-artery disease who were subdivided into high-risk subgroups defined angiographically, clinically, or by a combination of angiographic and clinical factors: (1) high angiographic risk (three-vessel disease and impaired left ventricular function) — at 7 years, 52 per cent in medically treated patients versus 76 per cent in surgically treated patients (P = 0.002); at 11 years, 38 and 50 per cent, respectively (P = 0.026); (2) clinically defined high risk (at least two of the following: resting ST depression, history of myocardial infarction, or history of hypertension) — at 7 years, 52 per cent in the medical group versus 72 per cent in the surgical group (P = 0.003); at 11 years, 36 versus 49 per cent, respectively (P = 0.015); and (3) combined angiographic and clinical high risk — at 7 years, 36 per cent in the medical group versus 76 per cent in the surgical group (P = 0.002); at 11 years, 24 versus 54 per cent, respectively (P = 0.005). Survival among patients with impaired left ventricular function differed significantly at 7 years (63 per cent in the medical group versus 74 per cent in the surgical group [P = 0.049]) but not at 11 years (49 versus 53 per cent).

The surgical treatment policy resulted in a nonsignificant survival disadvantage throughout the 11 years in subgroups with normal left ventricular function, low angiographic risk, and low clinical risk, and a statistically significant disadvantage at 11 years in patients with two-vessel disease.

We conclude that among patients with stable ischemic heart disease, those with a high risk of dying benefit from surgical treatment, but beyond seven years the survival benefit gradually diminishes. (N Engl J Med 1984; 311:1333-9.)

IN 1975 the Veterans Administration Cooperative Study of Surgery for Coronary Arterial Occlusive Disease first reported a statistically significant survival difference in favor of surgery in the subgroup of patients with left main coronary-artery disease.[1] Two years later, in a preliminary report[2] on patients without disease in the left main artery who were followed for a minimum of 21 months, no significant difference in survival was found between medical and surgical treatment groups either overall or in angiographically defined subgroups. Subsequently, a high-risk subgroup of patients without left main coronary-artery disease, defined on the basis of clinical risk factors alone, was reported to have a significantly reduced five-year cumulative mortality with surgery.[3]

This report compares 7-year and 11-year survival after assignment to medical and surgical treatment in patients who were followed for a minimum of 107 months. Survival results for the entire group as well as for risk groups defined by angiographic and clinical measures are also presented for patients without left main coronary-artery disease. Updated survival results for patients with such disease have been reported previously.[4]

Report prepared by Katherine M. Detre, M.D., D.P.H., Peter Peduzzi, Ph.D., Timothy Takaro, M.D., Herbert N. Hultgren, M.D., Marvin L. Murphy, M.D., and George Kroncke, M.D. Address reprint requests to Dr. Detre at the Veterans Administration Medical Center, West Haven, CT 06516. For a complete listing of participants, members of the Operations and Executive Committees, Coordinating Center staff, and consultants, refer to *Circulation* 1981; 63:1329 (Appendix C).

Supported by the Veterans Administration Cooperative Studies Program, Medical Research Service, Veterans Administration Central Office, Washington, D.C.

METHODS

The Veterans Administration cooperative study of coronary-artery bypass grafting is a randomized controlled trial of medical therapy versus medical plus surgical therapy for the treatment of patients with stable angina pectoris and angiographically confirmed coronary-artery disease. The study design, entry criteria, and base-line characteristics of the patient population have been described previously.[5] Briefly, between 1972 and 1974, 686 patients with stable angina pectoris of more than six months' duration who had been receiving medical therapy for three months and who had resting or exercise electrocardiographic evidence of myocardial ischemia were randomly assigned to medical or surgical therapy. Patients were excluded from randomization if they had had a myocardial infarction within six months or if they had refractory systemic diastolic hypertension (>100 mm Hg), left ventricular aneurysm or other serious cardiac disease, other organ-system disease making surgery inadvisable or limiting life expectancy to less than five years, unstable angina, or uncompensated congestive heart failure.

In the 1972-1974 cohort, 354 patients were randomly assigned to medical therapy, and 332 to surgical therapy, at a total of 13 clinical sites. The base-line distribution of risk factors (history, angiographic findings, electrocardiographic findings, and severity of angina) was comparable in the two treatment groups.[6]

Twenty patients randomly assigned to bypass surgery did not have an operation. Ninety-four per cent of those who underwent surgery did so within three months after random assignment. The average number of diseased vessels in surgically treated patients was 2.4, and the average number of grafts placed was 2.0. All 45 patients with single-vessel disease received at least one graft, and one fourth received multiple grafts. Of the 102 patients with two-vessel disease, 80 per cent received two or more grafts. Of the 163 patients with triple-vessel disease, 90 per cent received two or more grafts, and 37 per cent received three or more.

The overall 30-day operative mortality rate was 5.8 per cent. The incidence of perioperative myocardial infarction, calculated on the basis of the development of new Q waves, was 9.9 per cent. Vein-graft angiography was performed in 79 per cent of surgical patients (247 of 312) between 10 and 15 months after surgery, and 353 of 503 grafts placed (70 per cent) were patent at one year; 87 per cent of patients (214 of 247) had at least one patent graft. Five years after random assignment, 52 of the 312 patients had died, and 9 had had a second operation. Graft angiography was done at five years in 156 of the 251 remaining eligible patients (62 per cent), and the patency rate was 67 per cent. The one-year and five-year graft-patency rates for the 143 patients evaluated at both times were 74 and 67 per cent, respectively.

Of 354 patients randomly assigned to medical treatment, 133 (38 per cent) had bypass surgery during an average follow-up of 11.2 years. Of the 133, 22 had left main coronary-artery disease and crossed over to surgery on an elective basis in accordance with a protocol amendment.[7,8] Thirty-five (11 per cent) of the 312 patients randomly assigned to surgery who had coronary-artery bypass grafting have had repeat grafting.

Medical therapy consisted of nitrates, beta-blockers, and other medications administered to achieve symptomatic relief of angina. At one year, 26 per cent of medically treated patients were taking nitroglycerin or nitrates only, 3 per cent were using propranolol only, and 65 per cent were taking both types of medication. The corresponding rates at five years were 27, 4, and 57 per cent. At one year and five years, 6 and 12 per cent of patients, respectively, were not taking any medication. The surgical patients took less medication than the medical patients, but their use of medication increased between one and five years. At one year, 42 per cent took no medication, 45 per cent were taking nitroglycerin or nitrates only, and the remaining 13 per cent were taking both types of medication. The corresponding rates at five years were 25, 36, and 36 per cent. At five years 3 per cent of surgical patients were taking propranolol alone.

The average follow-up time was calculated as the average time from the date of random assignment to the date of the analysis. Included in the calculation were patients who died and those known to be alive but without current follow-up data except for survival status.

Cumulative survival rates were determined by the actuarial life-table method, with death from all causes used as the end point. The survival status for patients who did not return for scheduled follow-up visits was ascertained by a retrieval system known as BIRLS (Beneficiary Identification and Records Locator Subsystem, Austin, Tex.), which is unique to the Veterans Administration network. Telephone contact was used in the few cases in which BIRLS had no patient record. The survival status was known for all but one patient. At present, 99.9 per cent of study patients have completed 9 years of follow-up, 91 per cent have completed 10 years, and 73 per cent have completed 11 years. Life-table cumulative survival rates were calculated according to the original treatment assignment (treatment policy) from the date of randomization. Differences in cumulative survival between the two treatment groups were assessed by the Mantel–Haenszel test. Thus, the 7-year statistic represents the cumulative survival experience up to 7 years, and the 11-year statistic represents the cumulative experience up to 11 years. All P values reported are two-tailed and uncorrected for multiple comparisons.

In addition to the overall treatment results, survival was compared in angiographically and clinically defined subgroups of patients without left main coronary-artery disease. The angiographically defined subgroups were identified on the basis of the number of vessels diseased (one, two, or three) and left ventricular function. The presence or absence of left ventricular functional impairment was determined according to a central reading of base-line left ventriculograms performed at the Seattle Veterans Administration Medical Center under the supervision of Dr. Karl Hammermeister. Global ejection fractions and segmental contraction abnormalities were measured. Contraction abnormalities were graded as follows: 1, no abnormality; 2, minimal hypokinesis or akinesis involving less than 25 per cent of the heart border; 3, moderate hypokinesis or akinesis of 25 to 75 per cent of the heart border; 4, dyskinesia, left ventricular aneurysm, or paradoxical wall motion; and 5, severe generalized hypokinesis or akinesis of the entire heart border. Left ventricular function was considered to be impaired if the global ejection fraction was less than 50 per cent or if the contraction grade was over 2; otherwise, left ventricular function was defined as normal. By this definition, 55 per cent of the patients had impaired function. In previous reports[1-5,9] left ventricular function was defined as abnormal if there was cardiac enlargement, elevated end-diastolic pressure (>14 mm Hg), an ejection fraction under 45 per cent, or any degree of contraction abnormality, as evaluated by the individual participants. Central readings on left ventriculograms were done in 75 per cent of the patients. Base-line readings by the individual clinics were used to provide data on left ventricular function in the other patients, according to the new definition. The combination of three-vessel disease and impaired left ventricular function was classified as a high angiographic risk. All other combinations of one-, two-, or three-vessel disease and normal or impaired left ventricular function constituted a low angiographic risk.

Subgroups with a low, middle, or high clinical risk were defined on the basis of a multivariate risk function in order to predict five-year mortality,[3,10] using four established clinical-risk variables measured at base line: the New York Heart Association classification, a history of hypertension, a history of myocardial infarction, and an ST-segment depression on the resting electrocardiogram. Other risk factors, which were not uniformly measured in all patients at base line (e.g., positive exercise test) or which had a low prevalence in the study population (e.g., congestive heart failure), could not be considered for inclusion in this risk function. Patients in the low-risk subgroup included those with none or only one of the four risk factors except for ST depression. The high-risk subgroup consisted of patients with combinations of two or three of the strongest predictors (ST depression, a history of myocardial infarction, and a history of hypertension) — i.e., those with multiple clinical risk factors. The validity of this method for the classification of patients into clinical-risk groups has been established in an independent population.[10] Reviewers and others[11,12] have criticized such "post hoc" subgroups. However, the original protocol for the 1972-1974 Veterans Administration study clearly outlined the ana-

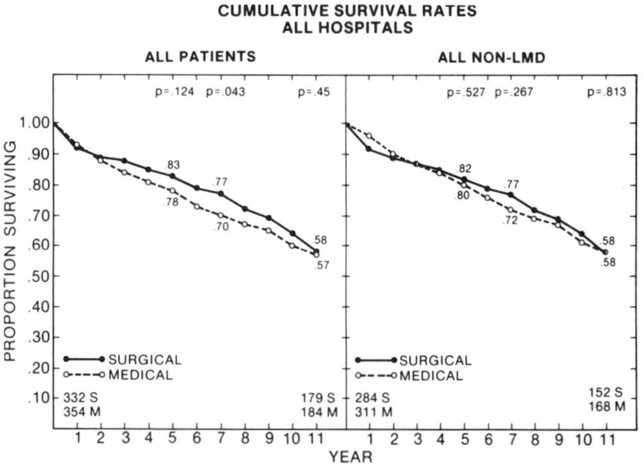

Figure 1. Eleven-Year Cumulative Survival for All Patients and for Those without Left Main Coronary-Artery Disease (non-LMD), According to Treatment Assignment. Numbers of patients at risk are given at bottom of figure. M denotes medical, and S surgical.

lytical steps for development of both the angiographic- and clinical-risk groups: "Regression analyses will be used to determine the effect [of base-line variables] on mortality and to determine groups with low and high mortality risk. . . . Analyses [life table] will be done for patients in low and high risk groups." Thus, the clinical-risk groups, defined by noninvasive base-line measures, were neither more nor less post hoc than the angiographic-risk groups, defined by such factors as left main coronary-artery disease or the combination of vessel disease and left ventricular function.

Survival analyses are based on data from all 13 hospitals, by treatment policy. In the Results we focus on the 7-year and 11-year cumulative survival rates. The five-year survival rates (early experience) are shown in the figures but are not discussed in the text, except in comparing this study with the European and the National Heart, Lung, and Blood Institute studies. All treatment comparisons are presented in reference to the medical treatment policy.

Results

Cumulative survival rates are shown in Figures 1 through 5. Patients with left main coronary-artery disease are excluded from the subgroup analyses shown in Figures 2 through 5.

Overall Results

Overall, excluding patients with left main coronary-artery disease, the treatment difference was not significant at seven years (72 per cent in the medical group versus 77 per cent in the surgical group, P = 0.267; Fig. 1). The medical and surgical survival curves converge when follow-up data are extended to 11 years (58 per cent in both groups, P = 0.813). During the first 7 years of follow-up the average annual mortality rates were 4.0 per cent for medical therapy and 3.3 per cent for surgery, including operative mortality, as compared with 3.5 and 4.8 per cent, respectively, between 7 and 11 years.

If patients with left main coronary-artery disease are included, the trends are similar, although the treatment difference in all patients was statistically significant at 7 but not at 11 years.

Vessel Disease

There was a nonsignificant trend toward improved survival with surgery at seven years in the subgroup of patients with three-vessel disease: 63 per cent with medical treatment vs. 75 per cent with surgical treatment, P = 0.061 (Fig. 2). The difference in the cumulative survival rates diminished after 7 years, resulting in only a 6 per cent difference at 11 years. At 7 years neither patients with single-vessel disease nor those with double-vessel disease had a significant difference in survival associated with treatment, although at 11 years surgically treated patients with two-vessel disease had a marginally significant disadvantage in survival (P = 0.045).

Left Ventricular Function

At 7 but not at 11 years, there was a significant difference in survival between medically and surgically treated patients with impaired left ventricular function (63 vs. 74 per cent, respectively; P = 0.049); survival rates at 11 years were 49 and 53 per cent, respectively (P = 0.249, Fig. 3). Among patients with normal left ventricular function, survival was 84 per

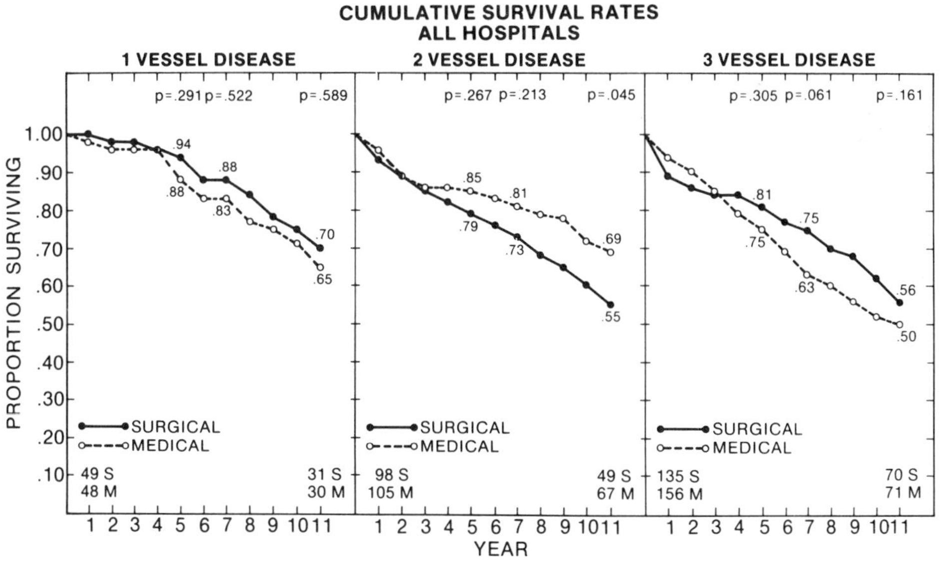

Figure 2. Eleven-Year Cumulative Survival for Patients without Left Main Coronary-Artery Disease Who Had Single-, Double-, or Triple-Vessel Disease.

Numbers of patients at risk are given at bottom of figure. M denotes medical, and S surgical.

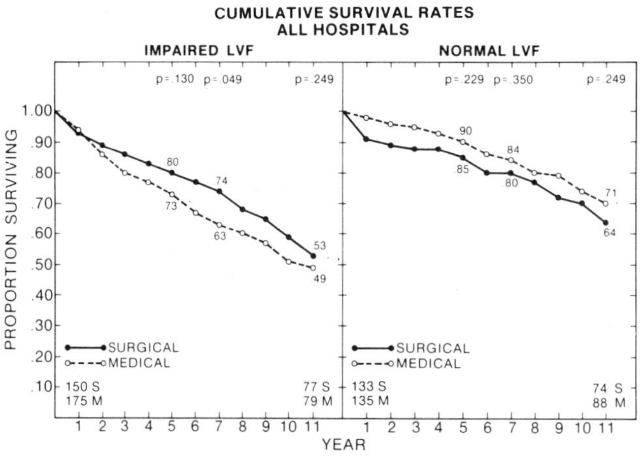

Figure 3. Eleven-Year Cumulative Survival for Patients without Left Main Coronary-Artery Disease, According to Whether Left Ventricular Function (LVF) Was Impaired or Normal.

Numbers of patients at risk are given at bottom of figure. M denotes medical, and S surgical.

cent in the medical group and 80 per cent in the surgical group at 7 years, and 71 and 64 per cent, respectively, at 11 years. These differences were not significant.

Risk Analysis

There was a statistically significant improvement in survival at seven years in surgically treated patients with a high angiographic risk (three-vessel disease with impaired left ventricular function); the rates were 52 per cent for medical treatment versus 76 per cent for surgical treatment ($P = 0.002$, Fig. 4). Although from 7 to 11 years, the marked difference in survival rates diminished from 24 to 12 per cent, the difference in cumulative survival up to 11 years remained significant ($P = 0.026$). In contrast, by 11 years, patients with a low angiographic risk had a survival rate of 68 per cent with medical therapy and 61 per cent with surgery ($P = 0.105$).

The Veterans Administration study reported a significant survival benefit with surgery at five years in patients with a high clinical risk and a significant benefit with medical therapy in patients at low risk.[3] The seven-year survival rates in the high-risk tercile were 52 per cent for the medical group and 72 per cent for the surgical group ($P = 0.003$, Fig. 5). Beyond seven years, survival remained higher in the surgical group, but the difference gradually diminished from 20 to 13 per cent by 11 years. The cumulative survival experience up to 11 years differed significantly between the two treatment groups ($P = 0.015$). In contrast, for patients in the low-risk tercile there was a 7 per cent survival disadvantage with surgical therapy at seven years (88 per cent in the medical group vs. 81 per cent in the surgical group, $P = 0.093$), which increased to 10 per cent at 11 years (73 per cent in the medical group vs. 63 per cent in the surgical group, $P = 0.066$). In the middle-risk tercile, there was no significant difference in survival at any time.

When survival in the subgroup of patients with a high angiographic risk was studied separately in the patients at low, middle, and high clinical risk, a statistically significant surgical benefit was observed only in patients who were at high risk not only angiographically but also clinically (Table 1). No significant difference in survival was observed in patients with a high angiographic risk who had a low or middle clinical risk. Although the survival experience was similar in all clinical-risk subgroups of surgically treated patients with a high angiographic risk, survival in medically treated patients decreased with increasing clinical risk at both 7 and 11 years, reflecting the strong

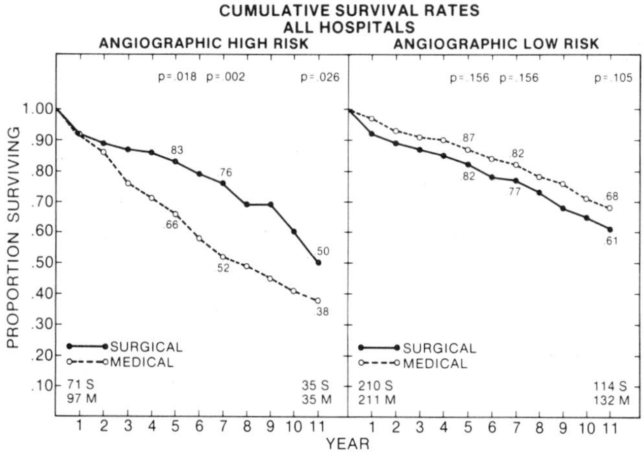

Figure 4. Eleven-Year Cumulative Survival for Patients without Left Main Coronary-Artery Disease, According to Angiographic Risk.

High risk was defined as three-vessel disease plus impaired left ventricular function, and low risk as one-, two-, or three-vessel disease plus normal left ventricular function or one- or two-vessel disease plus impaired left ventricular function. Numbers of patients at risk are given at bottom of figure. M denotes medical, and S surgical.

additional effect of clinical risk factors on the natural history of patients with a high angiographic risk.

Conversely, when survival in patients with a low angiographic risk was studied separately in the three clinical risk groups (Table 1), a disadvantage with surgery was observed at 7 and 11 years in patients who were at low risk by both measures; however, the differences were not significant. Again, the strong effect of the clinical risk factors on the natural history was evident.

Left Main Coronary-Artery Disease

The mortality rate for 48 patients with left main coronary-artery disease who were randomly assigned to surgical treatment increased after the seventh year of follow-up (data not shown). During the first seven years, the average annual mortality rate was approximately 3 per cent; thereafter, the rate increased to nearly 5 per cent. Comparison with the assigned medical group was futile, since 47 per cent of the original medical group crossed over and 44 per cent died, leaving only four patients with the original treatment assignment at seven years.

Discussion

Current survival results by treatment policy for all 13 hospitals with an operative mortality rate of 5.8 per cent (Fig. 1) indicate that for all patients and for those without left main coronary-artery disease, the cumulative survival experience up to 11 years did not differ significantly (at a two-tailed alpha level of 5 per cent) between medical and surgical treatment groups.

This overall result disregards the heterogeneous natural history of the subgroups. Consistent with the hypothesis that surgery could be advantageous for patients whose natural history was expected to be poor but would offer little or no advantage for those with a good prognosis, we found a range of treatment effects in subgroups, from a significant advantage to a borderline or nonsignificant advantage and even a disadvantage, with surgical therapy. In particular, the small group of patients who were at high risk both angiographically and by noninvasive clinical risk measures derived the greatest survival benefit from surgery (Table 1), second only to the benefit in patients with left main coronary-artery disease reported previously.[1,4] A statistically significant difference was also found when subgroups were defined by angiographic predictors alone — i.e., three-vessel disease and moderate to severe impairment of left ventricular function (Fig. 4) — or by the high-clinical-risk measure alone (Fig. 5). The surgical benefit was not significant at 11 years in the subgroups with three-vessel disease alone (Fig. 2) or with moderate to severe impairment of left ventricular function (Fig. 3), although a benefit of borderline significance appeared at 7 years ($P = 0.061$ and 0.049, respectively).

At the other end of the spectrum were the subgroups of patients with a good prognosis: those with one- or two-vessel disease (Fig. 2), normal left ventricular function (Fig. 3), a low angiographic risk (Fig. 4), and a low clinical risk (Fig. 5). With the exception of the group with two-vessel disease, for which the surgical survival rate was significantly worse ($P = 0.045$), the

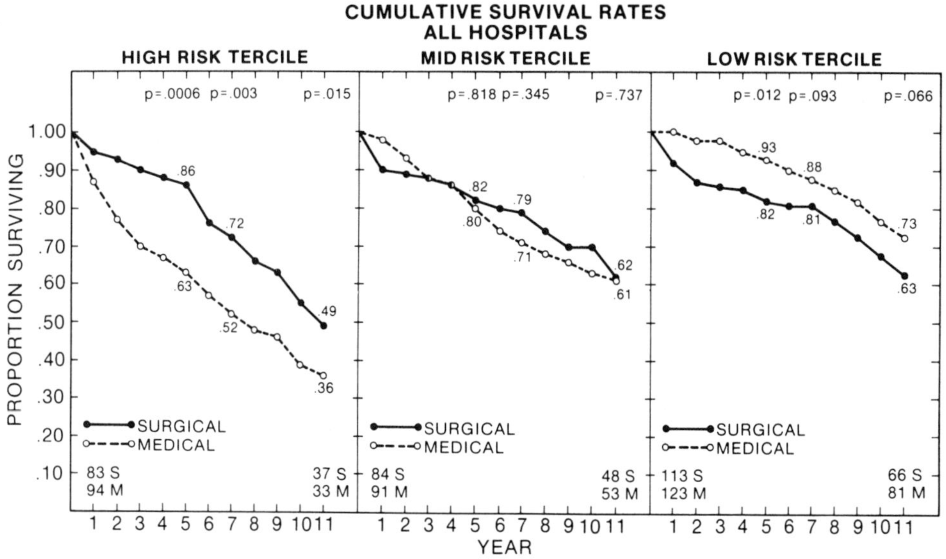

Figure 5. Eleven-Year Cumulative Survival for Patients without Left Main Coronary-Artery Disease, According to Clinical Risk. See text for definitions of high, middle, and low clinical risk. Numbers of patients at risk are given at bottom of figure. M denotes medical, and S surgical.

Table 1. Cumulative Survival Rates at 7 and 11 Years In Patients without Left Main Coronary-Artery Disease, According to Angiographic and Clinical Risk.*

		7-Year Rate (%)			11-Year Rate (%)		
	No.	Med †	Surg †	P	Med †	Surg †	P
		rate ±S.E.			*rate ±S.E.*		
High angiographic risk							
High clinical risk	67	36±7	76±9	0.002	24±7	54±10	0.005
Middle clinical risk	49	50±9	79±9	0.069	40±9	43±13	0.345
Low clinical risk	50	79±8	77±8	0.818	62±10	52±10	0.586
Low angiographic risk							
High clinical risk	108	67±7	70±6	0.531	46±7	46±7	0.732
Middle clinical risk	124	82±5	78±5	0.569	73±6	68±6	0.521
Low clinical risk	184	90±3	81±4	0.079	76±5	66±5	0.092

*A total of 13 patients could not be classified: 4 had missing data for the number of diseased vessels, 2 for left ventricular function, and 7 for the clinical-risk subgroup.

†Med denotes medical group, and Surg surgical group.

11-year survival disadvantage with surgical treatment was not statistically significant in the low-risk subgroups. The small survival disadvantage with surgery in these subgroups can probably be explained by the initial mortality associated with surgery.

Although the individual subgroup results reported here are weakened by the multiplicity of comparisons and the loss of power in some strata with small numbers of patients, the survival differences during the first seven years can generally be characterized by what is known about the natural history of chronic stable angina. Depending on the presence or absence of known prognostic indicators, the seven-year cumulative mortality in the medical cohort varied widely, from 10 to 64 per cent, yet mortality in the surgical cohort ranged only from 12 to 30 per cent. This resulted in a significant reduction of mortality for surgically treated patients with combinations of risk factors.

Two other large-scale randomized studies of coronary-artery bypass grafting have reported survival results: the European Coronary Surgery Study[13] and the National Heart, Lung, and Blood Institute's Coronary Artery Surgery Study (CASS).[14] Comparison of the three studies is difficult, because each enrolled different types of patients, and the periods of patient enrollment were different. For example, unlike the Veterans Administration study, CASS did not enroll patients with serious left main coronary-artery disease or with severe angina,[14] and the European study did not enroll patients with an ejection fraction under 50 per cent or with single-vessel disease.[13]

Probably in part because of differences in patient characteristics and in part because of improvement in both therapies, the five-year survival rates in medically and surgically treated patients without left main coronary-artery disease differed among the three studies. For medically treated patients the rates were 80 per cent in the Veterans Administration study, 85 per cent in the European study (calculated from reported data[13]), and 92 per cent in CASS; for surgically treated patients the rates were 82, 93 (calculated from reported data[13]), and 95 per cent, respectively. The corresponding percentage reductions in overall mortality for the surgical group as compared with the medical group were 10 per cent in the Veterans Administration study, 53 per cent in the European study, and 38 per cent in CASS. Neither the Veterans Administration result nor the CASS result was statistically significant.

The subgroups with the largest benefit from surgical treatment in the Veterans Administration study have no direct counterparts in the other two studies. The subgroup of patients in CASS that resembles most closely the Veterans Administration high-angiographic-risk group, the subgroup with three-vessel disease and an ejection fraction under 50 per cent, had a nearly significant benefit from surgery at five years ($P = 0.063$). On the other hand, the European study, which examined the joint effect of clinical and angiographic risk factors, concluded that "in the absence of [clinically defined] prognostic variables in patients with either two- or three-vessel disease the outlook is so good that early surgery is unlikely to increase the prospect of survival." Thus, all three studies point toward a possible surgical benefit in the presence of high risk — i.e., multiple risk factors that indicate a poor prognosis measured by angiography or by other means.

With data now available from the extended follow-up in the Veterans Administration study, long-term results of therapy can be studied. So far, the most important observation is that the mortality rate in all surgical subgroups increased between 7 and 11 years. During the first seven years of follow-up, the average annual mortality rate was 3.3 per cent for all surgically treated patients without left main coronary-artery disease, as compared with a rate of 4.8 per cent during the next four years. For medically treated patients without left main coronary-artery disease, the rates were 4.0 and 3.5 per cent, respectively. The increased mortality in the surgical group is consistent with the findings of the Montreal Heart Institute investigators who followed a series of patients for 12 years. They found that although angina had improved in 80 per cent of patients at 6 years, it remained improved in only 47 per cent of the 12-year survivors.[15] The annual graft-closure rate at 7 to 12 years was 5.2 per cent — more than double the 2.1 per cent rate between 1 and 7 years.[16] The Montreal Heart Institute predicted that because of late graft changes, long-term relief of symptoms and survival may be compromised. Our observation of accelerated mortality after seven years in surgically treated patients but not in those receiving medical treatment supports this prediction.

In conclusion, we found that in the Veterans Administration study population bypass surgery did not significantly improve overall survival among patients without left main coronary-artery disease. However, a survival benefit with surgery was observed at five to seven years in subgroups of patients with multiple clinical and angiographic risk factors. The observed benefit with surgery diminished gradually when follow-up was extended to 11 years.

References

1. Takaro T, Hultgren HN, Lipton MJ, Detre KM, et al. The VA Cooperative Randomized Study of Surgery for Coronary Arterial Occlusive Disease. II. Subgroup with significant left main lesions. Circulation 1976; 54: Suppl 3:III-107-17.
2. Murphy ML, Hultgren HN, Detre K, Thomsen J, Takaro T, et al. Treatment of chronic stable angina: a preliminary report of survival data of the randomized Veterans Administration cooperative study. N Engl J Med 1977; 297:621-7.
3. Detre K, Peduzzi P, Murphy M, et al. Effect of bypass surgery on survival of patients in low- and high-risk subgroups delineated by the use of simple clinical variables: Veterans Administration Cooperative Study of Surgery for Coronary Arterial Occlusive Disease. Circulation 1981; 63: 1329-38.
4. Takaro T, Peduzzi P, Detre KM, et al. Survival in subgroups of patients with left main coronary artery disease. Circulation 1982; 66:14-22.
5. Detre KM, Hultgren HN, Takaro T, et al. Veterans Administration Cooperative Study of Surgery for Coronary Arterial Occlusive Disease. III. Methods and baseline characteristics, including experience with medical treatment. Am J Cardiol 1977; 40:212-25.
6. Takaro T, Hultgren HN, Detre KM, Peduzzi P, Murphy M. Results of the VA randomized study of medical and surgical management of angina pectoris. In: Hammermeister KE, ed. Coronary bypass surgery: the late results. New York: Praeger, 1983:19.
7. Detre K, Peduzzi P. The problem of attributing deaths of nonadherers: the VA coronary bypass experience. Controlled Clin Trials 1982; 3:355-64.
8. Parisi AF, Peduzzi P, Detre K, Shugoll G, Hultgren HN, Takaro T. Characteristics and outcome of medical nonadherers in the Veterans Administration Cooperative Study of Coronary Artery Surgery. Am J Cardiol 1984; 53:23-8.
9. Takaro T, Hultgren HN, Detre KM, Peduzzi P. The Veterans Administration Cooperative Study of stable angina: current status. Circulation 1982; 65: Suppl 2:II-60-7.
10. Peduzzi PN, Detre KM, Chan YK, Oberman A, Cutter GR. Validation of a risk function to predict mortality in a VA population with coronary artery disease. Controlled Clin Trials 1982; 3:47-60.
11. Braunwald E. Effects of coronary-artery bypass grafting on survival: implications of the randomized coronary-artery surgery study. N Engl J Med 1983; 309:1181-4.
12. *Idem.* The treatment of coronary artery disease: lessons from clinical trials. Presented at the fifty-sixth annual meeting of the American Heart Association, Anaheim, Calif., November 16, 1983.
13. European Coronary Surgery Study Group. Long-term results of a prospective randomised study of coronary artery bypass surgery in stable angina pectoris. Lancet 1982; 2:1173-80.
14. CASS Principal Investigators. Coronary Artery Surgery Study (CASS): a randomized trial of coronary artery bypass surgery: survival data. Circulation 1983; 68:939-50.
15. Enjalbert M, Vaislic C, Lespérance J, Grondin CM, Bourassa MG, Campeau L. Relief of angina and survival 12 years after XOrtocoronary saphenous vein graft bypass surgery. Circulation 1983; 68: Suppl 3:III-116. abstract.
16. Campeau L, Enjalbert M, Lespérance J, Vaislic C, Grondin CM, Bourassa MG. Atherosclerosis and late closure of XOrtocoronary saphenous vein grafts: sequential angiographic studies at 2 weeks, 1 year, 5 to 7 years, and 10 to 12 years after surgery. Circulation 1983; 68: Suppl 2:II-1-7.

Reprinted from *The New England Journal of Medicine*
311:1333-1339 (November 22), 1984

APPENDIX B: Selected Papers

Guide to Comparative Clinical Trials

Clifford S. Goodman*

This guide is intended to help a reviewer evaluate reports of comparative experimental clinical trials. Such trials are a mainstay of medical technology assessment, but their worth depends on the care with which they are designed, implemented, and analyzed.

Experimental trials are prospective studies in that they entail the intentional application of a technology to an experimental group and then the observation of the effects of the technology. Comparative experimental clinical trials are typically used to compare the safety and effectiveness of a new technology with a standard treatment. Trials may have more than one experimental group. In the simple comparative trial, patients with a common condition are assigned to an experimental group or to a control group. The experimental group receives the new technology, and the control group receives no treatment, a placebo, a standard treatment, or a variation (e.g., a different dosage) of the experimental treatment. After a designated time, each individual in the experimental and control groups is assessed for a designated endpoint or outcome. Endpoints may be measured in qualitative terms (e.g., survived or died) or quantitative terms (e.g., blood pressure measurements).

The most definitive type of experimental clinical trial is the *randomized controlled clinical trial* (RCT). In an RCT, patients are randomly assigned to experimental and control groups. Randomization reduces bias that might otherwise be introduced by prognostic and other selection factors not accounted for in the design of the trial.

There are a number of design variations, which can be used in combination, to the simple comparative trial. Some of these are crossover, stratified, matched, and factorial designs.

In a *crossover* trial, patients are systematically switched from one treatment group to another during the trial, and outcomes in the same patient are contrasted. Switching may be determined by a time-dependent rule or a disease-state-dependent rule. In a self-controlled trial, which incorporates many of the same features of crossover studies, a sin-

* National Research Council Fellow, National Academy of Sciences, Washington, D.C.

gle treatment under study is evaluated by comparison of patient status before and after treatment. Louis et al. (1984) describe important factors in determining the effectiveness of crossover and self-controlled designs, e.g., crossover rules, and carry-over and sequencing effects.

In a *stratified* trial, patients are categorized according to characteristics which are thought to have prognostic significance (e.g., stage of disease), so as to isolate treatment effects from those of the prognostic factors. Stratification may be used in designing a trial, or it may be applied in data analysis after completion of the trial. *Matching* is an allocation process, used to gain statistical precision, of sorting patients into pairs matched according to significant prognostic factors, and then randomly assigning one member of each pair to the treatment group and the other to the control group. (For trials involving multiple treatment groups, patients can be matched into groups of the appropriate number.) In a *factorial* design trial, combinations of treatment factors are grouped and observed to determine independent and interactive effects of multiple treatments. For example, a 2 × 2 factorial design could be used to determine the effects of medication and dietary counseling for the treatment of hypertension in four treatment groups: medication and counseling, medication only, counseling only, and neither medication nor counseling. Experimental design and the design of clinical trials in particular are discussed extensively in the literature, e.g., in Campbell and Stanley (1963), Cook and Campbell (1979), Chalmers et al. (1981), Friedman et al. (1981), Mosteller et al. (1980), Peto et al. (1976, 1977), and Shapiro and Louis (1983).

Useful observations of the effects of technologies may be made under nonrandomized and nonexperimental conditions. Although this guide is written to accommodate the assessment of RCTs, other types of clinical trials are subject to most of the assessment criteria discussed here. Some trials use *historical control* groups selected from hospital charts or computerized data bases, or standard outcomes from reports in the literature (e.g., organ transplant survival curves or rejection rates following *N* years). In *observational studies* (including most epidemiological studies), assignment of patients to treatment and control groups is generally not under the control of the investigator, making it difficult to control for prognostic factors which might affect observed outcomes. These may include prospective studies as well as retrospective studies (i.e., those in which the investigator identifies treatment and control groups after their exposure and nonexposure to the technology in question). Although lacking the rigor of RCTs, observational studies are valuable in formulating hypotheses and in ruling out certain explanations for observed effects of technologies. Observational studies and those using historical controls may be useful in situations in which comparative experimental designs are impossible or precluded by ethical, financial, and other constraints. Examples of observational studies are *cohort* and *case-control* studies.

CLINICAL TRIAL REPORTING

No study can be adequately interpreted without information about the methods used in the design of the study and the analysis of the results. Instructive surveys of clinical trial reporting (e.g., by Chalmers et al., 1983; DerSimonian et al., 1982; Freiman et al., 1978; Lavori et al., 1983, and Louis et al., 1984) demonstrate the extent to which important methodological elements are reported in clinical trials and their bearing on findings.

DerSimonian et al. (1982) examined 67 clinical trials published in four prominent medical journals in 1979–1980 for 11 important aspects of trial design and analysis (e.g., method of randomization, blinding, and statistical methods). Of the 11 items for each of the 67 trials published in the four journals, 56 percent were clearly reported, 10 percent were ambiguously mentioned, and 34 percent were not reported at all. The method of randomization was reported in only 19 percent of the papers, and statistical power to detect treatment effects was discussed in only 12 percent. Table B-1 lists the percentage of articles that reported the 11 aspects of trial design and analysis in the four journals sur-

TABLE B-1 Percentage of Clinical Trial Articles in Four Journals Reporting 11 Important Aspects of Design and Analysis

Design and Analysis Aspects	Whether Reported[a]	Journal[b] (Number of articles) *NEJM* (13)	*JAMA* (14)	*BMJ* (19)	*Lancet* (21)	Total (67)
Eligibility criteria	R	77	36	21	29	37
	?	23	50	58	48	46
	O	0	14	21	24	16
Admission before allocation	R	85	64	63	29	57
	?	8	7	5	14	9
	O	8	29	32	57	34
Random allocation	R	100	71	95	71	84
	?	0	0	0	0	0
	O	0	29	5	29	16
Method of randomization	R	15	43	16	10	19
	?	23	0	11	0	7
	O	62	57	74	90	73
Patients' blindness to treatment	R	62	71	37	57	55
	?	0	21	21	5	12
	O	38	7	42	38	33
Blind assessment of outcome	R	46	43	26	14	30
	?	23	36	21	29	27
	O	31	21	53	57	43
Treatment complications	R	92	71	58	48	64
	?	0	0	5	5	3
	O	8	29	37	48	33
Loss to follow-up	R	100	93	74	62	79
	?	0	7	11	5	7
	O	0	00	16	33	15
Statistical analyses	R	92	79	100	95	93
	?	0	0	0	0	0
	O	8	21	0	5	8
Statistical methods	R	92	86	79	86	85
	?	0	0	5	0	1
	O	8	14	16	14	13
Power	R	15	36	5	0	12
	?	0	0	5	5	3
	O	85	64	89	95	85
Mean, all items	R	71	63	52	46	56
	?	7	11	13	10	10
	O	23	26	35	45	34

[a] R denotes item reported, ? item unclear, and O item omitted.
[b] *NEJM* denotes the *New England Journal of Medicine*, *JAMA* the *Journal of the American Medical Association*, *BMJ* the *British Medical Journal*.
SOURCE: R. DerSimonian et al. (1982).

veyed. Emerson et al. (1984) repeated the study on 84 clinical trials published in 1 year in six journals, and they found that 58 percent were clearly reported, 5 percent were ambiguously mentioned, and 37 percent were not reported at all.

Freiman et al. (1978) examined 71 published *negative* trials (i.e., those in which the outcomes of treatment groups were found to be no different than those of control groups) to determine whether investigators adequately addressed a particular element of trial design: power to detect important clinical differences between treatment groups.

The study found that of 71 papers on medical randomized controlled trials that reported no significant differences among treatment groups, only four of the trials were large enough to ensure a reasonable chance, in this instance a power greater than 0.90, of detecting a 25 percent improvement in patient outcomes. Only 30 percent of the trials had power greater than 0.90 for detecting a 50 percent improvement.

Chalmers et al. (1983) provide evidence for the seriousness of bias introduced by various methods of treatment assignment. Among 145 papers reporting controlled clinical trials of the treatment of acute myocardial infarction, they found significant differences in bias associated with the method of treatment assignment. At least one prognostic factor was maldistributed ($p < 0.05$) in 14.0 percent of the blind randomized studies (57 papers), in 26.7 percent of the unblinded randomized studies (45 papers), and in 58.1 percent of the nonrandomized studies (43 papers). Significant differences in outcome (case fatality rates) between experimental and control groups were reported in 8.8 percent of the blind randomized studies, in 24.4 percent of the unblinded randomized studies, and in 58.1 percent of the nonrandomized studies. These reporting rates among the three types of papers differed significantly ($p < 0.05$).

The major subjects addressed in this guide are

- basic descriptive material
- sample size
- selection of patients
- random allocation
- blinding
- treatments
- compliance
- withdrawals/loss to follow-up
- treatment complications
- tabulation of outcomes
- statistical methods and analyses
- power

These aspects of clinical trials should be closely examined before one combines the results of smaller trials, or generalizes the results of trials to other populations. This guide draws upon work of others in the reporting of clinical trials, especially that of Chalmers et al. (1981) and DerSimonian et al. (1982), from whom permission has been granted to use the same or similar wording in places. Table B-2 summarizes the items referred to in the text and may be used as a reviewer's checklist.

TABLE B-2 Checklist for Comparative Clinical Trials

Check or complete multiple entries where applicable[a]

1. Basic descriptive material
   a. Authors ____________________
   b. Title ____________________
   c. Journal/publication ____________________
   d. Date/volume ____________________
   e. Trial type
      ___Randomized ___Matched
      ___Simple comparative ___Factorial
      ___Crossover ___Historical control
      ___Stratified ___Not reported
      Observational (specify) ____________________
      Other (specify) ____________________
   f. Sources of financial support
      ___NIH ___VA ___Drug company
      ___Other ___Not reported
   g. Biostatistician cited as author or evaluator
      ___Yes ___No ___Not reported
   h. Start and end dates for trial given
      ___Yes ___No
   i. Peer reviewed
      ___Yes ___No ___Unknown
   j. Statement of significant findings
      Major endpoints
      ___ + + Statistically significant (treatment)
      ___ + Trend (treatment)
      ___ 0 No difference
      ___ − Trend (control)
      ___ − − Statistically significant (control)
      Minor endpoints
      ___ + + Statistically significant (treatment)
      ___ + Trend (treatment)
      ___ 0 No difference
      ___ − Trend (control)
      ___ − − Statistically significant (control)
      ___ None
      Side effects
      ___ + + Statistically significant
      ___ + Trend
      ___ 0 No side effects
      ___ na

TABLE B-2 *Continued*

2. Sample size
   a. Expected control group endpoint(s)
      ___Yes ___No ___Unclear ___na
   b. Improvement of clinical interest that should not be missed
      ___Yes ___No ___Unclear ___na
   c. Levels of risk given
      α: ___Yes ___No
      β: ___Yes ___No
   d. Prior estimate of numbers of patients required
      ___Yes ___No ___Unclear ___na
3. Selection of patients
   a. Patient sources
      ___University ___Public ___Private
      ___Clinic ___Industry ___Not reported
   b. Admission criteria description
      ___Yes ___No ___Unclear
   c. Rejection criteria description
      ___Yes ___No ___Unclear ___na
   d. Number of patients actually entering trial given
      ___Yes ___No
   e. Reject log reported
      ___Yes ___No ___na
4. Random allocation
   a. Method
      ___Envelope ___Pharmacy ___Telephone
      ___Not reported ___na
      Other (specify)________________
   b. Stratification/blocking
      ___Yes ___No ___na
   c. Blinding of random allocation described
      ___Yes ___No ___na
   d. Testing of randomization described
      ___Yes ___No ___na
5. Blinding
   a. Patients as to treatment assignment
      ___Yes ___No ___na
   b. Physicians as to treatment assignment
      ___Yes ___No ___na
   c. Physicians and patients as to trends of trial
      ___Yes ___No ___na
   d. Biostatisticians/other evaluators
      ___Yes ___No ___na
   e. Testing for blinding
      Physicians: ___Yes ___No ___na
      Patients: ___Yes ___No ___na
6. Treatments
   a. Description
      ___Yes ___No ___Unclear
   b. Patient number and treatment

	Number	Treatment
Controls	___	________
Group 1	___	________
Group 2	___	________
Group 3	___	________

   c. Placebo described
      ___Yes ___No ___Unclear ___na
7. Compliance
   a. Defined
      ___Yes ___No ___Unclear
   b. Accounted for all patients
      ___Yes ___Partial ___No
   c. Biological equivalent
      ___Yes ___No ___na
8. Withdrawals/loss to follow-up
   a. Listed
      ___Yes ___No ___na
   b. How analyzed
      ___Counted in original treatment group
      ___Counted as end result at time of withdrawal
      ___Counted as in both ways above, and other ways
      ___Discarded
      ___Counted in new group
      ___Not reported
      ___na
9. Treatment complications
   ___Described ___Not described
10. Tabulation of outcomes
   ___Given ___Not given
11. Statistical methods and analyses
   a. Statistical methods reported (specific tests, techniques, computer programs, etc.)
      ___Yes ___No
   b. Statistical analyses reported (beyond means, percentages, standard deviations)
      ___Yes ___No
   c. Test statistics given for endpoints
      ___Yes ___No ___Unclear
   d. Associated probability values given
      ___Yes ___No ___Unclear
   e. Confidence intervals given
      ___Yes ___No ___Unclear ___na
   f. Regression or correlation analyses
      ___Yes ___No ___Unclear ___na
   g. Statistical discussion of treatment complications given
      ___Yes ___No ___Unclear ___na
   h. Appropriate retrospective analysis of subgroups given
      ___Yes ___No ___Unclear ___na
12. Power addressed for negative trials
   ___Yes ___No ___na

[a] Yes means reported; unclear means inadequate, partial, or ambiguous information; no means not reported; na means inapplicability is reported or clearly implied.

Adapted from Chalmers et al. (1981).

Basic Descriptive Material

When assessing a published report of a clinical trial, the reviewer should note certain basic descriptive information, beginning with *authors*, *title*, *journal*, and *date of publication*.

The report of the clinical trial should include a description of the *trial design* (e.g., RCT, stratified-blocking). Other basic descriptive information includes the *sources of financial support* for the trial and whether or not a *biostatistician* has participated in the study (as an author, consultant, or reviewer). Studies should list the *starting and stopping dates* of the trial so that the results can be interpreted in the light of other changes in therapy that may have occurred. The paper should include a *statement of significant findings* as the author understands and interprets them.

It would be helpful for the reviewer of a published trial to know whether or not the report of the trial has been *reviewed by peers*. However, this often is not readily discernable, even among published papers that have been so reviewed. Although many journals use peer reviewers for most or all articles reporting scientific findings, these journals, as a matter of editorial policy, may not disclose whether or not a particular article was subject to peer review.

Sample Size

The numbers of patients in the trial affect the ability of the trial to detect differences between experimental and control groups. (The risks of making errors in detection of differences—α, the probability of the false-positive error, and β, the probability a false-negative error—are discussed below.) There should be evidence that a *prior estimate of the numbers of patients required* has been made.

A paper should list the *expected control group endpoint(s)*, the *improvement of clinical interest that should not be missed*, the *chosen levels of risk* (α and β), and the *number of patients required*. Here is an example from a trial of cyclosporine in cadaveric renal transplantation:

> Sample size was decided on the basis of a two-sided test of the hypothesis of equality of treatment groups for one-year graft survival. At the 5 per cent level of significance, the power of the test was set at 90 per cent for an expected difference between the two treatment groups of 20 per cent (55 vs. 75 per cent). The sample size was established at 100 patients per treatment group. Statistical analysis of the background variables was carried out to assess the balance between the two groups (Canadian Multicentre Transplant Study Group, 1983).

Regrettably, few studies do this (Altman, 1983). Only 12 percent of the trials reviewed by DerSimonian et al. (1982) reported calculations of power in planning sample size; Mosteller et al. (1980) found that less than 2 percent of the trials they reviewed did so.

Selection of Patients

The paper should provide a detailed description of the *criteria for admission and rejection of patients* to the trial, and should show that these criteria were applied before knowledge of the specific treatment assignment had been obtained. Without selection criteria, it is difficult to interpret and apply the findings of the trial. To the extent that study patients are not selected at random from a well-defined population (not to be confused with random allocation to treatment groups), doubt may exist as to whether trial findings may be generalized to that population, as well as to others. Thus, a mere statement that a certain number of patients with a given diagnosis were randomized is insufficient. First, admission criteria should be given which describe who was eligible for the study, e.g., patients with a particular diagnosis and treatment history, in a certain medical center, in a particular year, etc. Second, rejection criteria should be given which describe reasons why those who might otherwise have been admitted were ruled out of the study, e.g., diagnosis not confirmed by pathology, other serious illnesses, patient refusals, etc. The *number of patients actually entering the trial* should be given.

The description of the eligible patient population rejected for the trial can be as important as the documentation of the subjects studied. A log of those patients who are not allowed to enter the trial should be kept, including the reasons for their noneligibility. The primary use of such a *reject log* is to help identify bias in patient selection. An attempt should be made to compare the outcome of the rejected patients to the outcome of the trial subjects to detect any important selection biases, especially in instances in which cooperative studies are being undertaken at different centers.

Random Allocation

Random allocation of patients to treatment groups is a major bias-reducing technique in controlled clinical trials. The observed results of a trial may be affected (biased) by an uneven distribution to treatment groups of factors that affect prognosis such as age, disease state, or concurrent medical problems, as well as by the experimental treatment. (These prognostic factors may be referred to as *confounding variables* or *covariates*.) Proper randomization is an indifferent yet objective procedure which, among other benefits, tends to spread prognostic factors evenly among treatment groups.

A randomized study should provide information about the *method of random allocation* of patients, including information about the mechanism used to generate the random assignment and success in implementing it. A simple statement that a random assignment was made is insufficient, because some methods of random assignment may be effective but are poorly implemented, and some that appear to be random have serious weaknesses. In studies in which randomization was not possible, this should be noted.

Although random number tables or coin flipping may be unbiased in and of themselves, they may be used in ways which allow for the introduction of bias into a trial. Randomization should be verifiable as well as properly executed. Methods such as flipping coins, tossing dice, or drawing cards cannot be verified, and may lead investigators to interfere with the process. Some methods which are verifiable can also be too easily inspected by study personnel, providing opportunity for bias to influence acceptance and therefore treatment distribution. Examples are allocation by birth date, chart number, alternate cases, and an open randomization table.

Random numbers from one of the published random number tables or pseudorandom numbers generated by a well-studied computer method offer good sources of randomization. After being admitted into a trial, it is best that the patient is assigned to a treatment group by a central source. A preferred method of randomization uses carefully prepared, sealed, consecutively numbered opaque envelopes. In the case of a drug trial, drugs should be prepackaged and numbered for each patient before the time of randomization. Envelopes and packages should be returned to the biostatistician for verification of assignment.

Whereas simple randomization tends to spread prognostic factors evenly among treatment groups in trials with large numbers of patients, small studies are more vulnerable to imbalances of prognostic factors. To enhance the effect of randomization in studies with small sample sizes, the patient allocation process may include stratification and blocking. Patients are first classified according to one or more important prognostic factors (stratification), and then they are randomly assigned to experimental groups so that predetermined, appropriately fixed proportions of patients from each stratum receive each treatment (blocking) (see, e.g., Lavori et al., 1983). If used, the methods for stratification and blocking should be described.

Randomization should be *blinded* in that the investigator must not be able to deduce which treatment is next in line when a patient is accepted into the trial. It is especially important to *blind the randomization process* when the treatments are not blinded or trends in the study are known to the admitting investigator. An admitting investigator with a bias for or against a therapy that is thought to be next up for assignment may readily circumvent the patient in whom a suspected outcome might, in the view of the investigator, favor one treatment over another, or the investigator may delay admission until some other patient has been admitted. The informed consent procedure is an opportunity to inject this bias.

One method of *testing randomization* is the measurement of the prognostic factors of the groups being compared. Listing only demographic comparisons such as the usual age and sex distributions is usually insufficient.

If the distribution among the treatment groups of prognostic factors is disproportionate, the cause may be chance or a previously unsuspected bias; thus, the distribution of known prognostic factors by treatment category should be shown in tabular form. These data are critical in both assessing the efficacy of the blinding of the randomization (which, if in serious doubt, will generally result in a trial's results being discarded) and removing the unwanted effects of chance variation by using stratified analysis of a trial's results. Analysis-of-variance modeling of prognostic factors may be used to reduce bias and to increase precision of estimates of effects (Lavori et al., 1983). If the trial results are to be considered for use in combination with other trial results, the significance of known prognostic factors by treatment category may be important in deciding whether to do so.

Blinding

Blinding is a major bias-reducing technique in clinical trials. Many papers report that the therapy given was concealed from the patient or the physician or both (double blinding). However, many reports stop after using the term *blind* or *double blind* and leave the reader uncertain of exactly what has been concealed from whom. These terms are not sufficiently descriptive because the roles in the trial may not be limited to the patient and physician. Four or more parties may be involved with as many roles; each may be subject to hopes and prejudices about the trial. These are (1) the person(s) making the random allocations to treatment groups, (2) the patients, (3) the physicians or other providers, and (4) the biostatistician or other evaluators. Sometimes the physician makes the random assignment to treatment groups and/or is the evaluator. Such multiple responsibilities present further opportunities for bias which must be checked.

Persons making the random assignments who have knowledge of the assignments made for particular patients may have their own prejudices and hopes, which may bias the assignments. For scientific and ethical reasons, blinding of patients and physicians as to the ongoing results of the study is important. Of course, patients' attitudes toward their treatments may affect compliance, participation, and outcomes. The physician who gives or orders treatment naturally hopes for success and may treat patients differently, given knowledge of treatment assignments, such as providing extra attention to patients with the less-preferred treatment. If the treatments and randomization process are not adequately blinded, knowledge of the trial trends could lead the conscientious physician to alter the intake of patients to the trial or to influence withdrawals from the trial. From an ethical standpoint, the physician should no longer ask patients to join a study or to remain in it if the physician perceives an impressive trend. A *data-monitoring committee*, charged with studying the trial and notifying the investigators when a change in protocol should be considered or when the trial should be discontinued, is a proper inclusion in the informed consent procedure (Chalmers, 1976). Although such a committee would not dissolve the ethical considerations (which would be shifted in part to it), it would better enable the physician to act consistently in randomization and treatment. Evaluators who are aware of the treatments given may bias their findings, despite conscious efforts to be fair. When necessary, the statistician-evaluator who has properly participated in planning the trial may work with coded data.

As for randomization, the methods of achieving blindness should be reported to give the reader important information for judging the adequacy of a trial's protection from bias. Although not all types of blindness are feasible for all trials, every reasonable attempt should be made to achieve as many types of blindness as possible. This aspect requires careful consideration and reporting by the authors. Five aspects of a trial which should be blinded (Chalmers et al., 1981) are as follows:

1. the randomization process (discussed above under Random Allocation);
2. patients as to treatment assignment;
3. physicians as to treatment assignment;
4. physicians and patients as to trends/ongoing results of the trial; and
5. biostatisticians/other evaluators.

In certain trials, patients and physicians should be blinded to the timing of interventions, e.g., the point during crossover trials at which patients switch from one treatment group to another.

It is not sufficient to assume that a double-blind procedure is effective. In good studies the physicians and their patients are *tested for blinding* at the end of the study to determine whether or not they have guessed treatment assignments.

Treatments

All *experimental and ancillary treatment regimens* must be described well enough to allow interpretation of the results and replication in other studies or practice. This includes the timing and amount of treatments in the trial and all other allowable treatments.

If a trial used a *placebo*, it is insufficient merely to mention that a placebo was given. Identity of appearance and taste where applicable should be documented, and evidence for physician and/or patient ability to distinguish between placebo and experimental treatment should be noted.

Compliance

Objective methods of verifying that patients are conforming to the protocol should be described. For example, in a drug trial, pill counts would be acceptable. When subjective (indirect) assessments of compliance are used, the validity of the subjective measure should be addressed. *Biological equivalent* refers to a measure, where appropriate, of a therapeutic agent after absorption or injection, preferably in its active form. Examples are pre- and postvagotomy measurements of gastric acid output in therapeutic trials of peptic ulcer. Blood or urine levels of an active agent may also be used to measure compliance. Biological equivalent measurements are useful both as measures of compliance and in describing treatments.

In some trials the assessment of compliance is self-evident, such as in certain trials comparing surgical and medical treatments for a disease. Trials in which patients are to maintain regimens on an outpatient basis, especially over an extended period, present special problems in validating compliance. In some trials, a patient's compliance may be partial or temporary, as well as positive or negative. In any case, definitions for what constitutes compliance must be explicit, and compliance of all patients should be accounted for.

Withdrawals/Loss to Follow-up

In most reported trials, a number of subjects drop out or are withdrawn after the trial is under way. In trials with long-term follow-up, large trials, and trials with complicated protocols, some follow-up data are likely to be missing. Sometimes investigators cannot collect outcome data from all subjects because some die, move away, decline to continue to participate, or become lost from the study group for other reasons.

Information should be available regarding what happened to all the patients treated. *Dropouts should be listed* by diagnosis, treatment, reason for withdrawal, and whether withdrawal occurred as a result of patient or investigator initiative. It is usually important to report outcome in this group after the time of withdrawal, and they should be considered in the main analysis of the trial. When dropouts are properly reported, the reader can often assess the effect of missing data on the trial's conclusions; otherwise, the skeptical reader may conclude that the paper should be dismissed. Different kinds of withdrawals (i.e., in terms of prognostic characteristics) could bias the final makeup of each treatment group, thus diminishing the efficacy of the randomization procedure for obtaining similar kinds of patients in each treatment group.

Trials that do not mention withdrawals, or whose withdrawals exceed 5 percent, should be carefully scrutinized. Deletion of cases by the investigator after completion of the study raises strong concern over investigator bias and undermines any findings.

Universal application of a rule regarding counting of withdrawals without considering the nature of a trial and its objectives may give misleading findings (Sackett and Gent, 1979). Depending on the type of study, withdrawals are handled in different ways, for example, as follows.

1. Patients are considered as an end result for the group to which they were originally assigned regardless of what happens to them.
2. Patients can be counted as an end result at the time of withdrawal.
3. The results are analyzed with the dropouts handled as in both 1 and 2 and in other ways if appropriate. For instance, it may be useful to characterize treatment groups in terms of patient-years of treatment, to which even withdrawals, under certain well-defined circumstances, would make contributions.
4. Patients can be ignored or eliminated from the study at the time of withdrawal, and thus not be counted as an end result. Although this is often done, it is rarely defensible.
5. Patients may change groups, i.e., cross over, and be considered as an end result in the new group. Unless this is done as part of the planned protocol, it is not defensible.

Treatment Complications

The paper should provide information describing the presence or absence of *side effects* or complications after treatment. To determine the usefulness of a treatment, readers need to assess the nature and incidence of these side effects and their implications for patient care. The report should describe an active search for side effects or complications and discuss those that are found. If no side effects occur, this should be explicitly stated. As is done in the main analysis, *statistical analysis* should be made of side effects if the sample size warrants it, including comparisons of percentages with a statistical test of significance and the observed probability. Given no significant difference in side effects, the probability of the false-negative error (β) should be mentioned.

Tabulation of Outcomes

A good study will *tabulate all events employed as outcomes* (endpoints) so that the reader can check the calculations and use the data more effectively in combining the results of different studies. Data of trial results should not be aggregated to a level that would preclude the reader from conducting secondary analyses. For all discrete endpoints that are spread over time, such as mortality or morbidity, even for some trials of short duration, life table or time series analysis should be carried out. Some papers present outcome data as crude rates, e.g., a 5-year death rate. This may be useful summary information, but alone it may be inadequate for illustrating the course of treatment effects. The data should be presented in a form that would allow the reader to reproduce the survival curve or curves.

Statistical Methods and Analysis

The uncertainty associated with real-world sample sizes usually requires formal statistical inference to evaluate the effects observed in trials. When an author merely states that p was less than 0.05 without identifying the statistical test, readers cannot satisfy themselves that the methods were appropriate. The paper should include statistical analyses going beyond the computation of means, percentages, and standard deviations. The names of the specific statistical methods, i.e., tests, techniques, and computer programs (with program version) used for statistical analyses should be given. In the *analysis* of the data gathered in any clinical trial there are certain minimal procedures that are indicative of quality. These include, but are not limited to, *significance of major endpoints*, *confidence intervals*, and *regression or correlation analyses*.

The level of *statistical significance* is the probability of making a false-positive, or Type I, error, i.e., concluding that there is a difference between the experimental and control groups when in fact there is none. The probability of a Type I error is known as α. When significance is reported, it should be given in such a way that the reader can make the actual calculations. Both the test statistic and its associated probability values should be stated. If one is given without the other, the reader may have trouble verifying or understanding the statistical conclusions.

Confidence intervals should be provided for the measurements used as trial endpoints. Confidence intervals provide information that adds to the accept-reject findings of a hypothesis test. The confidence limits define the interval in which one can be reasonably confident (e.g., greater than 90 percent) that the true difference between treatments lies. If that interval includes zero, the null hypothesis of no true difference cannot be rejected. However, the location and width of the interval may suggest the direction of a true difference and the ability of a larger sample size to reject the null hypothesis. Confidence intervals that encompass clinically unrealistic measurements raise questions about the assumed distribution of measurements and should be discussed.

Regression or correlation analyses should be carried out for trials when it is of interest to know how treatment and outcome variables change or do not change together, such as when the critical response is a function of drug dosage or predetermined, quantifiable clinical factors.

When a trial is over, it is tempting and sometimes useful to select for analysis subgroups that were not stratified at the trial's outset. However, investigators and reviewers should realize that such post hoc study is subject to selection bias just as is any retrospective study, and that no rigorous conclusions can be drawn from them. *Retrospective studies* are useful to suggest new studies; may point out inadequacies arising from the random allocation process, dropouts, or compliance; and may help to estimate their effect on outcomes.

Although many papers state the specific objectives of the study, it is often very difficult to find results in the paper that apply directly to the specific objectives. A clear presentation of results should be made.

Power

The probability of making a false-negative, or Type II, error, i.e., of not detecting a difference between the experimental and control treatments when in fact one does exist, is known as β. *Power*, generally defined as $(1 - \beta)$, is the probability of avoiding Type II error, i.e., detecting that true difference. As discussed above, the paper should provide information describing the determination of sample size before the trial, which would enable the detection of clinically important differences.

Although confidence limits portray the uncertainty of a treatment effect, discussion of power denotes the strength of the conclusion. As illustrated in the study by Freiman et al. (1978) referenced above under Clinical Trial Reporting, small sample size frequently leads to trials with little power to detect differences among treatment groups. If the difference between the experimental and control groups is not statistically significant, then the false-negative error and its probability should be addressed. A well-designed trial with high power that detects no statistically significant difference between treatments can be convincing. But if no statistically significant difference is found and the power is low, or not discussed, the reader cannot dismiss the possibility that the study was not large enough to detect an important treatment effect. For a negative trial, it would be informative to estimate the number of patients that would have been required to document as significant the observed difference between treatment and control groups, assuming that that difference were to hold up with the larger sample size.

REFERENCES

Altman, D. G. 1983. Size of clinical trials. British Medical Journal 286:1842–1843.

Campbell, D. T., and J. C. Stanley. 1963. Experimental and Quasi-Experimental Design for Research. Chicago: Rand McNally.

Canadian Multicentre Transplant Study Group. 1983. A randomized clinical trial of cyclosporine in cadaveric renal transplantation. New England Journal of Medicine 309:809–815.

Chalmers T. C., and discussants. 1976. How to turn off an experiment. In J. D. Cooper and H. D. Ley, eds., Ethical Safeguards in Research on Humans. Washington, D.C.: Interdisciplinary Communications Associates.

Chalmers, T. C., P. C. Celano, H. S. Sacks, and H. Smith. 1983. Bias in treatment assignment in controlled clinical trials. New England Journal of Medicine 309:1358–1361.

Chalmers, T. C., H. Smith, B. Blackburn, B. Silverman, B. Schroeder, D. Reitman, and A. Ambroz. 1981. A method for assessing the quality of a randomized control trial. Controlled Clinical Trials 2:31–49.

Cook, T. D., and D. T. Campbell. 1979. Quasi-Experimentation: Design and Analysis Issues for Field Settings. Chicago: Rand McNally.

DerSimonian, R., L. J. Charette, B. McPeek, and F. Mosteller. 1982. Reporting on methods in clinical trials. New England Journal of Medicine 306:1332–1337.

Emerson, J. D., B. McPeek, and F. Mosteller. In press. Reporting clinical trials in general medical journals. Surgery.

Freiman, J. A., T. C. Chalmers, H. Smith, and R. R. Kuebler. 1978. The importance of beta, the Type II error and sample size in the design and interpretation of the randomized control trial. New England Journal of Medicine 299:690–694.

Friedman, L., C. Furberg, and D. deMets. 1981. Fundamentals of Clinical Trials. Boston: Wright-PSG.

Lavori, P. W., T. A. Louis, J. C. Bailar, and M. Polansky. 1983. Designs for experiments—parallel comparisons of treatment. New England Journal of Medicine 309:1291–1299.

Louis, T. A., P. W. Lavori, J. C. Bailar, and M. Polansky. 1984. Crossover and self-controlled designs in clinical research. New England Journal of Medicine 310:24–31.

Mosteller, F., J. Gilbert, and B. McPeek. 1980. Reporting standards and research strategies for controlled trials. Controlled Clinical Trials 1:37–58.

Peto, R., M. C. Pike, P. Armitage, N. E. Breslow, D. R. Cox, S. V. Howard, N. Mantel, K. McPherson, J. Peto, and P. G. Smith. 1976. Design and analysis of randomized clinical trials requiring prolonged observation of each patient, Part I. British Journal of Cancer 34:585–612.

Peto, R., M. C. Pike, P. Armitage, N. E. Breslow, D. R. Cox, S. V. Howard, N. Mantel, K. McPherson, J. Peto, and P. G. Smith. 1977. Design and analysis of randomized clinical trials requiring prolonged observation of each patient, Part II. British Journal of Cancer 35:1–39.

Sackett, D. L., and M. Gent. 1979. Controversy in counting and attributing events in clinical trials. New England Journal of Medicine 301:1410–1412.

Shapiro, S. H., and T. A. Louis. 1983. Clinical Trials: Issues and Approaches. New York: Marcel Dekker.

Information Needs for Technology Assessment

Morris F. Collen*

Technology assessment has been defined in this volume and elsewhere[1] as a complex process requiring a broad comprehensive base of data in order to permit evaluation of short- and long-term, intended and unintended, and direct and indirect consequences of the use of technology.

A technology assessment usually first defines the technology to be studied, identifies the alternative technologies with which it competes, describes the patients using the technology, and considers the goals of decision makers for whom the technology assessment is intended; then it evaluates the process and outcomes of using the technology for these patients. Accordingly, the information needs for a technology assessment include (1) descriptive information of the technology and how it is used; (2) descriptive information of alternative, competitive technologies; (3) descriptive data of the patient and population users of the technology; (4) evaluative data of direct, intended effects; and (5) evaluative data of indirect, unintended effects.

This section lists *what* information is usually needed for a comprehensive technology assessment. Information sources that can provide these data (such as registries and data bases), and how the data are acquired are considered in Chapter 3.

DESCRIPTIVE INFORMATION OF THE TECHNOLOGY

Definition of the Type of Technology

The different approaches to classification of technologies have been mentioned in Chapter 2, and different types of technology require different information for assessment. As a minimum, a technology can be classified using recommended standard terms when available as being a drug,[2] a technique or procedure,[3,4] a device or equipment, or a system.

Functional Specifications of the Technology

Information specifying *what* the technology is intended to do, its purpose or objectives, is necessary in accordance with the functional classification of the technology. Evaluation methodology is sufficiently different for the following functional groups to require detailed functional specifications of a technology when used for:

- Screening or diagnostic medicine, such as screening for fetal neural tube defects by the maternal serum alpha-fetoprotein test, computed tomographic (CT) scanning for the diagnosis of abdominal tumors, etc.
- Therapeutic, preventive, or rehabilitative medicine, such as cancer therapy, cardiac surgery, immunizations, prosthetics, etc.
- Supporting or coordinating medicine, such as a hospital computer system.

Technical Specifications of the Technology

An evaluation of *how* the technology works will usually require information as to the following:

- Technical description of the technology, its structure and operational characteristics, exact type of procedure, etc.
- Supporting resources needed, such as necessary specialized technical personnel and their training, supplies, facility site, and energy requirements.
- When appropriate, data on process quality control, reliability, preventive maintenance, and backup requirements.

Costs of Technology

Reliable cost data are difficult to obtain, but as a compromise, fees or charges to the

* Director, Technology Assessment, Department of Medical Methods Research, Kaiser-Permanente Medical Care Program, Oakland, California.

user are often used as substitutes for costs. Unless specific cost centers are established to identify the various expenses associated with the utilization of the technology, accurate costs will not usually be available. Information will be needed as to capital costs for equipment and facilities and direct operational costs including those for personnel, supplies, depreciation of equipment, etc.

Process information as to workload can then provide unit costs per procedure or per use of technology.[4] When appropriate, and if a defined population of users is available, then total expenditures can be derived for the technology per unit of population using the technology (e.g., per one thousand patients, or per one million population).

Alternative Technologies

Similar information as described above will need to be obtained for alternative competing technologies used for the same functional requirements. For example, for the diagnosis of abdominal body tumors, one will need information to assess alternative scanners (x-ray CT versus ultrasound versus nuclear medicine).

PROVIDER, PATIENT, AND POPULATION INFORMATION

Patient Workload

In order to evaluate cost-effectiveness, the following information will be needed:

- Number of patients using the device (equipment) or receiving the procedure, per unit of time (e.g., per episode of illness or per day) for specific conditions.
- Number of patients with the same condition receiving alternative technology.
- Criteria used for appropriate selection of patients for the alternative technologies.

Patient Demographic Information

For patients using the technology, information will be required as to number of patients (yet preserving patient confidentiality), age (date of birth), sex, race and ethnic group, occupation, and residence area (e.g., zip codes). Marital status, family status, and educational and financial information are important for some technologies such as those used for home or self-care. Health habits and life-styles may be important factors influencing patient outcomes.

Relevant Patient Medical Information

Diagnoses for which the technology is used must be available in detail as appropriate for the specific technology, indicating severity or staging of disease and using a standardized diagnosis code.[5-8] Also, information will be needed as to how often the technology was used for the specific conditions, such as total usage for an episode of illness and patient outcome from the use of the technology.

Linkage of medical data will be needed from multiple medical records (i.e., for multiple episodes of illness, office visits, and hospitalizations). Prior use of medical services may be important.

Relevant Population Medical Data

To determine rates of use of technology in the population that is served requires data as to the size of the targeted or user population and incidence and prevalence of the condition or disease in the population using the technology.

Provider Information

Health care provider specialty services that use the technology (e.g., cardiac surgery, obstetrics, nuclear medicine, etc.) will need to be identified. Also information will be needed as to the facility sites providing the services, such as (1) ambulatory care visits/encounters for technology used in the office, (2) hospital admission rates and days in hospital for technology used in the hospital, and (3) nursing home days and home care visits for technology used in these sites. Appropriate information will be needed for ancillary services, including pharmacy drug usage, clinical laboratory tests, x-ray procedures, electrocardiograms, electroencephalograms, cardiac catheterization, hemodialysis, etc.

Payments for Technology

Who pays for the use of a technology may influence its rate of diffusion and utilization.

Charges to patients for specific technology procedures[9] and sources of payment (self-pay, insurance, Medicare, etc.) will be needed.

EVALUATIVE INFORMATION

Intended Users of the Technology Assessment

Technology assessments are usually conducted for health care policymakers, but they may also be intended for use by administrators, physicians, and patients. Each of these groups has special interests that may require different information. Policymakers and administrators will be especially interested in comparative cost-benefit analyses for competing technologies, whereas patients will be primarily concerned with health care outcomes.

Evaluative Information for Direct, Intended Effects

Effectiveness Effectiveness measures how well the technology works, that is, the extent to which the technology achieves its specified intended objectives. Evaluation information usually includes measures of both patient outcome and the health care process.

Evaluation of clinical effectiveness for screening and diagnostic technology requires information on sensitivity, specificity, yield rates, etc. For therapeutic technology, effectiveness measures for individual patients usually include information on health status outcomes, functional disabilities which limit patients' return to work, etc. For population groups, information needs include the effects on health indexes; rates of morbidity, disability, and mortality; and average years of life gained.

Managerial or production effectiveness, such as for coordinating technology, will need information on throughput time, error detection rates, etc.

Clinical Safety Technology assessments usually need information as to clinical hazards, toxicity, adverse effects, etc.

Economic Analysis and Efficiency Efficiency measures will require information as to the resource costs used to achieve specified levels of technology effectiveness for clinical, medical, or outcome efficiency, such as unit cost per true positive test for diagnostic technology or cost per episode of illness for a therapeutic technology. Assessment of managerial, technical process, or production efficiency will require measures of unit cost of technology per unit of operational time, etc.

Effects of discount rates must be considered in valuing costs and benefits over time. Information should be obtained to assess the effect of organizational financial arrangements on costs, utilization, and rate of diffusion/replacement of technology when applicable (e.g., fee-for-service or cost-reimbursement versus health maintenance organization [HMO] capitation payments or prospective budgeting).

An assessment of benefits from the use of medical technology adds an additional extensive set of information requirements, including estimated value of extended years of life to individual patients[10] and to the group.[1] A cost-benefit analysis requires a basis for converting all benefits to monetary terms.

Similar information will be required for all competing alternative technologies, including data on appropriateness of patient utilization rates for the alternative technologies. It may be of interest to assess the actual (and appropriate) mix of competing technologies used per unit of population served (e.g., per one thousand patients or per one million population served).

EVALUATIVE INFORMATION FOR INDIRECT, UNINTENDED EFFECTS

An indirect or unintended consequence of the use of a technology may be very extensive, and usually the decision makers for whom the assessment is being prepared have special interests which will determine the specific information needed. As has been emphasized, different data may be needed for a technology assessment providing options for patient-consumers than may be needed for clinicians, for hospital administrators, or for government policymakers. Accordingly, the assessment of indirect consequences requires a correspondingly broad range of information needs, including, when appropriate, data as to societal effects, legal effects, ethical effects, and environmental effects.

RECOMMENDATION FOR A STANDARD MINIMUM DATA SET

Using the above guidelines and other published minimum data sets as models,[11–14] it is recommended that there be developed a minimum data set for medical records to better satisfy the basic information needs for their use in technology assessments. Such a minimum data set could contain essential and necessary data for many technology assessments. Of course, this could not provide sufficient comprehensive data for every assessment, and special data subsets could be developed for the different technology types and for those that require analytic methods. Nevertheless, it would encourage a more uniform approach to data collection and documentation which should increase the potential of using medical record data for technology assessment, facilitate data linkage, permit meaningful data comparisons, and support retrospective studies.

NOTES

[1] Office of Technology Assessment. 1980. The Implications of Cost-Effectiveness Analysis of Medical Technology. Washington, D.C.: U.S. Government Printing Office.

[2] American Hospital Formulary Services for Drug Classification.

[3] Current Procedural Terminology (CPT-4). American Medical Association.

[4] Blue Cross/Blue Shield Codes for Procedures.

[5] International Classification of Diseases, 9th Revision, Clinical Modification (ICD-9-CM).

[6] Systematized Nomenclature of Medicine (SNOMED). American Association of Pathologists.

[7] Classification of Reasons for Visits. National Ambulatory Care Survey (NCHS).

[8] International Classification of Health Problems in Primary Care (ICHPPC-2), World Health Organization of National Colleges, Academies, and Academic Associations for General Practitioners/Family Physicians (WONCA).

[9] California Relative Value Codes for Physician Reimbursement.

[10] McNeil, B. J. Values and Preferences of Patients and Providers (see p. 535 of Appendix B of this book).

[11] Uniform Ambulatory Medical Care. Minimum Data Set. DHEW Pub. No. (PHS) 81-1161. Washington, D.C.: U.S. Government Printing Office.

[12] Guidelines for Producing Uniform Data for Health Care Plans. DHEW Pub. No. (HSM) 73-3005. Washington, D.C.: U.S. Government Printing Office.

[13] Uniform Hospital Discharge Data. Minimum Data Set. DHEW Pub. No. (PHS) 80-1157. Washington, D.C.: U.S. Government Printing Office.

[14] Long-Term Health Care. Minimum Data Set. DHHS Pub. No. (PHS) 80-1158. Washington, D.C.: U.S. Government Printing Office.

Toward Evaluating Cost-Effectiveness of Medical and Social Experiments

Frederick Mosteller*
Milton C. Weinstein†

The United States has been increasingly concerned about costs of health care (Fuchs, 1974; Hiatt, 1975). One possible response to this concern is an accelerated strategy for evaluating the efficacy of medical practices, with the hope that identifying those practices that are not efficacious will lead to their abandonment and, therefore, to substantial savings in health care resources (Cochrane, 1972). An alternative response to the cost problem acknowledges that information on efficacy will not eliminate the need to face trade-offs between increasing incremental costs and diminishing incremental benefits. Moreover, information on efficacy will not resolve the highly individual and subjective judgments about the value of symptom relief or other aspects of improved quality of life.

These two responses to the health cost problem are not mutually exclusive, although they lead to different emphases. While we concentrate on evaluation of efficacy, we acknowledge—and, indeed, seek to elucidate—some of the limitations of evaluation of efficacy as a means of improving the public health or controlling costs.

Evaluation has its own costs, and so it needs to be considered how much different kinds of evaluation are worth and what their benefits may be. The long-term goal of the research that we outline here would be to develop and demonstrate a methodology for assessing these benefits and costs.

To oversimplify for a moment, two possible scenarios resulting from the evaluation of efficacy can be identified. In the first, a therapy or diagnostic method proved ineffective (or at least cost-ineffective) would be dropped by the profession, and the money saved would reduce the national medical budget without substantially impairing health. In the second scenario, a procedure is proved effective, and this leads to more widespread use and resulting health benefits. There are examples of both scenarios: gastric freezing for the first, and antihypertensive medications for the second.

Students of policy, however, will recognize both of these scenarios as idealized and unrealistic. Technological changes and changes in practice are ordinarily slow, except in crisis situations. For the first scenario, funds not used for one purpose are quickly and smoothly diverted to other uses, possibly ones that compensate for an abandoned procedure. Advocates of a procedure let go slowly and use ostensible (and sometimes legitimate) scientific arguments to cast doubt on the validity of the evaluation. For the second scenario, practitioners may be slow to adopt new procedures, even if proved efficacious, unless they perceive the benefits to be immediate and attributable to the intervention (a general obstacle to adopting preventive medical practices).

Although we recognize the difficulty of the task, we are reminded of the need for some rational basis for allocating resources to clinical experiments. Budgets for clinical trials at the National Institutes of Health (NIH) are under constant surveillance, and vigilant members of Congress will want to know that resources have been well spent. Administrators at NIH facing straitened budgets must choose carefully medical procedures in which to invest the resources for a clinical trial, recognizing that a trial done in one area means a trial not done in another. Can these administrators not only improve their decision rules for internal budget allocation but also determine whether additional resources spent on clinical investigations have a greater ex-

* Chairman, Department of Health Policy and Management, Harvard School of Public Health.

† Professor of Policy and Decision Sciences, Harvard School of Public Health.

pected return than resources spent at the margin elsewhere in the health sector? The economist's test of allocative efficiency (equal incremental return across and within sectors of the budget) has more than a little conceptual appeal in this domain, but the analytical tasks are formidable.

HOW ARE EVALUATIONS USED?

The value of an evaluation depends on how its results are translated into changes in practice. Consider three models of decision making in the presence of information from evaluations: the normative, the descriptive, and the regulatory.

In the normative model, the ideal, physicians act in the best interests of the society. They process new information rationally. They allocate resources according to the principles of cost-effectiveness analysis, electing the procedures that yield the maximum health benefits obtainable from the health care budget. Although some future reconfiguration of incentives in the U.S. health care system may move the United States closer to that state of affairs, the normative model of decision making is best thought of as an unattainable ideal; the value of information under this model is the best that can possibly be expected.

In the descriptive model, or models, an attempt would be made to assess what the response of physicians and other decision makers *would be* to the information from a trial. Here, past experiences must be relied on, as well as information from economic, sociologic, and psychologic theories. We need to learn how to predict when the response will be rapid, when it will be slow, when it will be nonexistent, and when it will be paradoxical. Perhaps a model can be developed, based on data from past history, that would identify the characteristics of the procedure, the type of study (e.g., randomized versus observational, large versus small, multicenter versus single institution), the nature of the medical specialty, and other variables that can be combined into a prediction of response.

In the regulatory model, the possibility of interventions (by government, by insurers, by professional societies) intended to make medical practice more responsive to information would be allowed. For example, reimbursement might be preconditioned on evidence of efficacy or otherwise linked to the state of information. Food and Drug Administration (FDA)-type procedures for practices other than drugs and devices would fall into this category. We recognize many problems inherent in such an approach: establishing criteria for efficacy when outcomes have multiple attributes (including survival and many features of the quality of life), and establishing criteria for efficacy to apply to a heterogeneous population when the procedure could not have been tested in all possible subpopulations. We are open to the possibility that more decentralized approaches to altering incentives for practice in response to information on efficacy—or even to collecting the information itself—may be possible.

WHAT IS BEING EVALUATED?

Initially the problem was defined as that of evaluating the worth of a randomized clinical trial (RCT). Inevitably, the question arose, "Compared with what?" One possible answer was: "Compared with what would have happened in the absence of an RCT." The possibilities are varied: perhaps observational studies of procedures after they are widely practiced, perhaps clinic-based or community-based studies, perhaps systematic efforts using data banks, perhaps NIH consensus development conferences, perhaps committee appraisals in the Institute of Medicine, or perhaps review papers in leading professional journals. Whatever the alternatives may be, we do not seem to be able to deal with the RCT, or other methods, in isolation. Obviously this necessity for breadth multiplies the research effort enormously.

AN ANALYTIC FRAMEWORK FOR ASSESSING COST-EFFECTIVENESS

We suggest a general conceptual model for evaluating the cost-effectiveness of medical evaluations, and illustrate its applicability to two particular clinical trials.

Cost-Effectiveness Analysis and Health Practices

Economists turn to cost-effectiveness analysis when resources are limited and when the objective is to maximize some nonmonetary output. This technique is well suited to the assessment of medical procedures in which outcomes do not lend themselves to monetary valuation. The cost-effectiveness of a medical procedure may be evaluated as the ratio of its resource cost (in dollars) to some measure of its health effectiveness (Weinstein and Stason, 1977; U.S. Congress, 1980; Warner and Luce, 1982). The units of effectiveness vary across studies, but years of life gained (perhaps adjusted or weighted for quality) are the most commonly used. The rationale for using such a ratio as a basis for resource allocation is as follows. Assume that the society's objective is to allocate its health budget to achieve the maximum total health benefit (setting aside, for the moment, equity concerns). Then the optimal decision rule is to rank order programs in increasing order of their cost-effectiveness ratios (C/E) and to assign priorities on this basis. The C/E ratio for the last program chosen under the budget constraint may be interpreted as the incremental health value (for example, in years of life, or quality-adjusted years of life) per additional dollar allocated to health care.

Although the cost-effectiveness model is far from being used as a blueprint for health resources allocated in practice, many studies along these lines have helped to clarify the relative efficiency with which health care resources are being, or might be, consumed in various areas of medical technology (Weinstein and Stason, 1976; Bunker et al., 1977; U.S. Congress, 1980).

A Cost-Effectiveness Model for Clinical Trials

In the above formulation, the net costs (C) and net effectiveness (E) are uncertain. For purposes of today's decision making, it may be reasonable to act on best estimates of these values, but the possibility that new information might alter perceptions of these variables must not be obscured, thus permitting reallocations of the budget in more health-producing ways. It is reasonable to ask what is the value of information about the effectiveness (or cost) of a medical procedure? Moreover, since resources for providing such information (e.g., for clinical trials) are limited, it is reasonable to ask what is the cost-effectiveness ratio *for a clinical trial*, where the cost would be the resource cost of the trial, and the effectiveness would be the expected increase in the health benefits produced, owing to the information. We would also want to take into account the possibility that, if the utilization of a procedure drops as a consequence of the trial (e.g., if the procedure is found not to be effective), that might have the effect of freeing health care resources for other beneficial purposes.

Thus, the cost-effectiveness ratio for a study would be represented as $C_{study}/[\Delta E - (\Delta C/\lambda)]$, where C_{study} is the cost of the study, ΔE is the net expected health gain (e.g., years of life gained) attributable to the study, ΔC is the net expected addition to health care cost attributable to the study, and λ is an "exchange rate" between health benefits and health care costs. Below are comments on each of these terms.

The net expected health benefit from the study (ΔE) depends on a number of factors, such as the following: the presumptive probability that the intervention being evaluated is more effective than the current intervention; the magnitude of the possible gain in effectiveness; the probability that the study will detect the effect, if present; the proportion of the population that will adopt the new intervention if the trial is conducted and under each possible study result; the proportion that will adopt the new intervention if no trial is conducted.

The net expected addition to health care cost could be positive (if the trial leads to adoption of a more-expensive intervention) or negative (if the trial leads to cost savings—for example, if the prevailing therapy is found to be no more effective than placebo).

The weighting factor λ reflects the equivalent health value society wishes to place on health resource costs. Under our idealized normative model, λ would equal the cost-effectiveness ratio for the lowest priority health program adopted under society's budget constraint. More realistically, it could reflect the cost-effectiveness ratio for the health programs that would, in fact, be forgone if the new intervention absorbed a share of available resources. Or, it could reflect society's explicit monetary valuation of health, in terms of willingness to pay, human capital, or other measures.

Finally, the numerator, C_{study}, represents the cost of the study itself. In order to express both numerator and denominator in comparable units of time (e.g., cost per year, benefits per year), they would both have to be either an annual value or a present value, according to appropriate accounting procedures.

Examples

Beta-Carotene The first example concerns an ongoing trial of beta-carotene against placebo, in which the hypothesis is that beta-carotene might prevent cancer. Background on this subject and details of the calculations of cost-effectiveness of the trial have been reported (Weinstein, 1983).

An expected annual benefit (ΔE) of 4,600 years of life saved was calculated as follows:

	0.1	(prior probability of effect)
×	0.15	(percent reduction in cancer mortality if effect is present and if intervention is universally adopted)
×	0.64	(probability that study will detect effect, if present)
×	0.10	(increase in proportion of population consuming more than 15 mg/day beta-carotene if study is positive, compared with no study)
×	400,000	(cancer deaths per year)
×	12	(years of life saved per number of cancer deaths averted).

An expected annual cost (ΔC) of $66 million was based on the assumptions that an additional 10 percent of the population would consume 15 mg/day at an annual cost of $30 (for a pharmacologic preparation), and that this would occur with a probability of 0.11 (allowing for the risk of a false-positive study result*).

The cost of the study (C_{study}) was estimated to be $4 million. Taking the value of this amount 15 years later, when the first cancer deaths would be avoided, and taking an annual value in perpetuity at 5 percent per annum leads to an annual equivalent of $420,000.

If the cost of treatment is ignored, therefore, the cost-effectiveness ratio for this study would be:

$$\frac{\$420{,}000/\text{year}}{4{,}600 \text{ years of life/year}},$$

or $91/life-year gained. If the cost of treatment is included and an opportunity cost of $50,000 per year of life is assumed, then the ratio becomes:

$$\frac{\$420{,}000/\text{year}}{4{,}600 \text{ years of life/year} - (\$66 \text{ million/year})/(\$50{,}000/\text{year of life})},$$

or $128/life-year gained. In either case, this trial appears to be an excellent investment.

This randomized trial was funded, after some controversy, as an add-on to a trial examining the relation between aspirin and myocardial infarction. The study, following more than 20,000 physicians over a 5-year period, is now in progress.

Mild Hypertension Calculation of the potential benefits and costs of a mild hypertension trial was made at the time such a trial was being considered by the Veterans Administration and the National Institutes of Health (Laird et al., 1979). First, the cost of the trial was estimated at $135 million, assuming that 28,000 subjects were followed

* If the study has a 64 percent chance of detecting a genuine effect and a 5 percent chance of detecting an effect when none is present, then the probability of a positive study is (0.1)(0.64) + (0.9)(0.05) = 0.109.

for 5 years. Next, the size of the population at risk was estimated to be 20 million, of which 10 percent was already being treated. To simplify, consider three possible results of the trial as viewed prospectively at that time: not efficacious, efficacious, and inconclusive. If the finding was that treatment is not efficacious, and if this finding is translated into practice, then 2 million persons per year would *not* spend an average of $200 on treatment, for a total of $400 million per year. Over 10 years, with discounting at 5 percent per annum, the present value would be $3 billion. Say that a 0.1 probability was assigned to the event that treatment is not effective and that a 0.2 probability was assigned that the study would show conclusively that the effect is either zero or small enough to be considered outweighed by risks and costs. (The latter estimate can be made more rigorous by considering study size, a prior distribution of the efficacy parameters, such as mortality rates, and the probability that each particular finding would result in reduced utilization.) Under these assumptions, the study appeared to have a 0.02 chance of saving $3 billion over 10 years, an expected value of $60 million. Therefore, this contingency would pay back half the cost of the study. Then the analysis would have to be repeated under the possibility that treatment is efficacious and that the study will demonstrate this. To do this, the health benefits would have to be estimated—as Weinstein and Stason (1976) have done—and the additional treatment costs owing to increased utilization would have to be added. It would also be necessary to consider the false-negative case (treatment is efficacious, but the study says it is not) and the false-positive case (treatment is not efficacious, but the study says it is). These estimates could be substituted into the cost-effectiveness model and the cost-effectiveness ratio of the study could be assessed.

The epilogue to this fable (although it is by no means over) is that this particular trial never was conducted, but another major trial reported its results in 1979 (Hypertension Detection and Follow-up Program, 1979). It reported a significant and important treatment effect, especially in the mildly hypertensive group. The controversy continues as to whether this community-based study was really measuring the effects of antihypertensive medication or whether other differences between the treatments could have accounted for the difference in mortality.

PROBLEMS IN ASSESSING COST-EFFECTIVENESS OF STUDIES

As the foregoing illustration suggests, the diversity and incomparability of situations forces us to tailor the evaluation to a particular study. Diagnosis, prevention, therapies, palliation, and health care delivery all fall within the scope of the studies that we might try to evaluate. RCTs can be used for any of them, or they may be a component of evaluation. For example, in considering the dissemination of a new, expensive technology, a RCT may be required to help measure the effectiveness of treatment as one component of an evaluation. Another component might be related to utilization patterns, and yet another might be related to costs. We will probably tend to focus on RCT as a method of providing information on efficacy and take information on other aspects of cost-effectiveness as given. However, we may also want to consider how to assess the value of information on costs or on patterns of use of medical procedures and facilities. In any event, the following tasks lie before us in virtually any attempt to evaluate a study positively.

How Decisions Will Be Made with the Experiment

We do not know very much about how decisions are actually made. We need a systematic set of historical studies that tells us the situation before, during, and after the evaluations. (The term *evaluations* is used because often more than one is available.) From these, it might be possible to identify the factors that tend to predict the impact of evaluations on practice. For example, how does the effect of a RCT on practice depend on the existence of an inventory of prior observational studies? Does it matter whether the RCT contradicts or confirms the previous studies?

Does the second, or third, RCT seem to make more of a difference than the first? Perhaps, as Cochrane (1972) suggested, we should systematically plan more than one trial, not just for scientific reasons, but because people will pay attention to the results.

How Decisions Will Be Made from the Literature

Suppose we take the observational study model in which an innovation comes into society, is practiced (or experimented on) for awhile, and reports appear. What is the course of events? We can draw upon the literature for theoretical insights, but the empirical data base is thin. We see no way to handle this except to obtain a collection of situations and try to trace them as cases and then to generalize some models. For example, by systematically reviewing a surgical journal through the years, Barnes (1977) has found examples of surgical innovations that later were discarded.

Measures of Efficacy

Acute and chronic diseases tend to give us different measures of outcome. In acute diseases we usually focus on proportion surviving, proportion cured, or degree of cure, rather than length of survival. Morbidity, measured perhaps by days in the hospital, gives another measure of efficacy. Ideally costs, risks, and benefits from the new treatment would be compared with those from the standard treatment.

In chronic disease, we may be especially concerned with length of survival and with quality of life. Although it is generally agreed that quality of life is important, indeed it is often the dominant issue, its measurement, evaluation, and integration into cost-benefit studies currently must still be regarded as experimental (Weinstein, 1979).

Heterogeneous Populations

Information on homogeneity of response to treatment across patients and providers tells about the uncertainty of improvements a therapy offers. If community hospitals get different results from teaching hospitals, or if various ethnic, age, or sex groups produce differing responses, then efficacy becomes difficult to measure. In these circumstances, there is difficulty in nailing down the amount of gain attributable to new information.

A trial may be valuable in describing who can benefit from a procedure and who can not. Such information could save lots of money, even if most procedures are beneficial for some people. But learning how to describe the subpopulations that can benefit may not be easy, especially if there is not a good predictive model when patients are allocated to treatments and it is decided how to stratify the study.

Assessing the Information Content of Studies

The precision of outcome achievable by various designs depends on their size, on their stratification, and on the uniformity of individual and group responses. In addition, the measurement technique sets some bounds on precision because simple yes-no responses may not be as sensitive as those achieved by relevant measured variables. When the outcome variables measured are not the relevant ones, but are proxies for them, both precision and validity and lost.

The RCT, however, is likely to give values for a rather narrow setting and would need to be buttressed by further information from before and after the investigation.

Nonexperimental designs run the gamut from anecdotes or case studies of single individuals through observational studies. Current behavior toward such studies is of great variety, ranging from ignoring them, to regarding them as stimuli for designing studies with better controls, to regarding them as being so true as to override contradictory results from better-controlled studies. The reasons given for these differing attitudes include the fact that physicians like the medical theory, that institutions like the implied reimbursement policy, that no one has a better therapy, that patients need something, that a new generation of physicians is required to understand the new biological theory, and that patients will not comply, but those do not help in developing a normative basis for judging the information content of the data from the studies.

Predicting the Demand for Procedures

By assessing numbers of patients with the disease and the rates with which the disease occurs and progresses, we can get an idea of the importance of a procedure and its value. The value of an innovation also depends on how soon another innovation that is at least as good comes along and is adopted.

Thinking about the course of diffusion over time raises another important question: At what point in time should a trial be conducted? We do not want to wait too long, because then the procedure will be established and practice will be hard to change. But we also do not want to do the trial too soon, because (1) the technology may not be technically mature and may yet improve over time (in which case nobody will pay attention to the trial if it shows no benefit), and (2) the innovation may turn out to be an obvious loser and sink into obscurity under its own weight.

Assessing Priors

Gilbert et al. (1977) took a small step in this direction by reviewing randomized clinical trials in surgery over a 10-year period. They estimated the distribution of the size of the improvements (or losses). They separated the experiments into two classes: those innovations intended to improve primary outcomes from surgery and anesthesia and those intended to prevent or reduce complications following surgery and anesthesia. They found the average gain across studies to be about 0 percent improvement, and the standard deviation for the gain in the primaries to be about 8 percent and for the secondaries to be about 21 percent. Such empirical studies help assess the prior probabilities of the size of an improvement by an innovation.

Costs and Risks of Studies

If we already have an experimental design, we are likely to be able to evaluate its direct costs. Although there can be quarrels about whether the cost of treatment, for example, should be allocated to the cost of the investigation, there should not be much difficulty evaluating the price of a given trial. On the other hand, in certain cancer trials, the incremental cost may be small because the fixed cost of a multicenter study group has already been paid. It is understood that incremental cost is the appropriate measure.

The question of risks is a thorny one that arises when human subjects are given a treatment that is less effective than the alternative (Weinstein, 1974). For treatments that may be applied to reasonably large numbers of patients, this should be considered a minor risk compared with the long-term value of knowing which is the better treatment. However, if horizons are short, these problems may be more important.

Other Benefits of Trials

One of the great values of combining well-founded facts with good theory resides in the bounds that can be set. Thus a study that gives solid information about death rates, recovery times, and rates of complications for a variety of treatment groups is likely to provide extra values that go beyond its own problem. The National Halothane Study, for example, not only studied the safety of anesthetics, generally, but also provided data used to design other studies, stimulated the further Study of Institutional Differences (in operative death rates), and acted as a proving ground for a variety of statistical methods and encouraged their further development. How shall such information be evaluated?

Another benefit of clinical trials is that they may reinforce a general professional awareness of the value of scientific evidence of efficacy.

CONCLUSION

This paper outlines a general program of research. Until such a program can be carried out, three observations seem likely to stand up to further scrutiny:

1. In planning a controlled trial, it would be valuable for people expert in effectiveness, costs, and other data in that health area to perform at least a rough, back-of-the-envelope calculation of potential benefits and cost savings. This sort of analysis cannot hurt unless we make major omissions or misallocations of costs, and even if we do not yet know how to implement a full-blown planning model of the type we have outlined, it may help.

2. Evidence of efficacy from controlled trials will not solve the health care cost problem and will not eliminate uncertainty from medical decisions. Value judgments related to outcomes with multiple attributes (including quality of life) will remain, as will uncertainties at the level of the individual patient. Moreover, the problems of what to do about procedures that offer diminishing (but positive) benefits at increasing costs will always be with us.

3. Clinical trials can help, however; and we need to learn what their value is and how to increase it. As a nation, we may try various institutional changes to encourage the use of information from trials by practitioners, perhaps by linking reimbursement to demonstrated efficacy, but more likely by providing incentives to be both efficacy-conscious and cost-conscious.

An earlier, longer version of this paper (Mosteller and Weinstein, 1985) was prepared for the National Bureau of Economic Research's (NBER) Conference on Social Experimentation, supported by the Alfred P. Sloan Foundation and held on Hilton Head Island, South Carolina, March 5–7, 1981. The authors are solely responsible for any opinions expressed in this paper.

The authors wish to thank John Bailar, Leon Eisenberg, Rashi Fein, Howard Frazier, Alexander Leaf, and Marc Roberts for their comments and suggestions. We are especially indebted to David Freedman, Jay Kadane, and other participants in the NBER conference for their thoughtful criticism.

This research was supported in part by a grant from the Robert Wood Johnson Foundation to the Center for the Analysis of Health Practices and by National Science Foundation Grant SES-75-15702.

REFERENCES

Barnes, B. A. 1977. Discarded operations: surgical innovations by trial and error. In J. P. Bunker, B. A. Barnes, and F. Mosteller, eds., Costs, Risks and Benefits of Surgery. New York: Oxford University Press.

Bunker, J. P., B. A. Barnes, and F. Mosteller. 1977. Costs, Risks, and Benefits of Surgery. New York: Oxford University Press.

Cochrane, A. L. 1972. Effectiveness and Efficiency: Random Reflections on Health Services. London: Nuffield Provincial Hospitals Trust.

Fuchs, V. R. 1974. Who Shall Live? New York: Basic Books.

Gilbert, J. P., B. McPeek, and F. Mosteller. 1977. Progress in surgery and anesthesia: benefits and risks of innovative therapy. In J. P. Bunker, B. A. Barnes, and F. Mosteller, eds., Costs, Risks, and Benefits of Surgery. New York: Oxford University Press.

Hiatt, H. H. 1975. Protecting the medical commons: Who is responsible? New England Journal of Medicine 293:235–241.

Hypertension Detection and Follow-up Program Cooperative Group. 1979. Five-year findings of the Hypertension Detection and Follow-up Program. Journal of the American Medical Association 242:2562–2755.

Laird, N. M., M. C. Weinstein, and W. B. Stason. 1979. Sample-size estimation: a sensitivity analysis in the context of a clinical trial for treatment of mild hypertension. American Journal of Epidemiology 109:408–419.

Mosteller, F., and M. C. Weinstein. 1985. Toward evaluating the cost-effectiveness of medical and social experiments. In J. A. Hausman and D. A. Wise, eds., Social Experimentation. The National Bureau of Economic Research. Chicago: University of Chicago Press.

U.S. Congress, Office of Technology Assessment. 1980. The Implications of Cost-Effectiveness Analysis of Medical Technology. Washington, D.C.: U.S. Government Printing Office.

Warner, K. E., and B. R. Luce. 1982. Cost-Benefit and Cost-Effectiveness Analysis in Health Care: Principles, Practice, and Potential. Ann Arbor, Michigan: Health Administration Press.

Weinstein, M. C. 1974. Allocation of subjects in medical experiments. New England Journal of Medicine 291:1278–1285.

Weinstein, M. C. 1979. Economic evaluation of medical procedures and technologies: progress, problems and prospects. In U.S. National Center for

Health Services Research, Medical Technology, DHEW Pub. No. (PHS) 79-3254. Washington, D.C.: U.S. Government Printing Office.

Weinstein, M. C. 1983. Cost-effective priorities for cancer prevention. Science 221:17–23.

Weinstein, M. C., and W. B. Stason. 1976. Hypertension: A Policy Perspective. Cambridge, Mass.: Harvard University Press.

Weinstein, M. C., and W. B. Stason. 1977. Foundations of cost-effectiveness analysis for health and medical practices. New England Journal of Medicine 296:716–721.

Technology Assessment in Prepaid Group Practice

Morris F. Collen*

Technology assessment (TA) as applied herein is the process of evaluating the extent to which a medical technology achieves its intended objectives and examining important unintended and indirect consequences from the use of the technology. The TA process, in general, follows that recommended by the Office of Technology Assessment (OTA),[1] and has been applied in prepaid group practice (PGP) to a variety of medical technologies, including procedures, equipment, or systems that are used for diagnostic, therapeutic, or coordinating patient care services.

A prepaid group practice (often called a health maintenance organization or HMO) is an organization of health care providers who by contract provide specified comprehensive services to a defined, voluntarily enrolled membership, financed primarily through periodic per capita payments of members' dues or premiums.

INCENTIVES FOR TECHNOLOGY ASSESSMENT

TA is a useful management tool for a prepaid group practice whose expenditures are largely limited by prospective annual budgets and whose revenues are primarily generated by periodic payments of fixed premiums from its defined membership.[2] Within the constraints of a fixed annual budget, the group is motivated to practice a level of quality care which satisfies its patients and retains its members. The PGP administrator strives to improve managerial efficiency by modifying care processes to decrease costs yet provide adequate services to satisfy and retain members, such as increased efficiency of scheduling systems, training lower-cost personnel for technical procedures, applying systems engineering to appropriate care processes (such as multiphasic health testing to save physician time), etc. PGP physicians are increasingly being encouraged on a micro-level to improve their clinical efficiency by using clinical analysis to arrive at the best diagnosis and treatment at the lowest cost.

Although a physician is traditionally trained to provide clinically effective care at a cost acceptable to the patient, prepayment reverses the traditional financial incentives of fee-for-service practice and encourages patients to seek *well care* in addition to *sick care*.[3] Under a fee-for-service or cost-reimbursement financial arrangement, a medical care provider's income is directly dependent upon revenues generated from the services provided to patients. In the PGP, the program profits primarily from its well members, and there is a direct financial incentive to provide to the sick appropriate, effective care at the lowest cost.

Within the PGP financing structure, an increase in the use of a technology often increases expenses and does not generate revenues as it might in a fee-for-service or cost-reimbursement program. Nor, in a non-profit program, are there any tax savings from the purchases of equipment that otherwise could increase cash flow. Accordingly, there exists in PGP significant incentives to acquire and employ only those technologies that maintain or increase the effectiveness of medical care yet contain or decrease costs. In the past, the competition to HMOs has been from fee-for-service practitioners. To survive under the newly increasing competition from other health maintenance organizations, a PGPs physician and management must prudently select cost-effective technology to sustain an appropriate balance between quality of medical care services to its patients and costs (premiums) to its members.

The peer pressures on physician specialists to acquire and use the same innovations in technology employed by others in their spe-

* Director, Technology Assessment, Department of Medical Methods Research, Kaiser-Permanente Medical Care Program, Oakland, California.

cialty must be balanced in a PGP by the financial constraints of the fixed budget. This requires prudent allocation of limited resources among competing alternative technologies and specialties which provides strong incentives to obtain the most cost-effective technology. Of course, this incentive is present in any hospital with a fixed annual budget, but the PGP cannot balance an overspent equipment budget by utilizing the new equipment to generate more revenues.

SELECTION OF TECHNOLOGY FOR ASSESSMENT

TA is an expensive process so it is usually done only when use of the technology requires sufficient resources to justify the cost of it. An existing technology may be selected for assessment because (1) physicians request a change in the established usage and there are insufficient data available to administration as to its comparative cost-effectiveness; (2) the aggregate expenditures from the use of the technology have reached a level that calls for a reassessment as to whether its utilization is appropriate; or (3) there exist alternative, competitive technologies and uncertainty as to which is the most cost-effective. For a new technology, a decision is required as to whether the technology is still investigational, or whether it should be provided to PGP members as a benefit.

A TA usually is funded by the PGP, but for large, expensive TAs some grant support may be solicited from governmental or nonprofit foundations. When the TA is entirely initiated and funded by a PGP, it is usually prepared for internal use only, and it is rarely published in the literature since it will likely be limited to specific organizational objectives.

If a TA is initiated or supported in whole or in part by an outside grant, it is then prepared to satisfy both internal and public distribution. Such a TA will be more comprehensive, and the document becomes one in the public domain through publication in the scientific literature.

When a technology has been selected for assessment, it is necessary first to define the technology precisely and determine its objectives for its specific applications, then to identify alternative technologies also used for the same applications.

A two-dimensional categorization of technology (complexity and clinical application) is often used since the process of assessment differs for a single procedure, an expensive equipment item, or a complex system; furthermore, the assessment varies for diagnostic, therapeutic, and coordinating (such as computer support) technology.

Specific medical conditions are defined for which the diagnostic or therapeutic technology is used, and the prevalence and incidence of these conditions are estimated in the population being served. It is a great advantage to a PGP that its defined population provides a denominator, so the rates of utilization of the technology for these conditions can be appraised to provide projections of workloads for the technology and requirements for the associated technical personnel.

TA METHODOLOGY

An evaluation of the extent to which the technology achieves its specified objectives involves an analysis of its effectiveness and cost and of the comparative cost-effectiveness for alternative technologies to achieve these same objectives. Appropriate evaluative data are used, when available, from studies conducted within the medical care program. Otherwise data are sought from the medical literature. For unavailable or controversial data, appropriately selected experts within the PGP are used for consensus development to provide substitute data, e.g., as was done to obtain probabilities of patient outcome after alpha-fetoprotein screening.

Effective analysis of the technology is conducted in accordance with its category; i.e., for a diagnostic technology, its sensitivity and specificity in achieving its intended diagnosis; for a treatment technology, its effects on morbidity, disability, and/or mortality; and for a coordinating technology, its having achieved its intended effects on efficiency or productivity. Analysis of effectiveness includes evaluation of safety and of known adverse effects. Effectiveness is then compared to that of alternative technologies used to achieve the same objectives.

Economic analysis is conducted to determine unit costs (or charges) and total costs (including both direct and indirect costs) for the specified uses of the technology. Economic analysis sometimes includes the impact of different payment modes for medical services, such as prepayment versus Medicare cost-reimbursement, purchase versus lease financing for capitalized equipment, etc.

Cost-effectiveness analysis provides comparative costs of employing alternative technologies to achieve similar, specified levels of desired effectiveness. The advantages and disadvantages of an alternative technology are specified (e.g., criteria or clinical indications for patient selection in the treatment of end-stage renal disease). Other benefits from the use of each technology are considered, although a formal cost-benefit analysis is rarely conducted due to methodological problems associated with subjective estimates of benefits, such as the value of added years of life, quality of life measures, etc.

A comprehensive TA requires an appraisal of important unintended consequences from using a medical technology, including any significant legal, ethical, organizational, social, or environmental effects.

Legal and legislative aspects are considered in almost every TA, such as licensing requirements for biofeedback therapists, legislative regulations for Medicare that affect selection of center versus home hemodialysis treatments, etc. Medical liabilities have been a worrisome consideration from the consequences of false-positive and -negative tests, as in the case of screening pregnant women for fetal neural tube defects by the alpha-fetoprotein test.

Ethical considerations are important in establishing criteria for selecting patients most suitable for a technology. This was of great concern for patients with end-stage renal disease before Medicare financed every patient with this condition.

Unintended consequences for a PGP can result, for example, from the increasing interest of surrounding community and health plan members in more self-care and holistic practices, including biofeedback. Environmental effects may be a serious consideration, perhaps for the effect of the location of shared-facilities technology on the accessibility to care, as, for example, the consideration of centralization versus decentralization of hemodialysis centers on transportation requirements for patients.

Most cost-effectiveness analyses are tested as to their sensitivity to potentially important variations in the data used. For example, differences in the characteristics of patients' ages and in the causes of end-stage renal disease greatly affect the optimal mix of alternative technologies required by a PGP.

EXAMPLES OF TA IN PGPs

Some PGPs were solicited for statements as to their experience with TA, and the following responses were obtained.

TA in Northern California by KPMCP

The Kaiser-Permanente Medical Care Program (KPMCP) in Northern California established in 1961 its Department of Medical Methods Research (MMR). Its purpose is to conduct research directed toward utilizing modern technology for the development of improved methods of providing and delivering medical care within the KPMCP.

MMR is professionally administered by its director under the Permanente Medical Group. All MMR grants and contracts are the financial responsibility of the Kaiser Foundation Research Institute, a nonprofit, tax-exempt corporation.

From 1968 to 1973, the federal government's National Center for Health Services Research and Development (NCHSR&D) awarded to MMR a Health Services Research Center grant with a technology focus. Its primary project was to develop a computerized pilot medical data system in the Kaiser-Permanente San Francisco hospital and to establish a medical data base for both patient care and health services research.

In 1979, the Division of Technology Assessment was established within MMR. The primary purpose of its technology assessments is to aid in the selection of the most cost-effective technology. This division has employed technology assessment for procedures, equipment, and systems used in diagnostic, therapeutic, and coordinative patient care services. The TA process, in general, first identifies for assessment an appropriate technology that uses substantial resources. The TA then determines the characteristics of the population utilizing the technology and determines the workloads for its utilization. Alternative technologies used for the same specified objectives are evaluated as to important intended and unintended consequences, with consideration of alternative mixes of competing technologies per million people. The TA has used epidemiological methods, controlled studies, medical record studies, literature reviews, consensus development, and sensitivity analysis. The intent is not to arrive at a single decision or recommendation, but to present the important consequences of appropriate alternative technologies so that management can make a more rational decision. Thus the TA attempts to decrease the uncertainty of decision making.

Technologies suitable for assessment have been identified at all organizational levels. The executive director requested a TA on biofeedback to assist in a policy decision as to whether it should be included as a prepaid benefit. Service chiefs had already requested a TA of alternative technologies for the treatment of end-stage renal disease, when administration also requested this after it was learned that Medicare, beginning January 1982, would decrease the reimbursement of costs. Pediatric geneticists requested a TA on alpha-fetoprotein screening because of impending legislation requiring it for pregnant women as a screening test for fetal neural tube defects. Technology procedures suitable for TA also have been identified by monitoring organizational gross expenditures; e.g., two-view chest x rays were the most frequently ordered diagnostic radiology procedure, so a TA was conducted to assess the consequences of alternative criteria for utilization of this technology.

Periodic surveys of chiefs of professional services have been conducted in order to attempt to identify as early as possible future substantial increases in capital-intensive equipment needs, e.g., as has just occurred for diagnostic imaging equipment.

Some TAs conducted by KPMCP's Division of Technology Assessment are summarized below:

Biofeedback A new treatment modality was advocated by physicians for chronically recurring headaches and other conditions. A TA was completed using data from three Kaiser-Permanente medical centers and from the literature. The consequences were assessed as they would relate to three alternative organizational decisions for providing biofeedback as a health plan benefit, namely, full biofeedback benefits, partial benefits for treatment of chronic headaches only, and no biofeedback benefits. Included was a sensitivity analysis of effects from a variety of biofeedback treatment schedules.

Utilization of Diagnostic X Rays Skull, chest, and upper gastrointestinal tract diagnostic x-ray procedures are leading radiological expenditures for ambulatory care services. A TA was completed analyzing clinical indications (i.e., referral criteria) for ordering these x-ray examinations and the effects of the radiologists; it reports on the diagnosis, treatment, and outcome of patients.[4] This study was supported in part by a grant from the Food and Drug Administration's (FDA) Bureau of Radiological Health.

Serum Alpha-Fetoprotein Increasing legislative interest in this procedure could require KPMCP to provide serum alpha-fetoprotein screening tests to 30,000 pregnant women each year, followed by a series of costly technical procedures (including ultrasonography and amniocentesis) when positive. A TA compares the consequences of screening versus no screening of this subpopulation.

End-Stage Renal Disease The increasing cost of institution-based or center hemodialysis, the decreasing cost-reimbursement from Medicare, and the alternative technologies now available for the treatment of end-stage renal disease (ESRD) patients make this an ideal TA for identifying the most cost-effective mix of alternative technologies, per one million KPMCP members, for the treatment of ESRD patients over a projected 10-year period.

Multiphasic Health Testing By comparing the use of a systematized process for providing periodic health examinations with the traditional health checkup mode and by conducting a long-term controlled study of effectiveness it was shown that a more comprehensive battery of tests are provided at a lower cost and that they use less physician time. The multiphasic approach was more effective in decreasing mortality from potentially postponable conditions, and the cost of care for 12 months after the checkup was less for those receiving the multiphasic checkup as compared to the traditional mode for similar groups of patients standardized by age, sex, and health status.[5] The study was supported by a grant from the National Center for Health Services Research (NCHSR).

Team Primary Care An alternative system for providing primary care employs a team of physicians, nurse practitioners, a health educator, and a mental health counselor, and includes a multiphasic type of health checkup in the initial entry visit. A TA is being conducted that compares cohort members randomly assigned upon joining the KPMCP to either the new team or to traditional primary care services. This is a follow-up study of a new approach to ambulatory care involving the entry of patients through a paramedically staffed health evaluation service.[6,7] This study is supported in part by a grant from the H. J. Kaiser Family Foundation.

Hospital Computer System A prototype hospital computer system was installed in one medical center and a patient computer medical record system was compared to a traditional hospital and outpatient record system.[8] This study was supported in part by a grant from the NCHSR.

TA in Oregon by KPMCP

The Kaiser-Permanente Medical Care Program (KPMCP) in Oregon has a Health Services Research Center, the primary aim of which has been to design, develop, and direct research and demonstration projects to add to knowledge about health and medical care.[9] The following briefly summarizes some of the projects that can be categorized as TA studies.

Do-Not Admit Surgery Study This study compared the costs, quality of care, and satisfaction with surgical services performed in hospital operating rooms on nonadmitted patients with similar services performed on hospital inpatients.[10]

Contraceptive Studies The purposes of contraceptive studies are to understand factors that determine the acceptability of various contraceptive methods (including contraceptive sterilization and new hormonal contraceptive methods for men), and to evaluate the long-term medical and psychosocial sequelae of various procedures (such as vasectomy).[11]

Alcohol Treatment Demonstration Project The purpose of this project was to implement and evaluate a new program for alcohol services. The evaluation included an analysis of the effect of a copayment on the use of alcohol treatment services, on patient functioning, and on nonalcohol-related utilization.[12]

Television for Community Health The overall objective is to develop and test a unique behavior change program directed at obesity and obesity-related behaviors. This study will use broadcast television and two levels of professional support: (1) regular mailings to participants and (2) regular mailings together with some direct assistance in the establishment of local mutual support groups and in the training of group leaders. In addition to assessing efficacy, the secondary objective is to estimate the costs of implementing a similar program in the context of any HMO and to produce the operations manual, educational materials, and support documents required to allow the ready implementation of such a program in other HMOs or other population organizations.

In addition, clinical drug intervention trials have been conducted, including participation in the Multiple Risk Factor Intervention Trial (MRFIT) and the Beta-Blocker Heart Attack Trial (BHAT)

TA In Southern California KPMCP

The Kaiser-Permanente Medical Care Program (KPMCP) in Southern California has taken a pragmatic orientation to TA.[13] Its efforts in this regard are to review new technologies with a major emphasis on whether they are ready for introduction and whether they work as reported. These efforts are an integral part of management decision making and operations. Specific areas in which these studies have been conducted include computed tomography (CT) scanners, nuclear magnetic resonance imaging, nuclear emission computerized tomography, intensive care unit monitoring systems, computerized arrythmia detection systems, and other mini- and microcomputer medical applications.

A second emphasis for technology evaluation has concerned operational effectiveness, productivity, and cost-effectiveness. Questions studied have included the following: Does the southern region have sufficient volume to effectively provide new technology or service or should the technology/service be centralized in one or a few medical centers or dispersed widely throughout the region? And what is the most effective way to staff and otherwise operate with the new technology?

Other studies in this area have included open heart surgery, bone marrow transplantation, and computerized systems such as outpatient pharmacy, appointment making, x-ray file management, electrocardiogram (EKG) interpretation, and admission/discharge/transfer.

A third level of effort incorporates the other efforts, as appropriate, to develop a southern region plan for implementing a technology or service for the benefit of our members. Questions concern the demand for the service, quality, cost, and other considerations. Areas that have been addressed include open heart surgery, CT scanning, radiation therapy, neurosurgery, hemodialysis, skilled nursing facilities, acute rehabilitation services, neonatal intensive care units, and chemical dependency rehabilitation.

In summary, the KPMCP southern region's efforts include not only the issues of hard technology that are usually considered as technology assessment, but also the assessment of human and management factors that have an impact on the ultimate value of the use of technology. Efforts are directed toward answering the following question: What is the most cost-effective approach to using existing and new technology for the benefit of our members?

TA in the Harvard Community Health Plan

In 1977, the Board of Trustess of the Harvard Community Health Plan (HCHP) established a fund for research at HCHP, to which would be donated 0.5 percent of the gross premium income of the plan each year.[14] A research department was established to implement this program, and contributions to research activities from HCHP are channeled through an HCHP foundation, which has its own board of trustees. The current plan contribution to research amounts to some $400,000 per annum and grows with the size of the plan's overall budget.

Research in the effectiveness and the cost-effectiveness of clinical practices at HCHP is represented in a number of projects, some of which are conducted wholly internally, some of which are conducted by outside investigators with HCHP as a passive site, and some of which represent truly collaborative investigations. What follows are brief summary descriptions of the major projects in this area currently under way at HCHP.

Laboratory Test Use Funded partially by the National Fund for Medical Education, this is an 18-month study of the utilization of 15 common laboratory tests in ambulatory centers. The study is directed at understanding variations in behavior within internal medicine practice groups. Interventions, including educational interventions and computer-based feedback, are being tested for their impact on interprovider variability. This study makes considerable use of an automated medical record system.

Studies of Mitral Valve Prolapse Patterns of use of diagnoses and management techniques for mitral valve prolapse are studied in an ambulatory population. The study will, among other things, attempt to determine variations in practice among providers and the impact of diagnostic and therapeutic interventions on the total well-being of the patient, including self-image, recreational behaviors, and medical management.

Nondiagnostic Uses of Ultrasound in Pregnancy This is an investigation of the ways in which ultrasonography in pregnancy affects the management of patients and alters their well-being in ways other than classic medical outcomes. The study involves interviews of women undergoing ultrasonography, as well as chart reviews and physician interviews about patterns of management.

Changes in Physician Test Ordering A study in cooperation with physicians at HCHP who have managed hypertension and other chronic conditions records interprovider variations in practice, and will compare HCHP-based practices to practices in settings with other forms of organization and financial incentives.

Efficacy Studies of Diagnostic X Rays This study is gathering prospective information on the use of intravenous pyelograms and upper gastrointestinal x-ray series. Clinical predictors of the outcomes of these tests are being assessed.

Cost-Effectiveness of Periodontal Therapy A randomized study is being conducted in HCHP's Dental Department of different ways of managing periodontal disease, comparing surgical and medical interventions.

Analysis of Hospitalization Costs Following a large increase in the cost of inpatient hospitalizations over the past 2 years, this study is a detailed review of hospital bills to determine areas of inflation of hospital costs. The study will attempt to understand what types of conditions and types of diagnostic and therapeutic procedures consume resources in hospitalized patients. A detailed substudy is being conducted with respect to costs of the neonatal intensive care unit.

Valued Outcomes in Chest X Rays This is an investigation of the reasons for use of chest x rays in the Kenmore Center of HCHP. Patients and physicians are being interviewed to determine what information each values, and what forms of information in general motivate the decision to order the test.

Cost-Effectiveness of Lead Screening A cost-effectiveness analysis of lead screening was begun at the Harvard School of Public Health and has been continued at HCHP.

Analysis of Diagnostic Skill This study uses a large data base consisting of physicians' estimates of the changes of positivity in their ordering of throat cultures and chest x rays in children. Receiver operating characteristic analysis is being employed to characterize the diagnostic skill of different physicians at different levels of training.

In addition to the above studies, work is under way in cooperation with Johns Hopkins University and with the Harvard School of Public Health to characterize the ways in which different clinical conditions at HCHP consume health care resources. Studies have also been conducted on clinical trials, such as prophylactic use of phenobarbital to prevent febrile seizures in children.

TA in Group Health Cooperative of Puget Sound

Group Health Cooperative of Puget Sound (GHC) is a member-owned health care cooperative founded in 1947 with the purpose of providing health care on a prepaid basis. The governance of Group Health Cooperative is constituted by the triad of board, management, and professional staff. It is through the collaboration of this triad that technology assessments and decisions based on them are made.[15]

Typically, in the past, technology assessment at GHC was explicit only when a new technology that required a considerable capital outlay was proposed. In these cases a medical staff proponent of the new technology, usually a specialist subgroup, would develop effectiveness and cost-effectiveness data with the assistance of management staff. The resultant proposal was presented to the professional staff executive council, and a recommendation was then sequentially forwarded to the board planning committee, the board fiscal and management committee, and finally to the board itself. Occasional technology assessments and resultant decisions have been made within the professional staff alone when the technology did not require significant capital outlay. For example, after assessment, ileojejunal bypass for obesity was discontinued as a matter of professional staff policy, on the basis of inadequate safety (due to metabolic complications) and unproved effectiveness. Similarly, certain unusual nutritional therapies were not allowed to begin.

Recently, under the stimulus of the need to maintain an attractive and appropriate benefit package and yet hold dues at a competitive level, technology assessment at GHC has become more explicit and systematic. The professional staff has formed and chairs a medical services committee, with representation from management and the board. Through this committee the professional staff fills what it sees as its responsibility to assess predominantly new but also old medical technologies and makes appropriate recommendations to the board.

The Medical Services Committee takes as its agenda requests for provision of new services or requests for evaluation of currently provided services. Such requests may originate with consumers, board, management, or professional staff. Technologies that are rapidly changing in their rate of utilization (at least 30 percent in 2 years or 50 percent in 5 years) are automatically considered by the committee. With staff assistance the proponents of a particular technology prepare a justification of the technology in question, specifically with answers to the following questions.

1. Is the technology *medically appropriate*, i.e., efficacious for the individual and/or effective for the population, or else an appropriately managed investigational technology? To answer this question the literature is examined regarding efficacy and effectiveness, and alternative technologies are reviewed. Unproved (investigational) technologies may be considered medically appropriate at GHC provided that (a) their utilization is part of a properly designed study, (b) GHC benefits by having participated in the study either directly by early access of results or indirectly, and (c) the cost of the technology is no greater than that of existing practice or any net increased costs are defrayed by funds from outside membership dues.
2. What is the cost of the technology to the health care organization? The cost in personnel and facilities is estimated, and a judgment is made as to whether this represents (a) cost savings through displacement of other technology or through cost-avoidance through improved health outcomes, (b) a break-even reallocation of funds through displacement of other technology, or (c) increased costs requiring new money.
3. What priority should this technology have among technologies competing for coverage under the budget for the benefit package? This is a value judgment based on the estimated cost and benefit to individuals and the population. If a technology is considered to have low priority but still to be medically appropriate, a recommendation to allow it to be provided on a fee-for-service basis may be made (with the fee going to the cooperative). Similarly, an investigational technology can receive no priority for coverage, but a recommendation may be made to allow it to be provided through the use of fee-for-service or research funds if it is provided as part of an appropriately designed study.

Examples of assessments made by the committee and the resultant decisions include the following:

Stool Occult-Blood Screening for the Secondary Prevention of Colorectal Cancer Coverage for this technology was originally proposed by members of the Family Practice Section. Such screening was judged by the committee to be medically appropriate as noninvestigatory and effective, to have estimated costs partially recovered from avoided costs of treatment with the remainder to be defrayed by an increase in membership dues, and to merit a high priority for coverage.

Penile Prosthesis for Selected Impotence Coverage for this technology was proposed by members of the Urology Section. The technology was judged to be medically appropriate as noninvestigational and effective, to have costs which would require new monies, and to merit a low priority for coverage. Because of its efficacy for selected individuals it was recommended that the service be provided on a fee-for-service basis until covered.

Scolitron, an Electrical Muscle Stimulator for the Correction of Scoliosis Proposed for coverage by orthopedists, this technology was judged to be medically appropriate only as an investigational, probably effective technology. As an investigational technology it could receive no priority for coverage. The scolitron was recommended for utilization only if it could pass the criteria for an investigational technology: that its utilization be part of an appropriate study, that the organization benefit from participation in the study, and that net costs be no greater than those for existing alternative treatments.

Insulin Pump for the Treatment of Diabetes Proposed for coverage by internists, this technology was judged to be medically appropriate only as an investigational technology of unknown effectiveness. It could receive no priority for coverage, and could be used only if it could pass the criteria for an investigational technology.

Mandibular Osteotomy for Malocclusion This technology is being provided currently and is covered. Review was requested by personnel responsible for benefits and coverage. The committee judged that the technology, although effective, could not be judged medically appropriate because it is a dental rather than medical technology. The committee recommmended that it be dropped from coverage, although it could be continued on a fee-for-service basis, for an estimated savings of $200,000 per year in an overall budget of approximately $130,000,000 per year.

Mammography This technology is currently provided and covered as medically appropriate for cases selected according to specific criteria. Mammography came to the attention of the committee because of its rapidly increasing utilization rate and a resultant request for additional radiologists. The committee determined that it was not known whether the increasing referrals for mammography followed the proper selection criteria, and therefore no judgment could be made as to medical appropriateness of hiring additional radiologists for this purpose. The question of whether the increasing utilization was medically appropriate was referred back to the professional staff committee.

Ultrasound for Diagnostic Assessment of Pelvic and Intrauterine Structures This technology is currently provided and covered as medically appropriate. It came under review because of a request by the obstetrical and gynecological surgeons for new ultrasound equipment. The committee determined that in the interest of avoiding duplication, the appropriateness of purchasing additional ultrasound equipment should not be considered until it was determined whether the radiologists or obstetrician/gynecologists should more appropriately provide the service.

The recommendations of the Medical Services Committee are passed on to the Management Benefits Committee, which structures benefits recommendations for the Fiscal and Management Committee of the board. It is the task of the Fiscal and Management Committee to integrate recommendations as to benefits together with all other budgetary recommendations for final review and decision by the board.

It is interesting to note that this medical technology assessment activity is carried on at GHC with no direct outside stimulation. (Indeed, it is not referred to as technology assessment.) Rather, it is the result of the internal perception that such assessment is a necessary part of doing business as a prepaid group practice.

NOTES

[1] Office of Technology Assessment. 1980. The Implications of Cost-Effectiveness Analysis of Medical Technology. Chapter 3: Methodological Findings and Principles. Washington, D.C.: U.S. Government Printing Office.

[2] Office of Technology Assessment. 1980. The Implications of Cost-Effectiveness Analysis of Medical Technology. Chapter 10: Health Maintenance Organizations. Washington, D.C.: U.S. Government Printing Office.

[3] Garfield, S. R. 1970. Multiphasic health testing and medical care as a right. N. Engl. J. Med. 283:1087–1089.

[4] Collen, M. F. 1983. Utilization of Diagnostic X-ray Examinations. Department of Health and Human Services, 83-82008. Washington, D.C.: U.S. Food and Drug Administration.

[5] Collen, M. F. 1979. A Case Study of Multiphasic Health Testing. Appendix C in Medical Technology and the Health Care System. A Study of the Diffusion of Equipment-Embodied Technology. A Report by the Committee on Technology Health Care, National Academy of Sciences. Also, Multiphasic Health Testing Services. 1978. New York: John Wiley.

[6] Garfield, S. R., M. F. Collen, R. Feldman, et al. 1976. Evaluation of an ambulatory medical care delivery system. N. Engl. J. Med. 294:426–431.

[7] Collen, M. F., S. R. Garfield, R. H. Richart, et al. 1977. Cost analysis of alternative health examination modes. Arch. Intern. Med. 137:73–79.

[8] Collen, M. F. 1974. Hospital Computer Systems. New York: John Wiley.

[9] Greenlick, M. R., Director, Health Services Research Center. Personal communication.

[10] Marks, S. D., M. R. Greenlick, A. V. Hurtado, J. D. Johnson, and J. Henderson. 1980. Ambulatory surgery in an HMO, a study of costs, quality of care and satisfaction. Med. Care 28:127–146.

[11] Weist, W., and members of the WHO Task Force on Psychosocial Factors in Family Planning. 1980. Acceptability of drugs for male fertility regulation: a prospectus and some preliminary data. Contraception 21:121–134.

[12] Hayami, D. E., and D. K. Freeborn. 1981. Effect of coverage on use of an HMO alcoholism treatment program, outcome, and medical care utilization. Am. Pub. Health 71:1133–1143.

[13] Ruml, J., Director, Benefit/Cost Analysis. Personal communication.

[14] Berwick, D. M., Research Director. Personal communication.

[15] Watkins, R., Staff Physician. Personal communication.

A Randomized Controlled Trial to Evaluate the Effects of an Experimental Prepaid Group Practice on Medical Care Utilization and Cost

Gerald T. Perkoff*

The Medical Care Group of Washington University (MCG), now the Medical Care Group of St. Louis, Missouri, was begun as a randomized controlled trial to compare prepaid group practice with fee-for-service practice for comparable groups of people to learn more about the effects of the organization of medical care upon utilization and costs. Although small, it was possible through the enrollment mechanism to develop prospective study and control groups and to obtain sound data on hospital and ambulatory services utilization and costs.

The MCG plan offered comprehensive family care by salaried internists, pediatricians, and obstetricians who provided primary ambulatory, hospital, emergency, and home services, and specialists on the full-time faculty of Washington University School of Medicine who provided consultations, surgery, laboratory, x ray, and other procedures and services. The primary care physicians received no instructions about delivery of care and practiced according to their own best judgment. Thus, the study was confined as much as possible to the effects of prepayment and organizational change upon utilization and costs. The potential favorable effects of a financial incentive were avoided purposely.

All MCG services were prepaid and were financed by an experimental insurance option which was added to the patient's group plan; hospitalization benefits remained unchanged. Control families were covered under a comprehensive major medical plan with the same hospitalization benefits as those of the patients in the study group.

Hospital utilization data were derived directly from bills paid by Metropolitan Life Insurance Company. While gynecologic services and costs were included, obstetrical hospital days and visits were excluded from both study and control data. Obstetrical utilization was thought unlikely to be influenced by the experimental design. Two systems were necessary for collection of ambulatory services data. An encounter form was used for MCG enrollees. For controls, analysis of insurance deductibles, claims and tax records, plus multiple telephone and questionnaire surveys were used. Information was obtained from 77 percent of the controls in these surveys. It was found that control enrollees were quite knowledgeable about insurance coverage and income tax deductions for medical care and most maintained detailed records for tax purposes. From these records and surveys, control ambulatory services utilization was estimated and compared to study group data. Since the control enrollees paid for services on a fee-for-services basis, a fee equivalent was recorded for prepaid group study patients. Costs of operation of MCG related to patient care were recorded separately from any research expenditures just as though MCG was a private group practice. Thus, exclusive of any research costs, the sums expended for professional and paraprofessional salaries, rent, supplies, biologicals, telephones, telephone answering services, data management, and administration were added together and considered the cost of operation.

Salaries paid to professional and paraprofessional personnel were prorated according to the actual time allotted to patient care in the MCG. This proration was the figure used in calculating the cost of operation, from which the cost per visit then was calculated for primary care MCG services. MCG paid the specialty departments and divisions of the medical school for specialty and laboratory services on a fee-for-service basis through the experimental period. Therefore, it was possi-

* Curators Professor & Associate Chairman, Department of Family & Community Medicine, and Professor of Medicine, University of Missouri School of Medicine, Columbia, MO 65212.

ble to determine the actual cost for each of these directly.

All services were expressed as services/100 person years (PY) where person years are:

$$(PY) = \Sigma \frac{\text{persons enrolled} \times \text{months enrolled}}{12}$$

RESULTS

Hospital utilization varied by type, age, and sex. For children, surgical admission rates were slightly higher among MCG patients than among controls. MCG children were admitted for nonsurgical conditions less often than were controls, and this difference was statistically significant ($p < 0.05$). Overall, a 33 percent reduction ($p < 0.01$) in hospital days utilized by children occurred.

For adults, a similar result was noted in nonsurgical admissions. MCG men were admitted at a rate 55 percent lower than that of control men ($p < 0.01$); MCG women's admissions were only minimally less. For both men and women considered separately or combined as all adults there was a statistically significant reduction in hospital days used ($p < 0.01$). Overall, nonsurgical admissions were significantly reduced for all subgroups, as were hospital days used, down 35 percent ($p < 0.01$). For surgical conditions, however, the converse was true; MCG men were admitted 68.5 percent more than control men ($p < 0.01$); surgical admissions of MCG women also were higher than those of the controls, but to a lesser extent than those of the men. The net result was little difference in surgical days used by the two groups. The reduced nonsurgical utilization was so striking that hospital days utilized by all groups combined still were statistically significantly lower for MCG compared with controls, down 23 percent ($p < 0.01$).

MCG patients had higher utilization rates for office visits and consultations, diagnostic x-ray and laboratory services, and preventive services. Adult women used the most office visits, even though the data exclude pre- and postnatal visits and associated laboratory services. There were other major contributors to increased MCG ambulatory service rates than office visits per se, especially diagnostic x-ray and laboratory services. The total rate for ambulatory services in MCG was severalfold that for controls ($p < 0.01$).

Certain aspects of the ambulatory services data utilization require special comment. The preventive services and consultations data were likely to be recorded completely for MCG patients by virtue of the specific data collection system set up to capture such information. For the control group, however, immunizations, other preventive health care examinations, and follow-up visits to consultants were not always clearly identifiable on physicians' bills, and therefore could not be reported accurately. This no doubt led to a systematic underreporting of these services in controls. However, even if both initial consultations and follow-up visits to consultants are considered as office visits in both groups, and all preventive services in MCG and in controls are excluded from the final data, the MCG ambulatory care rates still were 426 services/100 PY compared to 265 services/100 PY for controls ($p < 0.01$).

During the study period, only nine insurance claims were presented to the Metropolitan Life Insurance Company for nonemergency, out-of-plan hospital admissions. These admissions added only 3.1 hospital days/100 PY and represented only 5.8 percent of all hospital days used. Out-of-plan utilization would appear to have been minimal.

MCG actual costs and fee equivalents for diagnostic and therapeutic visits were quite comparable to those that were charged controls, as were actual costs/visit. For preventive visits, the MCG actual cost and MCG fee equivalent again were comparable. Both, however, were considerably greater than the total preventive fees that controls paid, primarily because many more preventive services were provided to MCG enrollees than to controls.

The cost per visit did not give a complete picture of ambulatory care provided, because MCG enrollees received more visits and services than did controls. When allowance was made for this difference, MCG showed greater cost per person year than did controls for each type of service, except for surgery and hospital charges.

Visits to specialists made up 28.7 percent of all diagnostic and therapeutic visits. Initial referrals were 11.3 percent of all visits or one referral for each 8.8 primary care visits. Charges for specialty consultations and laboratory and x-ray services were 31 percent of all costs, or almost 53 percent of the MCG costs exclusive of hospital charges. Together with those provided in MCG itself, then, cost of physician, laboratory, and x-ray services made up over 70 percent of all nonhospital costs incurred (Perkoff et al., 1976; Perkoff, 1979).

DISCUSSION

Within the limits of the methodology employed, the data presented appeared to support the major basic premise of the experiment. Hospital utilization by MCG enrollees was less than that of control enrollees for children and adults, and overall. This was almost entirely the result of reduced admissions for nonsurgical causes.

The ambulatory services corollary to reduced hospital use expected on theoretical grounds was observed in every major category. The changes in ambulatory services utilization were highly significant statistically, and were so large as to make it unlikely that the known deficiencies in methods for collecting the control data could account for the result. The major effect on ambulatory services provision was on ancillary services—x-ray, laboratory, and preventive services. Thus, while office visits did increase, there was no evidence of excessive demand for illness care. It should be noted that control health care utilization was low, but there is no evidence that this was an underserved group. Rather, the MCG plan resulted in increased utilization in an otherwise relatively healthy population.

The major difference between expected results and findings was that MCG surgical admissions were increased rather than decreased. One of the accepted explanations for reduced hospital utilization in a prepaid plan is that elimination of the fee incentive reduces unnecessary surgery. Details of the MCG surgical experience and discussion of possible explanations for the results have been published elsewhere (Perkoff et al., 1975). Suffice it to say here that no differences were found in the types of conditions for which surgery was done in the MCG enrollee group compared with controls, nor were there differences in the proportion of different operations, including those often thought of as elective or unnecessary.

These studies provided sound evidence for the often-stated belief that hospital utilization can be decreased and ambulatory services utilization can be increased by a system which combines prepayment for comprehensive medical care services with an organized medical care delivery system. The assumption always is made that such reductions in hospital utilization will reduce the cost of medical care by the substitution of less expensive ambulatory care for the most expensive hospital care. There are fewer data than assumptions on this important issue, and this study did not resolve the problem. It was not possible to know whether reduced hospital use resulted directly from increased ambulatory care or that both were results of change in care patterns for the same people. In any case, cost savings were spotty and much less than expected.

The study was designed to see whether the organization of medical care into a prepaid group practice could affect utilization and cost of care without any effort being made to control the practice of either the primary care or consultant physicians. Thus, only prepayment and organization of care varied among the study and control groups. Other factors that might have led to cost savings and that are characteristic of some prepaid group practices—i.e., limitations on the number of hospital beds available, extensive management systems, incentive plans, use of salaried specialty personnel, ownership of hospitals—were not part of the study. By measuring medical care utilization in both study and control groups; by accounting for expenditures in the study group on an actual cost and fee equivalent basis; and by paying full fees to the appropriate departments for all consultant, x-ray, and laboratory services provided by salaried physicians, it was hoped that the effects on utilization and cost of only two factors, prepayment and organization of care, could be isolated. Both commonly are considered to be remedies applicable to the present medical care system to yield cost savings. In addition, it was hoped that other potential areas for influencing medical care and medical care costs would be recognized. Within limits, these goals were reached.

In addition to examining the basic premise, the study suggested several other ways costs might be contained in prepaid group practice, or indeed, in the traditional system. Better training of primary care physicians in certain specialties surely could reduce referrals to several major specialties. Utilization of less expensive allied health personnel for various high-use and more routine services such as preventive care could lead to lower costs. In the area of prevention, more needs to be done to identify those procedures which truly are of value, with elimination of other less useful tests and examinations.

More important, however, are specific fiscal measures to reduce the cost of all needed services. Since physicians' services accounted for the majority of MCG nonhospital costs, any plan for controlling medical care costs will have to deal with this area of cost generation.

SUMMARY

Organization of medical care into an effective group with prepayment did lead to reduced hospital and increased ambulatory services utilization, but in and of itself did not lead to reduced medical care costs. Several other aspects of prepaid group practice were identified and may lead to cost control, especially reduced cost of physicians' services. Although special characteristics of MCG differed from those of larger prepaid group practices, the data did suggest that high expectations of cost savings from this method of medical care delivery may need to be modified as this concept is applied more broadly in varied private and public medical care settings.

REFERENCES

Perkoff, G. T. 1979. Changing Health Care: Perspectives from a New Medical Care Setting. Ann Arbor, Michigan: Health Administration Press, University of Michigan.

Perkoff, G. T., L. I. Kahn, W. Ballinger, and J. K. Turner. 1975. Lack of effect of an experimental prepaid group practice on utilization of surgical care. Surgery 77:619–623.

Perkoff, G. T., L. I. Kahn, and P. Haas. 1976. The effects of an experimental prepaid group practice on medical care utilization and cost. Med. Care 14:432–449.

The Metro Firm Trials: An Innovative Approach to Ongoing Randomized Clinical Trials

David I. Cohen*
Duncan Neuhauser†

Randomized clinical trials are said to be expensive, hard to organize, and fraught with ethical difficulties. The demand for more such trials persists, however, because of the need to definitively evaluate the large number of medical interventions of debatable or undemonstrated efficacy. If the difficulties in conducting these trials could be substantially reduced, it would greatly facilitate a more widespread evaluation of medical care.

The Department of Medicine at Cleveland Metropolitan General Hospital (Metro) is organized into four similar teams of physicians associated with similar 28-bed inpatient units and similar outpatient clinics (firms).[1] New patients are randomly assigned to one of these four firms. Experimental changes in the delivery of care are being carried out on an ongoing basis (trials). We think that this is one solution to some of the problems of conducting randomized clinical trials.

In this paper we shall describe the Metro firm trials in the context of the historical background from which this system arose. We shall then discuss the development of the system for the purpose of research, and briefly describe some of the trials which have been conducted in this setting. Practical issues including costs and human subjects review will be addressed. Finally, we shall discuss some of the unique methodologic issues which have arisen during the firm trials.

HISTORICAL BACKGROUND

Many hospitals have had arbitrary, haphazard, or rotational methods of assigning new patients to one of several similar teams of physicians. Such institutions include the Johns Hopkins Hospital, The Massachusetts General Hospital (internal medicine ward services), and the Sodersjukhuset in Stockholm, Sweden.

The earliest study known to us, and based on this kind of arrangement, is described by Haller.

> During the 1880's the Cook County Hospital in Chicago placed every fifth medical case and every fourth surgical case under homeopathic treatment. Comparative mortality statistics indicated a difference of roughly one percent, with the allopaths (regular physician) reporting a 7.2 percent mortality and the homeopaths 82 percent.[2]

Another example was the Boston City Hospital where all new patients were assigned on a rotational basis to either the Boston, Harvard, or Tufts University services. This arrangement was assumed to permit an equitable distribution of patients. As far as we know this arrangement was used for research purposes only once by Halperin and Neuhauser[3] who observed differences in treatment for elective inguinal herniorraphies among the three services. This rotational arrangement at Boston University took over complete teaching responsibility for the hospital.

In 1956 Thomas Chalmers reported a coordinated series of four studies he and others carried out during 1951[4] in the United States Army Hospital in Kyoto, Japan, which was designated the Hepatitis Center for American soldiers during the Korean War. Over

* Department of Medicine, Cleveland Metropolitan General Hospital, Case Western Reserve University.

† Department of Epidemiology and Community Health, Case Western Reserve University.

4,000 hepatitis patients were treated there, and 460 patients were entered into the studies. Patients with jaundice were randomly assigned to one of four inpatient wards (p. 1167 in note 4). Different regimens of diet, rest, and patients' conditions were compared. The patient was used as the unit of analysis. Chalmers et al. thus had a unique opportunity to study a large number of soldiers with the same disease.

With the Metro firm trials, we have purposefully developed a system and introduced a formal randomization procedure in order to create a laboratory for ongoing clinical and health services research.

THE METRO FIRMS

The firm system was developed by the late director of the Department of Medicine, Charles Rammelkamp, for several reasons. The system promoted continuity both between patients and their physicians and between house staff and their attendings. Both the former and current directors of the Department of Medicine have strongly supported the firm system and have advocated its use as a research laboratory. The Division of General Medicine has been established and is responsible for the four firms. It also has hierarchical control of the system. The combination of foresight, support, and control has allowed Metro to continue to develop this research model. Moreover, it provides a clear focus for general internal medicine within a department with strong subspecialty interests.

Initially, new patients were assigned to the firms on a rotational basis. Since 1980 new patients have been randomly assigned to the firms according to a computer-generated table listing the firms in random sequences of four. In this manner we ensure equal distribution of patients among firms.

Not only are new patients randomly assigned, but since July 1981, all new internal medicine residents have been randomly assigned to the firms by lottery. Both patients and resident physicians remain with their firm throughout their connection with the hospital in order to provide continuity of care. Subspecialty consultants come to the firms on request. Second-year residents rotate out of the firms for subspecialty training, and patients needing subspecialty care go to subspecialty clinics, although they return to their firm for general medical care.

TABLE B-3 Volume of Services and Staffing in the Four Metro Firms

	Number
Firms	4
Inpatients admitted per firm per month	80
New inpatients admitted per firm per month	55
Outpatient visits per firm per month	240
Inpatient beds in each firm	28
Number of physicians in each firm	18

EXAMPLES OF THE METRO FIRM TRIALS

It is not our purpose here to provide a detailed description of our completed trials or of those currently in progress. We will, however, briefly describe several studies that represent the sorts of issues that can be explored using the firm system.

Our first studies dealt with health services research issues concerning physician behavior. In the first trial, house officers in two firms were provided with information about charges for the inpatient laboratory tests they ordered. House officers in the other two firms were provided with charges for their inpatient x-ray test usage.[5] The feedback of this information resulted in an overall decline in test usage. However, this effect was greatest in those firms in which group leaders became interested in using the data. Moreover, the greatest effect was observed after feedback was discontinued.

The second study was undertaken to evaluate a program intended to improve physician compliance with the delivery of preventive interventions. In this trial, house officers in two randomly selected experimental firms were offered educational seminars and given checklists with the medical records of their patients to encourage the use of Pneumovax, influenza vaccines, and mammography.[6] House officers in the control firm were not given checklists, although they were invited to the seminars. The use of the experimental maneuvers of interest increased significantly (from 5 to 45 percent among eligible patients) in the experimental group while remaining unchanged among the controls.

A subsequent trial was of a more clinical nature. When intravenous therapy teams were introduced to the inpatient medical services at Metro, they were done so in a sequential manner, that is, one firm at a time. This enabled us to evaluate their efficacy in decreasing the incidence of phlebitis and more serious complications associated with intravenous therapy. Firms on which the intravenous therapy team was functioning were compared with those on which intravenous catheters were inserted and maintained by the house staff, as had been the traditional practice.[7] A clinically and statistically significant decrease in intravenous catheter-related complications was observed in those firms in which the intravenous therapy team was functioning, thus supporting its efficacy. A subsequent analysis of the data permitted a description of the natural history of intravenous catheter-associated phlebitis.[8]

PRACTICAL CONSIDERATIONS

The Metro firm trials are particularly appropriate for research on the organization and delivery of medical care. They may also be used to study highly prevalent medical conditions. The ongoing randomization within the firm system provides a setting in which such research can be conducted at a reasonable cost.

Costs

Although a determination of the real costs involved in conducting clinical trials is a complicated issue, the extra costs, requiring outside funding for the first three trials, totalled less than $100,000. Suffice it to say, these trials are not expensive in relation to many randomized clinical trails. Costs may be even further reduced with the availability of a computerized data base. Currently the hospital provides several independent noncommunicating computerized data bases. These provide basic sociodemographic data on each patient, lab test results, and financial information. We plan to develop a hospital-wide patient information system which will merge these data and permit retrieval at low cost. Within the year it is expected that computer terminals will be available in each firm's inpatient unit. We plan a series of trials related to computer introduction, data availability, and the use of decision models for patient care.

Human Subjects

The development of any clinical research laboratory requires the approval and cooperation of the Committee on Human Investigation. If one accepts the idea that small teams (firms) are a preferred type of organization, then we would propose that the best way to ensure equal access to good care is to randomly assign physicians and patients to firms. This is the approach that the human subjects committee has taken at this hospital. The first two trials were considered to be administrative changes which did not require their detailed attention. Human subjects committees are to some degree idiosyncratic for each hospital, and in another hospital the response might be different.

UNIQUE METHODOLOGIC ISSUES

The firm system has provided an excellent setting for research. However, our experience in conducting trials in this setting has given rise to some unique methodological issues and theoretical considerations which are considered below.

Randomization

Although we have attempted to ensure as complete a randomization process as is possible given the constraints of a teaching program, we have had to consider the theoretical possibility that there might be some decay of the process with time. For example, it is conceivable that some unique attribute of a firm may lead to greater or lesser retention of a given type of patient.

To date, we have not observed such a phenomenon, nor have we been able to detect differences in the sociodemographic characteristics of patients among the four firms. Nevertheless, because the possibility of a decay in the randomization process exists, we have taken the precaution of running two separate analyses of our data for each trial. The impact of an experimental intervention is first analyzed using only the patients newly randomized into the firms, and is then analyzed using all patients. If we can demonstrate the same effect in both groups, we can assume either that randomization decay has not occurred, or if it has, that it has not influenced our results. In this way we can gain the statistical power associated with the larger patient population.

Unit of Analysis

One particularly difficult problem in trials of therapeutic interventions and studies of the organization and delivery of medical care is the determination of the appropriate unit of analysis. For example, in the Veterans Administration multicenter trial comparing medical and surgical therapy for the treatment of patients with chronic stable angina, 596 patients were used as the unit of analysis.[9-11] However, one could argue that the unit of analysis might have been the 13 participating surgical teams. A similar issue may be considered in the case of the Burlington Trial of the use of nurse practitioners for primary patient care.[12,13] Although patients were used as the unit of analysis to compare the care provided by nurse practitioners and doctors, one might argue that the sample size was one group of doctors and one group of nurse practitioners in one clinic in one Canadian province. Another example is the evaluation of fluoridation of the water supply in two Michigan towns,[14,15] which is generally considered the best test of the effect of a fluoridated water supply on tooth decay. The unit of analysis was assumed to be patients; one could argue that the unit of analysis might have been the town. The running debate on this question of unit of analysis[16-18] has no simple resolution.

In the Metro firm trials the firms are randomly selected to serve as experimental or control groups, and physicians and patients are randomly assigned to firms. Thus, there are four potential levels of analysis: the experimental versus control firms, each firm as a separate entity, the physician within each firm, or the individual patients. Which, then, is the appropriate unit of analysis? The solution we propose is to use a hierarchical, or nested, k design in which firms are nested within intervention group, physicians within firms, and patients within physicians.

To some extent, the unit of analysis will vary depending upon the question being addressed in a study or may vary for multiple questions addressed in a single trial. In our second trial we paid particular attention to this issue. Because we were concerned with the delivery of preventive care to our patients, and because they had been a unit of randomization, they were treated as the unit of analysis for comparisons of the delivery of preventive procedures. However, to the extent that we were interested in the attitudes and behavior of house officers, and because they had also been a unit of randomization, they were also treated as a unit of analysis for these issues.

The Hawthorne Effect

In trials associated with staff education and group dynamics, the possibility exists that an educational intervention in one firm will be communicated to other firms. Results from the initial trials suggest that there was little, if any, cross-firm contamination given the fact that the experimental effects were so large. Comparisons between control and experimental firms and between pre-experimental and experimental conditions should allow us to monitor for any possible contamination phenomenon for each study.

The Hawthorne effect[19] could occur in intervention studies of medical care organization. Observed behavioral changes could be the effect of attention alone. One approach to controlling for this Hawthorne effect is to run two trials concurrently. In our first trial, two firms received information on laboratory test charges, while the other two firms were controls. Concurrently, the lab test control firms were the experimental firms for the feedback of x-ray test charges. The lab test experimental firms were the control firms for the x-ray charge feedback study. We thus planned interventions on both firms in an effort to control for the Hawthorne effect. Nevertheless, because we cannot accurately measure the Hawthorne effect independently for each experiment, we are unable to control for this problem in the manner possible for double blind drug studies.

Generalizability

A legitimate question exists as to the generalizability of data collected in one setting, particularly one as unique as Cleveland Metropolitan General Hospital which is both a public institution and a major academic unit of Case Western Reserve University. One means of overcoming this problem would be the development of cooperative multicenter studies with other similar institutions in which a similar system might be established.

CONCLUSION

The Metro Firm trials will not solve all the problems of medical care evaluation. However, we believe that the firms provide a unique model for conducting clinical and health service research efficiently and inexpensively. We hope that other hospitals will develop similar models, and look forward to cooperating with them in multicenter trials.

We are indebted to Drs. Thomas C. Chalmers, Frederick Mosteller, Mitchel Gail, and Harold Goldberg for their advice, encouragement, and criticisms.

NOTES

[1] Waggoner, D. M., J. D. Frengley, R. C. Griggs, and C. H. Rammelkamp. 1979. A "firm" system for graduate training in general internal medicine. J. Med. Ed. 54:556.

[2] Haller, J. S. 1981. American Medicine in Transition 1849–1910. Urbana, Illinois: University of Illinois Press.

[3] Halperin, W., and D. Neuhauser. 1976. MEU: A way of measuring efficient utilization of hospital services. Health Care Management Review 1(2):63–70.

[4] Chalmers, T. C., R. D. Eckhardt, W. E. Reynolds, J. G. Cigarroa, N. Deane, R. W. Reifenstein, C. W. Smith, and C. S. Davidson. 1955. The treatment of acute infectious hepatitis. Controlled studies of the effects of diet, rest, and physical reconditioning on the acute course of the disease and on the incidence of relapses and residual abnormalities. J. Clin. Invest. 34:1163–1235.

[5] Cohen, D., P. Jones, B. Littenberg, and D. Neuhauser. 1982. Does cost information availability reduce physician test usage? A randomized clinical trial with unexpected findings. Med. Care 20(3):286–292.

[6] Cohen, D., B. Littenberg, C. Wetzel, and D. Neuhauser. 1982. Improving physician compliance with preventive medicine guidelines. Med. Care 20(10):1040–1045.

[7] Tomford, J. W., C. O. Hershey, C. E. McLaren, D. K. Porter, and D. I. Cohen. 1984. Intravenous therapy team and peripheral venous catheter—associated complications: A prospective controlled study. Arch. Intern. Med. 144:1191–1194.

[8] Hershey, C. O., J. W. Tomford, C. E. McLaren, D. K. Porter, and D. I. Cohen. In press. The natural history of intravenous catheter associated phlebitis. Arch. Intern. Med. 144:1373–1375.

[9] Murphy, M. L., H. N. Hultgren, K. Detre, J. Thomsen, T. Takaro, and Participants of the Veterans Administration Cooperative Study. 1977. Treatment of chronic stable angina. N. Engl. J. Med. 297(12):621–627.

[10] Special Correspondence: A debate on coronary bypass. 1977. N. Engl. J. Med. 297(26):1464–1470.

[11] Detre, K., M. L. Murphy, and H. Hultgren. 1977. Effect of coronary bypass surgery on longevity in high and low risk patients. Lancet 2:1243–1245.

[12] Spitzer, W. O., D. L. Sackett, J. C. Sibley, R. S. Roberts, M. Gent, D. J. Kergin, B. C. Hackett, and C. A. Olynich. 1974. The Burlington randomized trial of the nurse practitioner. N. Engl. J. Med. 290:251–256.

[13] Sackett, D. L., W. O. Spitzer, M. Gent, R. S. Roberts, W. I. Hay, G. M. Lefroy, G. P. Sweeny, I. Vandervlist, J. C. Sibley, L. W. Chambers, C. H. Goldsmith, A. S. Macpherson, and R. G. McAuley. 1974. The Burlington randomized trial of the nurse practitioner: Health outcomes of patients. Ann. Intern. Med. 80:137–142.

[14] Arnold, F. A., Jr., H. T. Dean, P. Jay, and J. W. Knutson. 1956. Effects of fluoridated public water supplies on dental caries prevalence—Tenth year of the Grand Rapids-Muskingum study. Public Health Rep. 71(7):652–658.

[15] Dean, H. T., F. A. Arnold, Jr., P. Jay, and J. W. Knutson. 1950. Studies on mass control of dental caries with flouridation of the public water supply. Public Health Rep. 71(7):652–658.

[16] Simon, R. 1981. Composite randomization designs for clinical trials. Biometrics 37:723–731.

[17] Cornfield, J. 1978. Randomization by group: A formal analysis. Am. J. Epidemiol. 108(2):100–102.

[18] Williams, P. T., S. P. Fortmann, J. W. Farquhar, A. Varady, and S. Mellen. 1981. A comparison of statistical methods for evaluating risk factor changes in community-based studies: An example from the Stanford three-community study. J. Chronic Dis. 34:565–571.

[19] Rothlesberger, F. J., and W. J. Dickson. Management and the Worker 1939–1975. Cambridge, Mass.: Harvard University Press.

Values and Preferences in the Delivery of Health Care

Barbara J. McNeil*

Over the past 5 years many persons engaged in health care have become concerned with the need for increased incorporation of patient values regarding quality of life into medical decision making. They also have become concerned with major lacks in knowledge about the kinds of information that should be available to aid patients in making such value decisions. These concerns may have arisen, in part, as a natural evolution of emphasis from quantity of care to quality of care. They may also have arisen, in part, from studies like those of Cassileth and coworkers[1] indicating that an increasing fraction of younger individuals with cancer want more information about their disease and want to play a more active role in its management (Table B-4).

Whatever the origin, values and preferences are now important in an explicit fashion to many providers of health care and to their patients. This article will review some of the considerations facing each of these groups and will give, where possible, supportive data from the literature. The ethical issues involved in choosing between diagnostic strategies and alternative therapies will become clear.

PROVIDERS OF HEALTH CARE

Providers (taken to mean physicians, nurses, nurse practitioners, etc.) have two major tasks: (1) *obtaining* data on the results of medical interventions, with *results* including not only health outcomes themselves but also the functional implications of such health outcomes; (2) *presenting* data in as unbiased a fashion as possible so that the values and preferences of their patients can be assessed and incorporated into medical decisions. Providers must also worry about how to use these data to assess preferences; for logical emphasis, however, assessment techniques will be discussed as part of the patient's perspective.

Obtaining Data

In some diseases (e.g., hypertension) outcome states for both treated and untreated patients are well documented. The Framingham study on cardiovascular diseases and the Veterans Administration (VA) study on medical therapy for hypertension have, for example, provided a wealth of data on the incidence (as a function of age) of a large variety of sequelae (strokes, myocardial infarction, angina, etc.).[2-5] Such studies generally fail, however, to give the *functional* implications of these sequelae: how many patients with stroke return to work, are self-sufficient, need to change careers? How many patients with heart attacks return to work, worry unnecessarily about their disease, etc.? Data here are spotty at best (see notes 6 and 7 for typical examples), but if available, they would help health care professionals educate patients more effectively about the likely course of their disease.

In oncology, in which many alternative therapies exist and therefore patient values become increasingly important, the situation is even worse. Large strides have been taken and progress has been made to increase the life expectancy of patients with cancer. The End Results Reporting Data,[8] published every 4 years, and periodic updates in *CA*, a journal for clinicians, emphasize these changes. Data on the incidence of associated morbidities are less detailed and are not available so widely and easily. In addition, the functional implications of such morbidities—e.g., those for mastectomies, ileostomies, radical prostate surgery, etc.—are seldom available. Also, when available, their presentation is frequently skewed so that only

* Professor of Clinical Epidemiology and Radiology, Harvard Medical School and Brigham and Women's Hospital.

TABLE B-4 Participation and Information Preferences by Age Group

Preferences	Patients in the Following Age Groups (years) Selecting Response (%) (N = 256)			
	20–39	40–59	60+	*p* Value
Participation preferences				
Prefer participating in decisions	87	62	51	
Prefer leaving decision to M.D.	13	38	49	<0.001
Type of information desired				
Want all information—good and bad	96	79	80	
Want only minimal or good information	4	21	20	<0.05
Preferences for detailed information				
Prefer minimum	15	40	31	
Prefer maximum	85	60	69	<0.01

SOURCE: Ann. Intern. Med. 92:834, 1980.

data from patients with minimal functional sequelae are discussed.

Presenting Data

Studies of the effects of alterations in data presentation on both physicians and patients are new and preliminary. Their importance is great, however. Some physicians present data to their patients in terms of life expectancies, others in terms of survival rates, and others in terms of mortality rates. Some physicians give a great deal of data regarding the immediate (less than 30 days), short-term side effects of alternative treatments and others give less. Some physicians try to give a full picture of the associated morbidities; others give an abbreviated picture.

How do these styles influence the choice a patient might make between or among alternative therapies? Data from cognitive psychology have recently suggested that the way data are presented can have a major impact on treatment choice.[9] One pilot study illustrates this effect in medicine.[10]

Treatment for operable lung cancer can involve either radiation therapy (RT) or surgery, and the results of these can be expressed in terms of cumulative probabilities of being alive or dead at varying points in time (Table B-5); these data can also obviously be integrated so that a life expectancy figure is obtained. When students, healthy outpatients, and physicians were asked to choose between surgery or radiation therapy, assuming that they had lung cancer, major and systematic differences in the percentage of respondents choosing radiation therapy were observed (Table B-6). For example when these data were presented in terms of mortality, radiation therapy was favored; when they were presented in terms of life expectancy, surgery was favored. In addition other systematic effects were found by concealing the identity of the two treatments and calling them A or B instead. This maneuver systematically increased the likelihood of an individual's choosing radiation therapy.

The above study was designed to illustrate the effects of explicit perturbations of data presentation on treatment choice in an exper-

TABLE B-5 Cumulative Likelihoods for 60-Year Old Men (Percent)

	Dying		Living	
	Surgery	RT	Surgery	RT
During treatment	10	0	90	100
By 1 year	32	23	68	77
By 5 years	66	78	34	22

TABLE B-6 Percent Choosing RT Over Surgery (S)

Label	Dying	Living
S – RT	44	18
A – B	61	37

imental situation. In clinical situations the problems may get more complex and provide increasing problems for providers of health care. These providers must worry not only about the effects seen in Tables B-5 and B-6 but also about other more implicit effects. For example, whatever the data presented, it is possible in a real clinical situation for providers to present data *alone* or do providers always end up providing data *plus* some of their own values? A recent study in psychiatry[11] would suggest the latter.

Implications

Major efforts must be made to make known the side effects of health interventions and, more importantly, their functional implications. Also, extensive research needs to be done to understand the extent to which the framing of data influences our ability to assess values and preferences. In addition, remedies for systematic biases in data presentation and interpretation and hence in decision making should be developed.

THE PATIENT

The assessment of a patient's values and preferences pervades all areas of his health care system from screening for occult disease, to diagnosing suspected disease, to instituting treatment for disease. Two questions are pertinent here: (1) For each of the above stages (screening, diagnosis, and treatment) do we have prototypical examples showing the importance of incorporating patients' values? (2) When should such values be assessed? At the time of the screening, diagnostic, or therapeutic encounter or sometime before the need actually occurs? Both of these questions will be addressed in turn.

PROTOTYPICAL EXAMPLES

When providers and patients think of preferences and values in medicine, they generally think of their impact on therapeutic choices. In fact, the importance of values far exceeds decision making in therapeutic medicine and, as indicated above, covers the whole range of medical interventions. In general, whatever the specific area of medicine involved, that methodology involved in assessing preferences is complex and will not be mentioned here. Instead, we will discuss the kinds of data required for proper incorporation of values at different stages of the medical process and the type of results that might be expected at these stages. Perhaps the reader will think of other analogous examples.

Screening for Disease

One example of this category relates to the screening of pregnant women for neural tube defects, using the alpha-fetoprotein (AFP) assay.[12] The major problem with this screening device is the fact that it has false-positive results that can lead to amniocentesis, which, in turn, can lead to the accidental abortion of a normal fetus. Thus, the question becomes, "Is a prospective parent willing to run the risk of an accidental miscarriage to avoid the birth of a child with a potential neural tube defect?" Several pieces of data are required to make an optimal decision: (1) responses to the question, "At what risk of a pregnancy's producing a severely deformed child would you prefer the risk of an elective abortion to the risk of having a child born with a neural tube defect?"; (2) the risk of having a child with a neural tube defect; (3) the false-positive rate of the AFP assay; and (4) the accidental abortion rate. With these Pauker and Pauker[13] were able to determine that about 50 percent of prospective parents who were already undergoing genetic counseling would want to have the screening test done. This 50 percent figure is undoubtedly a high one because individuals undergoing genetic counseling probably place a lower cost on the burden of an elective abortion than does the population as a whole. Nonetheless, it does indicate the role that values have in either establishing a screening program or in applying it to an individual patient. Another example along these same lines relates to amniocentesis for the detection of Down's syndrome.

Diagnosing Disease

A graphic example in this category is, "Should patients with presumed operable lung cancer be investigated for occult metastatic disease, knowing that 20 to 40 percent of these patients have such disease?"[14] If tests produced perfectly correct diagnostic information involving the presence of occult metastatic disease, then performing such tests would always be in the patients' best interests. Yet, if false-negative results occur, some patients would have unnecessary surgery and its attendant mortality rate (average, 10 percent; range, 5 to 20 percent). If false-positive results occur, some operable patients would not be offered the benefit from potentially curative treatment from surgery. Patients' attitudes toward the importance of near-term versus far-term survival are thus important in this decision to do preoperative staging examinations.

When a detailed analysis of patient attitudes was made and incorporated into this decision (Figure B-1), the data in Tables B-7 and B-8 emerged. Specifically, the 5-year survival rate is equal for the no-test and the test strategies if a *perfect* test (sensitivity and specificity both equal to 100 percent) is used. The life expectancy is slightly increased if a perfect test is used. Under all other circumstances, however, it is obvious that preoperative testing for occult disease should never be done if maximizing the 5-year survival rate or life expectancy were the goal (Table B-7). When patient values were incorporated, however, a large fraction of patients would benefit from testing even if the false-positive and false-negative rates for the test were in the 5 to 20 percent range (Table B-8).

Treating Disease

Two recent examples highlight the importance of incorporating patient attitudes into treatment decisions. One, already mentioned, involves the choice between surgery and radiation therapy for operable lung cancer. As indicated in Table B-5 the importance of near-term versus far-term survival is criti-

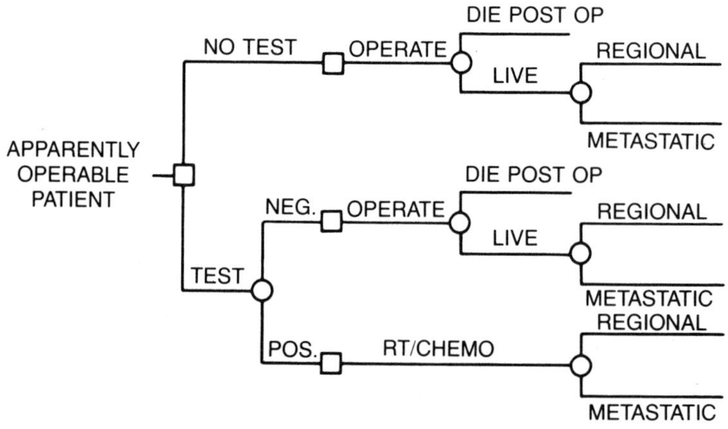

FIGURE B-1 Decision flow diagram comparing test and no-test strategies. In the no-test strategy (upper branch), patients with presumably operable bronchogenic carcinoma undergo surgery. Ten percent die perioperatively. Of the remaining patients, 80 percent have regional disease and are cured, while 20 percent have occult metastatic disease and are not cured. In the test strategy (lower branch), patients with presumably operable bronchogenic carcinoma are examined preoperatively in order to identify occult metastatic disease. Those patients with negative tests are treated surgically. Length of survival after operation depends on whether they have regional (true-negative test) or metastatic (false-negative test) disease. Those patients with positive tests are treated palliatively with radiation therapy or chemotherapy. Their length of survival also depends on whether they have regional (false-positive test) or metastatic (true-positive test) disease. (Reprinted with permission from Radiology 132:605, 1979).

TABLE B-7 Evaluation of Preoperative Testing in Patients with "Operable" Lung Cancer: Traditional Objective Approaches

Strategy	Sensitivity (%)	Specificity (%)	5-Year Survival (%)	Life Expectancy (years)	Optimal Decision
No preoperative testing			32.5	6.42	
Preoperative testing where test has:	100	100	32.5	6.43	Test
	90	95	32.0	6.36	No test
	90	90	31.5	6.29	No test
	80	95	32.0	6.35	No test
	80	90	31.5	6.29	No test
	80	80	30.5	6.15	No test
	50	90	31.5	6.28	No test

SOURCE: Radiology 132:608, 1979.

TABLE B-8 Evaluation of Preoperative Testing in Patients with "Operable" Lung Cancer: Incorporation of Patient Attitudes

Test Characteristics		Patients Who Should Be Tested (%)
Sensitivity (%)	Specificity (%)	
100	100	100
90	95	68
90	90	60
80	95	66
80	90	56
80	80	47
50	90	50

cal for this clinical problem. In a small study[15] that explored this problem using expected utility theory (i.e., assessing values or utilities individually and then integrating them with probability data*) the results suggested that at a 10 percent operative mortality rate 21 percent of 60-year-old men should have radiation therapy instead of surgery; 43 percent of 70-year-old men should have radiation therapy instead of surgery (Table B-9). At lower operative mortality rates these figures drop, and at higher rates they increase. These results are particularly striking when it is recalled that most therapeutic choices are not made on the basis of patient preferences as indicated here, but rather on the basis of absolute 5-year survival rates.

Data from the work of Torrance et al. have indicated that it is possible through the time trade-off technique[18] to determine, relative to perfect health, how individuals value various states of imperfect health.[19] On a scale of

TABLE B-9 Influence of the Measure of Therapeutic Efficacy on the Choice of Therapy when Excellent Surgical Results Prevail

Measure of Therapeutic Efficacy	Percent Who Should Receive Radiation Therapy Rather than Operation with Operative Mortality Rates of			
	5%	10%	15%	20%
At age 60:				
5-year survival	0	0	0	0
Expected utility	7	21	43	64
At age 70:				
5-year survival	0	0	0	0
Expected utility	14	43	50	71

SOURCE: N. Engl. J. Med. 299:1400, 1978.

* Note that this approach has been the traditional one advocated to date and involves assessing values, calculating expected utility, and then indicating what the patient *should* want.[16,17] It differs from the technique described in Tables B-5 and B-6, wherein a respondent is given the data and asked to make a *direct* choice. The relative advantage of each of these techniques needs to be explored.

TABLE B-10 Mean Utilities for Several States of Health in General Population and a Selected Subset

State of Health	Utility
Perfect health	1.00
Tuberculosis	0.68
Mastectomy for breast cancer	0.48
Depression for 3 months	0.44
Home dialysis for life	
By general population	0.39
By dialysis patients	0.56
Hospital dialysis for life	
By general population	0.32
By dialysis patients	0.52
Death	0.00

0 (death) to 1.0 (perfect health), they were able to obtain data for a variety of chronic health conditions (Table B-10). Using this same technique, McNeil and coworkers determined how people valued the state of having either no speech or artificial speech, caused by surgery for cancer of the larynx.[20] They then integrated this information with the results of alternative treatments for cancer of the larynx—surgery with high survival rates and no speech and radiation therapy with low survival rates and normal speech—and determined how many people so valued voice that they would want radiation therapy. The results indicated that about 20 percent of individuals fall in that category.

Implications

For a particular patient the weighing of quantity and quality of life may be important in choosing between alternative therapies for the same disease. Similarly, for society as a whole accurate weighting of quality and quantity of life may be important in developing a rank ordering of benefits achieved from various health interventions. Such an ordering would aid in an optimum allocation for health care resources. From these two perspectives and from the above prototypical examples, it should be clear that additional work is needed in two areas: (1) refinement of the methodology for assessing values and preferences, and (2) routine use of this methodology in the practice of medicine.

THE TIMING OF ASSESSMENTS

The methodology used in the assessments described above is detailed and complex and beyond the scope of this review (see notes 16–18 for a discussion of various methodologies). Suffice it to say that any kind of detailed questioning will be difficult to administer routinely in patients who have either become acutely ill or who have become recently aware of a long-term chronic problem about to afflict them. In addition, the validity of responses made under such circumstances could be questioned. These problems have led a number of individuals to suggest one or two courses of action. First, streamline questions and methodologic approaches so that they are no more complex than other activities a patient is asked to respond to. Second, identify a set of characteristics corresponding to optimal courses of action for a variety of patients and diseases; then, match a new patient to these characteristics and a course of action previously determined to be optimal for a similar individual. This second approach would require a "bank" of prototypical patients, each with an associated optimal decision.

Implications

Problems in timing value assessments are great. Their solution may depend in large part on the extent to which the methodology for value assessment is simplified. The easier the assessment technique the more likely that timely values can be obtained. The more cumbersome the technique the more likely a bank of prototypical values will be required.

Supported in part from a grant from the Henry J. Kaiser Family Foundation.

NOTES

[1] Cassileth, B. R., R. V. Zupkis, K. Sutton-Smith, and V. March. 1980. Information and participation preferences among cancer patients. Ann. Intern. Med. 92:832–836.

[2] Kannel, W.B., and T. Gordon. 1970. The Framingham Study: An Epidemiological Investigation of Cardiovascular Disease. Section 26. Some Characteristics Related to the Incidence of Cardiovascular Disease and Death: Framingham Study, 16-year Follow-up. Washington, D.C.: U.S. Government Printing Office.

[3] Kannel, W. B., and T. Gordon. 1970. The Framingham Study: An Epidemiological Investigation of Cardiovascular Disease. Section 25. Survival Following Certain Cardiovascular Events. Washington, D.C.: U.S. Government Printing Office.

[4] Veterans Administration Cooperative Study Group on Antihypertensive Agents. 1969. Effects of treatment on morbidity in hypertension: Results in patients with diastolic blood pressures averaging 115 through 129 mm Hg. J. Am. Med. Assoc. 202:1028–1034.

[5] Veterans Administration Cooperative Study Group on Antihypertensive Agents. 1970. Effects of treatment on morbidity in hypertension. II. Results in patients with diastolic blood pressures averaging 90 through 114 mm. J. Am. Med. Assoc. 213:1143–1152.

[6] Cary, E. L., N. Vetter, and A. Philip. 1973. Return to work after a heart attack. J. Psychosom. Res. 17:231–243.

[7] Weisbroth, S., N. Esibill, and R. R. Zuger. 1971. Factors in the vocational success of hemiplegic patients. Arch. Phys. Med. Rehab. 52:441–446.

[8] Axtell, L. M., S. J. Cutler, and M. H. Myers, eds. 1972. End Results in Cancer—Report No. 4 DHEW Publication No. (NIH) 73-272. Washington, D.C.: U.S. Government Printing Office.

[9] Tversky, A., and D. Kahneman. 1981. The framing of decisions and the psychology of choice. Science 211:453–458.

[10] McNeil, B. J., S. G. Pauker, H. C. Sox, and A. Tversky. 1982. On the elicitation of preferences for alternative therapies. N. Engl. J. Med. 306:1259–1262.

[11] Lidz, C. W. 1980. The weather report model of informed consent: Problems in preserving patient voluntariness. Bull. Am. Acad. Psych. Law 8(2):152–160.

[12] Pauker, S. G., S. P. Pauker, and B. J. McNeil. 1982. The effect of private attitudes on public policy: Prenatal screening for neural tube defects as a prototype. Med. Dec. Mak. 2:103–114.

[13] Pauker, S. P., and S. G. Pauker. 1977. Prenatal diagnosis: A directive approach to genetic counseling using decision analysis. Yale J. Biol. Med. 50:275–289.

[14] McNeil, B. J., and S. G. Pauker. 1979. The patient's role in assessing the value of diagnostic tests. Radiology 132:605–610.

[15] McNeil, B. J., R. Wichselbaum, and S. G. Pauker. 1978. Fallacy of the five-year survival in lung cancer. N. Engl. J. Med. 299:1397–1401.

[16] Keeney, R. L., and H. Raiffa. 1976. Decision Making with Multiple Objectives: Preferences and Value Tradeoffs. New York: John Wiley.

[17] Raiffa, H. 1968. Decision Analysis: Introductory Lectures on Choices Under Uncertainty. Reading, Mass.: Addison-Wesley.

[18] Torrance, G. W., W. H. Thomas, and D. L. Sackett. 1972. A utility maximization model for evaluation of health care programs. Health Services Res. 7:118–133.

[19] Sackett, D. L., and G. W. Torrance. 1979. The utility of different health states as perceived by the general public. J. Chronic Dis. 31:697–704.

[20] McNeil, B. J., R. Weichselbaum, and S. G. Pauker. 1981. Speech and survival: Tradeoffs between quality and quantity of life in laryngeal cancer. N. Engl. J. Med. 305:982–987.

New Federalism and State Support for Technology Assessment

George D. Greenberg*
Penny H. Feldman†

This paper considers the implications of new federalism for state government support of technology assessment. First we describe new federalism and related health policy initiatives of the Reagan administration. Second, we review the states' current involvement in technology assessment. Third, we examine state incentives and capacity to expand technology assessment efforts and their likely effectiveness should they choose to do so. Fourth, we discuss economic and political rationales for state involvement. Finally, we identify those aspects of new federalism, as well as concomitant changes in federal and state health policy, that we believe will be critical in influencing future state support for technology assessment.

NEW FEDERALISM AND HEALTH POLICY DEVELOPMENTS

At the outset of his administration, President Reagan asserted that his ultimate goal with regard to federalism was to sort out functional responsibilities between the federal and state governments and to turn back appropriate revenue sources and decision-making authority to the states (Cannon and Dewar, 1981; Reagan, 1982). The six block grants proposed as part of the fiscal year (FY) 1982 budget were to be a first step toward this ultimate goal, consolidating categorical grant programs in the areas of health, education, social services, energy, and emergency assistance. The block grants proposed for FY 1982 called for reduced federal funding and a minimum of federal strings, eliminating or reducing requirements for state matching funds, planning, reporting, maintenance of effort, and the like.

In the health field, the Reagan administration proposed two block grants, a health services block and a prevention block, funded at approximately 75 percent of FY 1981 program levels (Feder et al., 1982).[1] The administration also proposed to alter federal-state arrangements governing the $28 billion Medicaid program. For FY 1982 it proposed a 5 percent cap on federal Medicaid matching funds, so that the entire burden of future cost increases above the cap would fall on the states (Pelham, 1981a).[2] In conjunction with the cap proposal, states were to receive greatly expanded authority to restructure their Medicaid programs to achieve cost savings.

Congress substantially revised the administration's proposal in the Omnibus Budget Reconciliation Act of 1981. It created four health block grants instead of two, consolidating programs in the areas of primary care; maternal and child health; prevention; and alcohol, drug abuse, and mental health (Pelham, 1981b). The health blocks contained many more federal strings than the administration would have liked, but they did somewhat expand state discretion, particularly in the areas of maternal and child health and prevention. At the same time, they provided fewer federal dollars than previously. Furthermore, while Congress rejected the Medicaid cap, it voted to reduce federal Medicaid matching payments by 3 percent in 1982, 4 percent in 1983, and 4.5 percent in 1984; and it greatly enhanced states' flexibility to restructure their Medicaid programs.[3]

There have been no significant legislative advances toward new federalism since 1981, despite subsequent administration proposals

* Assistant Secretary for Planning and Evaluation, U.S. Department of Health and Human Services. Dr. Greenberg's contribution to this article was written in his private capacity. No official support or endorsement by the U.S. Department of Health and Human Services is intended or should be inferred.

† Harvard School of Public Health, Harvard University.

to federalize Medicaid (in exchange for state financing of the Aid to Families with Dependent Children and Food Stamp Programs) and to turn back a variety of domestic programs, including the four health block grants, to the states. Yet a variety of proposals to federalize all or large portions of Medicaid, to turn the remaining parts of the program over to the states to be funded through block grants, or to further alter and reduce federal matching payments for Medicaid remain on the administration's agenda to be moved forward pending the outcome of the 1984 presidential election (Grannemann and Pauly, 1983).

Complementing the administration's new federalism strategy in the area of health was its competition initiative. The goal of competition is to make consumers more cost-conscious by increasing cost sharing, in turn motivating health insurers and providers to promote more efficient health delivery systems to compete more effectively for the dollars of newly cost-conscious consumers. If competition were to succeed, the government's role at all levels would be reduced as government dollars were transferred to the private sector in the form of vouchers, tax credits, or the like. Private insurers, rather than federal or state government, would have the primary role in determining what health benefits beyond a minimum basic package should be included in their plans. Furthermore, private insurers, rather than federal or state government, would bear the burden of costs that exceeded the value of the government contribution. Major national legislation to promote competition has not yet been enacted by the Congress, despite the administration's FY 1984 proposals for caps on employers' tax deductible health insurance contributions, voluntary Medicare vouchers, and restructuring of Medicare Part A benefits to provide catastrophic coverage and impose cost sharing on the first 60 days of care. However, individual states are using the flexibility granted them under the Reconciliation Act of 1981 to introduce competitive incentives in their Medicaid programs.

The passage of hospital prospective payment for Medicare has been the administration's major accomplishment in the health care arena. Prospective payment has both regulatory and competitive aspects. It contains elements of regulation in that it establishes limits on budgetary resources that Medicare will pay for given diagnosis-related groups (DRGs) and requires elaborate governmental and intermediary monitoring to ensure that hospitals do not manipulate the system. Prospective payment is pro-competitive in that it provides incentives for hospitals to drop unprofitable services and compete with each other for patients in order to maximize their income. Whichever aspect of prospective payment is considered dominant, the DRG system should renew federal interest in technology assessment insofar as DRG rates are intended to reflect the real resource costs of medical technologies appropriate to specific diagnoses. Renewed federal interest may take the form of research support for the Prospective Payment Assessment Commission, a more narrowly conceived successor to the National Center for Health Care Technology.

The evolution of the DRG system, and associated federal support for technology assessment, will likely be as important as health block grants, Medicaid financing and reimbursement reform, and the success or failure of competitive incentive schemes in influencing future state support for technology assessment. Renewed federal interest in expanding technology assessment might obviate the role of the states, particularly in the context of a fully federalized Medicaid program. On the other hand, increased federal support for technology assessment might stimulate some states to expand their activities in this area, particularly in the context of Medicaid reform in which they were required to bear increased financial responsibility. Devolution of health program financing on the states can be expected to increase their interest in technology assessment as a means to promote cost control, while it erects political and financial barriers to actual state support of such studies. Finally, if competition were to succeed and Medicare/Medicaid expenditures were capped by means of vouchers or some comparable mechanism, technology assessment might become the concern of competing private insurers seeking to make more cost-effective decisions. We examine the implications of these scenarios in our concluding section.

STATE INVOLVEMENT IN TECHNOLOGY ASSESSMENT

By all accounts, current state involvement in technology assessment is minimal. The federal, state, and local governments spent $5.6 billion on health-related research in 1982. Nearly 90 percent ($5.0 billion) came from the federal government, and the rest came from states and localities (Gibson et al., 1983). Although estimates of government expenditures on technology assessment are sketchy, surveys by the U.S. Office of Technology Assessment (OTA; 1980) indicate that cost-effectiveness and cost-benefit analyses "are not frequently conducted or applied" by major federal health agencies, state and local governments, or nongovernmental organizations. It is quite likely then that only a small fraction of total health research spending is devoted to technology assessment; and, of course, an even tinier fraction is spent by state or local governments.

OTA (1980) reported that where cost-effectiveness or cost-benefit analyses had been conducted at the state or local level, their performance usually reflected the individual interests of government staff (and, by implication, not explicit policy directives of key decision makers). OTA (1980) found that most state and local analyses had been conducted in Massachusetts and New York. Those studies tended to focus on the costs and benefits or cost-effectiveness of various screening and other disease prevention programs. The difficulty of obtaining necessary data, the relatively high cost of comprehensive analyses—estimated at $381,000 by Coates (1972)—and a tradition of devoting relatively little money and staff to evaluation were cited as deterrents to state support for technology assessment (OTA, 1980).

If states are not devoting significant resources to conducting or contracting for technology assessment, they may nonetheless be using technology assessment results in a variety of reimbursement or regulatory decisions. Evidence of such action, however, is scanty and is largely anecdotal. As third-party payers, some states limit payment for experimental procedures under Medicaid. The definition of *experimental* may be drawn from federal Medicare/Medicaid guidelines (themselves drawn sometimes from formal evaluation and sometimes from expert opinion) or from the opinion of medical experts at the state level (OTA, 1980). As planners and regulators, states may draw on technology assessment to guide them in establishing standards or making particular certificate-of-need decisions. For example, Massachusetts originally granted certificate of need for computed tomographic (CT) scanners on the condition that hospitals participate in a formal evaluation of the technology, intended to inform future regulatory decisions.

States' use, as distinct from their financial support, of technology assessment is influenced by the availability of relevant studies produced under other auspices and, in the case of Medicaid, by a recent court ruling. Medicaid requires that states pay for all "medically necessary" services. In 1980, a federal court established that with regard to mandatory Medicaid services the individual physician's judgment determines medical necessity except where the state has an explicit policy limiting payment for experimental procedures. Otherwise the only permissible review of the physician's judgment is to determine whether there was a reasonable bias in fact for the diagnosis (*Rush* v. *Parham*, 1980). Thus under current court rulings, states' latitude in applying the results of technology assessment is apparently circumscribed.

POSSIBILITIES FOR MORE TECHNOLOGY ASSESSMENT BY STATES

In understanding states' minimal use of technology assessment today and in considering their possible future support for such activity, it is important to examine their incentives, capacity, and likely effectiveness should they expand technology assessment efforts. Why would a state want to conduct technology assessment and devote scarce resources to it? Do states have the money, staff, and technical know-how? Could states be successful if they tried?

Incentives

States have the constitutional authority to provide for the health and welfare of their citizens. In exercising this authority, they perform a variety of functions that provide potential incentives for supporting technology assessment: (1) they are responsible for traditional public health activities, including sanitation, communicable disease control, and the assurance of the quality of water and food supplies; (2) they provide institutional and ambulatory services for chronic conditions as well as for disease prevention and health promotion; (3) they invest directly in state hospitals, medical schools, and other health care facilities; (4) they engage in a wide set of regulatory activities ranging from institutional licensure and inspection to regulation of environmental hazards. In addition, as partners in the federal-state system, states act as third-party payers for personal health services for the Medicaid population (Wilson and Neuhauser, 1982). In theory, if not in practice, states could perform all of these functions better if their decision were informed by the results of cost-effectiveness or cost-benefit analysis. State incentives to expand efforts in a given area depend in part on what the federal government and the private sector are already doing and on whether the citizens of a state perceive they are adequately protected by the actions of federal agencies and private bodies.

Protection of the health and welfare of citizens involves states in the development and enforcement of standards of safety and efficacy. To the extent that federal agencies, such as the Food and Drug Administration, already develop and enforce such standards, state motivation to go beyond the federal minimum is reduced as long as federal agencies are not perceived as weak or ineffective. On the other hand, if new technologies appear to be beyond the control or authority of existing federal agencies, citizen fears may motivate states to act on their own. Dramatic incidents such as the recent Tylenol poisonings or perceived reductions in federal enforcement also can lead to renewed popular calls for state protections. For example, state regulation of environmental pollution may increase to the extent that the federal government deregulates this area, and state regulation of nuclear power production may also increase as public perception of the adequacy of Nuclear Regulatory Commission standards declines after incidents such as that at Three Mile Island.

The history of the passage of the Pure Food, Drug, and Cosmetic Act (1938) is illustrative of the dynamic and changing relationship between federal and state regulations. Calls for federal regulation in the early 1930s in response to cases of blindness from cosmetics and deaths resulting from dissolving sulfa drugs in carbon tetrachloride were blocked by business interests, until individual states began to enact very strict laws. Faced with strict regulation in some states, business helped enact a uniform national code in 1938, which preempted state action and preserved a national market (Jackson, 1969).

Health planning and cost-control programs enacted in the late 1960s and in the 1970s also illustrate the dynamic relationship among federal, state, and private actions. Approximately a half dozen states—including New York, Maryland, Connecticut, and Massachusetts—were the first to initiate health care regulation, using their constitutional powers to establish vigorous certificate-of-need and hospital rate-setting programs independent of federal mandates. The professional standards review and national health planning laws—enacted in 1972 and 1974, respectively—were intended by Congress to foster increased professional regulation and centralized resource allocation across the 50 states. National legislation provided political and financial incentives for previously inactive states and private groups to establish certificate-of-need agencies and peer review organizations where they had not before existed. On the other hand, associated federal rules and guidelines actually reduced the incentives for pioneering states to develop innovative regulatory programs.

In their role as service providers and third-party payers, state decision makers are similarly influenced by the degree of flexibility and the financial incentives embodied in federal law. As indicated above, Medicaid regulations governing medically necessary services, along with recent court rulings, provide a disincentive for states to independently evaluate the cost-effectiveness of Medicaid-reimbursable procedures. Furthermore, while the costs of conducting or contracting for cost-effectiveness or cost-benefit analyses are concentrated and not routinely reimbursed by the federal government, the costs of covering questionable medical procedures and equipment are relatively diffuse and—under current federal-state Medicaid matching arrangements—reimbursed by the federal government at rates ranging from 50 to 80 percent, depending on the state.

State investment in health facilities and equipment and state financing and provision of direct services are relatively free of federal constraints. However, state funding priorities are often subject to detailed scrutiny and approval by state legislatures. Technology assessment is an activity virtually devoid of popular appeal. Furthermore, knowing that affected interest groups and their legislative representatives tend to be highly resistant to cuts or changes in funding and service and that constituencies who bear the burden of efficiency measures are unlikely to be swayed by the results of cost-effectiveness analysis, decision makers in the state bureaucracy may be loath to divert scarce resources away from service provisions to support analytic studies. Given the unpopularity of benefit costs and negative coverage decisions and the often controversial nature of even the most authoritative cost-effectiveness studies, it is not surprising that technology assessment is not a high-priority item for state officials.

State Resources and Capacity

If states were motivated to expand technology assessment efforts, would they have the resources and technical capacity to do so? At a minimum, states would need the financial resources to adequately fund technology assessments. In addition, if they chose to conduct rather than contract for such assessments, they would require appropriately trained staff, adequate data bases, and the command of complex methodologies.

There has been general growth in state capabilities over the past 20 years. State fiscal capacity and strength grew significantly during the 1970s. States have upgraded and expanded their tax bases (Advisory Commission on Intergovernmental Relations, 1982).[4] Between 1960 and 1979, 11 states adopted personal income taxes, 9 enacted corporate income taxes, and 10 enacted general sales taxes. By 1979, 41 states had a broad-based income tax, 45 a corporate income tax, and 45 a general sales tax. A total of 37 states had all three levies in 1979 compared with only 19 in 1960 (Walker, 1981). The average tax bite by states rose from 7.6 percent of personal income in 1953 to 12.8 percent in 1977 (Walker, 1981). State and local receipts from their own sources rose from $105 billion in 1970 to $295 billion in 1980 (Walker, 1981). Although these trends do not speak to a specific state capacity to perform technology assessments, they argue against a hasty conclusion that states could not support expanded technology assessment efforts if they chose to do so.

On the other hand, after a period of growing surpluses, some state governments faced fiscal crisis in the early 1980s. Looming deficits resulted from the decline in the economy, federal cuts in intergovernmental aid, the enactment of tax or expenditure limits in several states, and past expansions in state services. A survey of state budget officers in the spring of 1981 indicated that state balances would drop to $2.3 billion or 1.5 percent of expenditures in 1982, enough to cover only 4 days of operations (Hamilton, 1982).[5] With previous surpluses depleted, many states faced constitutional limits against deficit financing. States reacted by reducing services and increasing taxes. These actions, along with an upswing in the economy, strengthened states' 1983 and 1984 fiscal position vis-à-vis the federal government. Combined state and local government surpluses of $15 billion were estimated for 1983, while the federal government faced a deficit of over $100 billion (Herbers, 1983). However, even in an improved fiscal environment, states' overall ability to finance expensive evaluative procedures is in question. The prospect of improved state finances raised the spector of further decreases in federal aid and highlighted the need for states to reestablish reserve funds rather than fund new priorities.

Furthermore, states such as New York, Massachusetts, Michigan, and California, with disproportionately high public health care expenditures in relation to tax capacity—i.e., those states that might benefit most from increased support for cost-effectiveness analysis in the long run—may be least able to finance it in the short run, while states with disproportionately low public health expenditures but high tax capacity (e.g., Texas, Florida, and Wyoming) may be disinclined to spend their money on technology assessment.[6] States cannot easily pool their resources to support expensive studies collectively. Thus their real capacity to support technology assessment is less than their combined tax capacity would suggest.

State personnel capabilities grew in the 1970s along with fiscal capacity. State governments have grown much more rapidly than the federal government. The number of federal employees remained roughly constant at 2.9 million between 1970 and 1980, while state employment increased from 2.8 to 36 million (Barfield, 1981). Between 1964 and 1978 the proportion of state agency heads with graduate degrees rose from 40 percent to 58 percent, and the proportion of state agency heads promoted from within the state civil service increased to over 50 percent (Broder, 1982). State health-planning and rate-setting agencies are one potential source of personnel with training and skills particularly well-suited to technology assessment. However, more to the point, university-based faculties and private consulting firms within a state can service state governments under contract as easily as they can serve the federal government. To the extent that neither the federal government nor the states currently have a large capacity to conduct technology assessments, future capacity can be built at either level, if funds are available.

To the extent that well-conducted technology assessments require access to large data bases, the conduct of large-scale clinical trials including diverse populations over long periods of time, and the development of complex methodologies, states' capacity to complete successful studies may be limited. For the most part, state agencies do not have access to or experience in amassing large data bases such as those used in studies supported by federal agencies such as the Health Care Financing Administration (HCFA) or the National Center for Health Services Research. Nor do states have experience in running clinical trials, such as those supported by the National Institutes of Health. Moreover, state data-processing and analytic capacities have been slow to develop. For example, in 1980, 9 years after the 1972 Social Security Amendments authorized 90 percent federal matching payments to states for the design, development, and installation of Medicaid Management Information Systems (mechanized claims processing and information retrieval systems), only 29 states had federally certified systems (HCFA, 1982). Of course, with data, as with staff, if states had funds available, they could contract for technology assessments from groups with the necessary administrative and methodological capacities. Whether or not studies under state sponsorship could achieve the level of data access (e.g., access to sensitive medical records) achieved by federally sponsored studies is an open question.

State Effectiveness

If states invest the resources, can they be effective? Relevant questions include the following: (1) Are parochial political forces in the state legislature more likely to overwhelm the judgments of scientists than they are in the Congress? (2) Could providers and patients escape the enforcement actions of states that regulate based on the conduct of stringent technology assessments by moving to states that do not? (3) Do states create economic and social chaos by basing regulatory actions on vastly different scientific standards? Unfortunately, there is little evidence available to answer these questions.

The political environment in each state is different. However, it can be reasonably predicted that coalitions of health policy analysts, scientists, and business groups concerned about rising health costs, who understand the potential role technology assessment can play, and who form the primary constituency in support of research, will be weaker on average in each of the 50 states than they are in Congress. Even in relatively proregulation states, state legislatures have supported local hospitals vis-à-vis state planning agencies by overturning certificate-of-need decisions with special legislation (Altman et al., 1981). To the extent that state legislatures are more responsive to coalitions of local providers than to various cost-control interests, scientific judgments may be less likely to be sustained.

Action by a single state always risks defeat if citizens can easily obtain desired services in nearby but unregulated environments in neighboring states. Just as physicians in some states purchased CT scanners for their offices to avoid certificate-of-need controls in hospitals, they might shift certain practices and procedures to nearby but out-of-town offices or institutions if those practices were judged non-cost-effective and nonreimbursable by a given state. The regulating state might experience some budgetary savings as a result of its application of cost-effectiveness analysis; however to the extent that non-cost-effective practices were shifted rather than deterred, its neighboring state might experience added costs. Systemwide savings would not accrue.

Finally, if state standards for aspects of research such as sample size, significance level, length of observation, etc., varied widely, state judgments as to safety and efficacy probably also would vary significantly. This could create significant uncertainty for patients and providers, shake public confidence in the integrity of regulatory decisions, and increase social costs in exchange for uneven budgetary savings.

CRITERIA FOR STATE ACTION

What is the appropriate role for the states in technology assessment? Is technology assessment one of those functions that should be decentralized via new federalism, or is it primarily a responsibility of the federal government? The literature on federalism offers several economic and political criteria for allocating responsibilities between federal and state governments.

A classic justification for federal action is the presence of serious externalities. A state may decide not to build a dam if only the costs and benefits to its citizens are calculated, but the federal government may be justified in building the dam if the benefits to citizens of another state downstream are added in. Similarly, federal intervention may be justified when states refrain from taking socially beneficial action for fear of putting themselves at a competitive disadvantage versus other states. For example, states may fear that tightening environmental controls unilaterally will simply drive businesses elsewhere or that raising welfare levels beyond the federal minimum may make them more attractive to nonproductive populations. Uniform federal action in such situations theoretically enhances the public good without sacrificing the interests of the individual states. A second consideration used to justify federal action is the fact that states may be in the position of a "free rider" vis-à-vis certain public goods. For example, Georgia cannot be defended from Soviet attack without also defending Florida. The citizens of a particular state might be tempted to provide less than their fair share if the federal government did not preempt the issue. Finally, when the scale of an enterprise is truly massive, when only the federal government can assemble the expertise or talent necessary to successfully complete a project, or when there are large economies of scale, the case for federal action is often considered strong. For example, the technical expertise and resources required to land a man on the moon were beyond the capacity of any single state. Hence federal action was considered necessary and appropriate by those who believed that the nation should develop space technology.

Although federal action is most often defended on grounds of equity of efficiency, state action is defended on grounds of preserving capacity for innovation, maintaining diversity and pluralism (the states constitute 50 laboratories), minimizing administrative complexity (fewer levels of government need to be involved), and maximizing democratic participation (state government is closer to the people). George Silver (1974) has argued that in the area of maternal and child health, federal grants have simply supported what states have wanted to do and federal action has always followed, not led, state action in that field.[7] Richard Elmore (1978) has reviewed a number of studies demonstrating that innovative programs tend to be successful when developed and implemented at the grass roots level by states and localities. Pressman and Wildavsky (1973) conclude that reducing layers of government and concomitant decision clearance points improves the prospects for program implementation.

On balance, we believe that the arguments supporting a primary federal role in financing, technical assistance, standard setting, and data gathering—if not in directly conducting—technology assessments are stronger than those supporting increased state responsibility. Technology assessment as such would probably benefit more from nationally accepted guarantees of scientific integrity and access to nationwide data sets than from innovation, diversity, or grass roots participation at the state level. Large federal deficits notwithstanding, the federal government is probably still better able to fund a major technology assessment effort than the states acting individually.

Furthermore, the findings of technology assessment have implications that extend beyond the boundaries of a single state. Hence there are significant externalities for states in conducting technology assessments and applying their results. Different state regulations with regard to technology may be self-defeating if providers and patients simply cross state lines to escape more stringent standards. Similarly, vastly different state action may make the marketing of new technologies so problematic that incentives for technological innovations are reduced. The payoff of the federal government will likely be greater than that to the states insofar as the impact of technology assessment can be maximized through uniform national policy. Yet in the context of reduced federal support for technology assessment, support by selected states or by the private sector is the only alternative to vastly diminished efforts in this area.

FACTORS IN STATE SUPPORT FOR TECHNOLOGY ASSESSMENT

Four factors, we believe, will largely determine the impact of new federalism on state support for technology assessment: (1) the availability of federal support for technology assessment, (2) the content of Medicaid financing and reimbursement reforms, (3) the allocation of block grant funds at the state level, and (4) the relative success or failure of competitive health care incentives.

Federal Support for Technology Assessment

Because technology assessment itself is expensive and technically complex, states have to be convinced that technology is cost-effective before making the investment. Even if states are convinced of the merits of technology assessments, the amounts they invest will depend upon what is already being spent at the national level, either by the federal government or privately funded institutes.

Just as technologies continue to develop and evolve, so do public attitudes and regulatory policies. In the 1960s and 1970s, expansion of the authority of federal agencies to deal with rapidly diffusing technologies discouraged and in some cases preempted state action. This situation might be reversed in the context of extensive deregulation and significant devolution of federal authority. States might be spurred to action if federal agencies did not or could not act, as citizens became concerned about possible harmful effects of increasingly unregulated technological development. So far this has not occurred in the health care sector.

Over time, under DRGs, the federal Health Care Financing Administration will establish rates for diagnosis-related groups that theoretically reflect the costs of technology appropriate to treating a given diagnosis. The perceived rationality and justifiability of changes in diagnosis-specific payment rates will presumably depend in part on the availability and persuasiveness of technology assessment studies relevant to technological advances in the treatment of illness. The potential role for federally sponsored technology assessment thus seems greatly enhanced under the DRG system.

Renewed and expanded federal commitment to technology assessment might obviate the role of the states. States acting alone may not be able to conduct large clinical trials, amass necessary data, or perform technically complex analyses. The federal government is generally better equipped to perform these functions. However, to the extent that the federal government provides financial support and technical assistance to states in developing methodologies and assembling the necessary data, the federal-state relationship could be stimulative and symbiotic rather than competitive. States' motivation to take advantage of federal support and assistance will depend in part on the degree of responsibility they bear for Medicaid financing and on the Medicaid reimbursement policies they pursue.

Medicaid Financing and Reimbursement Policies

Full federalization of Medicaid would eliminate the states' role as third-party payers and significantly reduce their financial stake in supporting a host of cost-containment efforts, among them technology assessment intended to promote more cost-effective medical care. State incentives might in fact be reversed if health care were federally financed but supply controls such as certificate of need remained a state responsibility under state licensing authority. For example, if services were fully financed by the federal government, states might have incentives to remove restrictions on bed supply since this would increase access of their own citizens to services while the bill would be paid by another level of government. Similarly, state incentives to invest scarce resources in technology assessment would be reduced if the bill for expensive technologies were fully paid at another level.

Alternatively, if Medicaid financing reforms took the form of federal caps or block grants to the states, states' financial stake in cost control would be maintained insofar as they were at risk for expenditures exceeding federal contributions. Under current matching arrangements, states pay between 25 and 50 percent of total Medicaid costs. Under a Medicaid block grant with fixed federal contributions, states' responsibility for costs above the federal contribution would rise to 100 percent. Significant devolution of Medicaid financing responsibility on the states can be expected to increase their interest in technology assessment as a means to support cost controls, but it also can erect political and financial barriers to their actually supporting technology assessment, as discussed in the section on block grants below. Furthermore, other cost-cutting actions, particularly reductions in Medicaid rolls or provider reimbursement rates, would likely be favored insofar as they offer quicker and large payoffs. Whether Medicaid financing is centralized or decentralized, federal and state choices about how to reimburse hospitals and other health care providers will affect interest in technology assessment.

As indicated above, a DRG form of payment might stimulate interest in technology assessment. On the other hand, payment systems—such as those in Massachusetts, Maryland, and New York—which impose global budgetary limits on hospitals or other providers would decentralize resource allocation decisions to the provider level and suggest a smaller role for government use of technology assessment as a cost-control vehicle. Yet given preset budgets and tight fiscal constraints, provider demand for more information on the cost-effectiveness of practices and technology might increase. Thus, under global budgeting systems there might be an important educative role for a central agency with a reputation for scientific integrity to guide individual providers in their resource allocation decisions. These effects would be similar to those of procompetitive schemes which also decentralize resource allocation decisions to the individual provider levels.

Block Grants

Consolidation of categorical programs—including Medicaid, if Congress chose that option—into block grants can be predicted to have several effects. First, block grants strengthen governors vis-à-vis their own state bureaucracies and enhance their ability to coordinate policy across state agencies.[8] Martha Derthick (1970) has pointed out how the most important factor in expanding the influence of the federal government is the creation of vertical linkages between federal and state professionals through the categorical grant system. Although federal influence may have fostered professionalism among state bureaucrats, it has also undermined the professionalism among state bureaucrats and has undermined the ability of the state executives to shift funds among program categories to increase policy rationality or cost-effectiveness. The relaxation of federal requirements through block grants should enhance states' interest in using the findings of technology assessment and other analytic studies to justify redistribution of formerly categorical dollars. As a result, block grants may increase state willingness to support such activities.

Second, another effect of block grants is to create political uncertainty. Power is shifted from Congress to 50 state legislatures. Interest groups with access to Congress must now win battles in 50 state legislatures to achieve the same results. Political outcomes will become less predictable given different political alignments and interest group strengths in each state. On average, certain industries are likely to be less dominant nationally than they are in the economy of a particular state (e.g., coal in Kentucky). And on average, state legislators are more likely to be responsive to a few local interests than are congressmen who represent larger constituencies where cross-pressures from different interests are more likely to be felt. Local coalitions of providers are alleged to have greater strength at the state level. This might reduce state effectiveness and interest in performing technology assessments if the technical judgments of state agencies were overturned by political forces in the legislature. Of course, cost-control and regulatory coalitions may be stronger in particular states than they are on average in the Congress. As noted above, legislation proposed in some states prior to the passage of the Pure Food, Drug, and Cosmetic Act of 1938 was much stricter than the law that ultimately passed the Congress with business support. On the whole, however, it seems unlikely that health policy analysts and other technology assessment advocates will be as influential in the individual states as they have been at the national level.

Third, block grants as enacted under the Reagan administration have increased fiscal constraints on currently funded programs and services. If Congress were to convert Medicaid from an open-ended entitlement program to a block grant, the fiscal impact on states would be far more severe than the fiscal impact of creating the existing health care blocks. The reduction in funds accompanying the creation of health block grants makes it unlikely that states will choose to divert resources to new functions such as technology assessment at a time when previously funded service programs are being cut back (Greenberg, 1981). The support for technology assessment within states will be further reduced by cutbacks in support for health planning agencies. In the past, national and state health planning programs created a national constituency of officials committed to analytical methods. To the extent that these programs have lost staff, the pool of talent within each state capable of performing technology assessment is reduced, as is an important impetus for cost-effective resource allocation.

However, should the federal government earmark special funds or undertake a major technical assistance effort to assist states in technology assessment, the combination of increased program flexibility and enhanced gubernatorial influence under block grants might induce states to look to technology assessment as a means for promoting efficiency and effectiveness in health care spending.

The Success or Failure of Competition

To date,the administration's competitive health care proposals have not received legislative endorsement. If the administration's competitive agenda were enacted, government involvement in medical resource allocation decisions could be expected to decline, and technology assessment would become less important than it is now as a government cost-containment vehicle.

On the other hand, to the extent that private insurers are motivated to influence the provision of health services in order to offer more competitive insurance premiums, they will have increased incentives to support technology assessment as a means to eliminate cost-ineffective services. They might choose to conduct their own studies (in order to gain a competitive advantage) or, given the externalities, to contribute funds to a central agency with a reputation for scientific integrity. The ability to eliminate third-party payment for previously covered but cost-ineffective procedures will depend in part upon consumer and physician acceptance of such changes. Therefore, the importance of a central agency (privately or publicly financed) which would develop methodologies and ensure integrity of studies might be enhanced under a competitive health care system, although such an agency would not directly influence or make coverage decisions. Whether the agency were located at the federal or state level would depend on the availability of federal funds, the degree of health care financing centralization or decentralization, and the extent to which competition became a national versus a state priority.

CONCLUSION

Distinguishing among state incentives to conduct technology assessments, state resources and capacity, and state effectiveness is a useful first step in assessing the effects of other developments in the health care system on state support for the development and application of technology assessment. Making these distinctions leads us to conclude that there are several factors that may lead states to assume a more active role in this area. In the first place, a minimum federal (or perhaps joint public-private) commitment to provide money for incipient state efforts, to secure data, and to ensure the scientific integrity of studies may be a precondition of expanded and effective state action. In addition, further decentralization of Medicaid, state adoption of DRG-type Medicaid payment systems, the expansion of health block grants, and the stabilization of state finances would promote state interest in technology assessment. In contrast, a major new federal initiative to conduct technology assessments, resulting, for example, from the need to administer the DRG payment system; the federalization of Medicaid; state adoption of global budgeting systems; the withering of block grants; and/or continued fluctuations in state fiscal conditions would probably undermine the modicum of existing state support for technology assessment.

NOTES

[1] The health services block grant would have consolidated 15 categorical programs, including community health centers; alcohol, drug abuse, and mental health programs; maternal and child health; and migrant health programs. The prevention block grant would have supplanted family planning, adolescent health services, hypertension, fluoridation, lead-paint screening, rodent control, and other preventive programs (Feder et al., 1982).

[2] According to the cap proposal, the federal government would have limited FY 1982 matching funds to a figure only 5 percent greater than the federal government's FY 1981 contribution to Medicaid (Pelham, 1981b).

[3] Several provisions of the 1981 Reconciliation Act are key in this regard. Specifically:

- States may eliminate certain recipient groups and/or services from their programs for the medically needy.
- States may limit recipients' freedom of choice to selected providers.
- States may add a wider list of health maintenance organizations (HMOs) to their list of Medicaid providers.
- States are no longer required to use Medicare's retrospective reasonable cost principles in paying hospitals under Medicaid. (While some states had already obtained federal waivers to experiment with prospective hospital reimbursement methods, such waivers should now be more widely available).
- States may use Medicaid dollars to substitute home and community-based services for long-term institutional care. The 1980 Budget Reconciliation Act had already relaxed the reasonable cost requirement for nursing home reimbursement (Pelham, 1981a).

[4] According to a recent study by the Advisory Commission on Intergovernmental Relations (ACIR), disparities across states in personal income have declined markedly, although disparities in tax effort have begun to grow again after a period of narrowing (ACIR, 1982).

[5] In fact, states and localities posted a combined operating deficit of $3 billion in 1982 (Herbers, 1983).

[6] Robert Pear (1982) presents data on disparities in

tax capacity and welfare/Medicaid spending for 10 states.

[7] Although Silver (1974) is critical of the lack of federal leadership in maternal and child health, the more general point is that the federal government often follows the leadership of the states.

[8] In some states, however, state legislatures are already working to limit the increased discretion of the governor.

REFERENCES

Advisory Commission on Intergovernmental Relations. 1982. Tax Capacity of the Fifty States: Methodology and Estimates. Publication No. M-134. Washington, D.C.

Altman, D., R. Greene, and H. Sapolsky. 1981. Health Planning and Regulation: The Decision-Making Process. Washington, D.C.: American Public Health Association Press.

Barfield, C. E. 1981. Rethinking Federalism. Washington, D.C.: American Enterprise Institute.

Broder, D. S. April 14, 1982. The "new federalism" fades away and with it an opportunity. Washington Post.

Cannon, L., and H. Dewar. March 10, 1981. Reagan asks $48 billion budget curb. Washington Post.

Coates, V. T. 1972. Technology and Public Policy, Summary Report. Prepared for the National Science Foundation. Washington, D.C.: George Washington University. Quoted in Steven A. Schroder and Jonathan A. Showstack. 1979. The Dynamics of Medical Technology Use: Analysis and Policy Options, p. 194 in Medical Technology: The Culprit Behind Health Care Costs? Stuart A. Altman and Robert Blendon, eds. DHEW Pub. No. (PHS) 79-3216. Washington, D.C.

Derthick, M. 1970. The Influence of Federal Grants. Cambridge, Mass.: Harvard University Press.

Elmore, R. 1978. Organizational models of social program implementation. Public Policy 26(2):185–228.

Feder, J., J. Holahan, R. Bovbjerg, and J. Hadley. 1982. Health. Pp. 271–305 in The Reagan Experiment, J. L. Palmer and I. V. Sawhill, eds. Washington, D.C.: The Urban Institute Press.

Gibson, R. M., D. R. Waldo, and K. R. Levit. 1983. National health expenditures 1982. Health Care Financing Review 5(1):1–31.

Grannemann, T. W., and M. V. Pauly. 1983. Controlling Medicaid Costs: Federalism Competition and Choice. Washington, D.C.: American Enterprise Institute.

Greenberg, G. D. 1981. Block grants and state discretion: A study of the implementation of the Partnership for Health Act in three states. Policy Sciences 13:153–181.

Hamilton, M. January 10, 1982. States must find ways to offset 'new federalism' cuts. Washington Post.

HCFA. 1982. Health Care Financing Program Statistics: The Medicare and Medicaid Data Book. 1981. Washington, D.C.: U.S. Department of Health and Human Services.

Herbers, J. 1983. Many states find sudden surpluses in their revenue. New York Times.

Jackson, R. O. 1969. Food and Drug Legislation in the New Deal. Princeton, N.J.: Princeton University Press, passim.

Pear, R. June 18, 1982. Many states still far from ready to go it alone. New York Times.

Pelham, A. 1981a. Health Program Spending Cut by 25 Percent. Congressional Quarterly August 15:1501–1504.

Pelham, A. 1981b. Medicaid Spending Cut, "Cap" Rejected. Congressional Quarterly August 15:1499–1500.

Pressman, J., and A. Wildavsky. 1973. Implementation. Berkeley: University of California Press.

Reagan, R. July 14, 1982. Excerpts from address to county officials' meeting. New York Times.

Rush v. *Parham*. 625 F. 2d 1150 (1980).

Silver, G. 1974. Report #1, Final Report of the Yale Health Policy Project. HRA Grant #S00900.

U.S. Office of Technology Assessment, Congress of the United States. 1980. The Implications of Cost-Effectiveness Analyses of Medical Technology. Appendix B, p. 145. Washington, D.C.: U.S. Government Printing Office.

Walker, D. 1981. Towards a Functioning Federalism. Cambridge, Mass.: Winthrop Publishers.

Wilson, F., and D. Neuhauser. 1982. Health Services in the United States, 2nd edition. Chapter 7. Cambridge, Mass.: Ballinger Publishing Co.

Government Payers for Health Care

Donald A. Young*

Between 1965 and 1980 the government replaced direct payment by consumers as the dominant source of the dollars used to purchase personal health care services and supplies. In 1980, a total of $217.9 billion was spent for personal health care in the United States. Government programs spent $86.4 billion and provided 39.7 percent of personal health care expenditures. Federal funds provided $62.5 billion, more than two-thirds of the public outlay. This compares dramatically with the situation in 1965 when the federal government paid only 10.1 percent of the bills for personal health care services and consumers paid 51.7 percent of the share. While the total expenditures for medical services has risen rapidly in this 15-year period, the percentage of the total outlay paid by the state and local governments and by private health insurance has remained relatively stable.

The dramatic increase in total governmental expenditures as well as the increasing share paid by the federal government makes governmental bodies significant parties with interest in health services delivery, the use of evaluative information, and making sound policy decisions regarding payment for medical services.

Although many governmental agencies expend funds for health services and supplies through an array of public programs, the Medicare and Medicaid programs are dominant, accounting in 1980 for $60.6 billion in personal expenditures, two-thirds of all public spending for personal health care, and financing nearly 28 percent of all personal health care expenditures. Other significant contributors to public spending for personal health care include veterans medical care, $5.8 billion; Defense Department medical care, $4.2 billion; worker's compensation, $3.9 billion; and outlays by state and local governments for hospital care, in addition to that provided to Medicaid recipients, $6.0 billion. Numerous other programs account for the remainder of the governmental medical care expenditures.

A brief overview of the largest governmental programs that provide medical services and benefits is followed by a more comprehensive examination of the Medicare program.

THE MEDICARE AND MEDICAID PROGRAMS

The Health Care Financing Administration (HCFA), through its Medicare and Medicaid programs, helps pay medical expenses of 50 million poor, elderly, disabled, and blind Americans. A total of 28 million people are Medicare beneficiaries and 23 million people are Medicaid beneficiaries. In 1980 $60.6 billion was paid for health services used by Medicare and Medicaid beneficiaries. This makes HCFA the single largest payer of health care services.

The Medicare program is a health insurance program. Like other public and private insurance programs, its purpose is to reduce the economic risk to beneficiaries of the cost of illness. The costs of the program are paid through Social Security tax payments, federal general revenues, and individual cost-sharing provisions. Although the program is administered by the Health Care Financing Administration, an agency of the Department of Health and Human Services (DHHS), the day-by-day claims processing and payment functions are carried out by fiscal agents under contract to HCFA. The contractors are generally public insurance organizations such as Blue Cross/Blue Shield or private commercial insurance companies. The processes of claims review and payment are, therefore, similar to the process used by these groups in the conduct of their private business.

The Medicare program differs from pri-

* Executive Director, Prospective Payment Assessment Commission, Washington, D.C.

vate health insurance, however, in that covered benefits are determined by Congress in statutory authority rather than contract and are subject to change by lawmakers and to interpretation by the executive branch of the government, which is charged with administering the program. Beneficiaries do not have the option of selecting from a range of benefit packages designed to meet their specific needs. Benefits available to one beneficiary are generally available to all beneficiaries subject to medical need for the services. In addition, in public and private insurance plans, premiums taken in plus administrative costs must equal or exceed over a period of time payments paid out. Because the Medicare program is funded by Social Security taxes and general revenues, there is no direct relationship between funds contributed by beneficiaries and funds paid for services provided to beneficiaries.

The Medicaid program differs in a number of respects from the Medicare program. The primary difference is that Medicaid is a voluntary, state-administered program. The federal government participates by sharing with the states the cost of providing care. In return, the government requires that a certain minimum level of services be made available as well as other requirements. Significant flexibility is given to the states in determining eligibility for medical assistance, benefits made available, and reimbursement amounts to be paid. Providers who participate in the program must accept Medicaid-determined reimbursements as payment in full and cannot bill beneficiaries. There is no beneficiary cost-sharing except for nominal copayments for a limited number of services. States may process claims themselves or contract with private organizations, and nearly half of the states currently contract out all or part of the claims processing functions.

DEPARTMENT OF DEFENSE

In 1980, the Department of Defense expended $4.2 billion for medical care for active duty personnel as well as retirees and military dependents. The greatest amount of this expenditure was for the direct provision of services in facilities owned and operated by the military. For military dependents, retirees and their dependents, and some other eligibility groups unable to obtain care in a medical facility, the federal government provides a medical benefits program, the Civilian Health and Medical Program of the Uniformed Services (CHAMPUS). It became effective December 7, 1956, and was amended in 1966 to include coverage for retired uniformed service personnel and their dependents as well as dependents of active duty personnel. CHAMPUS is provided by law (Title 10, United States Code, Chapter 55) and is operated in accordance with policies and procedures set forth by the Department of Defense in regulations.

Although it is not a health insurance program, CHAMPUS is similar in many respects to health insurance and especially to the Medicare program. Authorized medical services and supplies are cost shared by the government from money appropriated by the Congress to the Department of Defense for this purpose. The uniformed services to which CHAMPUS applies are the Army, Navy, Marine Corps, Air Force, Coast Guard, Commissioned Corps of the United States, Public Health Service, and Commissioned Corps of the National Oceanic and Atmospheric Administration.

Beneficiaries are encouraged, and in some circumstances required, to obtain medical care from uniformed services medical facilities, i.e., military (and Public Health Service) hospitals. Beneficiaries do, however, have the option of obtaining needed medical care from civilian sources when care is not available close to their homes or in emergency situations. For most medical care obtained from civilian sources, CHAMPUS requires that the beneficiary pay part of the expense through deductibles and cost-sharing. CHAMPUS program benefits are very similar to those provided by Medicare, and CHAMPUS also relies on contractors to receive and process the claims for service.

VETERANS ADMINISTRATION

The Veterans Administration (VA) health care system furnishes services to eligible veterans in 172 medical centers, 226 outpatient clinics, 92 nursing homes, and 16 domiciliaries. During 1980, VA treated approximately 1.25 million hospital inpatients; 15.8 million outpatient medical care visits were furnished directly by VA staff, and an additional 2.2 million visits were authorized by the VA payable to non-VA physicians authorized to render care on a fee-for-service basis. In addition, under an agreement with the Department of Defense, approximately 224,000 dependents of veterans were eligible to receive care under the Civilian Health and Medical Program of the Veterans Administration (CHAMPVA). The care was furnished in non-VA facilities.

HEALTH CARE FINANCING ADMINISTRATION

HCFA was established in 1977 to combine health financing and quality assurance programs into a single agency. It is responsible for the Medicare program, federal participation in the Medicaid program, and a variety of other health care quality assurance programs. As its mission statement indicates, HCFA views its responsibility to be much broader than simply paying medical bills.

The mission of HCFA is to administer the Medicare and Medicaid programs and related provisions of the Social Security Act in a manner that (1) promotes the timely and economic delivery of appropriate quality health care to eligible beneficiaries, (2) promotes beneficiary awareness of the services for which they are eligible and improves the accessibility of those services, and (3) promotes efficiency and quality within the total health care delivery system. To accomplish this mission, HCFA provides operational direction and policy guidance for the nationwide administration of the Medicare and Medicaid health care financing programs; the Professional Standards Review Organization (PSRO) and related quality assurance programs designed to promote quality, safety, and appropriateness of health care services provided under Medicare and Medicaid; quality control programs designed to ensure the financial integrity of Medicare and Medicaid funds; and various policy planning, research, and demonstration activities.

Medicare and Medicaid, along with other third-party payers, have an interest in containing administration and program costs and promoting efficiency in the delivery of services to beneficiaries while maintaining the availability of high-quality, medically necessary services. To make decisions regarding benefits, HCFA must have up-to-date medical, scientific, and health services research information. To understand how appropriate information influences benefit decisions in these programs, it is first necessary to review the authority, structure, and processes of the Medicare and Medicaid programs as they relate to benefit decision making.

Medicare

The Medicare program was established by Congress in 1965 with the enactment of Title XVIII of the Social Security Act and became effective on July 1, 1966. In 1972, major changes were made in the program's provisions, and the name of the Medicare program was officially changed to Health Insurance for the Aged and Disabled. The program provides payment for certain medical services for persons 65 years of age or over, disabled beneficiaries, and persons with end-stage renal disease. The program currently covers 24.9 million aged and 3.1 million disabled individuals.

In the title and opening sections of the Medicare statute, Congress indicated clearly that Medicare was to be an insurance program providing basic protection against the costs of medical care rather than a health services delivery program. In addition to stressing the insurance nature of the program, the opening sections of the statute prohibit any federal interference in the practice of medicine or the manner in which medical services are provided, guarantees beneficiaries free choice of qualified providers, and allows individuals the option of obtaining other health insurance protection.

The Medicare program consists of two separate but complementary insurance programs, a Hospital Insurance Program, known as Part A, and a Supplementary Medical Insurance Program, known as Part B. All persons age 65 or over who qualify for Social Security cash benefits, and individuals who have been receiving Social Security disability benefits for 24 months or more are automatically enrolled in Part A. Part A is financed by a payroll tax shared equally by employers and employees. Although Part A is called hospital insurance, covered benefits include medical services furnished in institutional settings including hospitals, skilled nursing facilities, or provided by a home health agency. Such institutions are termed *providers* by Medicare and must be certified as qualified providers of services and have signed an agreement to participate in the program. The Medicare law includes limits, based on the concept of a benefit period, on the services which may be covered in the various settings. The law also established cost-sharing by the individual through deductible and coinsurance payments. Part A providers of services are reimbursed directly by the program (for all reasonable costs) and generally cannot bill beneficiaries other than for applicable cost-sharing.

The Supplementary Medical Insurance Program (SMI), or Part B of Medicare, is voluntary for individuals who elect to be covered. It is financed from premium payments by enrollees together with contributions from appropriated general revenue funds. (Because of limits on premiums, the federal contribution has been increasing more rapidly than the premium. Currently, premiums finance about 30 percent of the program costs, with the remaining 70 percent coming from general revenues.) Medicare Part B covers medical services and supplies furnished by physicians or others in connection with physicians services, outpatient hospital services, and home health services. Physicians' services covered under the program include visits to the home, office, hospital, and other institutions. The program also pays for certain drugs and biologicals that cannot be self-administered, diagnostic x-ray and laboratory tests, purchase or rental of durable medical equipment, ambulance services, prosthetic devices, and certain medical supplies.

In contrast to Part A institutional costs reimbursement, benefits paid under Part B are usually reimbursed on a fee or charge basis. After the beneficiary pays an annual deductible, Medicare will pay 80 percent of the reasonable charge for most covered services for that year. Physicians and other suppliers, however, are allowed to charge beneficiaries an additional amount if the Medicare payment is less than their usual charge.

CLAIMS PROCESSING

The separation of the Medicare program into an institutional (provider) component (Part A) and a noninstitutional (medical services) component (Part B) was patterned after a program alignment used by Blue Cross/Blue Shield Associations in paying for services to their subscribers. In order to keep the federal health insurance program closely linked to the private sector, Congress decided that most claims-processing and administrative functions for both Part A and Part B of Medicare should be handled by public or private insurance organizations (commercial or Blue Cross/Blue Shield) acting as fiscal agents for the Medicare program.

The fiscal agents responsible for the administration of hospital insurance or Part A benefits are termed intermediaries. Institutional providers (hospitals, skilled nursing facilities, home health agencies) were initially allowed to select the intermediary of their choice; however, this is slowly changing. Intermediaries act as the link between the provider and the Health Care Financing Administration, which is responsible for the administration of the Medicare program. The major role of the intermediaries is to review and pay claims for the costs of providing care to beneficiaries. The intermediary makes these payments to providers for covered items and services on the basis of reasonable cost determinations following policies set by HCFA.

Under the SMI (Part B), the fiscal agents are called carriers. Carriers are selected on a geographical basis by the secretary of the Department of Health and Human Services; physicians and others furnishing Part B services have no say in selecting the carrier to process claims for these services. Since Part B services are reimbursed primarily on a reasonable charge (as opposed to reasonable cost) basis, one of the major functions of carriers is to determine the reasonable charges in their respective areas for each medical care service paid for under the program. Carriers are also responsible for reviewing and paying claims to or on behalf of beneficiaries for the services provided.

The functions performed by Medicare intermediaries and carriers in the adjudication of claims is similar for both their private and their government business. These functions include, in addition to claims review and processing, utilization review, beneficiary hearing and appeals, professional relations, and statistical activities. The final decisions regarding payment for services in their private insurance business is determined by a contract with beneficiaries or their representatives. The final decision in their Medicare business is determined by statutory authority, regulations promulgated by DHHS and program instructions, and guidance prepared by HCFA to implement regulations and statutory authority. In the absence of HCFA instructions concerning a specific service, authority is vested in carriers and intermediaries to make the benefit decisions. Medicare intermediaries and carriers are reimbursed for their administrative costs under the basic principle of no profit or no loss. Contractors are not at risk with respect to program benefit payments as these payments are entirely underwritten by the program. Contractors, however, are regularly evaluated as to their capability and efficiency in administering the program and are subject to loss of contract for poor performance.

Medicaid

The Medicaid program was also enacted by Congress in 1965. Title XIX of the Social Security Act, Grants to States for Medical Assistance Programs, succeeded earlier, welfare-linked medical care programs. Under the Medicaid program, states may enter into an agreement with the secretary of DHHS to finance health care services for certain categories of low-income individuals, primarily those eligible to receive cash payment under the Aid to Families with Dependent Children (AFDC) program and the Supplemental Security Income (SSI) program for the aged, blind, and disabled (categorically needy). In addition, many states have exercised the option to extend coverage to "medically needy" individuals who meet the AFDC or SSI categorical criteria but whose incomes are slightly above the welfare standards or individuals who have incurred substantial medical expenses. An estimated 22.5 million individuals are Medicaid recipients. The federal share of program costs is related to state per capita income, ranging from 50 percent in the highest per capita income states to 77 percent in the lowest per capita states. The federal contribution is referred to as Federal Financial Participation (FFP).

Federal law mandates that states cover hospital, physician, skilled nursing facility, family planning, home health, laboratory, x-ray, rural health clinic, and nurse midwife services for all eligible recipients, and early and periodic screening, diagnosis, and treatment (EPSDT) services for children under 21. States may also provide a variety of optional services, including intermediate care facility services, prescription drugs, dental care, eyeglasses, and other services.

States determine the scope of services offered and the reimbursement rate for these services subject to federal guidelines. They also exercise a great amount of control over the income eligibility level for Medicaid. The Omnibus Budget Reconciliation Act of 1981 further extended the states' flexibility in these matters. All of these variations in benefits offered, income standards, and levels of reimbursement mean that Medicaid programs differ greatly from state to state.

States are responsible for claims processing and other administrative functions for their Medicaid programs, although the federal government shares in the cost of these functions. Some states administer their Medicaid programs directly; others contract with the private sector to perform various functions. Fiscal agent contracts are currently used by the majority of states to process and pay claims for some or all services. Fiscal agents are reimbursed on either a cost-reimbursement or fixed-price basis. In some cases the state contracts with the same fiscal agent responsible for processing Medicare claims.

COVERAGE AND REIMBURSEMENT UNDER MEDICARE PROGRAM

This discussion will outline the current authority, criteria, and process by which decisions are made to pay for certain medical procedures and services within the Medicare program. The Medicare program pays for some or all of the cost of certain medical services furnished to eligible beneficiaries. In this regard, the Medicare program is similar to the insurance programs of other third-party payers such as Blue Cross and Blue Shield and commercial insurance companies. Individuals with such insurance plans are entitled to certain benefits under the conditions of their particular policy. Individuals, their employers, or other groups frequently negotiate with the insurance agent a package of benefits to be included in the policy, and subscribers are frequently given the opportunity to select from a range of different benefit packages the policy best suited to their needs, tastes, and income.

In the Medicare program, the benefits available to eligible beneficiaries are called *covered* services. Services not covered are not paid for with Medicare funds. The Medicare program differs from other insurance programs in that there is no negotiation between individual beneficiaries or their representatives regarding the content of a benefit package or selection of alternative benefit packages. Rather, all eligible beneficiaries may have partial or full payment made for those services which are covered if their medical condition and level of care is judged to warrant it.

In the following discussion, a distinction is made between issues related to *coverage* of services and issues related to *reimbursement* for services. Reimbursement, in terms of the Medicare program, deals with determining the methods and amounts of payment for services which are covered. Reimbursement issues become important only after it has been determined that a service is covered as a benefit. For example a new device may be developed which monitors the rhythm of the heart in a new way. After review, it may be determined that the device performs this function safely and effectively, and since heart rhythm monitors are covered services, the device is also covered. The question then becomes one of reimbursement. Should the level of reimbursement for the use of the device be the same as for devices previously used or is there reason for a different level of reimbursement? This discussion will focus on issues related to coverage rather than reimbursement of services, that is with determining the services to be paid for as benefits under the Medicare program rather than the method or level of reimbursement.*

Services covered by the Medicare program are determined by Medicare statute, regulations developed in keeping with the statute, program instructions included in a series of manuals used by those administering the program on a day-to-day basis, and interpretations of policy in response to specific inquiries.

Medicare Statute

The Medicare law specifically provides coverage for broad categories of benefits, for example, hospital benefits, skilled nursing facility benefits, home health benefits, physicians' services, ambulance services, laboratory services, durable medical equipment, and others. The Medicare statute also, to some degree, defines these broad categories of benefits. For example, *physicians' services* means ". . . professional services performed by physicians, including surgery, consultation, a home, office, and institutional call. . . ." The statute also lists some specific items which are covered such as diagnostic x-ray tests, surgical dressings, iron lungs, oxygen tents, wheelchairs, and others. In addition, the statute places some limitations, of a general and categorical nature, on the services

* This paper does not cover the new prospective payment system. See Chapter 5 of this book.

that can be covered when furnished by certain practitioners, such as dentists, chiropractors, and podiatrists. In addition to indicating what is covered, the law expressly excludes some categories and types of services from coverage, such as cosmetic surgery, personal comfort items, custodial care, and routine physical checkups.

The Medicare law does not, however, furnish an all-inclusive list of specific items, services, treatment procedures, or technologies covered. Thus, except for the listed examples of medical and other health services, the statute does not explicitly include or exclude coverage of most medical devices, surgical procedures, or diagnostic or therapeutic services.

The apparent intention of Congress, at the time the act was passed, was that Medicare should generally cover services ordinarily furnished by hospitals, skilled nursing facilities, and physicians licensed to practice medicine. However, it is also apparent that the Congress understood that questions as to coverage of specific items and services would invariably arise and would require a specific coverage decision by those administering the program. Thus, the Medicare law states:

> Notwithstanding any other provisions of this title, no payment may be made under Medicare for any expenses incurred for items or services . . . which are not reasonable and necessary for the diagnosis or treatment of illness or injury or to improve the functioning of a malformed body member.

This a key provision. First, by reason of the words "notwithstanding any other provision of this title . . ." this is an overriding exclusion, and may be applicable in a given situation despite the other provisions for coverage in the statute. Second, it provides the secretary of the Department of Health and Human Services considerable discretion and flexibility to respond to changes in the way health care is furnished, especially to the development and application of new medical practices, procedures, and devices.

Medicare Regulations

The regulations implementing the reasonable and necessary section of the Medicare law are also quite general [42 CFR 405.310(k)]. The term *reasonable and necessary* is not further defined in the regulation, nor does the regulation spell out a process for how this term is to be applied. The regulations do, however, contain a variety of specific exclusions and limitations on the benefits covered by Medicare. These exclusions include such things as routine physical exams, eyeglasses, cosmetic surgery, and dental services which were spelled out in the Medicare statute.

Program Instructions and Policy

The clearest formal operational definition of *reasonable and necessary* is contained in program instructions prepared by HCFA and sent to the fiscal agents (carriers and intermediaries) responsible for processing Medicare claims for services and administering the program on a day-by-day basis. This statement of policy translates the statutory and regulatory terms reasonable and necessary into a test of whether the item, service, or procedure in question is

1. generally accepted as safe and effective, or proven to be safe and effective;
2. not experimental;
3. medically necessary; or
4. furnished in accordance with accepted standards of medical practice in an appropriate setting.

Over the years, this test has been applied to many items and services resulting in a large collection of informal policy statements and accumulated decisions serving as precedents for current policy work. These policy statements are continuously undergoing change as medical services and procedures evolve and new research findings emerge.

Decisions on Individual Claims

The claim review process for the Medicare program is designed to identify services which may not be covered or about which there may be a question of medical necessity or reasonableness. Medicare's contractors (carriers and intermediaries) have discretion within the statutory, regulatory, and program instruction guidelines to decide coverage issues identified in the claims review process. All contractors have nurses on their claims review staffs and all have physicians available to provide advice and to consult with other physician specialists and peer groups in the community, in order to resolve coverage issues on the basis of sound medical judgment and information.

Medicare contractors are currently processing 200 million individual claims for service each year. Most of these are paid without serious questions being raised about whether the items and services are covered under Medicare. When questions are raised, they relate primarily to whether the service was medically necessary in the particular case and was furnished in an appropriate manner and setting, rather than to the broader issue of general coverage. However, at times an issue arises as to whether a procedure or item should be covered under any circumstance. These services are usually new procedures or new applications for existing procedures, although occasionally questions will arise regarding potentially outmoded services and items. Such questions are referred to the HCFA central office for further review and evaluation.

Although the claims review process is the major source of questions about coverage of procedures, items, and services, inquiries also come to HCFA from physicians and professional groups and with increasing frequency from manufacturers of medical equipment and devices. HCFA examines the question and is able to answer many referrals based on the statute, regulations, and existing policies and definitions concerning covered services. A few questions raise important new issues which HCFA cannot resolve without seeking additional professional and medical expertise.

If medical consultation appears necessary, HCFA will review the medical and scientific literature related to the service in question, gather appropriate articles and background material, and present the question to a panel of physicians employed by HCFA and other components of the department. The task of the panel is to sharpen and clarify the questions that need to be answered. For example, HCFA was asked recently if plasmapheresis (apheresis) was a covered service. After review and discussion, and with assistance from physician members on the panel from the Public Health Service (PHS), it was clear that apheresis had potential application for many diseases and conditions and that evaluations of this procedure were necessary based on the specific indications for its use. Currently, HCFA covers apheresis for a limited number of indications with additional evaluation under way. When the panel confirms the need for further expert medical opinion and evaluation, HCFA refers the question with the background information to PHS.

USE OF EVALUATIVE DATA IN COVERAGE DECISIONS

The criteria currently used to determine if an item or service is reasonable and necessary in terms of the Medicare program are as unspecific as safe and effective. HCFA may interpret the meaning of safe and effective in a very different manner from other groups. For example, in considering whether to approve new medical devices, the Food and Drug Administration (FDA) also uses the terms safe and effective. The process and specific criteria used by the FDA in evaluating the safety and effectiveness of a medical device for purposes of market approval, however, are very different from those used by HCFA to determine safety and effectiveness for the purposes of providing Medicare payment.

It is possible that a new device may be approved by the FDA based on a limited amount of research data focused on short-term safety and effectiveness of the device rather than longer-term safety and effectiveness in terms of improved health outcome necessary for Medicare coverage. Hence, certain devices or procedures may be approved by FDA but not covered as benefits under the Medicare program. Because both agencies use the terms safe and effective, the public may be confused by the seeming inconsistency.

The issue is further complicated by the language describing a service as either *generally accepted* as safe and effective or *proven* as safe and effective. There is no commonly accepted definition of these terms. For many new items, services, and procedures it may not be possible to make a decision based on general acceptability by the medical profession because the service has usually been provided by only a small number of physicians. Hence, the coverage decision will rest on medical evidence or judgments proving safety and efficacy. But even here, there is no clear agreement as to what constitutes an acceptable level of proof.

There are similar difficulties in determining if a procedure is still experimental. There are no accepted definitions or operational measures to indicate when a procedure or service has moved from a clear research phase, to an investigational phase, to accepted medical practice. In actuality, these stages overlap and research and investigation continue at the time a new procedure is gaining acceptance by practicing physicians. For example, studies of the diffusion of computerized axial tomography scanning indicate the diffusion of the procedure, and the growth of the investigative literature base proceeded in parallel. At what point has the procedure become generally accepted? The question is complicated further because the decision to pay is usually yes or no. It is generally not possible to pay for a service only in certain institutions or when performed by certain specially qualified physicians.

To date, HCFA and its medical and scientific advisors and contractors have not explicitly considered criteria beyond safety, efficiency, and research status in determining Medicare coverage policy. It is reasonable to assume, however, that other considerations such as economic, ethical, and social issues are at least implicitly considered as some procedures are evaluated for Medicare coverage. For example, coverage questions referred to HCFA for detailed evaluation frequently concern services or devices that have the potential for high program costs if covered. In such cases, economic considerations or issues of distribution of services and access to services may be an implicit factor in the decision to refer the issue to HCFA for evaluation or to initiate a thorough evaluation. Such considerations may implicitly affect the coverage decision if for no other reason than that a greater burden of proof may be required before a decision is made to cover the service as a Medicare benefit. To date, however, no safe and effective procedures have been denied coverage based on cost or social considerations.

Current Status of Coverage Decision Making

HCFA, its medical advisors, and the Medicare contractors have wide discretion in making coverage decisions concerning individual items and services. Although leaving significant room for flexibility and individual considerations and judgments by the medical profession, the lack of more explicit coverage criteria has also resulted at times in inconsistency from claim to claim or service to service. HCFA, in preparing national coverage instructions, which are binding on contractors, may also inconsistently apply the criteria in evaluating certain coverage questions. As noted above, a more rigorous burden of proof may be required for newly introduced services or costly services compared with established services which may be less safe or effective or more costly.

TECHNOLOGICAL INNOVATION, COVERAGE DECISIONS, AND MEDICAL PRACTICE

There is a belief that the technological research and development capabilities are exceeding the capacity of the health care delivery system and the individual practitioner to evaluate the medical research findings and appropriately apply them to patient care needs. Although drugs and some medical devices are subjected to scientific scrutiny by the FDA before marketing and wide availability, other medical procedures, devices, and services are accepted and widely applied by the medical community with little evidence regarding relative safety or effectiveness. For example, gastric freezing in the treatment of peptic ulcer disease and internal mammary artery ligation for coronary artery disease were widely used by medical practitioners before clinical studies demonstrated their lack of effectiveness. With the publication of evaluation studies, these procedures subsequently disappeared from the therapeutic armamentarium.

In addition, many medical devices and procedures are evaluated as individual items rather than in comparison with existing, alternative approaches to achieve similar medical outcomes. This is especially true for diagnostic studies in which new findings may be quickly applied and new tests are added to the array of those already available rather than replacing existing studies.

HCFA thus far has directed the bulk of its medical coverage evaluation resources to individual new devices and procedures. But innovations are also occurring in the patterns of health services delivery. Data are being gathered concerning the appropriate minimum numbers of procedures and distribution of services such as open heart surgery, the growth in numbers and appropriateness of coronary care and intensive care unit beds, home health and day care services, and so-called *unnecessary* surgery. Recently, there has also been a significant effort by the medical profession to move services from the traditional hospital setting to settings outside the hospital. Ambulatory surgical centers and free-standing cardiac rehabilitative facilities are examples of such movement of services. Medical and scientific evaluative information is also necessary to determine coverage policies in these areas.

For services that have long been accepted by the medical community, but frequently are unproved as to effectiveness, Medicare coverage policy has proceeded on administrative rather than medical judgments. For example, concerning home health or rehabilitation services, administrative decisions are usually made in terms of the Medicare statute, regulations, and policy. Only on occasion do new medical research findings or technological innovations lead to a change in policy.

The failure to use medical and health services research for assistance in determining coverage policy in the service area is understandable. Questions regarding the appropriate applications of new technologies or the existing patterns of health services delivery are complex and highly value-laden. Furthermore, there are very significant differences in delivery of medical care services in different areas of the country. A physician evaluating alternative approaches and selecting those services that best serve the needs of an individual patient will draw upon very different information and values than will a policy analyst evaluating information to determine if a service qualifies as reasonable and necessary and, therefore, will be paid for by the Medicare program.

Evaluative information is necessary for the physician and patient to select the proper mix of services. It is also necessary for the public policy official charged with the responsible administration of a publicly funded program. The absence of a sound information base as well as the potential conflict between the needs of an individual patient and the needs of third-party payers to exercise a fiduciary responsibility in behalf of all beneficiaries is the source of a major conflict surrounding benefit coverage decision making.

Frequently a test, procedure, or service is considered necessary by a physician if it is likely to make any difference at all in the diagnostic process or therapeutic outcome. The economic concepts of marginal gain and marginal cost may not be applied by practitioners in the care of individual patients, particularly when third-party payers such as Medicare are picking up most of the bill. In this case, the apparent costs to the individual approach zero and the service or test is ordered even if its value also may approach zero. For example, in evaluating a patient with coronary artery disease, many different tests and procedures are available. Are all the tests or only certain selected ones necessary for an individual patient? There are no clear research findings to answer the question, and because physicians are trained to acquire all the possible data available to minimize uncertainty, the tests are ordered and usually paid for by the Medicare or other third-party payers.

When either physicians or third-party payers turn to the medical and health services delivery research data for guidance on questions similar to this, they find it may fail to provide the information needed. Sound information and consensus on the safety and effectiveness of alternative methods of diagnosis, treatment, and delivery of services frequently do not exist as part of an accepted body of knowledge. Many procedures and services commonly used and accepted in medical practice have not been evaluated by means of carefully planned, well-designed, controlled clinical studies. Nevertheless, Medicare generally pays for these commonly accepted procedures and services when ordered by a licensed physician. It is the new procedures or new applications for accepted procedures that are currently subject to evaluation by the Medicare program.

The medical profession contends that an assessment of the risks and costs as well as the benefits of services and procedures has been central to the exercise of good medical judgment for decades and that such analysis and judgments are better made, and are being responsibly made, within the medical profession. An alternative view holds that an individual physician frequently does not have available all the information needed to make a sound decision regarding the safety and effectiveness of complex new procedures, although from the physician's own experience with the procedure it would appear to be working out well. Such might have been the case with carotid artery ligation or gastric freezing.

One view placing high weight on the judgment of individual physicians might be that if a physician orders any procedure or service Medicare should pay for it. An opposite view could require that payment be made only for those services that have been evaluated with evidence as to safety and efficacy. In practice, the Medicare program looks to the judgment, experience, and opinion of physicians and to sound scientific evidence.

Index

R

S

T